with the assistance of

R. M. F. FARRER-MESCHAN, M.B., B.S. (Melbourne, Australia), M.D.

Clinical Assistant Professor, Department of Obstetrics and Gynecology and
Associate in Radiology, Bowman Gray School of Medicine of
Wake Forest University, Winston-Salem, North Carolina

*With the assistance in selection of materials from the
three-volume text and editing by*

ANNE G. OSBORN, M.D.

Formerly Resident-Fellow in Neuroradiology at the Bowman Gray
School of Medicine of Wake Forest University, and now Assistant
Professor of Radiology, University of Utah, Salt Lake City, Utah

Synopsis of Analysis of Roentgen Signs in General Radiology

ISADORE MESCHAN, M.A., M.D.

Professor and Director of the Department of Radiology
at the Bowman Gray School of Medicine of Wake Forest
University, Winston-Salem, North Carolina; Consultant
Walter Reed Army Hospital; Chairman Committee on Radiology,
National Research Council, National Academy of Sciences, 1974–75

W. B. SAUNDERS COMPANY • Philadelphia • London • Toronto

W. B. Saunders Company: West Washington Square
Philadelphia, PA 19105

1 St. Anne's Road
Eastbourne, East Sussex BN21 3UN, England

1 Goldthorne Avenue
Toronto, Ontario M8Z 5T9, Canada

Synopsis of Analysis of Roentgen Signs in General Radiology   ISBN   0-7216-6301-X

Last digit is the print number: 9   8   7   6   5   4   3

To the memory of our parents

Preface

The present text is intended as a synopsis of a three-volume text, which emphasizes "the compilation and illustration of major roentgen signs in general radiology, their classification and correlation with clinical diagnosis and practice."

This *Synopsis* will provide the student with a condensation of diagnostic radiology, a field which is so vast that, even in the three-volume text, choices had to be made, and certain omissions were necessary. In this *Synopsis,* therefore, the selectivity of content has been doubly abbreviated, and it is hoped that the student, resident, practitioner, or radiologist might use this book as an initial guide to the larger text whenever he deems it necessary.

An attempt has been made to standardize the classification of roentgen signs by cataloguing them, as far as possible by (1) changes in size, contour, density, number, architecture, both internal and external, function, and position, on the one hand, and (2) changes in relation to time and treatment on the other.

Such standardization, in my judgment, permits a student to study the radiologic signs of a patient more objectively, and thereafter, to amalgamate these findings with the clinical facts so that a more intelligent differential diagnosis may be achieved. It is conceivable that such standardization might lend itself eventually to computerization and to greater statistical study of the absolute significance of certain roentgen signs, which admittedly are now based on judgment and experience. This still presents a possibility for the future.

I have continued to use the "midget exhibit" technique in teaching; the questions at the end of each chapter permit the student an element of self-instruction to reinforce his knowledge.

The chapter bibliographies in the three-volume text have not been repeated here, since the student may obtain these volumes in most medical libraries if he so desires. This omission is, of course, a space and economy measure, necessitated by the severe restrictions involved in reducing three volumes to one.

Finally, in this *Synopsis,* we have tried to define, by thoughtful limitation of the material to be included, a "body of knowledge" or "core curriculum," which in our experience has proved most essential to the generalist student or practitioner in his use of diagnostic radiology — so that, at least in the radiologic framework, he may begin to feel like the "complete physician."

ISADORE MESCHAN, M.D.

January 9, 1976

Acknowledgments

My acknowledgments for help received for the *Synopsis* are, of course, much the same as those indicated in the three-volume text and need not be repeated here. I continue to be eternally grateful to my wife, Dr. Rachel Farrer-Meschan, who was an "assistant author" of the larger original text and has continued to give unstintingly of her time and critical advice throughout this production as well.

Our secretarial staff, consisting primarily of Mrs. Edna Snow and Mrs. Betty Stimson, continues to be responsible for the typing of each draft of the manuscript, with great perseverance. The original typing of the index was done by Mrs. Edna Snow, Miss Victoria Vogler, and Mrs. Donna Ring. The index was further condensed and edited by the publishers. I continue to be tremendously grateful to the publishers and their several editors for their meticulous care in the reproduction of the illustrations, the editing, and the accuracy of production.

Last, but not least, even though Dr. Anne Osborn is named on the title page as an assistant in the selection of material from the three-volume text, I would once again like to express my indebtedness to her for her great help in selecting specific subjects from a great body of knowledge, so that this book would more closely approximate the "core curriculum" requirements of the medical student, the general practitioner, and the newer generation of young radiologists who might require an "overview" of general radiology.

This book, like other previous volumes, continues to emphasize my deep debt to my associates and to the various members of the Department of Audio-Visual Aids at the Bowman Gray School of Medicine, who were in the first instance responsible for so many of the illustrations. To all of these and many others, I continue to owe gratitude, credit, and acknowledgment. Ultimately, however, I must assume full responsibility for what appears in this text. I can only hope that it will fulfill its purposes.

ISADORE MESCHAN, M.D.

January 9, 1976

Contents

Background Fundamentals
for Diagnostic Radiology

SPECIAL PROPERTIES OF X-RAYS WHICH
PERTAIN TO DIAGNOSTIC RADIOLOGY

The special properties of x-rays which make them so very useful to diagnostic radiology are: (1) their *ability to penetrate* organic matter; (2) their ability to produce a *photographic effect* on photosensitive film surfaces; and (3) their ability to produce a *phosphorescence* (fluorescence) in certain crystalline materials.

Penetrability of Tissues and Other Substances by X-rays. Tissues and other substances with medical applications may be classified into the categories indicated in Figure 1–2 on the basis of their density and atomic structure. At one end of the spectrum are the *radiolucent* materials, through which the x-rays pass readily; at the other end are the *radiopaque* substances in which the x-rays are absorbed to a considerable degree in their passage so that little radiation escapes.

The x-rays which penetrate an anatomic part may be spoken of as the "remnant rays." These are the rays which ultimately affect the x-ray film or fluorescent screen and are responsible for the gradations of black and white on the image. Thus, in Figure 1–3, x-rays are shown diagrammatically to be traversing the cross-section of a forearm. The gradations of black, gray, and white as shown on the film beneath the forearm are due to the "remnant radiation" after the rays have been absorbed by the interposed tissues such as subcutaneous fat, muscles, and bone.

Unfortunately, in the process of passage through an anatomic structure the x-rays (and the secondary electrons produced within the anatomic part) are scattered in all directions, depending upon the energy of the primary x-ray beam. Such *scattered radiation* causes a loss of detail. Special devices must be interposed between the x-ray source and the film to eliminate the scattered rays from the ultimate image. *Coning devices, stationary and moving grids (Potter-Bucky diaphragm),* which help eliminate such scattered radiation will be described later.

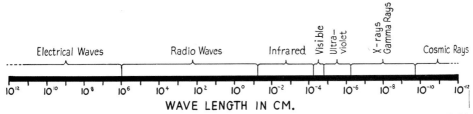

Figure 1–1 Diagram of the electromagnetic spectrum, illustrating the part of this spectrum occupied by x-rays.

VERY RADIOLUCENT	MODERATELY RADIOLUCENT	INTERMEDIATE	MODERATELY RADIOPAQUE	VERY RADIOPAQUE
Gas	Fatty tissue	Connective tissue Muscle tissue Blood Cartilage Epithelium Cholesterol stones Uric acid stones	Bone Calcium salts	Heavy metals

Figure 1–2 Classification of tissues and other substances with medical application in accordance with five general categories of radiopacity and radiolucency.

Photographic Effect of X-rays. Just as visible or ultra-violet rays alter light sensitive photographic emulsion, so do roentgen rays, so that when appropriately "developed," "fixed," and "washed," a permanent image is produced. The film employed for this purpose is ordinarily made with a thicker emulsion, although this is not absolutely necessary. The utilization of intensifying fluorescent screens (to be described below) has largely obviated such "direct radiography," since less x-irradiation is necessary for radiography by intensification techniques. However, when the body part under study (such as an extremity) is not large, when optimum detail is required, and when it is desired to allow no possibility for the interposition of an artefact on the roentgen image, such direct radiography is employed.

Fluorescent Effect of X-rays. When roentgen rays strike certain crystalline materials, a phosphorescence results. The spectrum of light so produced will vary with the crystalline substance—at times, it is largely ultraviolet, at other times, largely visible light. The ultraviolet light has proved to be most advantageous in respect to x-ray film emulsion. Intensifying screens consist mostly of a thin coating of such crystals on a cardboard surface. Their function is to provide a brighter image than would be provided by the direct photographic effect of the x-rays alone.

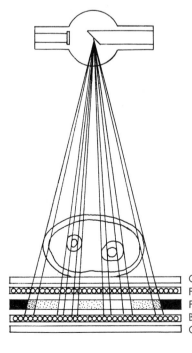

CASSETTE
FRONT FLUORESCING SCREEN
FILM WITH LATENT IMAGE
BACK FLUORESCING SCREEN
CASSETTE

Figure 1–3 Diagram illustrating x-rays from the target of an x-ray tube striking the forearm and passing through a cassette containing film. The remnant radiation passes through the forearm, producing a latent image upon the film.

Contrast Media

A body part may be visualized radiographically on the following bases:

1. The naturally occurring fatty envelope (or fascia)
2. Its naturally occurring gaseous content (lungs; gastrointestinal tract)
3. The naturally occurring mineral salts, such as the calcium salts of bone
4. By abnormally occurring gas, fat, or calcium salts
5. By the introduction of a contrast agent, which may be either *radiolucent* or *radiopaque*, into or around the body part. Such contrast agents should be physiologically inert and harmless.

Commonly Used Radiopaque Contrast Media

BARIUM SULFATE is particularly useful in studies of the gastrointestinal tract. It is inert, is not absorbed, and does not alter the normal physiologic function. At times it is used in colloidal suspension to obtain a particular type of coating of the mucosa, more effective for demonstration of small filling defects.

ORGANIC IODIDES, which are *predominantly excreted by the liver* and concentrated in the biliary tract, include: Telepaque, Priodax, Teridax, and Monophen, which may be given orally; and Cholografin (Biligrafin), which may be given intravenously.

ORGANIC IODIDES, which are *predominantly excreted or secreted selectively by the kidneys,* include: Hypaque (sodium diatrizoate), Renografin (Meglumine diatrizoate), and Iothalamates, such as Conray or Angioconray. These compounds are also widely favored for visualization of blood vessels. In low concentrations, they may be used for visualization of hepatic and biliary radicles by T-tube and operative cholangiography.

ORGANIC IODIDES *in suspension* may be particularly useful in visualization of oviducts (hysterosalpingography) (Sinugrafin) or the urethra (Salpix, Skiodan Acacia, Cystokon, and Thixokon).

IODIZED OILS, *slowly absorbable,* are used in myelography (Pantopaque); or in bronchography (Dionosil Oily).

Radiolucent Contrast Substances are *gases:* air, oxygen, helium, carbon dioxide, nitrous oxide and nitrogen. These are commonly used for visualization of the brain (pneumoencephalograms and ventriculograms), joints (arthrograms), and occasionally the subarachnoid space surrounding the spinal cord (myelograms). Air may also be used in the pleural space, peritoneal cavity, and pericardial space. Carbon dioxide is of particular value since it is well tolerated and very rapidly absorbed.

FUNDAMENTAL GEOMETRY OF IMAGE FORMATION AND INTERPRETATION

Penumbra Formation, Distortion, Magnification.   The manner in which an object placed in the path of the x-ray beam is projected depends on five factors: (1) **the size of the light source (effective focal spot size); (2) the alignment of the object with respect to the focal spot of the x-ray tube and the screen or films; (3) the distance of the object from the focal spot; (4) the distance of the object from the screen or film; and (5) the plane of the object with respect to the screen or film.**

When an image is projected from a pinpoint light source or focal spot, its borders are sharp. However, if the light source is a larger surface, the image is ill-defined at its periphery owing to "penumbra" formation (Figure 1–5).

In order to reduce the penumbra as much as possible the following measures must be taken: (1) the focal spot must be as small as possible; (2) the object-to-film distance must be as short as possible; (3) the object-to-focal-spot distance must be as distant as is practicable (Figure 1–5 B and C).

When the object is not centrally placed with respect to the central ray its image will be distorted, sometimes considerably (Figure 1–4). At times this distortion is unavoidable if one is to visualize an anatomic part (Figure 1–7), and in some of the radiographic positions this distortion brings into view a part which otherwise would be hidden. The phenomenon of projection may therefore be utilized to good advantage.

The problems of magnification must also be taken into consideration. Teleroentgenograms are "long distance radiographs," which diminish magnification. A minimum target-to-film distance of 6 feet is utilized for this purpose and even under these circumstances magnification of 10 to 15 per cent may be obtained for structures at a considerable distance from the film.

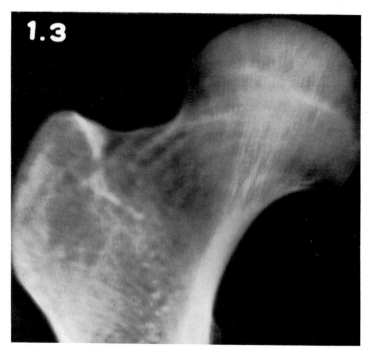

Figure 1–4 Radiograph showing blurring of an anatomic part caused by faulty relationship of the x-ray tube to the part being radiographed. In this instance the object-to-film distance was increased to 30 inches, but even though a relatively small focal spot was used and the other factors were correct, there is a significant blurring of the trabecular pattern of the head and neck of this femur. Roughly, a times 3 magnification was obtained, as the focal-film distance was 40 inches.

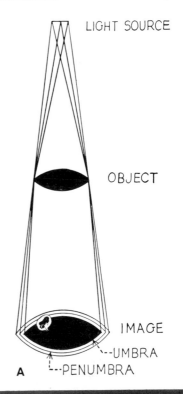

Figure 1–5 *A.* The smaller the focal spot the sharper the image. The illustration shows penumbra and umbra formation from a "surface" light source rather than a "point" source. Most x-ray targets are surface sources even though they are a fraction of a millimeter in size. A 0.12 mm. focal spot, if available, is useful in some magnification procedures, since it has virtually no penumbra. Most x-ray images are made with effective focal spot sizes of 0.6 mm. to 2 mm. *B.* Radiograph of a femur obtained at a focal-film distance of 72 inches and contact of the femur with the film (hence, object-to-film distance is zero), with a 1.3 mm. target size. Note that at this distance, with close contact of the object to the film, the trabecular pattern as visualized is excellent. (Courtesy of C. Ritchie, Winston-Salem, N.C.) *C.* Radiograph of the same femur again taken at 72-inch focal-film distance and a 0.3 mm. focal spot size. Notice that the trabecular pattern also appears distinct. At this long focal-film distance with good contact of the object with the film no particular gain is obtained at 0.3 mm. focal spot size.

Illustration continued on the following page

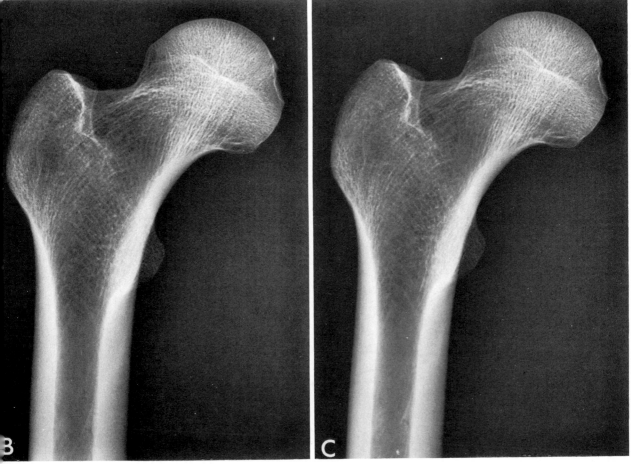

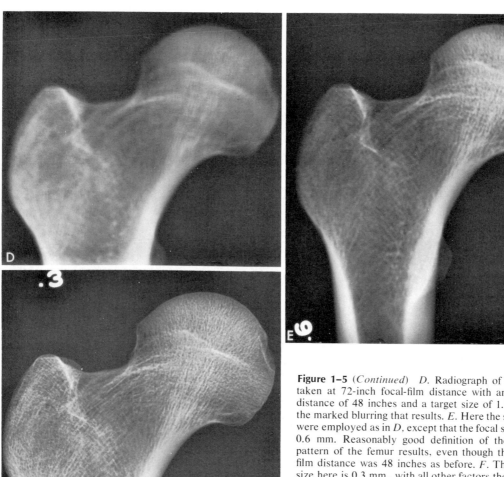

Figure 1–5 (*Continued*)   *D*. Radiograph of same femur taken at 72-inch focal-film distance with an object-film distance of 48 inches and a target size of 1.3 mm. Note the marked blurring that results. *E*. Here the same factors were employed as in *D*, except that the focal spot size was 0.6 mm. Reasonably good definition of the trabecular pattern of the femur results, even though the object-to-film distance was 48 inches as before. *F*. The focal spot size here is 0.3 mm., with all other factors the same. This is the optimum target size for detail when such long object-film distances are necessary. The magnification in *D*, *E*, and *F* is approximately times 3.

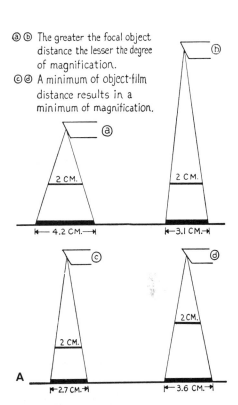

ⓐ ⓑ The greater the focal object distance the lesser the degree of magnification.

ⓒ ⓓ A minimum of object-film distance results in a minimum of magnification.

Figure 1–6 *A.* Effect of focal-object distance and object-film distance on magnification.

B and *C.* Radiographs of a femur showing the magnification that occurs when an anatomic part is placed at some distance from the film in relation to the total distance of the target to the film. In *B*, the object-to-film distance was 0 (good contact), whereas in *C* it was 30 inches. In both instances a very small focal spot size (0.3 mm.) was employed so that good detail was obtained even at a magnification of times 3 in *C*. (Courtesy of C. Ritchie, Winston-Salem, N.C.)

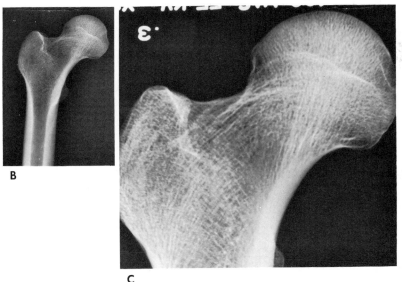

B

C

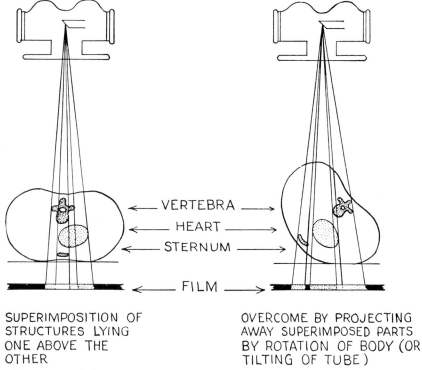

VERTEBRA

HEART

STERNUM

FILM

SUPERIMPOSITION OF
STRUCTURES LYING
ONE ABOVE THE
A   OTHER

OVERCOME BY PROJECTING
AWAY SUPERIMPOSED PARTS
BY ROTATION OF BODY (OR
TILTING OF TUBE)

Figure 1–7 *A.* Utilization of projection to overcome superimposition of anatomic parts.

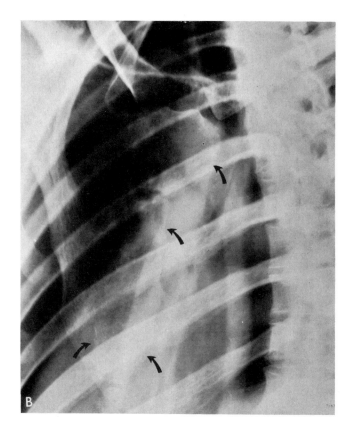

B. Radiograph showing how to obtain the oblique projection of the sternum without interference of spine and heart, thus affording a clear visualization of the sternum.

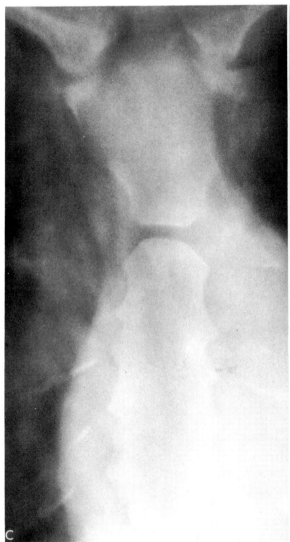

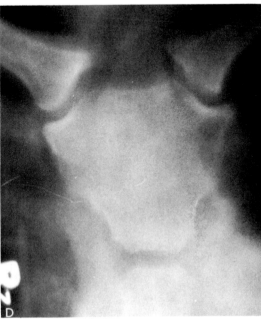

Figure 1–7 (*Continued*) *C*. Tomogram of the sternum showing improvement of detail that results. *D*. Similar improved detail in the manubrium.

2

Protective Measures in X-Ray Diagnosis

Quantification of Ionizing Radiation. Ionizing radiations are radiations consisting of alpha, beta, gamma, neutron rays (or particles) and x-rays which produce biological effects because they ionize, or separate, electrons from their parent atoms in compounds in the body. The *roentgen* (Figure 2–1) is the internationally

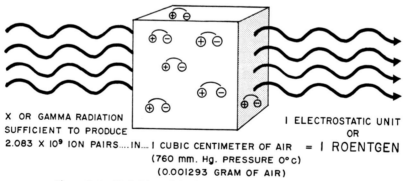

X OR GAMMA RADIATION SUFFICIENT TO PRODUCE 2.083 X 10⁹ ION PAIRS....IN.... I CUBIC CENTIMETER OF AIR = I ROENTGEN (760 mm. Hg. PRESSURE 0° C) (0.001293 GRAM OF AIR) / I ELECTROSTATIC UNIT OR

Figure 2–1 Definition of the "roentgen" in diagrammatic form.

accepted unit for quantity of ionizing radiation. It is defined as *"the quantity of x- or gamma radiation such that the associated corpuscular emission per 0.001293 grams of air produces, in air, ions carrying one electrostatic unit of quantity of electricity of either sign."* In everyday radiological practice it requires approximately 200 to 300 roentgens of x-radiation in the diagnostic quality range to produce a skin erythema. This occurs usually after a latent period of several days. Although the long term hazards of repeated exposure to x-rays are great for the technician and the physician, exposures of this order are seldom necessary for patients; hence, an erythema resulting from a diagnostic roentgenologic procedure is almost never observed in a patient.

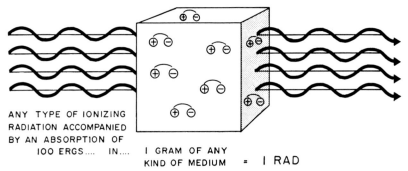

ANY TYPE OF IONIZING
RADIATION ACCOMPANIED
BY AN ABSORPTION OF
100 ERGS.... IN.... I GRAM OF ANY
KIND OF MEDIUM = I RAD

Figure 2-2 Diagram of the rad.

The *rad* (a word derived from "*r*oentgen *a*bsorbed *d*ose") (Figure 2-2) *is the dose of any type of ionizing radiation accompanied by an absorption of 100 ergs of energy per gram of absorbing material.* In contrast to the roentgen, which is a measure of "ionization in air," the rad is a measure of absorbed dose in terms of ergs of energy. Wherever feasible the *rad* is a more meaningful unit of quantification of ionizing radiation, since it is the absorbed dose which is most significant in the ultimate analysis of biological effect.

Radiation Dose Received by the Skin and Gonads in Radiographic Examinations. Table 2-1 summarizes interesting dose data in relation to commonly employed diagnostic radiologic procedures, with usual exposure times and numbers of films. The estimated dose to the ovaries ranges between 0.1 and 0.3 roentgens for the examination of the upper gastrointestinal tract, and 0.1 to 0.8 roentgens for barium enema study of the colon. It is important to know the physical factors employed: thus, in comparing a fluoroscopic technique with a target-to-tabletop distance of 30 inches without added filtration and one with a distance of 46 inches and 3 mm. added filtration, it becomes evident that a dosage ratio of almost 10:1 exists at the surface. At 10 cm. depth, however, this difference is minimized.

The dose range for single abdominal films to the mid-pelvis was found to fluctuate between 0.05 and 0.1 R for each exposure.

It is apparent from study of the accompanying table that the exposure most important for consideration is that related to the lumbar spine, the pelvis, the abdomen, excretory urography, and fluoroscopy.

TABLE 2–1   RADIATION DOSE RECEIVED BY THE SKIN AND GONADS IN RADIOGRAPHIC EXAMINATIONS (per film)

Examination	Kv.	mAs.	Focus-film Distance	Added Filtration	Dose per Exposure (with Back Scatter)		
					SKIN DOSE (MR)	MALE GONAD DOSE (MR)	FEMALE GONAD DOSE (MR)
Sinuses	80	40	27 in.	3 mm. Al	1040	0.1	0.05
Hand and wrist, postero-anterior	46	50	27 in.	3 mm. Al	100	0.04	0.01
Chest, postero-anterior	90	3	27 in.	3 mm. Al	8	0.01	0.02
Chest, tomogram (apices) antero-posterior	85	12B	100 cm.	3 mm. Al	110	0.01	0.02
Dorsal spine, antero-posterior	75	80B	110 cm.	3 mm. Al	480	1.0	1.3
Lumbar spine, antero-posterior	75	80B	110 cm.	3 mm. Al	480	0.5*	95.0
Lumbar spine, lateral	85	300B	110 cm.	3 mm. Al	2000	2.25	270.0
Lumbar sacral joint, lateral	90	400B	110 cm.	3 mm. Al	3000	2.0	350.0
Pelvis, antero-posterior	75	80B	110 cm.	3 mm. Al	480	20.0*	80.0
Abdomen, antero-posterior	75	60B	110 cm.	3 mm. Al	360	0.5*	75.0
Abdomen, B meal, prone (H.V.)	90	20B	110 cm.	3 mm. Al	130	1.5	20.0
I.V.P. renal, antero-posterior	75	80B	110 cm.	3 mm. Al	480	0.5*	95.0
I.V.P. bladder, antero-posterior	75	80B	110 cm.	3 mm. Al	480	10.0*	80.0
Knee, antero-posterior	82	25B	110 cm.	3 mm. Al	180	1.25	0.4
Ankle, antero-posterior	70	30B	36 cm.	1 mm. Al	200	0.1	0.025
Duodenal cap series, postero-anterior (H.V.)	90	15G	18 in.	5 mm. Al + TT	130	0.05	0.05
Fluoroscopy chest (I.I.)	75	90G (3 min.)	18 in.	5 mm. Al + TT	900	3.0	3.0
Fluoroscopy B meal (I.I.)	75	150G (5 min.)	18 in.	5 mm. Al + TT	1500	5.0	5.0

MR — 1/1000 R.

*Lead rubber protection.

B — Bucky.

G — Stationary grid.

H.V. — High voltage screen–Ilford Red Seal film. Other examinations Par Speed screens and Red Seal film extremities.

Ilfex film.

I.I. — Image intensifier, tube current, 0.5 to 1.0 Ma.

From Ardran, G. M., and Crooks, H. E.: Gonad radiation dose from diagnostic procedures. Brit. J. Radiol., *30*:295–297, 1957.

COMMON SENSE APPROACH TO THE PROBLEM OF HAZARDS DUE TO DIAGNOSTIC RADIOLOGY

The dose levels administered to the skin and gonads in radiographic examinations are usually so low that general effects of irradiation such as superficial injuries, hematopoietic injury, induction of malignant tumors, reduction in life span, or other effects such as lenticular cataract and sterility, are not observed. This is true, assuming that appropriate precautions are employed. However, the genetic aspects of roentgen exposure are important for consideration (Meschan; Norwood).

Webster has calculated that the saving of lives by discovery of tuberculosis and cancer by routine chest radiology far exceeds the hazards of the irradiation encountered when good technique is employed. So long as physicians have proper indication for the examinations chosen in a given patient, and so long as physicians who handle radiation use this valuable tool with the greatest of precision and precaution to themselves and their patients and personnel, the medical usage of radiation in the future is not likely to be deleterious to mankind.

Questions — Chapters 1 and 2

1. Draw a table with five columns with the following terms at the head of each column in sequence: Very radiolucent; moderately radiolucent; intermediate radiolucency; moderately radiopaque; very radiopaque. Under each column list as many substances as you know that are appropriate for the column. Define the terms radiopaque and radiolucent.

2. Draw a diagram illustrating how radiation affects a film when it passes through various anatomic parts differing in radiolucency and/or radiopacity.

3. Why does a cassette need special care? Why is it so easy to introduce artefacts on x-ray film when an x-ray cassette is employed?

4. What is the effect of a small focal spot *vs.* a large focal spot? How is this related to the process of magnification?

5. Define the following terms:
   a. The roentgen.
   b. The rad.

6. Describe doses received by the skin and the reproductive organs by radiographic and fluoroscopic study of the colon.

3

General Terms
and Concepts
Regarding Diagnostic
Radiology

DEFINITION OF TERMS WITH SPECIAL
RADIOGRAPHIC USAGE

Increased Density. Denotes a lighter or whiter shadow on the x-ray film, as produced by substances of greater density or thickness.

Decreased Density. Denotes a darker or blacker shadow on the x-ray film. It is produced by substances of low density or slight thickness.

Increased Radiolucency (Hyperlucency). Implies greater penetrability by the x-rays, and has the same connotation as decreased density.

Increased Radiopacity. Implies diminished penetrability by the x-rays and has the same connotation as increased density.

Antero-posterior and Postero-anterior. Indicates that aspect of the patient first in contact with the x-ray beam and thereafter the beam exit surface. Thus, the patient is in the postero-anterior position when the x-ray beam strikes the posterior aspect of the patient first and the anterior part of the patient is next to the film. The patient is in the antero-posterior position when the beam strikes the anterior aspect of the patient first.

Laterality. In describing the laterality of the patient relative to the x-ray beam, one always names the lateral or oblique projection according to the side of the patient closer to the film. Thus, a *right lateral film* is one taken with the right side of the patient next to the film. A *left lateral* is the reverse.

Obliquity. The oblique projections are named according to the side of the patient which is closer to the film. Thus, a *right anterior oblique* film is taken with the right anterior aspect of the patient closest to the film. A *right posterior oblique* film is obtained when the right posterior aspect of the patient is closest to the film. There are also the left anterior and left posterior oblique positions. The patient or part is usually at an angle of 45 degrees unless otherwise specified in these oblique views.

Recumbency.   Indicates that the patient is lying down when the film is taken. He may be either *supine* (on his back) or *prone* (on his abdomen). The beam in these cases is vertical with respect to the patient.

Decubitus Films.   The patient is in the *decubitus* position when he is lying on either side while an antero-posterior or postero-anterior film is taken. The beam in these cases is always horizontal. Thus, *right lateral decubitus* means that the right side of the patient is uppermost. *Left lateral decubitus* is the reverse. A more accurate terminology is desirable as follows: (1) Horizontal beam study, antero-posterior, with the patient on right (or left) side. (2) Horizontal beam study, postero-anterior, with the patient on right (or left) side. (3) Horizontal beam study, with patient supine (or prone) and right (or left) side nearest film.

Erect Position.   In this position the patient or the anatomic part is upright and the beam is horizontal. An erect chest film may be obtained with the patient standing or sitting.

Semirecumbent (Also Called Semi-erect).   This term implies that the vertical axis of the part being radiographed is at an angle of approximately 45 degrees with the horizontal.

Filling Defect.   A space-occupying mass within a hollow organ.

Niche.   In the wall of a hollow organ a recess which tends to retain contrast media. This term usually implies ulceration. A niche, in contrast to a diverticulum, has a broad, wide neck fusing imperceptibly with the contour of the lumen of the organ, whereas a diverticulum has a narrow neck.

Fluid Level.   The interface between fluid and air; it always assumes a horizontal appearance. The air above the fluid level is of diminished density, while the fluid itself is of intermediate density.

Bone Sclerosis.   An increase in the density of bone so that its radiographic appearance is much whiter than normal.

Eburnation of Bone.   Same as bone sclerosis.

Osteoporosis.   A pathologic state in which there is a diminished number of ossified trabeculae, so that the bone appears more radiolucent. The trabeculae which remain are normal bone.

Osteomalacia.   A pathologic state characterized by diminished bone density due to loss of bone mineral content. The protein content of the bone is less impaired or may not be impaired at all.

Hyperlucency of Bone.   A radiographic appearance of either osteoporotic or osteomalacic bone. This term should be utilized in description of the radiographs unless the true pathologic state is known.

Lipping.   A small osteophyte formation on the margins of the articular surfaces of bones. This is also called bony spur formation, although the latter term is commonly reserved for nonarticular bone.

Artefacts.   Changes on the film which do not have an anatomical basis directly related to the part being radiographed but are introduced by some technical fault, such as dirt in the cassette, or static electrical charge. Occasionally artefacts are introduced by items of clothing, immobilization devices, or even hair braids projected over the part.

Comparison Films.   Films taken of the side opposite to the one in question for comparison with the suspected abnormal side. These are very useful, particularly in children, and should be taken whenever possible.

Serial Films.   Films taken in sequence, either during a single study or after longer intervals of time, such as days or weeks.

Description of Radiographic Pathology

Radiographic pathology can be classified into the following categories in practically all instances: abnormality in (1) *position* of an organ or part; this includes the relationship to adjoining structures; (2) *size;* (3) *contour or shape;* (4) *density;* (5) *architectural pattern,* either a. *"edge"* pattern ("margins of lesion") or b. *internal* pattern; (6) *function;* (7) *number;* (8) *time sequence* (seconds, minutes, days, weeks, months, or even years); (9) *changes in response to treatment.* Additional descriptive categories may be applied in special circumstances to certain regions, organs, or organ systems.

> ### RADIOGRAPHIC PATHOLOGY—ITS GENERAL UNIVERSAL DESCRIPTION
>
> **Abnormality of:**
>
> Position and positional relationships
> Size
> Contour or shape
> Density (increased or decreased)
> Architectural pattern
>   Internally
>   At margins
> Number
> Function
> Time sequence
> Response to treatment

For example, in respect to the skeletal system, *alignment* of bone fragments with respect to one another and to the normal line of weight-bearing is important. Alignment of bones in respect to a joint is also important.

In the skeletal system, as in the lungs, the exact position of the abnormality must be described. In the long bones, is it epiphyseal, metaphyseal, or diaphyseal? In the lungs, is it in the upper lobe, middle lobe, or lower lobe?

In each area of the body a routine for study will be recommended.

Architectural Description concerns the "edge" or "marginal pattern," and the "internal appearance," in respect to the abnormal anatomic part, or the roentgen pathology per se. If a margin is present, there may or may not be a discrete "white line," suggesting a capsule or reaction in the adjoining bone. The "white line," if present, may be continuous, discontinuous, thin (less than 1 mm. ordinarily), moderately thick (1 to 2 mm.), or thick (approximately 3 mm. or more). Lung lesions may be ill-defined, nodular, linear, or lucent. If circumscribed and lucent, the margin may be thin or thick; if thick, it may be shaggy or regular. Each of these descriptive terms has special significance in relation to probable pathology, since the thin line may suggest a thin-walled cyst, while the thick wall suggests either tumor or abscess. The internal architectural appearance is of equal significance whether it is homogeneous, mottled, reticular, linear, lucent, or has water density, calcific density, or even greater than calcific density. Moreover, if there is a calcific density present, the size, shape, and position of the density are also important.

TERMS OFTEN USED IN ARCHITECTURAL DESCRIPTION

Margin	*Internal Appearance*
Well-defined and sharp	Homogeneous
a. No line of demarcation	Mottled
b. Thin line of demarcation	Reticular
c. Moderately thick demarcation	"Bubble-like"
d. Thick and "shell-like" demarcation	Linear-vertical
Ill-defined	Linear-horizontal
Shaggy	Lucent { gas / fat
Scalloped (or undulating)	
Laminated	
"Lacelike"	Water density
"Hair-on-end" or spiculated	Calcific density
"Maplike" or geographic	Speckled
"Picture-frame-like"	Punctate
"Spadelike"	"Popcorn-like"
"Applecore-like"	Metallic

The study of the architecture of the organ or part will often require the introduction of a contrast agent. Thus, the study of the intricate architecture of the brain may require pneumographic visualization of the ventricles or angiographic visualization of the blood vessels of the brain. A study of the architecture of the kidney, for example, will require not only excretory urography for visualization of the kidney cortex, the kidney calyces, pelves and adjoining ureters, but also renal arteriography and renal venography. The performance and study of these specialized procedures are often outside the scope of the present text, but appropriate mention will be made of them as necessary.

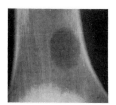 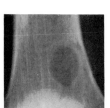 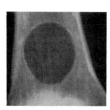 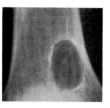 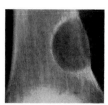

NO "RADIOLOGIC" CAPSULE

MALIGNANT TUMOR METASTASES

MULTIPLE MYELOMA

EOSINOPHILIC GRANULOMA

LIPOID DYSCRASIA

GIANT CELL
TUMOR   USUALLY
            SOAP-
ANEURYSMAL BONE   BUBBLE
CYST   INTERIOR

DISCONTINUOUS THIN
"RADIOLOGIC" CAPSULE

OSTEITIS FIBROSA CYSTICA
("BROWN TUMOR")

GAUCHER'S DISEASE

BRODIE'S ABSCESS

CONTINUOUS THIN
"RADIOLOGIC" CAPSULE

BRODIE'S ABSCESS

THICK "RADIOLOGIC" CAPSULE

CHRONIC GRANULOMA
OR ABSCESS

FIBROUS DYSPLASIA

BRODIE'S ABSCESS

THICK "RADIOLOGIC" CAPSULE
CORTICAL

FIBROUS CORTICAL DEFECT

FIBROMAS (CHONDROMYXOID)

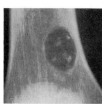

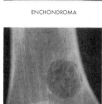

BONE CYST

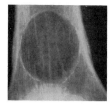

ENCHONDROMA

HEMANGIOMA

Figure 3–1   Analysis of solitary radiolucent lesions of bone by their marginal ("radiologic capsule") and inner architecture.

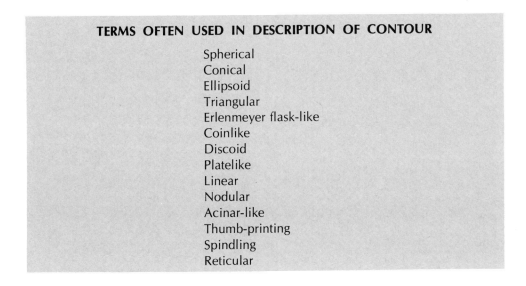

TERMS OFTEN USED IN DESCRIPTION OF CONTOUR

Spherical
Conical
Ellipsoid
Triangular
Erlenmeyer flask-like
Coinlike
Discoid
Platelike
Linear
Nodular
Acinar-like
Thumb-printing
Spindling
Reticular

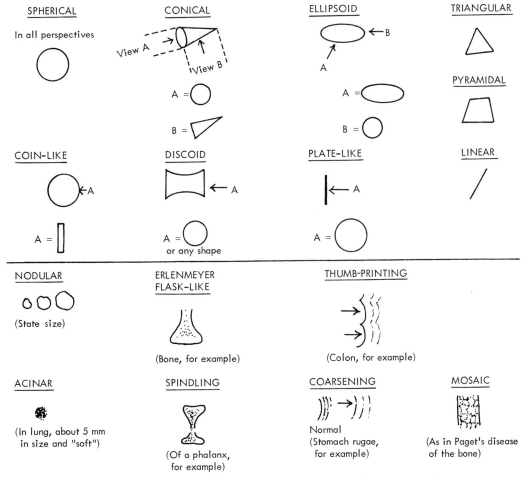

Figure 3–2   Diagram illustrating terms often used in description of contour or architecture.

Integration of the Radiographic Pathology with the Other Clinical Data

In essence, the various steps in radiologic diagnosis include: (1) *identification of the problem;* (2) *analysis,* to the extent that all facets are objectively separated one from the other and clearly defined; (3) *synthesis of diagnosis* by the integration of the available clinical facts and objective roentgen criteria.

This final synthesis involves a knowledge of disease patterns and of statistical incidence of disease in relation to age, sex, race, geography, familial tendency, occupational history, symptomatology, and clinical signs.

Questions – Chapter 3

1. Define the following terms:
    a. Increased radiographic density.
    b. Decreased radiographic density.
    c. Increased radiolucency.
    d. Increased radiopacity.
    e. Postero-anterior position.
    f. Antero-posterior position.
    g. Right lateral film.
    h. Right anterior oblique film.
    i. Supine film.
    j. Prone film.
    k. The decubitus position.
    l. Filling defects.
    m. Niche.
    n. Fluid level.
    o. Bone sclerosis.
    p. Eburnation of bone.
    q. Osteoporosis.
    r. Lipping of bone.
    s. Artefacts.
    t. Comparison films.
    u. Serial films.
2. List nine general factors for description of radiographic pathology.
3. What factors enter into the description of "architecture" in radiographic terminology?
4. What is a good systematic approach to the development of an opinion in respect to a radiographic problem?

4

Introduction to the Musculoskeletal System

THE CORRELATION OF THE BONE RADIOGRAPH WITH THE PHOTOMICROGRAPH

Normal Bone. In the normal healthy state, bone is a constantly changing organ, and bone formation and bone resorption are in equilibrium with one another except as required by growth and repair.

The accompanying radiograph, low-power photomicrograph (Figure 4–1) and diagram (Figure 4–3) show the following:

The dense, white zones (Figure 4–1) immediately adjoining the epiphyseal plate, shown in (4) and (6), represent zones of compact bone in the former, and calcified cartilage and osteoid in the latter (the zone of provisional calcification). The compact bone (2) is readily differentiated from the spongy bone of the diaphysis (7).

The articular cartilage is of intermediate radiolucency and blends with the surrounding intermediate-density soft tissues; it cannot be seen distinctly on the radiograph unless a contrast agent is introduced into the joint. When this is done, the examination is described as *arthrography*. Positive contrast agents, such as sodium or meglumine diatrizoate (Hypaque or Renografin), may be used, or gases such as air or oxygen, or double contrast techniques involving a combination of both. The epiphyseal plate (5) is similarly of intermediate density.

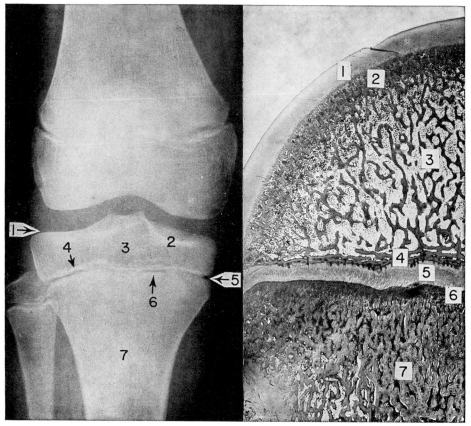

Figure 4–1 Antero-posterior radiograph of the knee and low-power photomicrograph of the end of a long bone with related areas labeled. (From Pyle, S. I., and Hoerr, N. I.: *Radiographic Atlas of Skeletal Development of the Knee*. Springfield, Charles C Thomas, 1955.)

Radiologic Terms

1. Articular cartilage does not show in a film.
2. White outline of subarticular margin of epiphysis.
3. Epiphysis.
4. Increased density of terminal plate; inner bone margin of epiphysis.
5. Epiphyseal line; strip of lesser density; epiphyseal plate; diaphyseal-epiphyseal gap. Radiographically, these terms exclude the recently calcified cartilage, which appears as part of the metaphysis.
6. Metaphysis; includes both calcified cartilage and newly-formed bone. (Zone of provisional calcification.)
7. Diaphysis or shaft.

Histologic Terms

1. Articular cartilage.
2. Compact bone of subarticular margin.
3. Epiphysis, spongy bone.
4. Terminal plate.
5. Epiphyseal disk; growth cartilage. Histologically, these terms include the calcified cartilage.
6. Metaphysis; includes only newly formed bone of primary ossification.
7. Spongy bone of diaphysis.

BONE PATHOPHYSIOLOGY AND BIOCHEMISTRY

Bone Composition. Bone is composed of 25 per cent water, 30 per cent organic substances, and 45 per cent inorganic substances. The organic content of bone consists mainly of proteins; the inorganic consists of 85 per cent calcium phosphate and 10.5 per cent calcium carbonate. The latter mineral substances are radiopaque and give bone its radiographic density.

The osteoblast is capable of extracting albumin and forming osteoid as its metabolic product. Osteoid is a collagenous substance which contains specific binding sites for bone minerals.

Factors Affecting Bone Formation (Figure 4–2). Bone may be laid down in accordance with predetermined congenital pathways (Barnhard and Geyer). It is probable that trabeculae usually develop according to prevailing stress (Feist). Systemic factors which play an essential role in bone formation are shown in Table 4–1.

Phosphatase is found consistently at sites of new bone formation as well as in

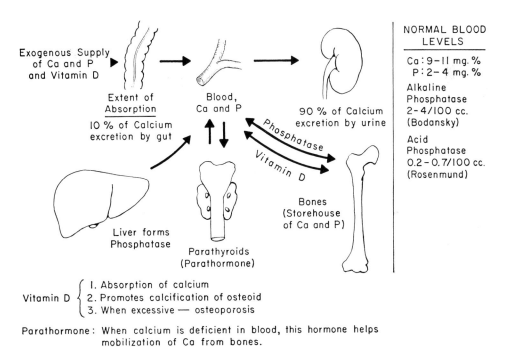

Figure 4–2 Factors governing calcium metabolism.

bone osteolysis. In an acid medium, phosphatase splits bone salts and returns the salt into the solution; in an alkaline medium, phosphatase activity promotes osteogenesis by liberating phosphate ions and precipitating calcium salts. Acid phosphatase is otherwise confined within the intact prostate gland, from which it may be released by invasive carcinoma.

Calcitonin is secreted in response to hypercalcemia in the thyroid gland (and possibly parathyroid gland as well), and its function seems to be to depress serum calcium levels by inhibiting bone resorption (Aliapoulios, Berstein and Balodimos; Foster).

Parathyroid hormone functions principally in the maintenance of a proper level of calcium in the blood by mobilization of calcium. A decrease in the level of serum calcium causes an increase in parathyroid hormone secretion. Parathormone exerts its effects at three distinct levels:

1. Inhibition of phosphate resorption at the renal tubular level, thus leaving a relative excess of calcium ions in the circulation;

2. Promotion of absorption of calcium and phosphorus at the intestinal mucosa level;

3. Direct stimulation of osteoclasts in bones to mobilize calcium.

Hyperparathyroidism is "primary" if it is due to a functioning adenoma of the parathyroid glands, or to diffuse hyperplasia; it is "secondary" when parathyroid stimulation results from intestinal malabsorption or renal malexcretion. "Autonomous" hyperparathyroidism (also called "tertiary") (Kleeman) is seen in those patients with chronic and overwhelming renal failure without adequate subsidence after institution of adequate treatment by dialysis and correction of electrolyte balance.

Vitamin D has three essential roles:

1. Absorption of calcium from the ileum;

2. Promotion of tubular phosphate excretion much like parathormone in the kidneys;

3. Direct action on bone by potentiating the osteoclastic activity stimulated by parathormone.

As a fourth possible function it may tend to catalyze bone calcification.

TABLE 4–1 FACTORS AFFECTING BONE FORMATION

Exogenous	Gastrointestinal Tract		Blood Serum Levels	Bone	Kidneys
Dietary calcium	Acid chyme	Favor absorption	Calcium	Storehouse for calcium and phosphorus	Glomerular function
Phosphorus	Adequate vitamin D		Phosphorus		Tubular function
Vitamins	Alkaline chyme		Phosphatase*		
A. C. D*	Excessive phosphates, fatty acids, soaps and carbonates	Impair absorption	Vitamins		
Proteins	Fluoride		Hormones		
			Pituitary (growth)		
			Calcitonin*		
			Adrenal corticosteroids (anabolic and catabolic)		
			Estrogens		
			Androgens		
			Parathormone*		

*See accompanying text.

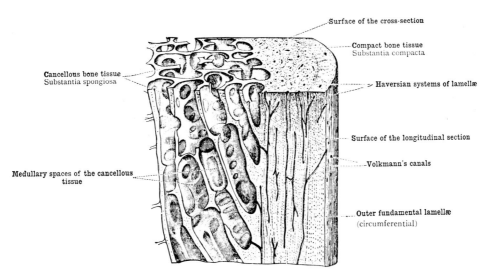

Figure 4–3 Diagram to illustrate the structure of bone. (From Toldt, C.: *An Atlas of Human Anatomy for Students and Physicians*. New York, Macmillan Co., © 1926.)

TABLE 4–2 RADIOGRAPHIC PATHOLOGY OF BONES*

Periosteum	Cortex	Trabeculae of Medulla	Disease States
1. Normal	Thin	Thin subnormal	Osteoporosis from multiple diseases
2. Normal	Thin	Trabeculae coarse; demineralization	Osteomalacia, rickets, hypophosphatasia Hypervitaminosis D Vitamin D resistant rickets
3. Normal	Subperiosteal resorption	Demineralization	Hyperparathyroidism
4. Normal	Normal	Trabeculae increased in number, thickness, or even density	Marrow disorders
5. Increased	Increased	Normal	Infantile cortical hyperostosis Treated rickets
6. Normal	Increased thickness	Trabeculae increased in thickness	Osteopetrosis Hypoparathyroidism Hyperphosphatasemia Vitamin D intoxication Idiopathic hypercalcemia
7. Increased	Increased	May be normal	Fluorosis (Adams and Jowsey; Carbone, et al.; Cohen; Rich and Ivanovich)
8. Normal	Increased but mosaic and bizarre	Decreased and increased, intermixed and mosaic	Osteitis deformans (Paget's disease)
9. Normal	Increased in thickness	Increased in number	Acromegaly

*Modified from Feist, J. H.: Radiol. Clin. N. Amer., *8*:182 (No. 2) 1970; and Meschan, I.: *Atlas of Normal Radiographic Anatomy*. 2nd ed. Philadelphia, W. B. Saunders Co., 1959.

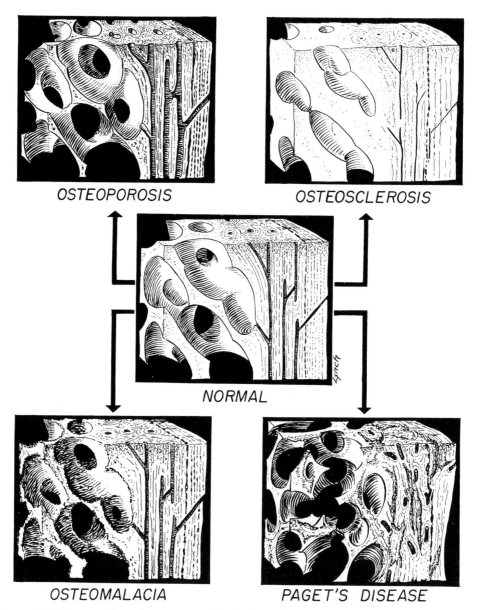

Figure 4–4 Diagrams illustrating gross morphologic changes in bone with osteoporosis, osteosclerosis, osteomalacia, and Paget's disease. On each diagram cancellous bone is represented on the left side and compact on the right. The haversian systems are shown to be widened in osteoporosis and osteomalacia, narrowed in osteosclerosis, and bizarre in configuration in osteitis deformans (Paget's disease).

TABLE 4–3 ROENTGEN APPEARANCES OF BONE CORRELATED WITH BIOCHEMISTRY*

General Roentgen Appearances	Disease Suggested	Serum			Urine	
		Calcium	Inorganic Phosphorus	Alkaline Phosphatase	Calcium	Phosphorus
Diffuse hyperlucency of bone. Occasional "pseudocystic" lesions of bone (brown tumors). Cortical resorption—middle and distal phalanges. Resorption lamina dura around teeth. Soft tissue and renal calcifications. Peptic ulceration duodenum.	Hyperparathyroidism: Primary					
	Early	↑	N	S↑	↑	N
	Advanced	↑	→↓	↑	↑	↔→
	Terminal	↑	↑	↑	↑	→
	Secondary	N-↓	↑	R↑	↑	N
Increased density of bones at times. Short metacarpals or metatarsals, especially fourth and fifth.	Hypoparathyroidism (Seabright Bantam)	→↓	←↑	N-→	→↓	→↓
	Pseudohypoparathyroidism	→↓	←↑	N-→	→↓	→↓
	Pseudo-pseudohypoparathyroidism	N	N	N	N	N
Hyperlucency of bone occasionally	Hyperthyroidism, marked	N	N	↑	↑	←↑
Usually no change in adults. In *child* delayed ossification of epiphyses, retarded growth, and "stippled" epiphyses. Dwarfism. Vertebrae diminished in height.	Hypothyroidism	N	N	N	N	N
Severe radiolucency of bone generally. Aseptic necrosis of heads of femora and humeri. Vertebrae partially collapsed. In *child*, accelerated ossification and closure of epiphyses leading to dwarfism. Peptic ulceration duodenum.	Hypercortisonism (Cushing's disease or syndrome)	N	N	N	↑	↑
Diffuse hyperlucency of bones. Biconcave endplates of vertebrae ("fish-like") with collapse.	Senile osteoporosis	N	N-O↓	N	N	N

Table 4–3 continued on following page

TABLE 4-3 ROENTGEN APPEARANCES OF BONE CORRELATED WITH BIOCHEMISTRY* (*Continued*)

General Roentgen Appearances	Disease Suggested	Serum			Urine	
		Calcium	Inorganic Phosphorus	Alkaline Phosphatase	Calcium	Phosphorus
Hyperlucency of bone distal to fracture (disuse atrophy).	Fracture healing (multiple and severe disuse atrophy)	↑	↑	↑	↑	N
Hyperlucency of bones. Expansion of metaphyses—"frayed" metaphyseal ossification, markedly diminished. Delayed ossification of epiphyses. Pathologic fractures and deformed bones under stress.	Hypovitaminosis D child rickets—active	↓	↓	↑	N	N
Marked hyperlucency of all bones—Biconcave appearances in vertebrae with partial collapse.	Adult—osteomalacia	N-↓	↓	↑	N	N
Hyperlucency of bones with some periosteal thickening. Soft tissue ectopic calcification.	Hypervitaminosis D	↑	N-↑	↑	↑	N
Hyperlucency of bone. In *child*, lucent strips in metaphyses with somewhat dense strip adjoining. Small spurs of bone at metaphyseal margins, which may be fractured. Epiphyses poorly ossified with white line around epiphyseal margins.	Hypovitaminosis C (untreated)	N	N	↓	N	N
Subperiosteal hemorrhages previously not manifest become calcified.	Healing scurvy	N	N	↑	N	N
Bizarre trabeculation of bones with thickened trabeculae interlaced with lucency—bones appear broadened, enlarged, and may be deformed.	Osteitis deformans (Paget's) mild—few bones Generalized and active	N N R↑	N N R↓	S-↑ ↑	N N N	N N N

Disease	Description					
Multiple myeloma Uncomplicated With renal involvement	Early, there may be no changes. Circumscribed, indiscriminately scattered, lucent foci, or diffuse hyperlucency. Pathologic compressions and fracture.	↑ ↑	N-↑ ↑	R↑ R↑	N-↑ ↑	↑ ↓
Osteosarcoma	Destroyed bone with reactive periosteal zone, and some bizarre calcification (in tumor osteoid).	N	N	↑	N	N
Tumor, metastatic to bone	Circumscribed, indiscriminately scattered lucent or sclerotic foci, or both. Pathologic fractures. With some metastatic tumors, bones may be diffusely "white" (i.e., metastatic carcinoma of prostate).	N-↑	N	O↑	N	N
Polyostotic fibrous dysplasia	Pseudocystic conglomerate foci with coarsened trabeculae and "shell of bone" appearance on margins of involved areas.	O↑	N	O↑	N	N

Code: N = Normal   O = Occasionally
       ↑ = Increased   S = Slight
       ↓ = Decreased   R = Rarely

Sources:
1. Bondy, P. K.: *Duncan's Diseases of Metabolism.* 6th Ed. Philadelphia. W. B. Saunders Company, 1969.
2. Aegerter, E. and Kirkpatrick, J. A., Jr.: *Orthopedic Diseases.* 3rd Ed. Philadelphia, W. B. Saunders Company, 1968.
3. Singleton, E. B. and Teng, C. T.: Pseudohypoparathyroidism with bone changes simulating hyperparathyroidism. Report of a case. Radiology, 78:388–393, 1962.

*Amalgamation of laboratory findings, courtesy of Dr. James L. Quinn, III.

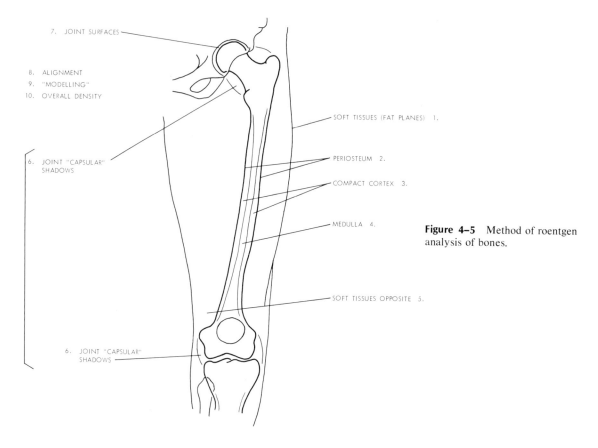

7. JOINT SURFACES

8. ALIGNMENT
9. "MODELLING"
10. OVERALL DENSITY

6. JOINT "CAPSULAR" SHADOWS

SOFT TISSUES (FAT PLANES) 1.

PERIOSTEUM 2.

COMPACT CORTEX 3.

MEDULLA 4.

SOFT TISSUES OPPOSITE 5.

6. JOINT "CAPSULAR" SHADOWS

Figure 4–5 Method of roentgen analysis of bones.

METHOD OF ROENTGEN ANALYSIS OF BONES (Figure 4–5)

1. Always have at least *two perpendicular views and one joint view.*
2. Determine whether or not *single or multiple foci* are involved by a bone survey wherever necessary. A *bone survey* consists of: two views of skull; two views of lumbar or thoracic spine; antero-posterior view of pelvis; and antero-posterior views of arms and thighs.
3. Make *comparison studies* of the two comparable sides of the body when appropriate.
4. Know *age and sex* of patient.
5. Know *hereditary factors, occupational history,* and, whenever possible, *clinical and laboratory data.*
6. *Study bones in sequence* (Figure 4–5).
    a. Systematically review general roentgen pathology, such as alterations in *position, size, contour, density, architecture* (internal and marginal), *number, function, changes occurring over a period of time,* and *changes resulting from treatment.*
7. *Classify objective roentgen* in respect to:
    a. *Monostotic vs. polyostotic*
    b. *Increased density vs. hyperlucency*
    c. *Overgrowth vs. undergrowth*
    d. *Architecture* of lesion or lesions (1) *internal,* and (2) *marginal*
    e. *Soft tissue or periosteal involvement*
    f. *Joint involvement*
8. Integrate available clinical facts (such as age) and objective roentgen signs to arrive at differential diagnosis.

BONE AGE VERSUS CHRONOLOGICAL AGE: MATURATION OF THE SKELETON

Major Factors Studied in Skeletal Maturation

1. *Ossification of the long and short bones* (usually complete *in utero*)
2. *Onset of ossification of the epiphyses*
3. *Completion of ossification* with fusion of the epiphyses and metaphyses
4. *Maturation indicators* in the wrist, hand, tarsus, foot, and knee (patella)

Epiphyses begin to appear at birth and are ordinarily complete by puberty. Ossification is usually complete by the 20th year in the female and the 23rd year in the male.

Author's Recommended Method

1. Radiographs are obtained of regions depending upon the chronological age of the child.

2. In these regions, onset of ossification and completion of ossification (fusion) are studied. The "age-at-appearance" percentiles for major postnatal ossification centers can be determined.

3. Maturation indicators are studied in the hand, wrist, tarsus, foot, and knee as indicated by the age of the child. These are tabulated in relation to the mean age given plus the standard deviation.

4. All of these data are interrelated to give the most probable age. Three radiographs can usually suffice. At puberty, however, more attention must be given to the centers of the hip, iliac bones, and the sesamoids of the thumb and other fingers.

General Rules for Use of Bone Age Data*

1. For children from birth to five years: registration of skeletal age by the time of appearance of centers of ossification.

2. For children five to 14 years of age: study maturation factors, and penetration of cartilaginous areas by reference to standards.

3. For children 14 to 25 years of age: register skeletal age by epiphyseal-diaphyseal union and reference to "Completion of Ossification" tables.

---

*Modified from Watson, E. H., and Lowrey, G. A.: *Growth and Development of Children.* 5th Ed. Chicago, Year Book Medical Publishers, 1967.

Usefulness of Skeletal Maturation Studies

1. Diagnosis and management of certain endocrine disorders
2. Evaluation of fetal maturity
3. Ability to anticipate onset of puberty
4. Ability to predict growth potential

However, the following factors must be taken into consideration:
1. Hereditary, individual, sexual, and population factors
2. Anatomic variations
3. Socioeconomic status
4. Contemporary data, since there is a general trend toward earlier skeletal maturation (Graham)

Disorders Which May Cause Small Stature*

Nutritional
  Malnutrition
  Hypervitaminosis D
Bone diseases
  Achondroplasia
  Hurler's syndrome
  Osteogenesis imperfecta
  Rickets

Central nervous system disorders
  Cerebral palsy
  Microcephaly
  Mongolism
  Porencephalia
  Postencephalitis
Chronic infections
  Bones, kidneys, or lungs
Congenital heart disease
Endocrine disorders
  Addison's disease
  Adrenogenital syndrome

Cretinism
Diabetes
Gonadal dysgenesis
Renal disorders
Hepatic disorders
  Atresia of bile ducts
  Cirrhosis
  Disorders of glycogen storage
  Galactosemia
Pulmonary disorders
  Asthma
  Cystic fibrosis
  Bronchiectasis
Blood diseases
  Severe anemia
Intestinal disorders
  Celiac syndrome
  Diaphragmatic hernia
  Fat or starch intolerance
  Gastrointestinal allergy

Disorders Which May Cause Large Stature*

Pituitary hyperfunction
Testicular hypofunction
Adrenal cortex adenoma or carcinoma
Genital hyperfunction
Pineal tumors
Tumors of hypothalamus

*From Watson, E. H., and Lowrey, G. H.: *Growth and Development of Children.* 5th Ed. Chicago, Year Book Medical Publishers, 1967.

TABLE 4-4 ABNORMALITIES OF SKELETAL DEVELOPMENT*

Legend: N = normal   ↑ = advanced   ↓ = retarded
(N) = probably normal   (↑) = possibly advanced   (↓) = possibly retarded

Condition	Skeletal Maturation	Growth and Stature	Comments
Central and General			
Hyperpituitarism (giantism)	N or (↓), may fuse late	↑ ↑	eosinophilic adenoma, acromegalic if late
Hypopituitarism (pan-, pituitary dwarfism)	↓ ↓, may never fuse	↓ ↓	? "normal" early
Primordial dwarfism (genetic, constitutional)	N or (↓)	↓	? bone maturation "scattered"
CNS disorders			(2° to neoplasm or other disease)
Pinealoma	↑	↑, adult? N	especially males
Fibrous dysplasia	↑	↑, adult? N	especially females
Craniopharyngioma	↓	↓	
Hypothalamic dysfunction	↑ or ↓	↑ or ↓	many associations, i.e., obesity
Exogenous obesity	N or (↑)	N or (↑), adult N	
Malnutrition and/or chronic disease	(↓)	(↓), adult may be N	
Chondro-osseous dysplasias and syndromes	↓ usually	↓ ↓ usually	rarely advanced, many die early
Gonads			
Hypergonadism (hyperplasia, neoplasm)	↑ ↑, fuse early	↑ ↑. adult ↓	(may be 2° to gonadotropin ↑ ↓)
Hypogonadism			
Eunuchoidism	N or (↓), fuse late	↑, long extremities	intrinsic, castration, 2° to disease
Pituitary	N	↓	not panhypopituitarism
Gonadal "dysplasias"			
Turner's syndrome	N or (↓), fuse late	↓	XO types, hypomineralization
Kleinfelter's syndrome	N or (↓), fuse late	↑, long extremities	XXY types
Abnormal sexual differentiation	(N)	(N)	pseudohermaphrodite types
Sexual developmental variations			
Delayed adolescence	(↓), then N	↓, adult N	
Premature pubarche	(↑), then N	↑, adult N	
Premature thelarche	N or (? ↑)	N	
Constitutional precocity	(↑), then N	↑, adult N	
Adrenals			
Cortical insufficiency (Addison's disease)	(↓)	(↓)	like a chronic disease (may be 2° to ACTH ↑ ↓)
Cortical hyperactivity (Cushing's disease)	(↓)	↓	cortisol ↑, hypomineralization
Adrenogenital syndrome (hyperplasia, neoplasm)	↑ ↑ ↑. fuse early	↑ ↑, adult ↓	usually masculinizing, rarely feminizing
Thyroid			
Hypothyroidism			(may be 2° to TSH ↑ ↓)
Congenital (cretinism)	↓ ↓ ↓ ↓	↓ ↓ ↓, infantile	epiphyseal dysgenesis hypermineralization
Acquired	↓	↓	
Hyperthyroidism	(↑)	(↑), adult N	? hypomineralization
Parathyroids			
Hyperparathyroidism (1° or 2°)	(N)	(N)	hypomineralization
Hypoparathyroidism	(N)	(N)	hypermineralization
(Pseudohypoparathyroidism)	(N)	↓	associated with XO types

*From Graham, C. B.: Personal communication, 1970.

Questions—Chapter 4

1. Draw a diagram of a high-power micrograph with a longitudinal section cut through the upper end of a long bone. The diagram should demonstrate the growing end of the epiphyseal plate as well as the adjoining metaphyses.

2. What three main groups of substances comprise the chemical constitution of bone?

3. List the various factors governing calcium metabolism and describe the interrelationship of these factors.

4. Where is phosphatase found and how does it act physiologically?

5. What is the principal function of parathyroid hormone (parathormone)?

6. What are the essential roles of vitamin D in respect to bone metabolism?

7. Indicate an example of a disease process in which there are circumscribed foci of trabecular thickening or increase in number of trabeculae.

8. Draw a diagram of a long bone and indicate a method of roentgenologic analysis which will ultimately allow a description of all the basic roentgenologic pathology.

9. Indicate where serum calcium and inorganic serum phosphorus are elevated or depressed in the following conditions: (a) primary hypoparathyroidism; (b) osteomalacia untreated; (c) menopausal osteoporosis; (d) multiple myeloma; (e) metastatic skeletal carcinosis; and (f) hyperthyroidism.

10. What is the main purpose in clinical medicine for the determination of bone age as compared with chronological age; and what is the system which was developed for radiographic determination of bone age?

11. Define osteoporosis and differentiate this condition from osteomalacia.

12. Describe some of the changes in bone which may be related to adjoining structures, and indicate by it the importance of studying structures adjoining bone.

13. Summarize some of the causes of retarded or accelerated bone development.

14. Outline the system which the author has developed for consideration of bone radiology in the final synthesis of diagnosis.

5

Fractures and Dislocations of the Extremities

INTRODUCTION

Description of "Minimal" Study

The radiographs for a suspected fracture or dislocation must be made in a minimum of two planes at right angles to each other, and special views must at times be utilized.

The areas studied must be large enough to include at least one joint and preferably two joints if the bone in question lies between two joints.

The mechanism of trauma or injury must be understood so that the part being radiographed will include adjoining areas which may have undergone secondary injury. Thus, for example, in injuries involving a fall on the outstretched hand, the elbow or clavicle may also sustain a fracture in addition to the wrist.

An understanding of the routine radiographic examinations employed is fundamental. Although the routine radiographic studies for each anatomic part are summarized in greater detail in the author's other texts, a brief review will be rendered here because of its importance.

Major Items for Analysis on Radiographs of Extremities for Fractures. Assuming that appropriate radiographic views are in hand, *four major items require careful analysis:*

1. The degree of apposition of the fragments
2. The alignment of the fragments with respect to the line of weight-bearing and movement of joints—diagrams in Chapter 11
3. The degree of torsion of the fragments with respect to one another
4. The degree of shortening of the bone as a whole

The radiographic method provides excellent data regarding the extent of the actual bone injury, the type of fracture (whether it is simple or comminuted, transverse, oblique, longitudinal, spiral, T-, V-, or Y-shaped), and whether there has been penetration by a pointed missile.

Some inferential information may also be gained: (1) Is there soft tissue caught between the fragments? (2) What is the associated soft tissue injury? (3) How much injury has been sustained in the periosteum? (4) How much cartilaginous or joint injury has been sustained?

The complete extent of associated soft tissue injury cannot be evaluated radiographically by simple radiographs and may sometimes require special arterial angiograms and neurological study.

> **Time Intervals Between Radiographic Studies.** Following the *initial diagnostic study,* films should be obtained as follows:
> 1. *Post-reduction and post-immobilization*
> 2. *One or two weeks later, if position has changed*
> 3. *After approximately six or eight weeks for primary callus*
> 4. *After each plaster cast or traction change*
> 5. *Before final discharge of the patient*

TYPES OF FRACTURES

The various types of fractures of the extremities are summarized in Figure 5–1. The following special comments are warranted regarding fracture types:

Avulsion- or Chip-type Fractures are often associated with forcible tearing of ligaments, tendons, or muscle attachments. This is the most serious aspect of this type of fracture.

The Most Important Consideration in the Oblique, Spiral, or Screwlike Fracture is the fact that soft tissue may be interposed between the fragments.

If interposition of soft tissues has occurred, impairment of the healing process may ensue.

Epiphysiolysis and Epiphyseal Injuries are classified into five types according to the Salter-Harris classification (Figure 5–2). Comparison films of the opposite uninvolved side should be obtained whenever possible. Significant disturbances in bone growth occur in only about 10 per cent of epiphyseal injuries because of the relationship of the usual fracture line to the epiphyseal plate and epiphyseal blood supply (DePalma; Rogers).

Types 4 and 5 in the Salter-Harris classification are most important to distinguish if at all possible. A minimum of two years is considered necessary before the possibility of shortening or deformity can be excluded. Radiographic evaluations should be performed at three to six month intervals, including comparison views with the opposite extremity.

Insufficiency, March, or Stress Fractures are also called "fatigue fractures," since they practically always occur at sites of maximal strain on bone, usually in connection with a type of unaccustomed activity. The second, third, or fourth metatarsals are frequent sites of occurrence, often without any demonstrable trauma. Another frequent localization is the upper third of the tibia.

Pathological Fractures are fractures superimposed upon an underlying pathological process in bone, such as metastatic disease, bone tumors or chronic osteomyelitis.

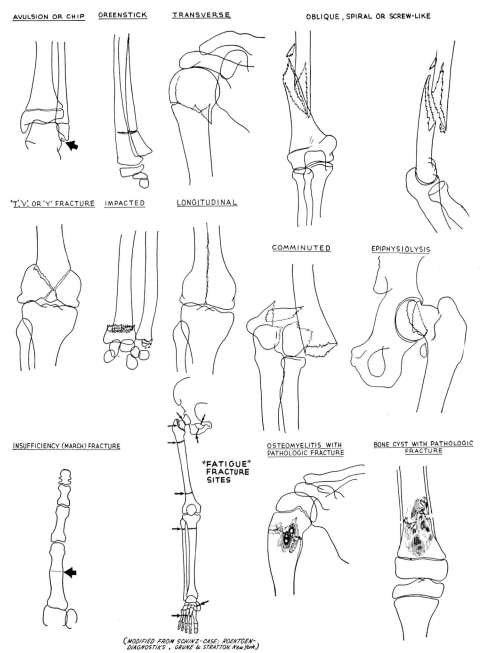

Figure 5–1 The various types of fractures of the extremities.

TYPE I

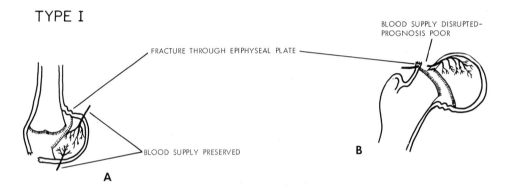

FRACTURE THROUGH EPIPHYSEAL PLATE

BLOOD SUPPLY DISRUPTED-
PROGNOSIS POOR

BLOOD SUPPLY PRESERVED

A

B

TYPE II

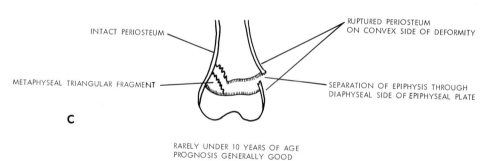

INTACT PERIOSTEUM

RUPTURED PERIOSTEUM
ON CONVEX SIDE OF DEFORMITY

METAPHYSEAL TRIANGULAR FRAGMENT

SEPARATION OF EPIPHYSIS THROUGH
DIAPHYSEAL SIDE OF EPIPHYSEAL PLATE

C

RARELY UNDER 10 YEARS OF AGE
PROGNOSIS GENERALLY GOOD

Figure 5–2

Illustration continued on the opposite page

TYPE III

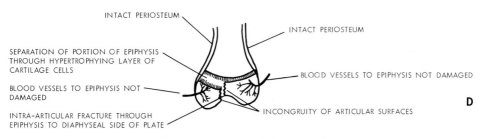

INTACT PERIOSTEUM

INTACT PERIOSTEUM

SEPARATION OF PORTION OF EPIPHYSIS THROUGH HYPERTROPHYING LAYER OF CARTILAGE CELLS

BLOOD VESSELS TO EPIPHYSIS NOT DAMAGED

BLOOD VESSELS TO EPIPHYSIS NOT DAMAGED

INCONGRUITY OF ARTICULAR SURFACES

INTRA-ARTICULAR FRACTURE THROUGH EPIPHYSIS TO DIAPHYSEAL SIDE OF PLATE

D

GENERALLY INVOLVES UPPER AND LOWER TIBIA.
PROGNOSIS GENERALLY FAVORABLE.

TYPE IV

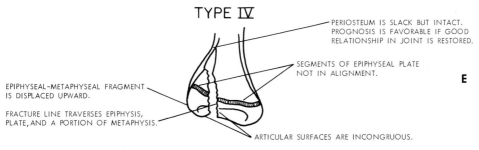

PERIOSTEUM IS SLACK BUT INTACT. PROGNOSIS IS FAVORABLE IF GOOD RELATIONSHIP IN JOINT IS RESTORED.

SEGMENTS OF EPIPHYSEAL PLATE NOT IN ALIGNMENT.

EPIPHYSEAL-METAPHYSEAL FRAGMENT IS DISPLACED UPWARD.

FRACTURE LINE TRAVERSES EPIPHYSIS, PLATE, AND A PORTION OF METAPHYSIS.

ARTICULAR SURFACES ARE INCONGRUOUS.

E

MOST COMMON IN LATERAL CONDYLE OF HUMERUS UNDER AGE 10.
INTERNAL FIXATION OFTEN NECESSARY.

TYPE V

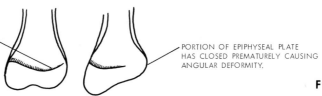

INJURY TO EPIPHYSEAL PLATE. NOTE: NO DISRUPTION OF ARCHITECTURE OF EPIPHYSIS OR METAPHYSIS OCCURS. SERIOUSNESS OF LESION MANIFESTS ITSELF AFTER A PERIOD OF GROWTH.

PORTION OF EPIPHYSEAL PLATE HAS CLOSED PREMATURELY CAUSING ANGULAR DEFORMITY.

F

KNEE AND ANKLE - 12 TO 16 YEARS.
ROENTGENOGRAMS ARE OFTEN NEGATIVE.
PROGNOSIS IS POOR - SHORTENING AND JOINT DEFORMITY RESULT.

TYPES 4 AND 5 ARE, THEREFORE, MOST IMPORTANT TO DISTINGUISH IF AT ALL POSSIBLE. A MINIMUM OF 2 YEARS IS CONSIDERED MINIMUM BEFORE ONE CAN EXCLUDE THE POSSIBILITY OF SHORTENING OR DEFORMITY. RADIOGRAPHIC RE-EVALUATION SHOULD BE PERFORMED AT 2 TO 6 MONTH INTERVALS, INCLUDING COMPARISON VIEWS WITH THE OPPOSITE EXTREMITY.

Figure 5–2 (*Continued*)

SYSTEMATIC REVIEW OF SOME CLINICALLY IMPORTANT APPENDICULAR SKELETAL FRACTURES AND DISLOCATIONS

Clavicle

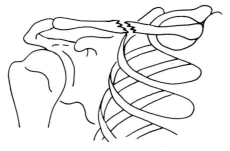 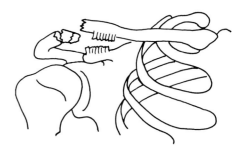

MOST FREQUENTLY
ENCOUNTERED FRACTURE
OF CLAVICLE
(IMPORTANT
COSMETICALLY)

FRACTURE MAY BE ASSOCIATED WITH RUPTURE OF CAPSULAR
LIGAMENTS AND CORACOCLAVICULAR LIGAMENTS.
FRACTURES DISTAL TO CORACOCLAVICULAR LIGAMENTS
FREQUENTLY FAIL TO UNITE.

Figure 5–3 Fracture of the middle and outer third of the clavicle. Fracture distal to the coracoclavicular ligaments with disruption of all ligaments usually requires surgical intervention.

Shoulder

X-RAY OF RECURRENT
SHOULDER DISLOCATION

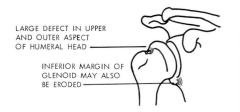

LARGE DEFECT IN UPPER
AND OUTER ASPECT
OF HUMERAL HEAD

INFERIOR MARGIN OF
GLENOID MAY ALSO
BE ERODED

(WHEN PRESENT, THIS LESION MAY BE
DIFFICULT TO DEMONSTRATE UNLESS
X-RAY IS TAKEN WITH ARM IN A 50 TO
80 DEGREE INTERNAL ROTATION)

Figure 5–4 Most frequent changes noted with recurrent shoulder dislocation.

Humerus

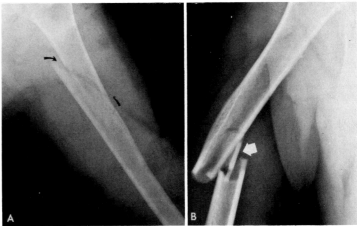

Figure 5–5 *A.* Spiral fracture of the humerus. *B.* Transverse comminuted fracture of humerus.

Elbow

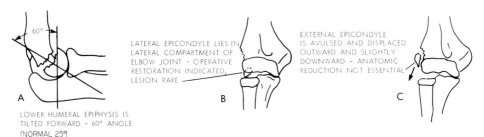

60°

A

LOWER HUMERAL EPIPHYSIS IS
TILTED FORWARD - 60° ANGLE
(NORMAL 25°)

LATERAL EPICONDYLE LIES IN
LATERAL COMPARTMENT OF
ELBOW JOINT - OPERATIVE
RESTORATION INDICATED,
LESION RARE

B

EXTERNAL EPICONDYLE
IS AVULSED AND DISPLACED
OUTWARD AND SLIGHTLY
DOWNWARD - ANATOMIC
REDUCTION NOT ESSENTIAL

C

Figure 5–6 Epiphyseal fractures of the lower humerus. (After Watson-Jones, R.: *Fracture and Joint Injuries.* 4th Ed. Baltimore, Williams & Wilkins Co., 1955.)

Head and Neck of Radius

Care must be exercised to recognize loose bone fragments within the elbow joint. Fractures of the radial head may conveniently be subdivided into (1) those which may be treated by conservative methods, and (2) those requiring excision of the radial head (DePalma) (Figure 5–7B).

Generally *those requiring excision of the radial head involve the articular surface with some displacement or tilt* of either a fragment of the head or the·complete head of the radius. An impacted fracture of the neck of the radius can usually be treated conservatively.

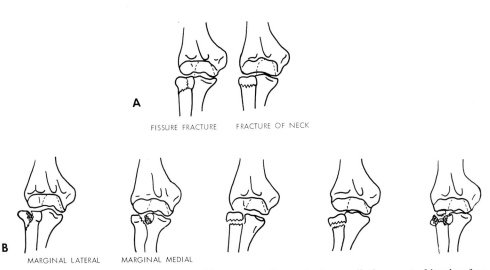

A

FISSURE FRACTURE   FRACTURE OF NECK

B

MARGINAL LATERAL   MARGINAL MEDIAL

Figure 5–7 *A.* Types of fractures treated by conservative methods—no displacement of head or fragment.
B. Types of fractures requiring excision of the radial head—displacement of head or fragment.

Ulnar Shaft

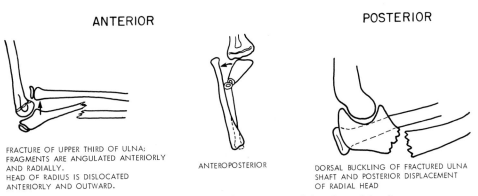

ANTERIOR

POSTERIOR

FRACTURE OF UPPER THIRD OF ULNA;
FRAGMENTS ARE ANGULATED ANTERIORLY
AND RADIALLY.
HEAD OF RADIUS IS DISLOCATED
ANTERIORLY AND OUTWARD.

ANTEROPOSTERIOR

DORSAL BUCKLING OF FRACTURED ULNA
SHAFT AND POSTERIOR DISPLACEMENT
OF RADIAL HEAD

Figure 5–8 Varieties of Monteggia fractures or dislocations of the elbow.

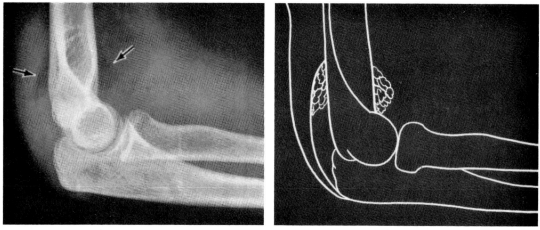

Figure 5–9   Lateral radiograph of 13 year old girl who fell on her elbow, incurring a traumatic bursitis. No fracture was demonstrated. Arrows indicate anterior and posterior radiolucencies representing respectively displaced anterior and posterior fat pads. Note the concavity inferiorly in the posterior fat pad due to the impression of the distended synovial sac; also the rounded posterior contour of the triceps tendon. (From Bledsoe, R. C., and Izenstark, J. L.: Radiology, *73*:720, 1959.)

Distal Forearm

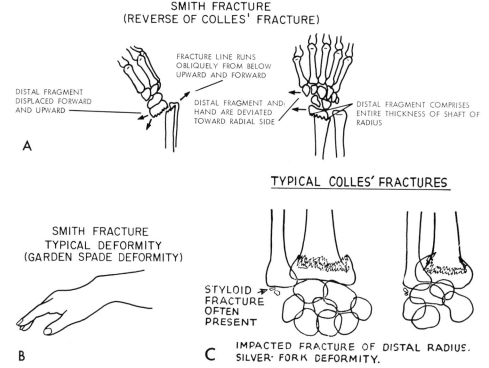

Figure 5–10   Diagram to illustrate Colles' and Smith fractures of the distal forearm. If the interosseous membrane is involved, pronation and supination may be impaired.

Wrist

Fractures of the Scaphoid (navicular) (Figure 5–12) are most frequent among the carpal bones of the wrist. *Healing depends much on the integrity of the blood supply.* This may readily be interrupted by certain types of fractures. *The arteries enter the scaphoid on the dorsal surface in the region of the tubercle and in the waist of the bone or midposition.* When separated from this blood supply, avascular necrosis may result.

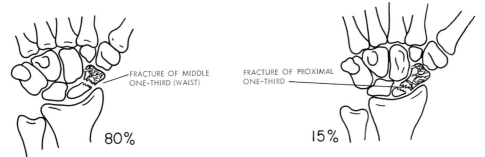

FRACTURE OF MIDDLE ONE-THIRD (WAIST)

FRACTURE OF PROXIMAL ONE-THIRD

80%

15%

FRACTURE THROUGH THE WAIST (MIDDLE THIRD), MAY LEAD TO ASEPTIC NECROSIS PROXIMAL FRAGMENT

FRACTURE THROUGH THE PROXIMAL THIRD

SOME OF THE ASSOCIATED INJURIES ARE:
DISLOCATION OF RADIOCARPAL JOINT.
DISLOCATION BETWEEN THE TWO ROWS OF CARPAL BONES.
FRACTURE-DISLOCATION OF DISTAL END OF RADIUS.
FRACTURE OF BASE OF THUMB METACARPAL (BENNETT'S FRACTURE).
DISLOCATION OF LUNATE.

NOTE: THERE MAY BE ANY COMBINATION OF THESE AND OCCASIONALLY A SEGMENTAL FRACTURE OF SCAPHOID OCCURS

Figure 5–11   Classification of the most frequent fractures of the scaphoid carpal bone.

Lunate and Perilunate Dislocations

VOLAR DISLOCATION OF THE LUNATE

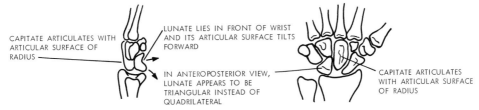

CAPITATE ARTICULATES WITH ARTICULAR SURFACE OF RADIUS

LUNATE LIES IN FRONT OF WRIST AND ITS ARTICULAR SURFACE TILTS FORWARD

IN ANTEROPOSTERIOR VIEW, LUNATE APPEARS TO BE TRIANGULAR INSTEAD OF QUADRILATERAL

CAPITATE ARTICULATES WITH ARTICULAR SURFACE OF RADIUS

Figure 5–12

DORSAL PERILUNAR DISLOCATION

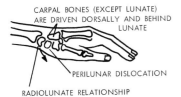

CARPAL BONES (EXCEPT LUNATE) ARE DRIVEN DORSALLY AND BEHIND LUNATE

PERILUNAR DISLOCATION

RADIOLUNATE RELATIONSHIP IS PRESERVED

Figure 5–13

DORSAL DISLOCATION OF THE LUNATE

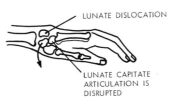

LUNATE DISLOCATION

LUNATE CAPITATE ARTICULATION IS DISRUPTED

Figure 5–14

VOLAR PERILUNAR DISLOCATION

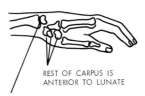

REST OF CARPUS IS ANTERIOR TO LUNATE

LUNATE RETAINS ITS NORMAL POSITION WITH RADIUS
NOTE: FRACTURE OF SCAPHOID MAY ALSO OCCUR WITH THIS MECHANISM.

Figure 5–15

Proximal Femur

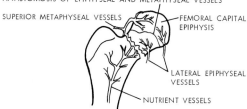

BLOOD SUPPLY OF THE FEMORAL CAPITAL EPIPHYSIS AND NECK OF THE FEMUR IN CHILDHOOD

EPIPHYSEAL PLATE – THIS PLATE PRECLUDES ANASTOMOSIS OF EPIPHYSEAL AND METAPHYSEAL VESSELS

SUPERIOR METAPHYSEAL VESSELS

FEMORAL CAPITAL EPIPHYSIS

LATERAL EPIPHYSEAL VESSELS

NUTRIENT VESSELS

NOTE: BLOOD SUPPLY COMING THROUGH LIGAMENTUM TERES AT THIS AGE IS VERY INADEQUATE AND CONFINED TO A SMALL SEGMENT OF EPIPHYSIS

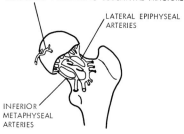

BLOOD SUPPLY OF THE FEMORAL HEAD

ARTERY OF LIGAMENTUM TERES, (NOT VERY SIGNIFICANT ORDINARILY, BUT MOST IMPORTANT FOLLOWING SUBCAPITAL FRACTURES)

LATERAL EPIPHYSEAL ARTERIES

INFERIOR METAPHYSEAL ARTERIES

Figure 5–16

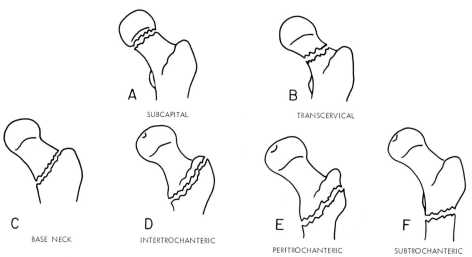

A — SUBCAPITAL

B — TRANSCERVICAL

C — BASE NECK

D — INTERTROCHANTERIC

E — PERITROCHANTERIC

F — SUBTROCHANTERIC

Figure 5–17   Fractures of the proximal femur—classification.

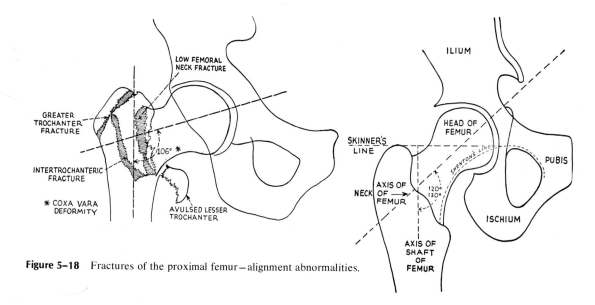

GREATER TROCHANTER FRACTURE

LOW FEMORAL NECK FRACTURE

INTERTROCHANTERIC FRACTURE

106° *

* COXA VARA DEFORMITY

AVULSED LESSER TROCHANTER

ILIUM

HEAD OF FEMUR

SKINNER'S LINE

SHENTON'S LINE

AXIS OF NECK OF FEMUR

120°
130°

PUBIS

ISCHIUM

AXIS OF SHAFT OF FEMUR

Figure 5–18   Fractures of the proximal femur—alignment abnormalities.

Shaft of the Femur

Classification. These may be transverse, oblique, spiral, or severely comminuted. In children occasionally they are greenstick.

Distal Femur

Lower End

1. Lateral or medial condylar
2. Supracondylar
3. Intercondylar, T-, V-, or Y-fractures
4. Supracondylar with marked posterior angulation as a result of the pull of the gastrocnemius muscle.

   In children there may be various types of epiphyseal fractures or displacements in accordance with the previously described Salter-Harris classification (Figure 5–24).

   Intercondylar fractures of the femur are always complicated by severe soft tissue damage and massive hemarthrosis.

Knee

1. Anterior tibial tubercle
2. Patella (with or without separation of fragments)
   a. With or without dislocation
   b. With or without tear of adjoining ligaments

   In the interpretation of fractures of the patella, various anomalies of the patella must be borne in mind. Thus, the *bipartite* and *tripartite patella* contain incomplete ossified segments of the patella. The unfused portions of the patella in these instances are in the *upper outer quadrant of the patella on its internal aspect in the lateral views.*

3. Fractures of the condyles of the tibia
   a. Fractures of the medial condyle (rare)
   b. Depression of the central portion of the tibial plateau
4. T- or Y-fractures of the upper end of the tibia, usually with downward depression of the tibial condyles.

   Chip or avulsion fractures of the tibial eminence are often associated with and indicative of anterior or posterior cruciate ligament tears. The associated ligamentous injuries are by far the most serious consequences of this fracture. Internal derangement of the knee may also be associated, such as in meniscal tears and fractures. These can be diagnosed radiographically with the aid of special contrast studies (contrast arthrography).

Tibia and Fibula

Union is notoriously slow and nonunion frequent. Ordinarily fractures of the upper shaft of the fibula can be disregarded, provided good alignment in the shaft of the tibia for weight bearing is obtained.

Fractures of the lower shaft of the fibula are often associated with fracture dislocations of the ankle.

A fracture in the lower shaft of the tibia is very often accompanied by a contre-coup upper shaft fracture in the fibula.

Ankle

Generally, injuries of the ankle are grouped into: (a) *inversion injuries* (Figure 5–20), and (b) *eversion injuries* (Figure 5–21). An effort is made, from the x-ray picture, to predict the ligamentous injury which has resulted.

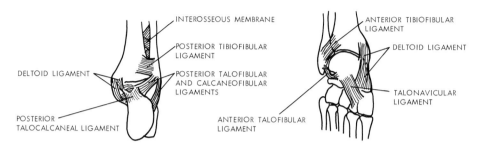

Figure 5–19   Diagrams demonstrating the major ligamentous structures of the ankle.

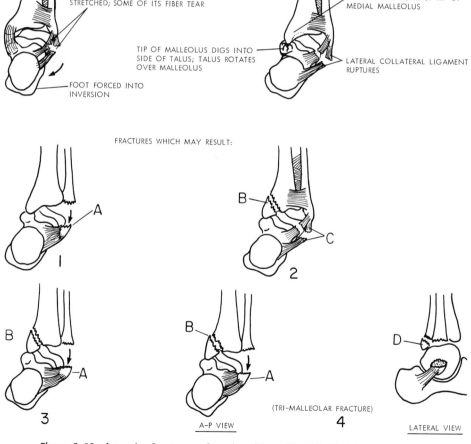

Figure 5–20   Inversion fractures and sprains of the ankle. (Modified from DePalma.)

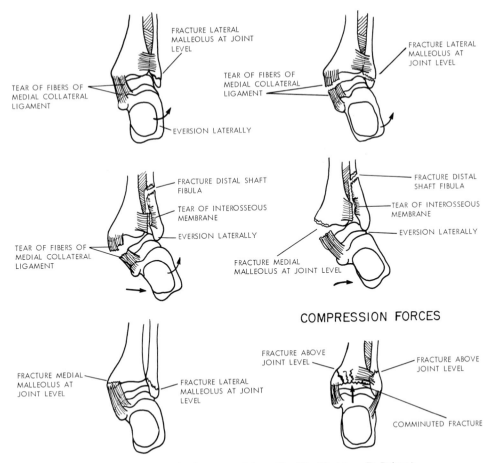

Figure 5–21 Eversion fractures of the ankle. (Modified from DePalma.)

Sesamoid Bones of the Foot and Ankle (Figure 5–22). Sesamoid bones of the foot and ankle occasionally may be confused with avulsion-type fractures and they may not necessarily be symmetrical on both sides of the body. Nevertheless, comparison films of the opposite side are recommended. The most common sesamoids are os trigonum, os peroneum, and the accessory navicular.

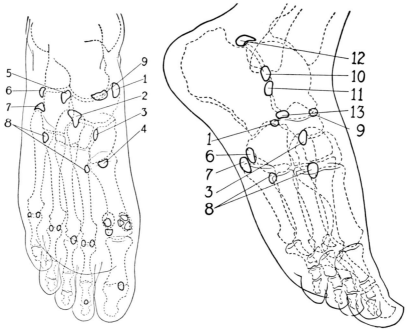

Figure 5–22 Schematic diagram to show sesamoid bones and supernumerary bones of the foot. (1) Os tibiale externum; (2) processus uncinatus; (3) intercuneiforme; (4) pars peronea metatarsalia I; (5) cuboides secundarium; (6) os peroneum; (7) os vesalianum; (8) intermetatarseum; (9) accessory navicular; (10) talus accessorius; (11) os sustentaculum; (12) os trigonum; (13) calcaneus secundarius. The most common of these are 1, 6, 7, 9 and 12. (From McNeill: *Roentgen Technique*. Springfield. Charles C Thomas, 1947.)

Questions—Chapter 5

See end of Chapter 6.

6

Fracture Healing, Complications From Fractures, and Methods of Treatment from the Radiologic Standpoint

THE MAIN HISTOLOGIC STEPS IN FRACTURE HEALING AND CORRELATED RADIOGRAPHS

Main Steps in Fracture Healing (Figure 6–1). The main histologic steps in fracture healing may be summarized in the following outline:
1. Formation of hematoma
2. Organization of hematoma
3. Formation of fibrous callus
4. Replacement of fibrous callus by primary bony callus
5. Absorption of primary bony callus and transformation gradually to secondary bony callus
6. Functional reconstruction of the bone in accordance with line of stress and adaptation by bone "modeling"

Every change in the position of fragments during the process of repair disturbs the formation of callus and therefore disturbs the repair process. If, in the course of healing, hyaline cartilage develops at the fracture margin, an actual false joint may in turn develop and nonunion ensue. The false joint is called a "neoarthrosis" and can be recognized by the formation of dense eburnated bone beneath the hyaline cartilage at the fracture margin (Figure 6–4).

Correlation of the Six Phases of Repair with Radiographic Appearances. The successive radiographic appearances in the process of fracture healing may be visualized as follows (Figure 6–3):

1. When the hematoma is formed there is considerable *soft tissue swelling* in the immediate vicinity of the fracture.

2. During the process of organization of the hematoma, there is shrinkage of the swelling and the formation of fibrous callus with *progressive radiolucency of the bone surrounding the fragments*. There may be some resorption of bone along the fractured cleft, producing *the widened cleft*.

In the case of comminuted fractures, if there should be a devitalized fragment the surrounding bone will tend to become radiolucent, whereas the devitalized fragment will retain its original density and will thus be readily identified as a *sequestrum*.

3. The *primary bone callus* is visualized as a faintly calcified area surrounding the fracture site. The time of appearance of bony callus is very variable and depends to a great extent upon the age of the patient and the fracture site. In young persons the bony callus is formed very rapidly, and in the newborn, massive bony callus may be visible by the end of one week.

4. The *primary bony callus becomes denser* and more sharply circumscribed and the bony cleft itself begins to be filled in by visible callus.

5. There is a *gradual and sharper delineation of the primary bony and periosteal callus* and actually a diminution in the size of the periosteal callus.

6. There is a gradual reformation of the normal appearing bony trabeculae and contour of the bone.

STEPS IN THE HEALING OF FRACTURES

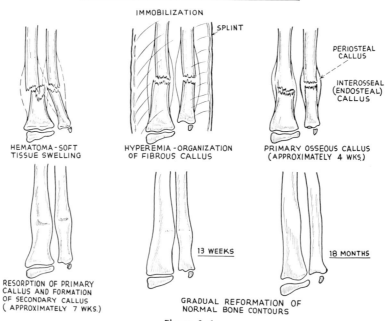

IMMOBILIZATION

SPLINT

PERIOSTEAL CALLUS

INTEROSSEAL (ENDOSTEAL) CALLUS

HEMATOMA-SOFT TISSUE SWELLING

HYPEREMIA-ORGANIZATION OF FIBROUS CALLUS

PRIMARY OSSEOUS CALLUS (APPROXIMATELY 4 WKS.)

RESORPTION OF PRIMARY CALLUS AND FORMATION OF SECONDARY CALLUS (APPROXIMATELY 7 WKS.)

13 WEEKS

GRADUAL REFORMATION OF NORMAL BONE CONTOURS

18 MONTHS

Figure 6–1

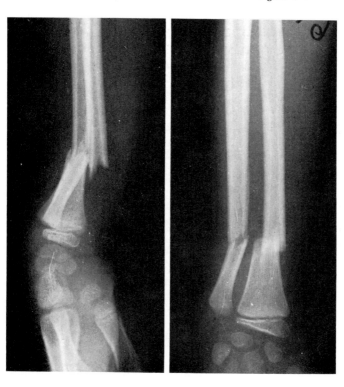

Figure 6–2   Hematoma, soft tissue swelling.

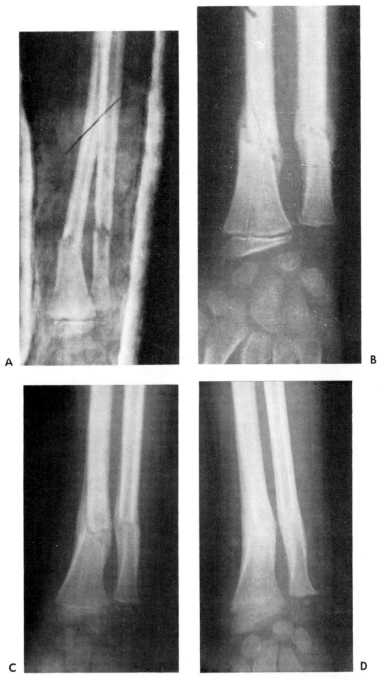

Figure 6–3 *A*. Hyperemia, organization of fibrous callus. *B*, Primary osseous callus (approximately 4 weeks). *C*. Resorption of primary callus and formation of secondary callus (approximately 7 weeks). *D*. Gradual reformation of normal bone contours (13 weeks).

Pathogenesis of Delayed Union (with Pseudoarthrosis Formation) or Nonunion (Neoarthrosis). Normally primary bony callus consists of a metaplasia of fibrous granulation scar tissue to fibro- and hyaline cartilage with some calcification. The greater the development of hyaline cartilage (from motion of fragments or delay in repair), the more protracted is lamellated bone formation, and the more likely is *pseudoarthrosis.*

If an actual cleft forms in this pseudoarthrosis, and the hyaline cartilage fails to calcify, *neoarthrosis* is formed with calcification deposition adjoining the hyaline cartilage. This may be recognized radiographically by a dense line of compact bone adjoining the fracture line (Figure 6–4).

Questions—Chapters 5 and 6

1. What radiographic views are minimal requirements in suspected fracture or dislocation?

2. How large an area should be studied in any suspected fracture?

(*Questions continued on page 54*)

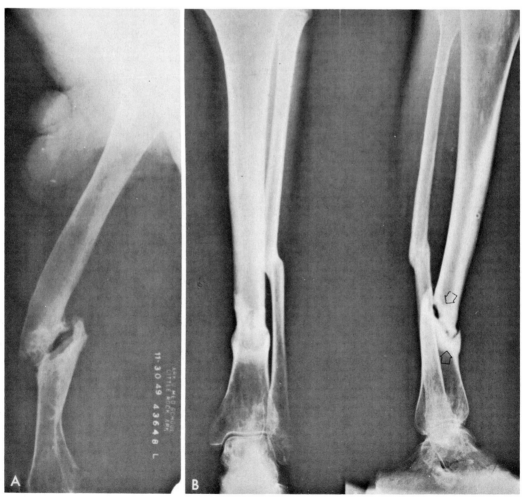

Figure 6–4 *A.* Radiograph demonstrating pseudoarthrosis. *B.* Radiograph demonstrating neoarthrosis. Note the eburnated smooth bone at the fracture margin.

COMPLICATIONS OF FRACTURES

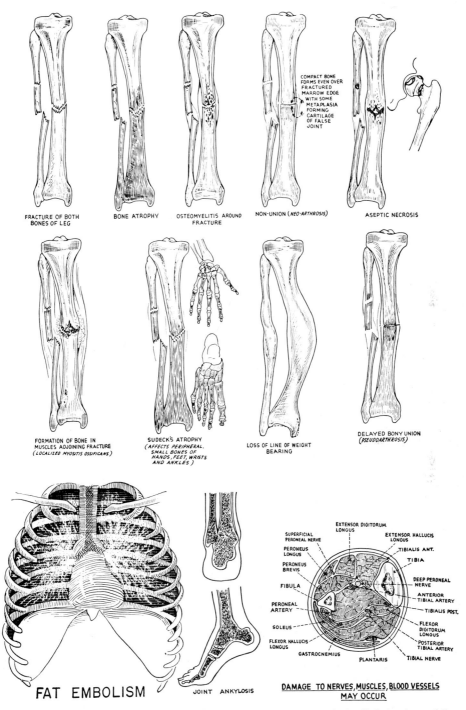

FRACTURE OF BOTH BONES OF LEG

BONE ATROPHY

OSTEOMYELITIS AROUND FRACTURE

NON-UNION (*NEO-ARTHROSIS*)

COMPACT BONE FORMS EVEN OVER FRACTURED MARROW EDGE WITH SOME METAPLASIA FORMING CARTILAGE OF FALSE JOINT

ASEPTIC NECROSIS

FORMATION OF BONE IN MUSCLES ADJOINING FRACTURE (*LOCALIZED MYOSITIS OSSIFICANS*)

SUDECK'S ATROPHY (*AFFECTS PERIPHERAL, SMALL BONES OF HANDS, FEET, WRISTS AND ANKLES*)

LOSS OF LINE OF WEIGHT BEARING

DELAYED BONY UNION (*PSEUDOARTHROSIS*)

FAT EMBOLISM

JOINT ANKYLOSIS

DAMAGE TO NERVES, MUSCLES, BLOOD VESSELS MAY OCCUR

EXTENSOR DIGITORUM LONGUS
SUPERFICIAL PERONEAL NERVE
EXTENSOR HALLUCIS LONGUS
PERONEUS LONGUS
TIBIALIS ANT.
PERONEUS BREVIS
TIBIA
FIBULA
DEEP PERONEAL NERVE
ANTERIOR TIBIAL ARTERY
PERONEAL ARTERY
TIBIALIS POST.
SOLEUS
FLEXOR DIGITORUM LONGUS
FLEXOR HALLUCIS LONGUS
POSTERIOR TIBIAL ARTERY
GASTROCNEMIUS
PLANTARIS
TIBIAL NERVE

Figure 6–5 Complications of fractures diagrammatically illustrated. It is implied that loss of line of weight-bearing also indicates excessive deformity.

3. What are the four major items requiring careful analysis in respect to fractures of extremities?

4. What are the recommended time intervals between radiographic studies following a fracture?

5. Indicate the various types of fractures by classification.

6. What is the importance of an avulsion- or chip-type fracture?

7. Indicate the Salter-Harris classification of epiphyseal injuries. What is the significance of these five types and their relative incidence?

8. Define "pathologic fracture."

9. From the standpoint of potential complications, what is the most important site for fracture of the clavicle?

10. What are the potential dangers in respect to vascular or radial injuries in fractures of the humerus and where are such fractures noted within the humerus?

11. What is Volkmann's ischemic contracture and with what fracture is this frequently found?

12. What is the importance of the carrying angle, especially in children?

13. What is the importance of recognition of chip fragments around the elbow in association with the joints of the elbow?

14. Why is it important to recognize loose bone fragments or altered configuration in fractures of the head and neck of the radius?

15. What is the importance of detection of the fat plane in the region of the elbow? What is the "displaced fat pad sign"?

16. Why is it important to attempt to visualize with clarity the position of the interosseous membrane?

17. Which are the most important fractures and dislocations of the carpal bones?

18. What is the blood supply of the scaphoid carpal bone and how does this relate to potential complications? Wherein does frequent complication arise?

19. What is the difference between lunate and perilunate dislocation? How many types of perilunate dislocations do we recognize?

20. What are the various types of fractures of the acetabulum?

21. How is the blood supply of the femoral capital epiphysis and neck derived?

22. Classify the dislocations of the hip.

23. What is acetabular dysplasia and what is its importance?

24. Why is it important to rotate the foot internally if possible in obtaining antero-posterior views for potential fracture of the neck of the femur?

25. What is the most frequent deformity in fracture of the neck of the femur?

26. What is Shenton's line? Skinner's line? What is the importance of these lining techniques?

27. Describe the basic ligamentous anatomy of the ankle and its importance in respect to fractures in this injury.

28. What injuries may result in inversion injury of the ankle?

29. What injuries of the ankle may result in eversion injuries?

30. What are the routine views for suspected injury to the calcaneus?

31. What is the tuber or critical angle of the calcaneus and what is its importance?

32. What are march fractures?

33. What are the most frequent sesamoid bones of the foot encountered?

34. What are the six main steps in fracture healing?

35. What is meant by pseudoarthrosis and neoarthrosis and how may they be recognized radiographically?

36. What are the various phases of repair in bone healing following fractures, as recognized radiographically?

37. List the various complications from fractures.

38. What are the major items for analysis on radiographs of extremities for fractures?

39. At what time intervals should fractured extremities be studied following the initial x-rays?

40. Outline the general principles for definitive treatment of fractures.

7

Congenital and Hereditary Abnormalities of the Skeletal System

Introduction

The subject of congenital and hereditary abnormalities has become exceedingly complex and extends far beyond the scope of this text. Inborn errors of metabolism are more and more being identified as specific metabolic disorders which in turn may be related to genetic mutations or chromosomal aberrations.

This section is included so that the student may formulate a systematic approach to these problems from the radiologic standpoint, and so that he may utilize the outlined material as a framework around which he may build a concept of the complexity of the field and its detailed parts.

We may divide this group of disorders into *four major categories:*

1. *Underdevelopment of a bone or extremity*
2. *Overdevelopment of single bones or an extremity or duplication of parts*
3. *Maldevelopment of a skeletal part*
   a. *Regional* — localized in one part of the skeleton
   b. *General* (systemic in skeletal system — possibly associated with abnormalities in other systems)
      (1) Skeletal abnormalities in relation to known *chromosomal aberrations*
4. *Diseases of bone* related to a *defect extrinsic* to the bone but involving the bone secondarily

TABLE 7–1 CLASSIFICATION OF CONGENITAL AND HEREDITARY OSSEOUS MALFORMATIONS

Underdevelopment	Overdevelopment, Sclerosis, or Duplication	Maldevelopment				Primarily Extrinsic to Bone
		Regional	General			
			Epiphyseal	Metaphyseal	Bones or Tissues Diffusely	
Brachydactylia	Hyperphalangism	Syndactylia	Congenital stippled epiphyses	Ollier's disease	Achondroplasia	Sprengel's deformity
Oligodactylia	Arachnodactylia (Marfan's syndrome)	Perodactylia	Dysplasia epiphysialis multiplex	Diaphyseal aclasis	Polytopic enchondral dysostosis (Morquio's; Pfaundler-Hurler; Leri)	Myositis ossificans progressiva
Aplasias and phocomelias	Klinefelter's syndrome	Peromelia		Metaphyseal dysplasia (Pyle's disease)	Osteogenesis imperfecta	Neurofibromatosis
Cleidocranial dysostosis	Melorheostosis	Madelung's deformity		Hypophosphatasia (hereditary) (see Chap. 8)	Acrocephalosyndactylia	Lipoid storage disease
Idiopathic familial osteolysis	Partial gigantism	Vertical talus			Mandibulofacial dystostosis (Francescheti's syndrome) (Treacher-Collins syndrome)	Hematopoietic disorders
Absent patella—fingernail syndrome (hereditary arthro-osteo-onycho-dysplasia)	Marble bone disease*				Congenital dysplasia of face and extremities	
	Engelmann's disease or hereditary multiple diaphyseal sclerosis (Ribbing)*				Craniometaphyseal dysplasia	
	Osteopoikilosis*				Chondroectodermal dysplasia (Ellis-van Creveld)	
	Osteopathia striata (Voorhoeve)				Familial metaphyseal dysplasia (Pyle's syndrome)	
	Epiphyseal dysplasia†			Known chromosomal aberrations	Mongolism (trisomy 21)	
	Congenital stippled† epiphyses (chondroangiopathia calcificans congenita)				Trisomy 16-18 (possibly trisomy 13-15 or triploid mosaicism)	

*See Chapter 7 (sclerosis of bone).
†See also fourth column of this table.

UNDERDEVELOPMENT OF A BONE OR EXTREMITY
(EXAMPLE)

Cleidocranial Dysostosis (Figure 7–1)

Radiographic Features. Aplasia of clavicles; delayed closure of the sutures of the skull; delayed and sometimes absent ossification in the bones of the pelvis, particularly in the pubes and ischia; curious shape of the phalanges; and moderately severe osteoporosis throughout.

The skull ordinarily contains numerous wormian bones in the vicinity of the lambdoid suture, deficient ossification of the bones of the cranial vault, large fontanelles, and a limited union of the frontal bone centrally. Usually there is also a deficient ossification in the symphysis of the mandible. The thorax often appears compressed from both sides.

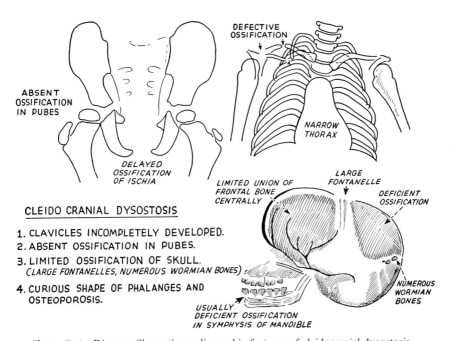

CLEIDO CRANIAL DYSOSTOSIS

1. CLAVICLES INCOMPLETELY DEVELOPED.
2. ABSENT OSSIFICATION IN PUBES.
3. LIMITED OSSIFICATION OF SKULL.
   (LARGE FONTANELLES, NUMEROUS WORMIAN BONES)
4. CURIOUS SHAPE OF PHALANGES AND OSTEOPOROSIS.

Figure 7–1 Diagram illustrating radiographic features of cleidocranial dysostosis.

OVERDEVELOPMENT OF A PART OR SUPERNUMERARY PARTS, OR OVERPRODUCTION OF BONE-PRODUCING SCLEROSIS (EXAMPLE)

This group of disorders includes those in which the bones are too numerous, too broad, or too long; or in which there are foci of sclerotic bone, suggesting overproduction. In this latter group the *sclerosis may be diffuse (marble bones), concentrated throughout the shaft (Engelmann's disease), or striated or spotted* in the bones.

Arachnodactylia (Figure 7–2) merely refers to long slender fingers but is often associated with a systemic syndrome called *"Marfan's hereditary syndrome."*

Clinical Features.   This is a rare, hereditary, congenital growth disturbance affecting the musculoskeletal, cardiovascular, and ocular systems. The individual is often tall and slender, and all the long bones may be elongated. The arch of the palate is usually high and there may be a double row of teeth. The head is apt to be dolichocephalic, the thorax funnel-shaped, and the muscles, tendons, and ligaments of poor tone and hypermobile.

A thumb protruding beyond the confines of the clenched fist appears to be a confirming sign of the Marfan syndrome (Steinberg); it has been proposed as a screening test for this syndrome.

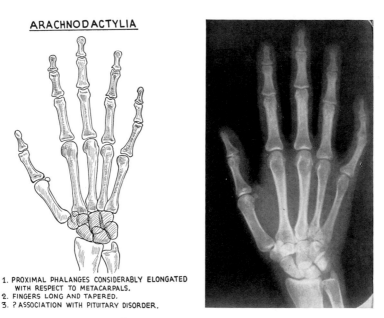

ARACHNODACTYLIA

1. PROXIMAL PHALANGES CONSIDERABLY ELONGATED
   WITH RESPECT TO METACARPALS.
2. FINGERS LONG AND TAPERED.
3. ? ASSOCIATION WITH PITUITARY DISORDER.

Figure 7–2   Arachnodactylia.

The most *common cardiovascular malformation is aneurysm formation,* usually of the dissecting type. However, *patent foramen ovale, mitral stenosis, or aortic insufficiency* may also be present.

Dislocation of the ocular lens is frequent and vision may be poor.

MALDEVELOPMENT OF AN ANATOMICAL PART—REGIONAL

The most important entities of this group are:

Syndactylia, or fusion of the fingers, in which the soft tissues or bones or both may be fused.

Perodactylia, in which the fingers appear to be amputated.

Peromelia, in which the extremities appear "flipperlike" and malformed.

Madelung's Deformity (Figure 7–3) (Paus), a hereditary overgrowth of the ulna, in which it extends distally and dorsally to the radius. There is also a bayonet-like projection of the distal end of the radius and the two bones tend to cross one another in lateral projection.

The Roentgenologic Criteria of Madelung's deformity may be summarized as follows:

A double lateral and dorsal bowing of the radius which involves the entire diaphysis but is most marked at the distal end.

A variable widening of the interosseous space due to the lateral curvature described above.

Shortening of the radius as compared with the normal standards for age and the relation to the size of the other bones of the upper extremity.

An alteration of the contour of the distal radius so that the articular surface of the epiphysis faces in an ulnar and palmar direction.

Premature fusion in the ulnar half of the epiphyseal line of the distal radius which contributes to accentuation of the deformity in early adolescence.

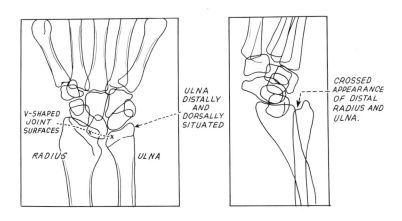

MADELUNG'S DEFORMITY

Figure 7–3

A change in the inferior radial articular surface with modification of the relationship of the carpal bones wedging them between the deformed radius and protruding ulna and giving them a triangular configuration with the lunate at the apex.

An arched curvature of the carpal bone which is a continuation of the arch of the dorsal bowing of the radial diaphysis (Langer).

MALDEVELOPMENT OF AN ANATOMICAL PART—GENERAL

Maldevelopments involving several extremities or the axial skeleton may be related to an inherited (genetic) disorder or to an intrauterine fetal affection. We shall briefly review these under four headings:

1. *Those predominantly involving the epiphyses*
2. *Those predominantly involving the metaphyses*
3. *Those affecting the bones and tissues generally,* often involving the axial skeleton as well
4. *Those diseases related to a defect extrinsic to the bone but involving the bone secondarily*

Predominant Epiphyseal Involvement

The two most important entities of this group are *congenital stippled epiphyses* and *epiphyseal dysplasia.* The latter is shown as an example.

Epiphyseal Dysplasia (Figure 7–4)

Radiographic Findings. Irregularity and hypoplasia of the developing ossification centers of the epiphyses, usually bilateral. The appearance suggests a "mulberry" deformity, due to separate centers arising and blending together. Their density eventually becomes normal but the deformity is permanent and causes some restriction of motion.

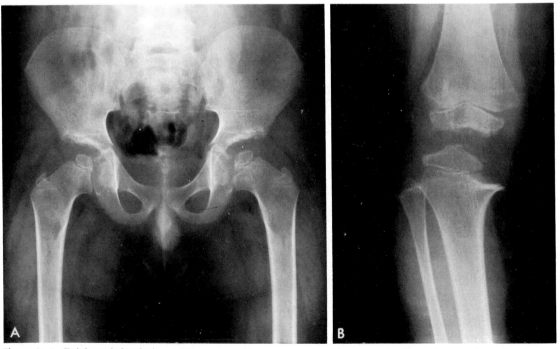

Figure 7–4 Epiphyseal dysplasia. *A.* Antero-posterior roentgenographic view of pelvis. Note small capital femoral epiphyses, wide joint space, and wide femoral necks. Acetabular margins are irregular. *B* and *C.* Antero-posterior and lateral views of the right knee showing fragmentation of the femoral and tibial epiphyses with lateral subluxation of the tibia. *D.* Antero-posterior view of right hand. Note short, broad metacarpals and phalanges. Ossification centers of capitate and hamate bones are irregular. (From Kaufman, E. E., and Coventry, M. B.: Proc. Mayo Clin., *38*:115, 1963.)

Predominant Metaphyseal Involvement

There are five major entities in this group. Chondrodysplasia is shown as an example.

1. *Chondrodysplasia* or *Ollier's disease*
2. *Multiple cartilaginous exostoses* or *diaphyseal aclasis*
3. *Metaphyseal dysplasia (Pyle's disease)*
4. *Hereditary hypophosphatasia (see Chapter 7)*
5. *Infantile familial or hereditary hypophosphatemia (see Chapter 8)*

Chondrodysplasia (Dyschondroplasia) or Ollier's disease is a disorder of the metaphyses primarily.

Radiographic Findings. Cartilaginous enchondromata appear as irregular, vaguely delimited defects and radiolucencies within the metaphyses. These are due to masses of cartilage in these sites. The bone may develop tumor-like swellings and may be short, thick and angulated, and there may be an osteolysis of the bony cortex of the metaphyses (Figure 7–5). Exostoses may also occur. Apart from the four extremities, the other involved areas are the pelvis, ribs, and rarely, the base of the skull. These enchondromatous masses may ultimately become almost completely, or at least partially, calcified.

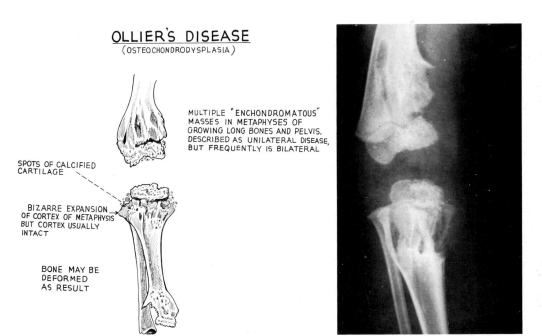

OLLIER'S DISEASE
(OSTEOCHONDRODYSPLASIA)

MULTIPLE "ENCHONDROMATOUS" MASSES IN METAPHYSES OF GROWING LONG BONES AND PELVIS. DESCRIBED AS UNILATERAL DISEASE, BUT FREQUENTLY IS BILATERAL

SPOTS OF CALCIFIED CARTILAGE

BIZARRE EXPANSION OF CORTEX OF METAPHYSIS BUT CORTEX USUALLY INTACT

BONE MAY BE DEFORMED AS RESULT

Figure 7–5

Diffuse Affection of Bones or Tissues

Only a few of the diseases in this category will be described, since so many groups and subgroups can be identified.

Achondroplasia or Chondrodystrophy (Maroteaux and Lamy) (Figure 7–6*B*). This is a congenital growth disturbance of endochondral bone associated with dwarfism. All the bones of cartilaginous origin, such as the pelvis, spine, shoulder girdle, skull, and extremities, are usually affected. The bones tend to grow circumferentially.

Radiographic Findings. (1) Marked shortening of bones of the extremities and the base of the skull. (2) Narrowed interpediculate distance of the vertebral bodies. (3) "Champagne-glass"-shaped pelvis (Figure 7–9). The ileum appears rectangular. (4) Decreased acetabular angles. (5) "Bullet-shaped" vertebrae (see Chapter 14). (6) Progressive stenosis and narrowing of the spinal canal. (7) Epiphyseal ossification centers are incompletely developed and deformed. Some of the epiphyseal plates close prematurely.

Many classifications of the bone dysplasias have been rendered but these are outside the scope of the present text (Table 7–3).

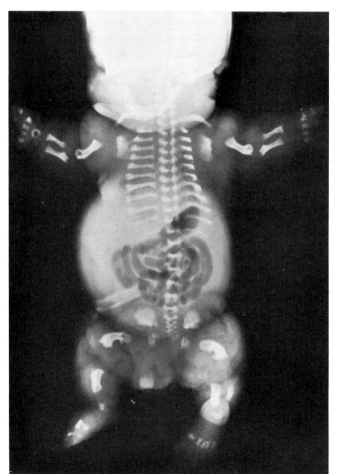

Figure 7–6 *A*. Thanatophoric dwarf, anteroposterior view. See text for description.

A

Diastrophic Dwarfism

Diastrophic dwarfism resembles achondroplasia clinically in that the pelvic configuration is similar (Langer, 1965).

In addition, the **most characteristic changes of diastrophic dwarfism are in the hands and feet, where the first metacarpal is small and the other metacarpals are broad with the distal end wider than the proximal end. In the spine the interpediculate distance increases from the level of L-1 to L-5 and is not narrowed as in the case of achondroplasia.**

Thanatophoric Dwarfism (Keats et al.) This type of dwarfism resembles a severe form of achondroplasia. The features distinguishing it from achondroplasia are the following:

1. Extreme flatness of the vertebral bodies, with excessive dimensions of the intervertebral spaces
2. Tubular bones very short and bowed, particularly in the lower extremities
3. Metaphyseal areas irregular in contour and frequently cupped

Whereas achondroplasia is transmitted as an autosomal dominant hereditary trait, with ominous genetic implications, this type of dwarfism is a dominant mutation apparently without a hereditary influence.

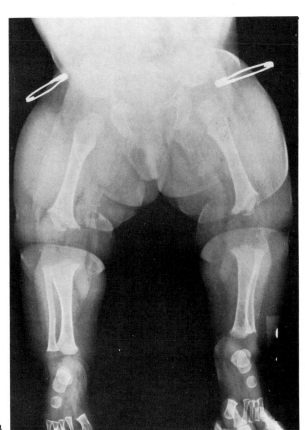

Figure 7–6 *Continued* *B*. Achondroplasia, pelvis and lower extremities. See text for description.

B

In Morquio's Disease (Figure 7–7) there is a severe disorder of epiphyses and enchondral bone formation, and a severe kyphosis in the mid-dorsal or dorso-lumbar region. An abnormality of mucopolysaccharide metabolism has also been demonstrated in the urine in a high percentage of patients (Robbins, Stevens, and Linker).

Radiographic Findings. The **arms are often very long** in contrast to those characteristic of achondroplasia, sometimes reaching to the knees, and in many cases they are held in valgus position. The knees are in genu valgum. The **skull is enlarged,** the frontal and parietal bones protrude, and saddle nose is frequently encountered.

The spine is composed of shallow vertebral bodies with a "beaking" of the vertebra immediately caudad to the kyphotic site. Morquio-Ullrich disease may be a variant of gargoylism (Hurler's disease) or Morquio's disease. The skeletal changes of Morquio's disease are present but only a few of the extra-skeletal abnormalities are seen (Goidanich).

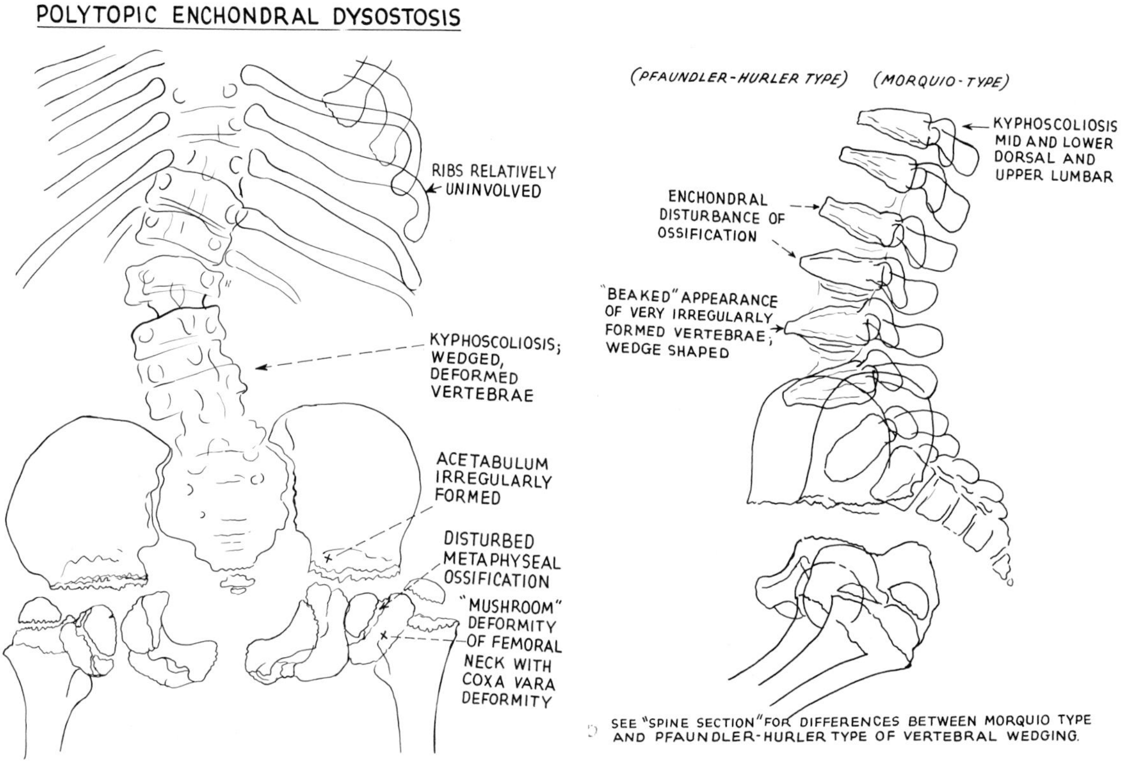

POLYTOPIC ENCHONDRAL DYSOSTOSIS

(PFAUNDLER-HURLER TYPE)   (MORQUIO-TYPE)

RIBS RELATIVELY UNINVOLVED

KYPHOSCOLIOSIS; WEDGED, DEFORMED VERTEBRAE

ACETABULUM IRREGULARLY FORMED

DISTURBED METAPHYSEAL OSSIFICATION

"MUSHROOM" DEFORMITY OF FEMORAL NECK WITH COXA VARA DEFORMITY

KYPHOSCOLIOSIS MID AND LOWER DORSAL AND UPPER LUMBAR

ENCHONDRAL DISTURBANCE OF OSSIFICATION

"BEAKED" APPEARANCE OF VERY IRREGULARLY FORMED VERTEBRAE; WEDGE SHAPED

SEE "SPINE SECTION" FOR DIFFERENCES BETWEEN MORQUIO TYPE AND PFAUNDLER-HURLER TYPE OF VERTEBRAL WEDGING.

Figure 7–7   Polytopic enchondral dysostoses. Tracings of abdomen and spine in Morquio's disease.

Pfaundler-Hurler's Disease (gargoylism; dysostosis multiplex)

Both Morquio's disease and Pfaundler-Hurler's disease have been referred to as "polytopic enchondral dysostosis" with many subgroups identified, or as the "mucopolysaccharide disorders."

Osteogenesis Imperfecta (Fragilitas ossium, Lobstein's disease, Van der Hoeve's syndrome)

Clinical Features. Three clinical types are distinguished:
1. Osteogenesis imperfecta congenita
2. Osteogenesis imperfecta tarda (osteopsathyrosis or Ekmann-Lobstein disease)
3. An additional form of the latter syndrome in which the fractures, which first appear at two to three years of age, seem to decline in frequency at about puberty.

Typically there is a high frequency of blue sclerae as a result of the abnormal thinness of the usually tough white supporting tunic of the eyeball and deafness from otosclerosis.

Hydrocephaly and congenital heart defects may coexist (McKusick; Elefant and Tosovsky; Caniggia et al.).

Radiographic Findings. The bone shafts are extremely thin, deficient in mineral structure, subject to frequent fractures, and highly deformed after healing of fracture has occurred.

In the skull there are multiple wormian bones that give a "jigsaw puzzle" pattern at sutural junctions. Hydrocephaly and congenital heart defect may also be found.

The roentgenographic features of osteogenesis imperfecta in the adult have been summarized by Levin as follows: (1) undermineralization of the bones; (2) biconcavity of the vertebral bodies; (3) multiple fractures which heal normally but with persistent deformity; (4) platybasia of the skull; (5) a tendency to a decrease in the trabecular pattern of most bones; (6) no dwarfism.

Chondroectodermal Dysplasia (Ellis-Van Creveld's disease) (Ellis and Andrew)

Clinical Features. This disease consists of *ectodermal dysplasia, chondrodysplasia, polydactylism,* and *congenital cardiac abnormalities.* The ectodermal dysplasia is characterized by defective nails and dentition and alopecia. The chondrodysplasia produces dwarfing and synostosis of the calvarium. The cardiac abnormalities are usually manifested by cyanosis, with patency of the interventricular or interatrial septa and transposition of the major blood vessels. Polydactyly is constant but fusion of the capitate and hamate bones is pathognomonic.

Radiographic Findings. The long bones are generally thickened and coarse, with acceleration of maturation of the secondary centers of ossification, and retardation of the primary centers of ossification. In the distal tibiae and fibulae there may be areas of osteosclerosis intermingled with rarefaction, somewhat similar to chondrodysplasia. **Peaking of the proximal ends of the tibiae,** described by Caffey as pathognomonic, is often found. There is often a curvature of the humeri. The thorax is narrow with horizontal clavicles and the third cuneiforms are often absent in both feet.

Acrocephalosyndactylia (Apert's syndrome) is a disease state consisting of *oxycephaly* (acrocephaly) and *syndactyly* of the fingers or toes. Often there are supernumerary metatarsals or phalanges. The *sella turcica tends to be enlarged* with an *accentuated digitate pattern* throughout the calvarium and premature fusion of the coronal or sagittal sutures. The skull tends to be "tower-shaped." The orbits are shallow, coexisting with hypertelorism and exophthalmos. The hard or soft palate is often malformed. *A single nail is common to the fused second, third, and fourth hand digits and is typical of Apert's syndrome* (Blank).

THE PELVIS AS A GUIDE IN NEONATAL AND CONGENITAL DISEASES OF BONE

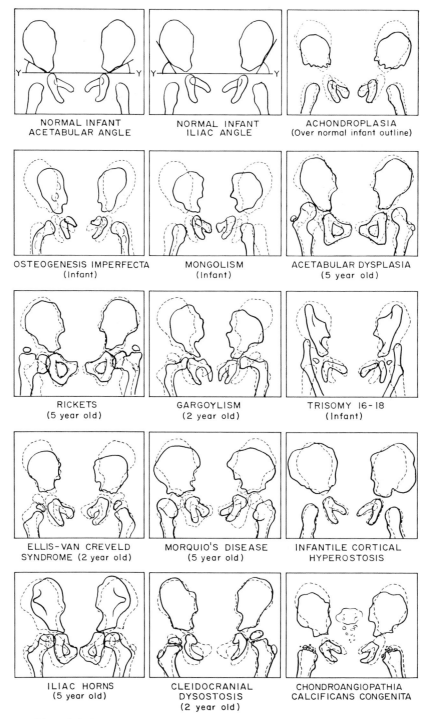

Figure 7–8 The pelvis in normal, neonatal, and congenital diseases. In each instance the equivalent normal pelvis is shown in dotted lines superimposed upon the abnormal.

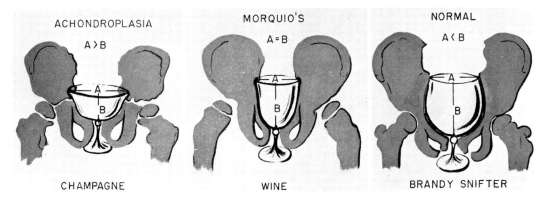

Figure 7–9 The inner pelvic contour as represented by different types of wine glasses. In achondroplasia, the pelvic width exceeds the depth due to decreased growth of the iliac base. The resulting appearance of the inner contour is that of a champagne glass. In spondyloepiphyseal dysplasia, the width and depth are equal and this results in a wine-glass shaped pelvis. The normal inner pelvic contour resembles a brandy snifter, the width of the pelvic inlet being less than its depth. The pelvis in multiple epiphyseal dysplasia corresponds to the normal.

(From Rubin, P.: *Dynamic Classification of Bone Dysplasias.* Chicago, Year Book Medical Publishers, 1964.)

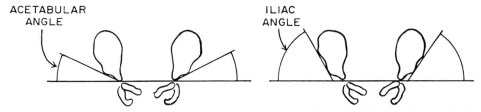

Figure 7–10 Diagrams illustrating the method of measurement of the acetabular and iliac angles. For range of normal values, see Table 7–2.

TABLE 7–2 RANGE OF NORMAL VALUES FOR ILIAC AND ACETABULAR ANGLES (From Caffey, 1967)

Category	Mean Acetabular Angle	SD	± 2 SD	Actual Range
Young normal infants less than 3 months of age	28°	4.7	37–18	44–12
Normal infants 3–12 months of age	22°	4.2	30–14	34–8
	Mean Iliac Angle			
Less than 3 months	81°	8.0	97–65	97–68
3–12 months	79°	9.0	96–60	101–62

TABLE 7–3 PRINCIPAL CHONDRODYSPLASIAS DETECTABLE AT BIRTH*

	Clinical Features in the Newborn	Extremities	Thorax	Vertebrae	Radiological Features in the Newborn		Misc.	Inheritance
					Pelvis	Skull		
Disorders incompatible with life.								
Thanatophoric dwarfism	Severe micromelia Narrowness of the thorax	Short, bowed (especially lower) Metaphyses irregular and cupped	Narrowness, but long trunk Ribs short	Platyspondyly Reduction of interpedicular distances of last lumbar	Iliac wings small and square Narrow sacro-sciatic notch	Shortened base Prominent frontal bone and depressed nose		Mutation
Achondrogenesis	Severe micromelic dwarfism	Micromelic		Severe dwarfism Defects in ossification, especially vertebrae				?
Disorders compatible with life.								
Achondroplasia	Micromelic dwarfism with characteristic craniofacial changes	Short, thick tubular bones – proximal bones worst Trident deformities – hands Epiphyses normal	Flat chested Ribs – club-shaped	Platyspondyly Reduction of lumbar interpediculate distances	Iliac wings square; sacro-sciatic notch acute	Short base, acute angle, hydrocephalus face small, prognathism		Dominant
Pseudoachondroplasia		Long bones short and thick Epiphyses irregular Brachydactyly Severe arthritis	Ribs normal with full round chest	Vertebra plana and platyspondyly	Iliac crests flared	Normal base and odontoid		
Chondrodysplasia punctata	Micromelic dwarfism, often asymmetrical cataract Ichthyosis	Micromelia; asymmetrical cataract often Small areas of calcification in joints Diaphyses normal	Stippling at anterior ribs and sternum	Small areas of calcification in vertebral bodies Vertical cleft in vertebrae	Stippling at iliac crests	Normal or head may be large		
Chondro-ectodermal dysplasia (Ellis-Van Creveld)	Polydactyly Ectodermal abnormalities Cardiac malformation	Polydactyly Metaphyseal notching Peripheral shortening of tubular bones Lateral defect in epiphysis of tibia leading to peaking	Narrow Clavicles horizontal		Horizontal acetabular roof with lateral spur projecting	Poorly developed	Ectodermal abnormalities Cardiac malformations in one-third of cases	Autosomal recessive

Asphyxiating thoracic dysplasia	Narrowness of the thorax Shortness of the limbs	Shortness of limbs	Narrowness and asphyxiation Shortened ribs		Similar to Ellis-Van Creveld		Third cuneiforms often absent in feet	Autosomal recessive
Diastrophic dwarfism	Micromelic dwarfism Club foot Cleft palate Deformity of the external ear (at 1 or 2 months of age)	Micromelia Clubfoot (cuboid feet and hands) Changes in epiphyses and metaphyses Epiphyses appear late Joint luxations Short and massive tubular bones	Normal	Scoliosis but vertebrae normal	Normal	Cleft palate Deformed external ear Normal skull otherwise		Autosomal dominant
Metatrophic dwarfism	Micromelic dwarfism Kyphoscoliosis	Micromelia Widened metaphyses		Kyphoscoliosis Reduction in height of vertebral bodies				Autosomal recessive
Mesomelic dwarfism	Micromelia with selective involvement of the forearm and leg	Micromelia selectively involving forearm and leg Incurvation of radius Aplasia of fibula						Autosomal recessive
Spondylo-epiphyseal dysplasia (congenital)	Dwarfism with shortness of the trunk	Delay in ossification Epiphysis irregular Diaphyses narrow Brachydactyly	Ribs normal in length	Platyspondyly Hypoplasia of T_{12}, L_1 with an anterior tongue Odontoid process hypoplastic	Broadness of the base of the iliac wings Acetabuli protrusio	Normal or platybasia May be enlarged Saddle nose		Dominant
Gargoylism (Hurler's syndrome) May be a variant of Morquio's		Pinching of metaphyses and shortening with stunting Tapering of distal ulna and radius Tapered metacarpals with apex at wrist	Ribs narrow medially and broadened distally, resembling a "caveman's club"	Hypoplasia D_{12}, L_1 with stepping defect anteriorly	Stenosis of iliac base and proximal femoral necks	Scaphocephaly "Shoe-shaped" sella turcica		Progressive, leading to shortened life span Hereditary error in metabolism of mucopolysaccharides

*Based on data from Maroteaux, 1969; P. Rubin, 1964; Langer, 1965; Keats et al., 1970.

HEREDITARY OR CONGENITAL DISEASES OF BONE RELATED TO A DEFECT EXTRINSIC TO THE BONE BUT INVOLVING THE BONE SECONDARILY

For the most part this group of disorders has an inherited metabolic basis. Since the separate diseases are more readily discussed in conjunction with their objective roentgen appearances in Chapters 8, 9, and 10, discussions of the lipoid storage diseases, hematopoietic disorders, neurofibromatosis, and endocrine disorders will be deferred to these later chapters.

SKELETAL ABNORMALITIES IN RELATION TO KNOWN CHROMOSOMAL ABERRATIONS

For a more detailed discussion and glossary, the student is referred to the companion text *Analysis of Roentgen Signs*.

As an example, Turner's syndrome is demonstrated.

Turner's Syndrome (gonadal dysgenesis or agenesis)

Radiographic Findings

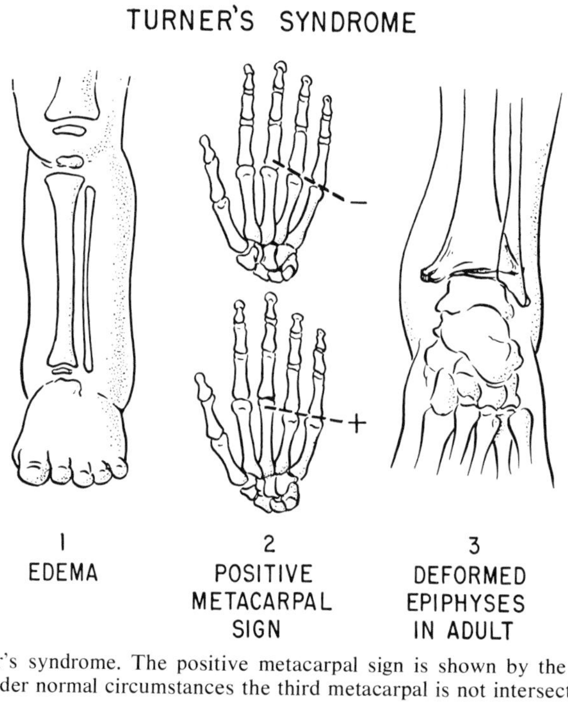

TURNER'S SYNDROME

| 1 | 2 | 3 |
| EDEMA | POSITIVE METACARPAL SIGN | DEFORMED EPIPHYSES IN ADULT |

Figure 7-11 Turner's syndrome. The positive metacarpal sign is shown by the line intersecting the third metacarpal. Under normal circumstances the third metacarpal is not intersected.

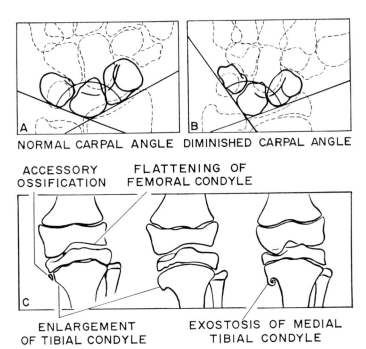

Figure 7–12 *A* to *C*. Further radiographic manifestations with Turner's syndrome (according to Kosowicz). Other radiologic manifestations are: (1) small and ridged sella turcica; (2) basilar impression of the skull; (3) increase in the carrying angle of the elbow (cubitus valgus); (4) changes in the spine resembling osteochondrosis; (5) hypoplasia of C-1 vertebral body; (6) male characteristics in the pelvis; and (7) thinness of lateral aspects of the clavicles and posterior aspect of the ribs.

The normal carpal angle is 131.5 ± 7.2°. (In arthrogryposis this angle is increased.)

8

Radiolucent Bone Diseases of Multiple Extremities or Regions

INTRODUCTION TO CHAPTERS 8 THROUGH 10

A diagrammatic representation of a spectrum of bone diseases is shown in Figure 8–1, beginning with uniform lucency and ending with uniform sclerosis (Chapter 10).

DIAGRAMMATIC REPRESENTATION OF RADIOGRAPHIC CATEGORIZATION OF BONE DISEASES

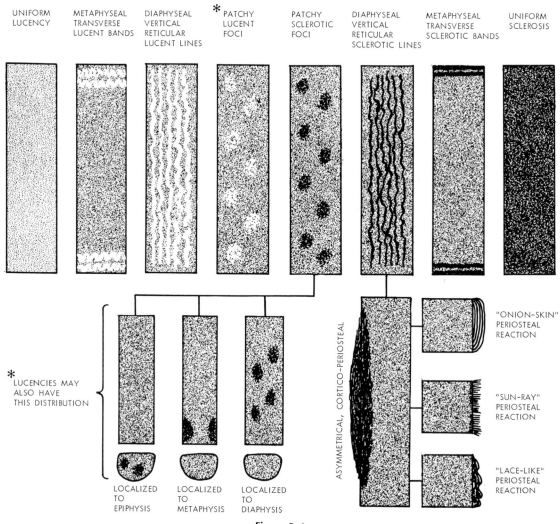

UNIFORM LUCENCY

METAPHYSEAL TRANSVERSE LUCENT BANDS

DIAPHYSEAL VERTICAL RETICULAR LUCENT LINES

*PATCHY LUCENT FOCI

PATCHY SCLEROTIC FOCI

DIAPHYSEAL VERTICAL RETICULAR SCLEROTIC LINES

METAPHYSEAL TRANSVERSE SCLEROTIC BANDS

UNIFORM SCLEROSIS

*LUCENCIES MAY ALSO HAVE THIS DISTRIBUTION

LOCALIZED TO EPIPHYSIS

LOCALIZED TO METAPHYSIS

LOCALIZED TO DIAPHYSIS

ASYMMETRICAL, CORTICO-PERIOSTEAL

"ONION-SKIN" PERIOSTEAL REACTION

"SUN-RAY" PERIOSTEAL REACTION

"LACE-LIKE" PERIOSTEAL REACTION

Figure 8–1

DIFFUSE RADIOLUCENT BONE DISEASES OF MULTIPLE EXTREMITIES

A classification of the lucent side of this spectrum is shown in Figure 8–2.

MULTIPLE OSTEOLYTIC LESIONS
OF MULTIPLE EXTREMITIES

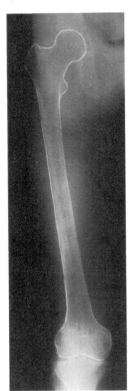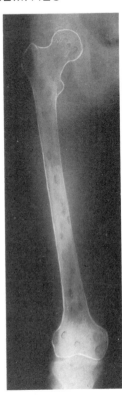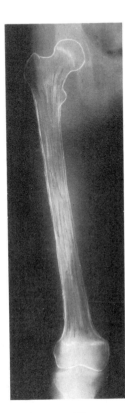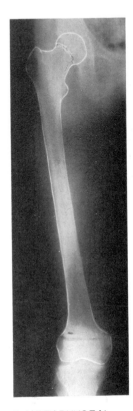

1. UNIFORM
   RADIOLUCENCY

2. CIRCUMSCRIBED
   MULTIPLE AREAS
   OF RADIOLUCENCY

3. FIBRILLAR
   OSTEOPOROSIS
   WITH COARSENING
   OF TRABECULAE

4. METAPHYSEAL
   TRANSVERSE
   OSTEOPOROSIS

Figure 8–2 Classification of radiolucent bone diseases of multiple extremities.

Polyostotic Diseases Characterized by Uniform Radiolucency

The entities in this group may be classified as shown in Figure 8–3.

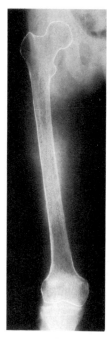

UNIFORM RADIOLUCENCY

1. OSTEOMALACIA
2. CALCIUM DEFICIENCY DUE TO INTESTINAL DISTURBANCES
3. RENAL RICKETS (RENAL OSTEODYSTROPHY) (SECONDARY HYPERPARATHYROIDISM)
4. FANCONI'S SYNDROME
5. PROTEIN DEFICIENCY OSTEOPATHY
6. ENDOCRINE OSTEOPATHY
7. RAYNAUD'S DISEASE
8. HYPOPHOSPHATEMIC–VITAMIN D REFRACTORY RICKETS
9. HYPERPARATHYROIDISM
10. SENILE OSTEOPOROSIS

Figure 8–3 Diseases characterized by uniform radiolucency.

The radiolucency in these disease entities may be due to:

1. *Insufficient osteoid matrix,* upon which the calcium salts may be laid (osteoporosis).

2. *Insufficient calcium salts* (osteomalacia).

3. *Active osteoclastic activity* which has removed the mineral as well as the osteoid component of bone, transforming much of the compact bone to a cancellous variety. New osteoid may be deposited around the old cannibalized trabeculae, but these may remain unossified owing to a deficiency of any of the following: vitamin D; calcium; phophorus in the diet; disturbances of absorption of calcium or vitamin D; or excessive serum phosphorus loss from the kidneys.

Renal Rickets (Figure 8–4)

Radiographic Findings

A **frayed appearance of the metaphysis** adjoining the epiphyseal plate, in the child or adolescent.

Increased radiolucency of the bones, generally with thinness of the cortex, and some bending or fracturing in the bone.

Subcortical erosion of the phalanges and pointing of the tufted ends of the distal phalanges.

Ectopic calcium deposition in all tissues where chloride or carbon dioxide ions are found in relative abundance, such as the lung alveoli, renal tubules,

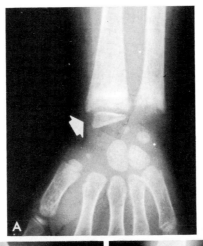

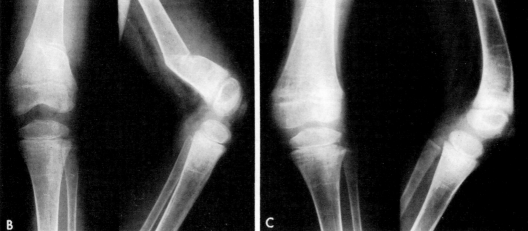

Figure 8–4 Renal rickets. *A*. P-A view of the wrist and hand demonstrating the great similarity of this process to avitaminosis D. *B*. A-P and lateral views of the right knee showing a diffuse osteoporosis as well as a pathologic fracture in the distal shaft of the femur. Note the typical frayed appearance in the distal metaphysis of the femur. *C*. Somewhat similar appearance of the left knee, although a pathologic fracture is not present. Note the marked anterior bowing, however, of the distal shaft of the femur (called "renal osteitis fibrosa cystica" by Albright and Reifenstein).

gastric mucosa, media of the medium-sized arteries throughout the body, and interstitially everywhere. In the kidney there is a characteristic **nephrocalcinosis** with calcium deposit in the renal pyramids (see section on primary hyperparathyroidism).

In some bones there are **circumscribed areas of lucency** suggesting "cystic" or "pseudocystic" appearances in the bone. (Osteitis fibrosa cystica with its so-called "brown tumors.")

Endocrine Osteopathies Producing Generalized Radiolucency. The hormones, in general, exert the following influences on the skeletal system: (1) determination of the rate of growth of the long bones; (2) the maturation of bones; (3) the time of closure of the epiphyseal plate. This establishes the absolute overall length of the bone, growth and thickness of the bone, and mobilization of the calcium salts from the bones to the blood and vice versa.

The radiolucent skeletal diseases which have their origin in disturbances in various endocrine glands are:
1. *Pituitary dwarfism*
2. *Hypothyroidism (cretinism)*
3. *Primary hyperparathyroidism*
4. *Secondary hyperparathyroidism*
5. *Adult hypogonadism*
6. *Pancreatic osteoporosis* in association with diabetes mellitus
7. *Diabetic dwarfism*
8. *Steroid therapy* may result in severe *skeletal osteoporosis, pathological fracture* and abnormal callus formation. The skull, ribs, pelvis, and vertebrae may be particularly affected. Pathological fracture, however, with the appearance of *aseptic necrosis* occurs especially in the heads of the femora and humeri (Figure 8–5).

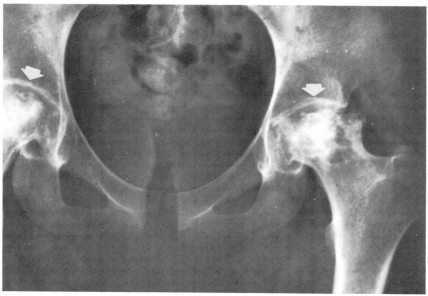

Figure 8–5   Aseptic necrosis resulting from steroid therapy combined with severe osteoporosis. The effect upon the heads of the femora is shown. Similar findings were evident in the heads of the humeri.

Hyperparathyroidism (Figure 8–6). In hyperparathyroidism arising from either parathyroid adenoma or hyperplasia, there is an excessive excretion of calcium and phosphate in the urine associated with high calcium and low phosphate levels in the blood. The increased calcium requirements of the blood may or may not call upon the bones for satiation; thus, *not all cases of hyperparathyroidism are associated with changes in the bones* (perhaps 40 per cent or more). If the exogenous supply of calcium is deficient, the bones of the body may show any degree of change, from osteoporosis to marked osteitis fibrosis cystica, and the appearances are illustrated in Figure 8–6.

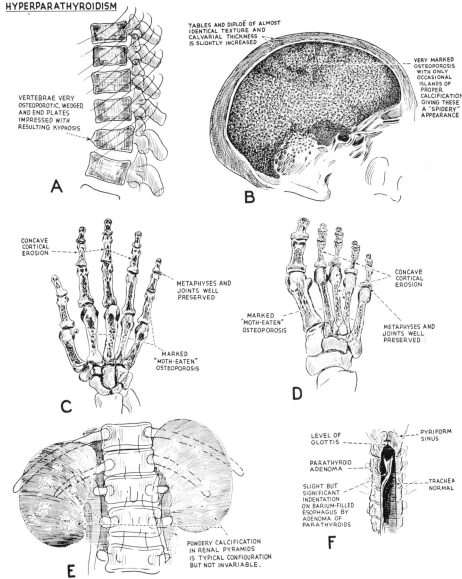

Figure 8–6 Hyperparathyroidism due to a parathyroid adenoma. *A* to *F*. Labeled tracings of the spine, skull, hand, foot, kidney areas, and neck region respectively in patient with a parathyroid adenoma. Note the extremely slight displacement of the esophagus by the adenoma. Note also the powdery calcification in the renal pyramids rather typical of the type of nephrocalcinosis which occurs in this condition.

Illustration continued on the following page

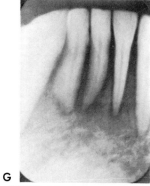

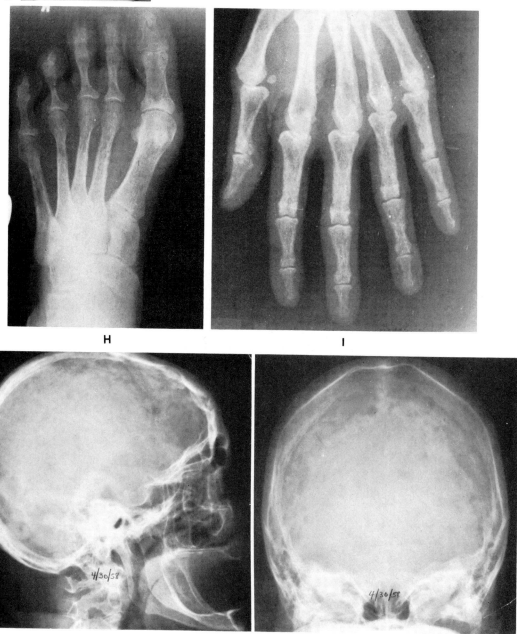

Figure 8–6 *Continued   G.* Loss of lamina dura in the alveolar ridges adjoining the teeth. *H* and *I.* Corticoperiosteal erosion of middle phalanges especially with diffuse hyperlucency of bones. *J* and *K.* Representative lateral view and Towne's view of the skull.

DISEASES CAUSING MULTIPLE AREAS OF CIRCUMSCRIBED, PATCHY RADIOLUCENCY, WITH NO SCLEROTIC MARGIN

Some diseases included in this group are listed and partially illustrated in Figure 8–7. We shall limit our discussion to just a few of these entities.

Of the entities mentioned, the most frequent in this category are:

Metastatic bone tumors, including multiple myeloma

The histiocytoses or reticuloendothelioses, including the lipoid storage diseases even though these are not related

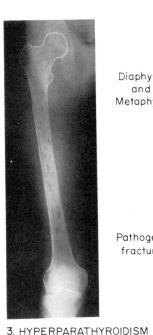

Diaphysis
and
Metaphysis

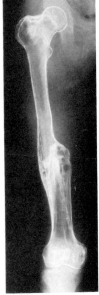

Pathogenic fracture

1. ACUTE DISSEMINATED INFECTIONS OF BONE–OSTEOMYELITIS
2. "ROUND CELL" TUMORS
   A–MULTIPLE MYELOMA
   B–EWING'S TUMOR
   C–NEUROBLASTOMA
   D–RETICULUM CELL SARCOMA
4. LIPOID GRANULOMATOSES AND HISTIO-CYTOSES, OR RETICULOSES
5. NEUROFIBROMATOSIS WITH BONY INVOLVE-MENT. BONE IS INVADED FROM WITHOUT IN RIB CAGE PARTICULARLY
6. METASTATIC BONE TUMORS–INTERMEDIATE NUMERICALLY BETWEEN I AND 2
8. OXALOSIS

3. HYPERPARATHYROIDISM (may be confined to "moth eaten" appearance of epiphysis)

7. POLYOSTOTIC FIBROUS DYSPLASIA

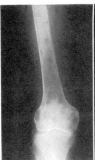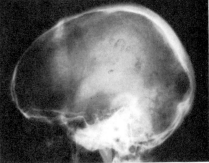

Figure 8–7 Diseases causing multiple areas of circumscribed radiolucency (intensified).

9. MULTIPLE MYELOMA–DISCRETE PUNCHED OUT AREAS–NO REACTIVE SCLEROSIS

Metastatic Bone Tumors

General Comment. The most common metastatic lesions come from the breast, lung, prostate, thyroid, and kidney. (Prostatic carcinoma usually produces sclerotic metastases—see Chapter 10.)

In a child, the most probable cause of osteolytic metastases is neuroblastoma.

The lytic metastases from carcinoma of the kidney and thyroid often produce a somewhat "bubbly" appearance (Greenfield).

Metastases distal to the elbows and knees are rare but do occur.

Metastatic Bone Tumors Which May Evoke a Periosteal Response. The metastatic bone tumors which are most apt to react in this manner include neuroblastoma and tumors that arise in the colon and prostate. Only about one-third of the metastases from lung carcinoma and 20 per cent from kidney carcinoma produce a periosteal reaction. Metastases from prostatic carcinoma are usually osteoblastic (Chapter 10), with dense periosteal new bone formation.

By comparison, some primary osseous tumors which elicit a periosteal response are: Ewing's sarcoma, 100 per cent; fibrosarcoma, 100 per cent; osteogenic sarcoma, 91 per cent; reticulum cell sarcoma, 85 per cent; chondrosarcoma, 50 per cent; and the malignant lymphomas, only 20 per cent.

Radiographic Findings. Metastatic osteolytic bone tumors have a variable appearance radiographically, ranging from only a **fine granularity** of the bones **to well-defined areas of osteolysis** in many bones of the body.

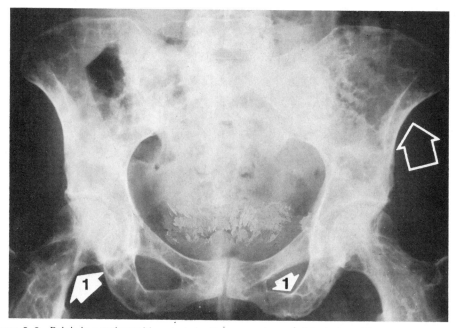

Figure 8–8 Pelvis in a patient with metastases from a carcinoma of the breast. The open arrow points to a lytic lesion in the left iliac bone. The large arrow (1) points to large lytic lesions extending into the neck and upper shaft of the right femur, and the small arrow (1) points to lytic metastases in the left pubis and ischium.

Multiple Myeloma (Plasma Cell Myeloma, Myelocytoma, Erythroblastoma, Lymphocytoma) (Figure 8–9)

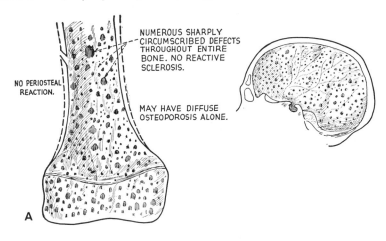

NUMEROUS SHARPLY CIRCUMSCRIBED DEFECTS THROUGHOUT ENTIRE BONE. NO REACTIVE SCLEROSIS.

NO PERIOSTEAL REACTION.

MAY HAVE DIFFUSE OSTEOPOROSIS ALONE.

A

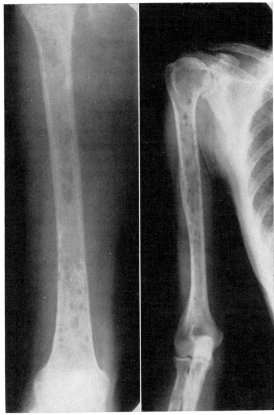

B

Figure 8–9 *A.* Diagrammatic representation of the most frequent radiographic appearances in the long bones and the skull. *B.* Antero-posterior view of the arm showing the "punched out" lesions in the humerus.

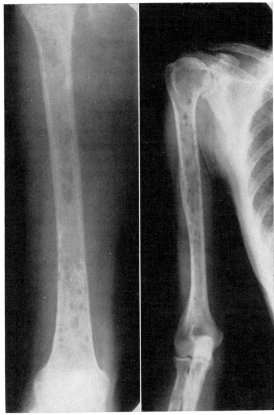

Illustration continued on the following page

Radiographic Findings

Numerous sharply circumscribed defects throughout the bone with no reactive marginal sclerosis.

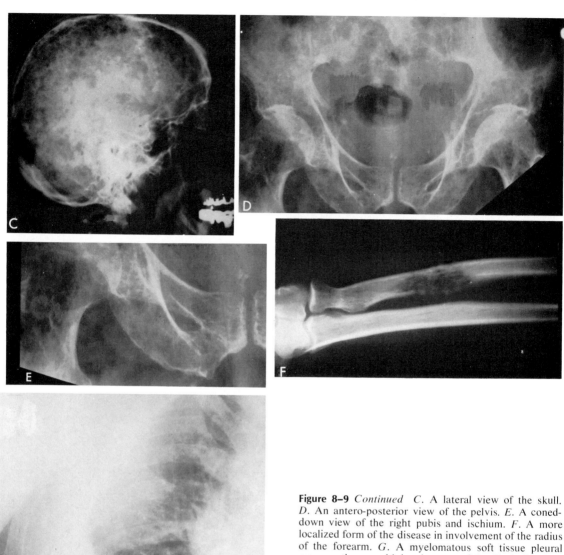

Figure 8–9 *Continued   C*. A lateral view of the skull. *D*. An antero-posterior view of the pelvis. *E*. A coned-down view of the right pubis and ischium. *F*. A more localized form of the disease in involvement of the radius of the forearm. *G*. A myelomatous soft tissue pleural mass contiguous with involvement of the ribs in the chest wall.

There may also be a diffuse osteoporosis with no particular punched-out area. Usually there is no periosteal reaction.

Some cases show no radiographic changes.

In the flat bones of the pelvis and occasionally in the ribs or sternum, the plasmocytoma may appear as an expanding radiolucent lesion with a thin coating of compact bone surrounding the lesion. Incomplete trabeculae may traverse the lesion.

The radiographic differential diagnosis must always include metastatic carcinosis and hyperparathyroidism. Often these entities are indistinguishable.

Neuroblastoma in Bone (Figure 8–10)

General Comments. This tumor may arise from the sympathetic nervous system anywhere in the body. *Half the cases have their origin in the adrenal medulla. Next to leukemia, neuroblastoma is the most common malignant disease in infancy and childhood,* the onset frequently occurring *before the age of seven.*

Radiographic Findings

Bone lesions are moderately well-demarcated **osteolytic** processes with a strong tendency to symmetry of involvement. Thus the lower portions of **both** femurs are apt to be affected. There are often three or more bones involved simultaneously at the time of discovery, and the lesion has a corticoperiosteal appearance when an isolated lesion is seen. The **multiplicity of these lesions,** however, is noteworthy.

The **bony cortex is usually destroyed** with a periosteal reaction which may assume a "**sunburst" appearance,** although this is not pathognomonic for neuroblastoma.

In the skull there is often separation of the **skull sutures (diastasis)** due to increased intracranial pressure from metastatic tumors or meningeal involvement.

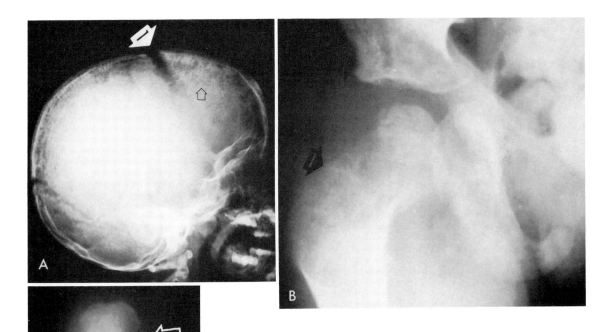

Figure 8–10 Neuroblastoma of bone. *A.* Lateral view of the skull showing diastasis of the suture with invasion of the calvarium usually from involvement of the meninges. *B.* Antero-posterior view of the right hip showing diffuse neuroblastomatous metastases involving the femur and the acetabulum. *C.* Metastases from the neuroblastoma to the os calcis in this same patient.

Reticuloendothelioses, Reticuloses, or Histiocytosis (the Lipid Granulomatoses) (Figure 8–11)

General Clinical Considerations. This group of diseases is basically due to histiocytic proliferation with lipid deposits in the sites of histiocytosis.

The Hand-Schüller-Christian complex consists of: Letterer-Siwe disease, Hand-Schüller-Christian disease, and eosinophilic granuloma (Robbins), perhaps all part of a continuous spectrum, with rapid proliferation in the very young (Letterer-Siwe disease), and slower and focal proliferation in older persons (eosinophilic granuloma). These disorders probably represent inflammatory histiocytic proliferation in various organs, sometimes with the accumulation of cholesterol as a secondary phenomenon.

In contrast, Niemann-Pick disease and Gaucher's disease are probably constitutional defects in the metabolism of complex lipids, i.e., sphingomyelin in Niemann-Pick disease and kerasin in Gaucher's disease. Since all of these have lipid deposits in the sites of histiocytosis, they can be considered as a group (Robbins).

Radiographic Findings

HAND-SCHÜLLER-CHRISTIAN COMPLEX

In Letterer-Siwe disease bone lesions are absent when the disease is first recognized, but may appear in the course of several months.

The roentgenologic features of the Hand-Schüller-Christian complex may be summarized as follows:

1. The bone defects are sharply demarcated, large, and "map-like" (Figure 8–9), especially in the skull. Both the inner and outer tables of the cranial vault seem to be equally affected, with no evidence of periosteal reaction, repair, or a sclerotic margin.

2. In particular, the mandible (in the infant) is frequently involved, producing the "floating tooth" appearance.

3. Pathologic fractures are frequent. Collapsed vertebrae (vertebra plana) may assume a sclerotic pattern.

4. Bone lesions may be absent from about 20 per cent of cases of Hand-Schüller-Christian disease. The exophthalmos and diabetes insipidus, when they occur in about half of these cases, are associated with bony lesions in the skull and orbit (forming the "classic triad" of this disease).

NIEMANN-PICK DISEASE

In this disease the bones are involved in a diffuse fashion, unlike the focal characteristics of the Hand-Schüller-Christian complex or Gaucher's disease.

GAUCHER'S DISEASE

In the infant, this condition may be indistinguishable from Letterer-Siwe disease. When the long bones are affected (Figure 8–11) a metaphyseal expansion of the bone often occurs, giving it an Erlenmeyer-flask contour around a large lytic focus; this may have a thin sclerotic margin or even a periosteal reaction.

The trabecular texture of the pelvis may be altered, with a tendency to sclerotic change in the vicinity of the pubis and sacroiliac joints.

With ischemic necrosis of the femoral heads, a mixed lysis and sclerosis may ensue. The most frequent sites of bone involvement are: femora; spine; hips; shoulders; tubular bones generally; and pelvis. The bones of the thoracic cage and skull are also often involved (Greenfield).

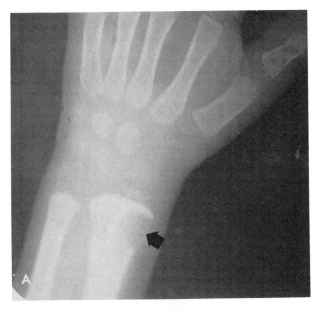

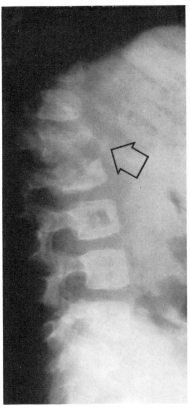

B

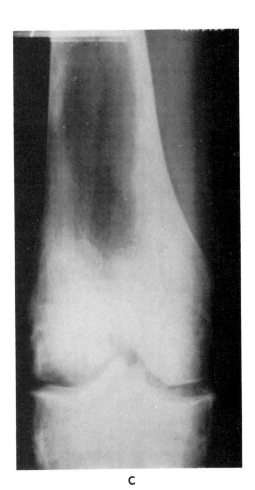

C

Figure 8–11 *A*. Histiocytosis X affecting the radius. *B*. The spine in Letterer-Siwe's disease. Magnified view of the upper lumbar vertebrae demonstrating the circumscribed lytic process coupled with irregular collapse of involved vertebrae. There is a tendency to diffuse flattening of vertebral bodies so involved. *C*. View of distal femur in a patient with Gaucher's disease, demonstrating Erlenmeyer-flask appearance.

DISEASES CAUSING MULTIPLE "RETICULAR" OR "FIBRILLAR" AREAS OF OSTEOPOROSIS WITH COARSENING OF THE TRABECULAE (Figure 8–12A)
(For irregular mosaic admixture of lucency and sclerosis as found in osteitis deformans or Paget's disease of bone, see Chapter 10)

The hemolytic anemias, anemias due to marrow hypofunction, and the bone changes resulting from leukemic and lymphomatous infiltration of bone all have certain changes in common in their radiographic appearances (Figure 8–12A).

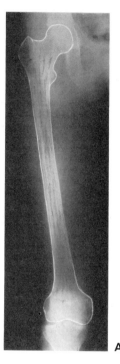

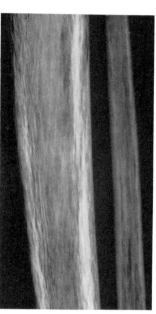

1. HEMOLYTIC ANEMIAS
   A–THALASSEMIA
   B–SPHEROCYTIC ANEMIA
   C–SICKLE CELL ANEMIA

2. LEUKEMIAS, LYMPHOMAS

3. CHRONIC POISONING, OR HORMONAL EFFECT

Figure 8–12 *A.* Intensified diagrammatic radiograph. *B.* "Fibrillar" appearance of the trabeculae in a patient with chronic monocytic leukemia.

A

B

Sickle Cell Anemia

Radiographic Findings

1. Coarse osseous trabeculation and demineralization
2. Vertebral end-plate ("fish") deformity. Anterior notching also
3. Splenomegaly (incidence decreases with age); hepatomegaly; cardiomegaly
4. Pulmonary infarction
5. Impaired renal function; renal papillary necrosis
6. Gallstones
7. Dactylitis
8. "Hair on end" pattern in skull (occasionally)

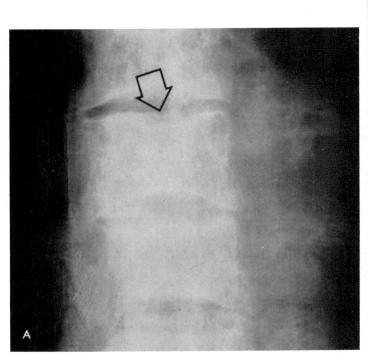
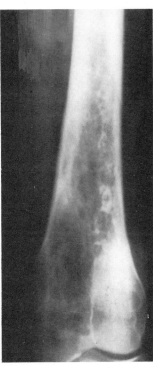

Figure 8–13 Sickle cell anemia. *A.* The vertebral body shows the squared-off appearance of the indented end-plate thought to be due to infarction immediately beneath the nucleus pulposus involving the end-plate and immediately adjoining the vertebral body. *B.* Infarction of the distal shaft of the femur in sickle cell anemia.

"Acute" (-Blastic) Leukemias

Pathologic Considerations and Radiographic Findings. Bone changes are frequently seen in individuals younger than ten years old. An incidence of over 80 per cent of bone lesions has been reported in this group. Bone changes with acute leukemias in children are related to (1) the **destruction of the marrow** by the proliferating reticulocytic elements; (2) a **tendency for the marrow to proliferate** (Figure 8–13A) in an effort to overcome cellular deficiencies; and (3) the **invasion of the periosteum** by the neoplastic elements, causing a periosteal elevation, proliferation, and so-called **"sun-ray striations"** of the periosteum or "hair-on-end" appearance. (4) Commonly there is a **transverse line of radiolucency** at the ends of the long bones beneath the metaphysis (Figure 8–14B). This occurs in over one-half the cases (Willson). Osteolytic lesions occur in 38 per cent, and periosteal reactions have been noted in 19 per cent (Karpinski and Martin; Kalayjian et al.).

The changes described show a predilection for the areas of most rapid bone growth, such as the knees, wrists, ankles, and shoulders. Because of this transverse appearance in the metaphyses, this entity must be mentioned in the next category for discussion.

RADIOLUCENCIES OCCURRING PRIMARILY TRANSVERSELY IN MULTIPLE METAPHYSES

The diseases which fall readily into this category are illustrated in Figure 8–15. In general, these disturbances occur in childhood, causing an interruption of the

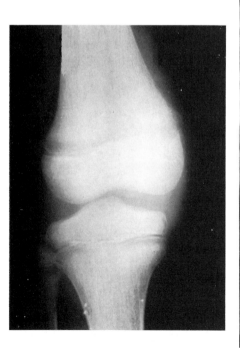

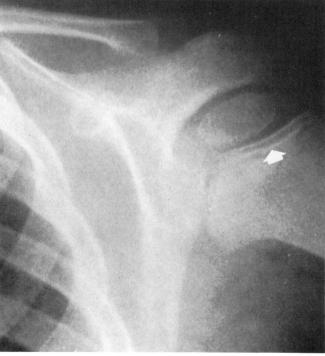

A   B

Figure 8–14 Bones in acute leukemia. *A.* The adjoining metaphyses of the femur and tibia around the knee show the broad lucent zone in a young individual with acute leukemia. *B.* Antero-posterior view of the shoulder in an infant with acute leukemia.

normal bone growth sequences at the epiphyseal plate and metaphyseal junction. As noted, they include the following disorders:

Newborn
    1. Hypophosphatasia
    2. Phenylketonuria
    3. Congenital syphilis
    4. Congenital rubella syndrome
    5. Acute leukemia of infants

Up to two years of age
    6. Hypervitaminosis A (excessive osteoclastic activity in metaphysis, with active proliferation of new bone in diaphysis)
    7. Hypovitaminosis C (scurvy)
    8. Hypovitaminosis D (rickets)

Older children
    9. Chronic renal osteodystrophy or renal rickets

METAPHYSEAL TRANSVERSE OSTEOPOROSIS

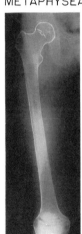
1. ACUTE LEUKEMIA (CHILDHOOD)
2. HYPERVITAMINOSIS A
3. HYPERVITAMINOSIS D
4. HYPOVITAMINOSIS D

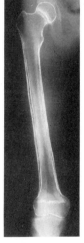
Increased zone of rarefaction

Subperiosteal new bone formation

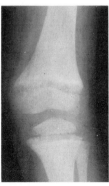
Cartilage zone increased and no calcification of epiphysis

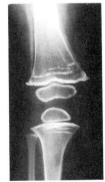
Increased zone of radiolucency proximal to zone of increased calcification

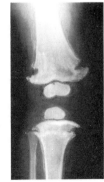
Transverse zone of no calcification

Slipped epiphysis

Poorly ossified spongiosa

4. RENAL RICKETS
7. HYPOPHOSPHATASIA
8. PHENYLKETONURIA

5. SCURVY

6. SYPHILIS

Figure 8–15 Radiolucent diseases characterized by osteoporosis arranged transversely, predominantly in the region of the metaphysis.

Osteomalacic Disorders

These include vitamin D deficiency in the adult or child, renal tubular acidosis (renal tubular defect), the chronic renal insufficiency diseases, and the hereditary disorders predisposing to osteomalacia—familial vitamin D resistance; Fanconi syndrome; and hypophosphatasia, an abnormal reduction in the activity of alkaline phosphatase in serum, many tissues, and bone. In all these disorders, there is a

Rickets

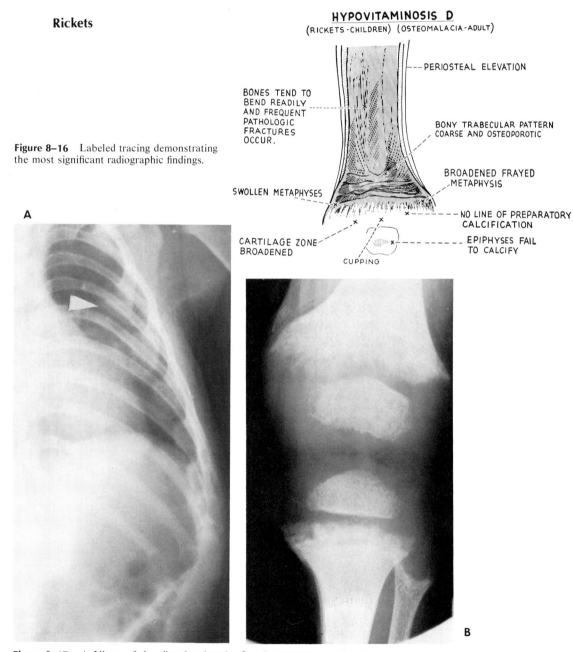

Figure 8–16 Labeled tracing demonstrating the most significant radiographic findings.

HYPOVITAMINOSIS D
(RICKETS-CHILDREN) (OSTEOMALACIA-ADULT)

---PERIOSTEAL ELEVATION

BONES TEND TO BEND READILY AND FREQUENT PATHOLOGIC FRACTURES OCCUR.

BONY TRABECULAR PATTERN COARSE AND OSTEOPOROTIC

BROADENED FRAYED METAPHYSIS

SWOLLEN METAPHYSES

NO LINE OF PREPARATORY CALCIFICATION

CARTILAGE ZONE BROADENED

EPIPHYSES FAIL TO CALCIFY

CUPPING

A

B

Figure 8–17 *A.* Views of the ribs showing the flared appearance at the costochondral junctions corresponding with a rachitic rosary.

B. Close-up view of the knee showing the frayed expanded appearance of the metaphyses of the femur and tibia and the irregular poorly ossified epiphyses of the femur and tibia.

defective mineralization of the osteoid matrix and a slowing down of matrix formation. The bones are fragile and subject to fracture, bending forces, and stress.

Scurvy

Pathophysiology

Vitamin C deficiency in infants causes a drop in the alkaline phosphatase activity as well as osteoid formation by the osteoblast. Cement substance necessary to maintain the integrity of capillary walls is also deficient, and underlies the hemorrhagic diathesis characteristic of this condition. The chondroblastic activity at the metaphyseal-epiphyseal junction proceeds well and the zone of provisional calcification can be identified, but the osteoblasts are incapable of forming osteoid. Resorption of the cartilage fails or slows down and at times the cartilage "overgrows," giving rise to bulbous enlargements at the costochondral junctions.

Radiographic Findings

The formation of new osteoid matrix on the degenerating cartilage and zone of provisional calcification is lacking, but when this zone persists somewhat, a **striped appearance** results.

The poorly "cemented" capillaries rupture and hemorrhage takes place alongside small fractures in the deficient bone. Because the periosteum is loosely attached (owing to the lack of cement substance), extensive **subperiosteal hemorrhages** are common. Following the administration of vitamin

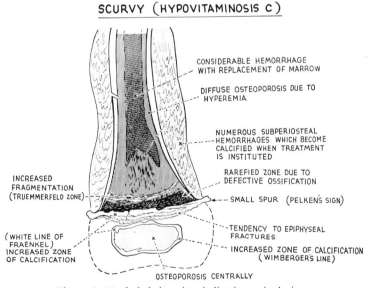

SCURVY (HYPOVITAMINOSIS C)

CONSIDERABLE HEMORRHAGE WITH REPLACEMENT OF MARROW

DIFFUSE OSTEOPOROSIS DUE TO HYPEREMIA

NUMEROUS SUBPERIOSTEAL HEMORRHAGES WHICH BECOME CALCIFIED WHEN TREATMENT IS INSTITUTED

RAREFIED ZONE DUE TO DEFECTIVE OSSIFICATION

INCREASED FRAGMENTATION (TRUEMMERFELD ZONE)

SMALL SPUR (PELKEN'S SIGN)

(WHITE LINE OF FRAENKEL) INCREASED ZONE OF CALCIFICATION

TENDENCY TO EPIPHYSEAL FRACTURES

INCREASED ZONE OF CALCIFICATION (WIMBERGER'S LINE)

OSTEOPOROSIS CENTRALLY

Figure 8–18 Labeled tracings indicating major lesions.

C, these subperiosteal hemorrhages undergo calcification and then reveal marked elevation and distribution of the entire periosteal envelope of a long bone.

There is a **bulbous enlargement at the costochondral junction.** The bulbous enlargement of the ends of the long bones and ribs in "renal rickets" is not nearly as great as with hypovitaminosis C and D, since affected children are older and the bones are growing in length more than circumference in these age groups.

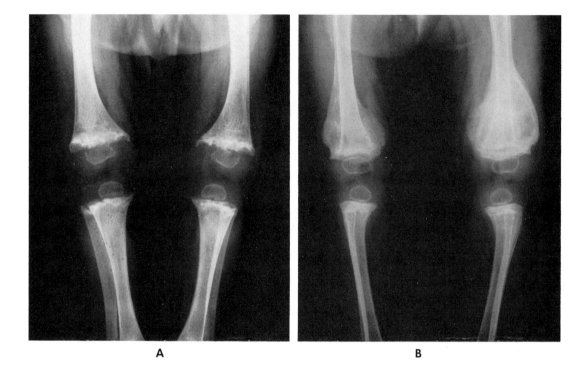

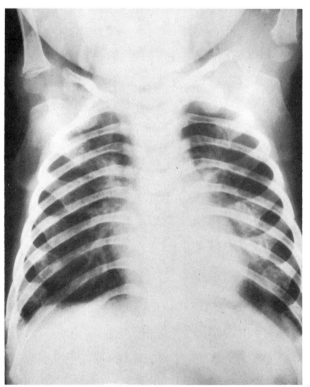

Figure 8–19 *A.* Femur and tibia around the knee in scurvy, before treatment. *B.* Same patient following treatment with large doses of vitamin C. Note the tremendous subperiosteal calcification in areas of previous hematoma formation. *C.* Chest in scurvy showing the scorbutic "rosary" at the costochondral junctions of each of the ribs. Note the marked flaring and the increased density of the metaphyses immediately adjoining the epiphyseal plates. A somewhat similar "rosary" is noted with rickets except that the increased density adjoining the metaphyses is not present.

Congenital Syphilis

Radiographic Findings

1. <u>INFANTILE</u> (APPEARS AT OR SHORTLY AFTER BIRTH AND DISAPPEARS SPONTANEOUSLY IN ABOUT 6-MONTHS)

TARSAL BONES HAVE POORLY DEVELOPED SPONGIOSA WITH DOUBLE RINGS – BONES SHOWN DIAGRAMMATICALLY WELL FORMED BUT ACTUALLY ARE NOT.

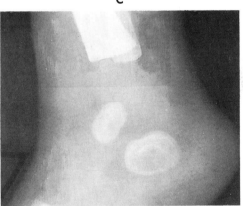

BILATERAL PERIOSTITIS (FEMUR, TIBIA, AND HUMERUS)

NO OSTEOPOROSIS

NO OSSIFICATION

OSTEOCHONDRITIS WITH BROAD CARTILAGE ZONE

INDENTED AREAS OF DESTRUCTION

WIDE SINGLE OR DOUBLE ZONE OF CALCIFICATION

WEAKENED ZONE SLIPPED EPIPHYSIS

POORLY OSSIFIED SPONGIOSA

GREATLY THICKENED OSSIFYING PERIOSTITIS PRODUCING APPEARANCE OF "SABER SHIN"

2. <u>JUVENILE</u> APPEARS TOWARD END OF FIRST DECADE – PERSISTS INTO ADULTHOOD, ESPECIALLY OF TIBIA, FEMUR, AND SKULL.

(ALSO SEE CHAPTER 10)

A

C

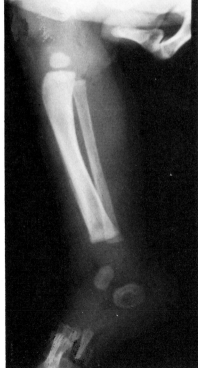

B

Figure 8–20 Congenital syphilis. *A*, Diagram.
  B. The leg in congenital syphilis, showing the periosteal elevation and concentric lamination of the tarsal bone.
  C. Close-up view of the concentric ossification and/or lamination of the ossification of the os calcis.

Additional findings may include:
  Slipped epiphyses
  Some resorption of the nasal bones at the bridge of the nose

Congenital Rubella Syndrome (Figure 8–21)

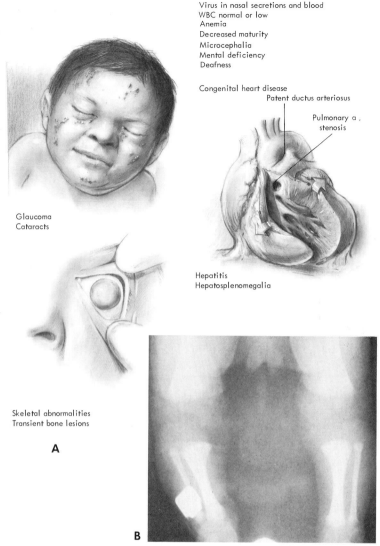

Virus in nasal secretions and blood
WBC normal or low
Anemia
Decreased maturity
Microcephalia
Mental deficiency
Deafness

Congenital heart disease
Patent ductus arteriosus

Pulmonary a.
stenosis

Glaucoma
Cataracts

Hepatitis
Hepatosplenomegalia

Skeletal abnormalities
Transient bone lesions

A

B

Figure 8–21 *A.* Diagram illustrating some clinical and radiographic findings in congenital rubella syndrome.

B. Congenital rubella syndrome. The lesions tend to disappear over a period of two to three months, or the zone of provisional calcification may remain inordinately dense. These changes are apparently due to a defect in the deposition and mineralization of the osteoid, and to defective calcification (in the zone of provisional calcification) of the cartilage prior to engulfment (Aegerter and Kirkpatrick; Singleton et al.; Rabinowitz et al.).

The degree of damage to the fetus depends primarily on the time of infection of the mother in relation to the pregnancy. When infection occurs early in gestation, more than 50 per cent of pregnancies end in abortion, stillbirth, or fetal malformation (Rubin). If infection occurs at the end of the first trimester, the probability of malformation is only slightly higher than for an uncomplicated pregnancy.

Radiographic Findings

The most striking manifestations are in the long bones, and the **bones at the knee are most frequently involved.** There are alternating transverse zones of lucency and sclerosis in the metaphyses, with an irregular density and contour of the zone of provisional calcification. At times there is only the broad band of lucency in the metaphysis.

There are linear and ovoid areas of radiolucency alternating with coarse trabeculae. The zone of provisional calcification is absent, thus creating a demineralized ragged appearance or splaying at the margins of the metaphysis, an appearance which to some extent resembles rickets or hypophosphatasia.

Questions – Chapter 8

1. What four main categories of radiolucent bone diseases of multiple extremities do we distinguish in our method of classification?

2. What are the main radiolucent diseases occurring in the epiphyseal-metaphyseal junction area?

3. What are the main nutritional disorders of growing children and how may they be differentiated radiographically?

4. What are the main radiographic features of acute leukemia in children?

5. What are the main radiographic features of renal osteodystrophy in children?

6. What are the main radiographic features of congenital syphilis?

7. What main disease categories are characterized by generalized radiolucency that is not sharply demarcated?

8. What is the basic defect in osteomalacia and what are the various types of osteomalacia?

9. What are some of the main endocrine osteopathies which produce generalized radiolucency?

10. What is meant by hypophosphatasia and what are some of its radiographic and clinical features?

11. Name the main categories of disease that are characterized by generalized radiolucency in scattered foci throughout the bony skeleton.

12. What malignancies are mainly believed to cause metastatic bone tumor?

13. What are the main clinical and radiographic features of primary hyperparathyroidism?

14. What are the main bone entities characterized by generalized radiolucency with a linear coarsening of the trabecular pattern of bone?

15. Indicate at least two and, if possible, three diseases of the systemic group which are characterized by lucency of epiphyses.

16. Indicate at least four diseases characterized by radiolucency of metaphyses in this systemic category.

17. Indicate several diseases which are characterized by widespread radiolucency involving epiphyses and metaphyses to a great extent.

18. Indicate several diseases characterized by elevation of the periosteum where the elevation is also combined with radiolucency of the bones. Indicate whether the elevation of the periosteum is more likely to appear "layered," "lacelike," or "spiculated."

19. Indicate those systemic radiolucent diseases which are accompanied by one or another form of metaphyseal expansion.

20. How would you characterize the skeletal findings in the so-called "reticuloendothelial marrow disorders"?

21. What is the "congenital rubella syndrome" and how does it affect the fetal skeleton?

9

Radiolucent Bone Diseases of a Single Extremity

The following classification will be followed (Figure 9–1):
1. *Diseases affecting the epiphyses* primarily
2. Radiolucent bone diseases affecting both the *metaphyses and epiphyses*

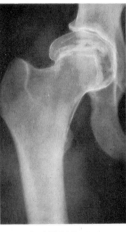

1. AFFECTING
   EPIPHYSIS
   PRIMARILY

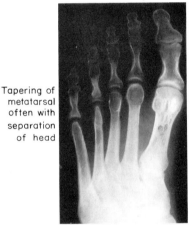

Tapering of
metatarsal
often with
separation
of head

Punctate
"honey
combing"

2. AFFECTING
   EPIPHYSIS AND
   METAPHYSIS

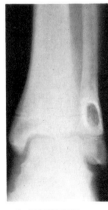

Marginal
sclerosis

Sharply
demarcated
area of
reabsorption

No sequestrae

3. AFFECTING
   METAPHYSIS
   WITH MARGINAL
   SCLEROSIS

Elevation of
periosteum
by exudate

Area of
absorption
in shaft

Infection
enters via
nutrient
shaft

4. AFFECTING
   METAPHYSIS
   PRIMARILY

   NO MARGINAL
   SCLEROSIS

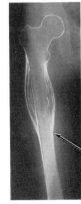

"Onion skin"
effect of
Ewing's

Codman's
triangle

5. CORTICO–PERIOSTEAL
   LESIONS

Figure 9–1 Classification of radiolucent bone diseases tending to remain localized to a single extremity or region. (Radiographs intensified.)

3. Radiolucent bone diseases affecting the *metaphyses primarily with thick or thin marginal sclerosis*
4. Radiolucent diseases affecting the *metaphyses primarily without marginal sclerosis*
5. *Diaphyseal corticoperiosteal radiolucent* lesions

DISEASES PRIMARILY AFFECTING THE EPIPHYSES
(Figure 9–2)

The most important entities in this category are illustrated in Figure 9–2.

The Osteochondroses (Focal Aseptic Necrosis of Bone). Osteochondrosis is a focal aseptic necrosis of the centers of ossification. The etiology is unknown but the disease is not of inflammatory origin. No epiphysis is immune from an osteochondrosis. Sometimes there are multiple foci of involvement.

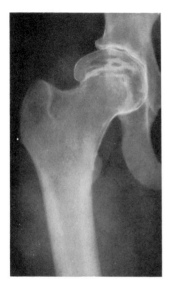 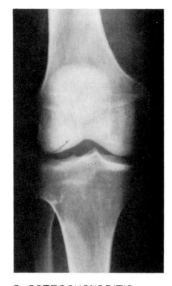 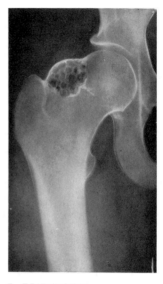

1. FOCAL ASEPTIC NECROSES OR THE OSTEOCHONDROSES
   DEFORMED FEMORAL HEAD OF LATE PERTHES' DISEASE

2. OSTEOCHONDRITIS DISSECANS OF KNEE

3. EPIPHYSEAL CHONDROBLASTOMA
   NUMEROUS CALCIFIC FOCI IN EPIPHYSIS AND ADJOINING METAPHYSIS

Figure 9–2 Diseases primarily affecting the epiphyses (radiographs intensified).

Radiographic Findings

1. With the onset of necrosis, subarticular lucencies appear in isolated foci
2. These necrotic foci increase in density
3. Fragmentation and fissuring of subchondral area occur
4. Flattening and deformity of epiphysis follow
5. Ultimately the bone reverts to its normal trabecular appearance, but marked deformity of the epiphysis persists
6. Epiphyseal closure occurs
7. Broadening and shortening of femoral neck with varus deformity usually follows
8. Degenerative, secondary arthritis may ensue

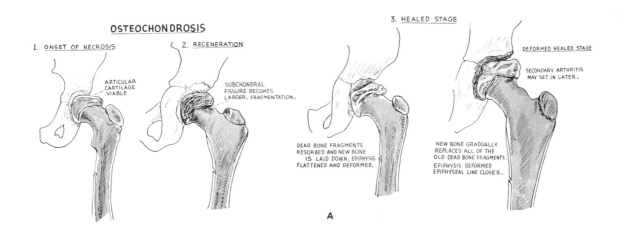

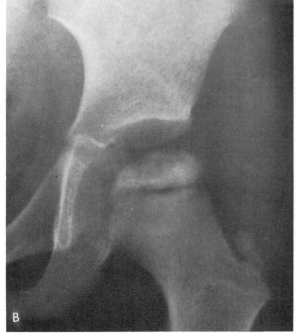

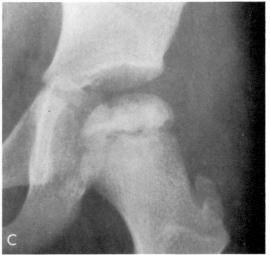

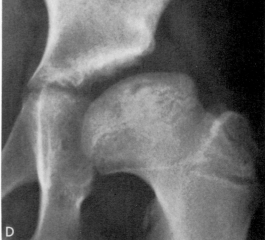

Figure 9–3 *A*. The pathogenesis of osteochondrosis as presented in the femoral head.

B, C, and *D*. Radiographs of three stages of osteochondrosis of the hip. The film in *B* was obtained on June 7, 1963; that in *C* was obtained on December 31, 1963, approximately 7 months later. *D* shows a much more advanced healing stage of osteochondrosis of the femoral head, demonstrating the marked flattening of the head of the femur with widening and mushrooming of the adjoining neck as well.

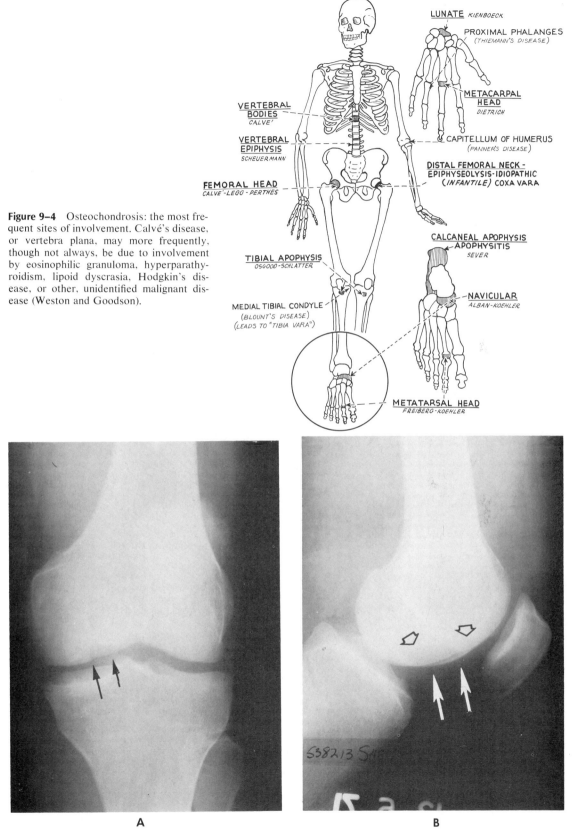

Figure 9–4 Osteochondrosis: the most frequent sites of involvement. Calvé's disease, or vertebra plana, may more frequently, though not always, be due to involvement by eosinophilic granuloma, hyperparathyroidism, lipoid dyscrasia, Hodgkin's disease, or other, unidentified malignant disease (Weston and Goodson).

Labels in figure:

LUNATE *KIENBOECK*
PROXIMAL PHALANGES *(THIEMANN'S DISEASE)*
METACARPAL HEAD *DIETRICH*
CAPITELLUM OF HUMERUS *(PANNER'S DISEASE)*
DISTAL FEMORAL NECK – EPIPHYSEOLYSIS-IDIOPATHIC *(INFANTILE)* COXA VARA
CALCANEAL APOPHYSIS APOPHYSITIS *SEVER*
NAVICULAR *ALBAN-KOEHLER*
METATARSAL HEAD *FREIBERG-KOEHLER*
VERTEBRAL BODIES *CALVE'*
VERTEBRAL EPIPHYSIS *SCHEUERMANN*
FEMORAL HEAD *CALVE'-LEGG-PERTHES*
TIBIAL APOPHYSIS *OSGOOD-SCHLATTER*
MEDIAL TIBIAL CONDYLE *(BLOUNT'S DISEASE) (LEADS TO "TIBIA VARA")*

A   B

Figure 9–5 *A* and *B*. Osteochondritis dissecans of the knee, involving the medial femoral condyle. This is a well-circumscribed osteolysis or sequestration of subchondral bone and overlying cartilage of a portion of an epiphysis. The dissected fragment may become totally separated from the rest of the bone, drop into the joint as a loose body, or retain a small particle of connection from which it derives its blood supply. A degenerative arthritis may supervene.

RADIOLUCENT BONE DISEASES PRIMARILY AFFECTING THE METAPHYSIS AND EPIPHYSIS

Neurotrophic or Neurovasculotrophic Osteopathy (Figure 9–6)

NEUROTROPHIC OSTEOPATHY

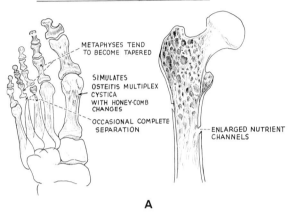

METAPHYSES TEND TO BECOME TAPERED

SIMULATES OSTEITIS MULTIPLEX CYSTICA WITH HONEY-COMB CHANGES

OCCASIONAL COMPLETE SEPARATION

ENLARGED NUTRIENT CHANNELS

A

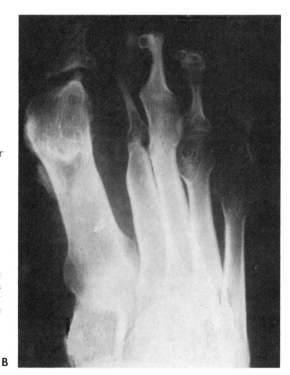

B

Figure 9–6 *A.* Line tracings of various types of neurotrophic osteopathy, *B.* Radiograph representing neurotrophic lesions of both feet. Note that the toes have not as yet completely sloughed away despite the very considerable osteolysis of the distal metaphysis of the metatarsals.

These findings are seen in:
1. Syringomyelia
2. Diabetes
3. Burns, frostbite, electrical injuries
4. Raynaud's phenomenon
5. Familial acro-osteolysis
6. Massive osteolysis and angiomatosis ("vanishing bone disease of Gorham")
7. Sudek's atrophy
8. Arthritis mutilans (rheumatoid arthritis, psoriatic arthritis. See Chapter 11.)

RADIOLUCENT OSSEOUS LESIONS AFFECTING METAPHYSES PRIMARILY WITH MARGINAL SCLEROSIS

These lesions include:
1. Brodie's abscess (Figure 9–7)
2. Enchondromata (Figure 9–8)
3. Chondromyxoid fibroma (Figure 9–9)
4. Solitary bone cyst (Figure 9–10)
5. Fibrous dysplasia (Figure 9–11)
6. Fibroxanthoma (nonosteogenic fibroma) (Figure 9–12)
7. Aneurysmal bone cyst (Figure 9–13)
8. Benign osteoblastoma (giant osteoid osteoma) (Figure 9–14)
9. "Chondromyxosarcoma"

Brodie's Abscess

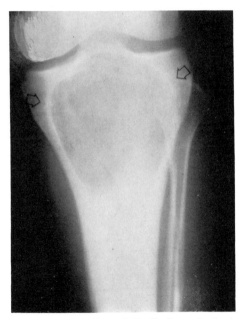

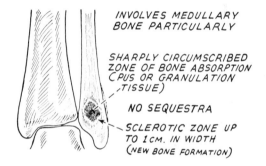

INVOLVES MEDULLARY BONE PARTICULARLY

SHARPLY CIRCUMSCRIBED ZONE OF BONE ABSORPTION (PUS OR GRANULATION TISSUE)

NO SEQUESTRA

SCLEROTIC ZONE UP TO 1 CM. IN WIDTH (NEW BONE FORMATION)

PATHOGENESIS: RELATIVELY AVIRULENT INFECTION AFFECTING MEDULLARY BONE WITH ONLY MODERATE LOCAL SYMPTOMS AND SIGNS OF INFLAMMATION

CLINICALLY: MAY OR MAY NOT HAVE SYSTEMIC SYMPTOMS

Figure 9–7 Radiograph of upper shaft of tibia with Brodie's abscess.

Enchondromas (Figure 9–8).   Solitary enchondromas are found mainly in persons over 20 years of age, in contrast to enchondromatosis (Ollier's disease), which occurs in younger people in a congenital pattern (Aegerter and Kirkpatrick). These are slow-growing cartilage masses which gradually replace the metaphyses of cylindrical bones, especially the short bones of the hands and feet. The humerus and femur may also be sites of involvement.

Radiographic Findings

There is a lucent replacement of the medullary trabeculae of the short bones so involved and a thin shell of cortex can be identified.

When the cortex becomes very thin, pathologic fracture may ensue. No periosteal reaction can be identified until a fracture induces callus formation.

Osteoblastoma (giant osteoid osteoma), although more frequently affecting the neural arch and processes of the spine, may also affect the small bones of the hand and foot in an identical fashion (Figure 9–14).

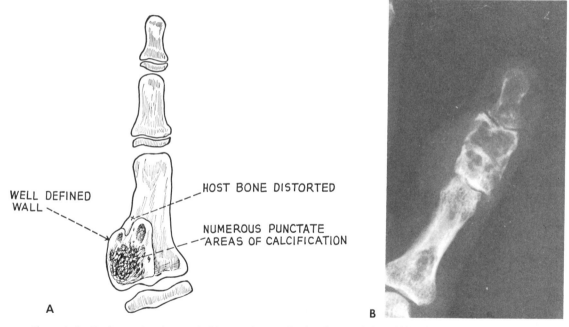

WELL DEFINED
WALL

HOST BONE DISTORTED

NUMEROUS PUNCTATE
AREAS OF CALCIFICATION

A   B

Figure 9–8   Benign enchondroma. *A*. Line tracing. *B*. Enchondroma of the middle phalanx of the fifth finger.

Chondromyxoid Fibroma

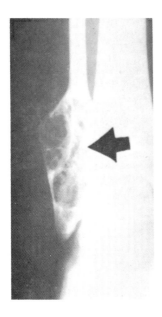

Sites: Long tubular bones
        Small tubular bones
        Flat bones
Size: 3 × 2 × 2 cm. to 8 cm. diameter
Radiographic appearance:
1. Overlying cortex expanded and thin due to pressure
2. Smooth border with lobulation
3. Well-defined medullary border
4. Occasional rim of sclerosis
   Absent periosteal reaction
5. Punctate calcification, limited by periosteum
6. Pseudoseptae inside: coarse trabeculation
7. Usually in metaphysis proximal to epiphyseal plate
8. Eccentric with respect to medulla

Figure 9–9 Chondromyxoid fibroma of the distal shaft and adjoining epiphysis of the fibula. (Courtesy of the Armed Forces Institute of Pathology, Washington, D.C.)

Solitary Bone Cyst

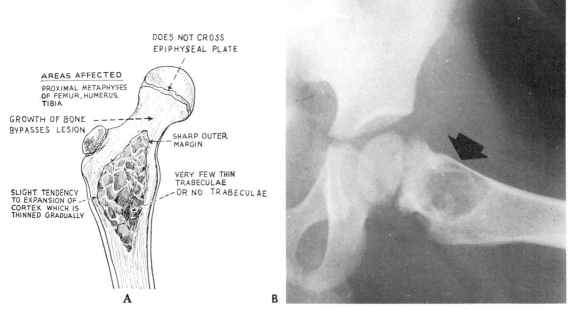

Figure 9–10 Diagram and radiograph illustrating a solitary bone cyst.

Fibrous Dysplasia of Bone

Clinical Considerations. Fibrous dysplasia may be monostotic or polyostotic. Any bone in the skeleton may be involved, particularly the long bones of the extremities, ribs, skull, and facial bones.

When *polyostotic,* clinical considerations frequently conform to a syndrome described by Albright: (1) The bone lesions tend to be unilateral in distribution; (2) There are often scattered areas of melanotic pigmentation of the skin, usually on the side of the bone lesions; (3) The syndrome occurs especially in young females with precocious puberty.

Pathology

The lesions in the bone are characterized by focal areas of fibrous replacement of bone with *metaplastic* formation of irregular bone.

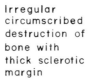

Irregular circumscribed destruction of bone with thick sclerotic margin

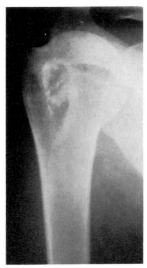

Figure 9–11   Fibrous dysplasia.

Radiographic Findings

"Ground glass" appearance, but **because of irregular masses of poorly woven bone internal to** the lesion, **fibrous dysplasia at times appears sclerotic rather than radiolucent.** (Some of the lucency may be related to coexisting arteriovenous malformations.)

Bending of the involved bone because of softening and pathologic fractures with marked proliferation of periosteal callus are common.

When the **facial bones** are involved, the **marked thickening and opacity** of the bones appear to predominate. Marked prognathism occurs with involvement of the mandible. Exophthalmos occurs with involvement of the orbit.

Encroachment upon the normal facial or cranial spaces is noteworthy.

Bony protuberances occur with involvement of the paranasal sinuses (see Chapter 12).

The lesions are practically always covered by a thick or thin bony cortical shell (Figure 9–11), since the cortex of the bone appears to be eroded from within and the periosteum deposits a thin shell of bone to compensate.

Fibroxanthoma (Nonossifying Fibroma of Jaffe); Fibrous Cortical Defect
(Figure 9–12)

General Considerations. This lesion is most frequently seen in the lower part of the femoral shaft near the epiphyseal plate. Less often, it occurs in the upper shaft of the tibia, the upper or lower part of the fibular shaft, and, far less frequently, in the shafts of the humerus, radius, ulna, or short tubular bones.

Radiographic Findings. The lesion appears as a radiolucent **cortical** defect near one end of the affected bone shaft. The long axis tends to parallel the long axis of the shaft and it ranges in size from 1 to 4 cm. In some instances it appears to be lobulated. There is ordinarily a very thin reactive shell around this lesion.

Jaffe believes that the fibroxanthoma is a later stage in the development of the fibrous cortical defect.

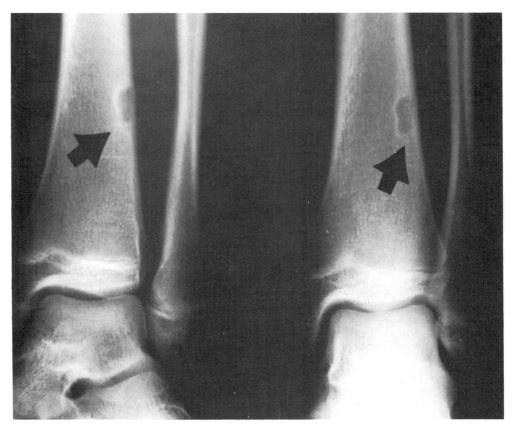

Figure 9–12   Nonosteogenic fibroma of Lichtenstein and Jaffe. (Courtesy of Colonel William L. Thompson, Armed Forces Institute of Pathology.)

Aneurysmal Bone Cyst (Figure 9–13)

Pathology. The cyst is a saccular protrusion of the bony cortex—a "blister of bone." Any bone of the skeleton may be involved. One-quarter of the cases occur in vertebrae (Aegerter and Kirkpatrick). It most often affects the ends of long bones but may affect the diaphysis, pushing the contiguous periosteum outward, which reacts by laying down a thin shell of bone. This thin shell may fracture, causing an extravasation of blood into the adjoining tissues. Occasionally the short tubular bones of the hands or feet may be affected. Children and adolescents are often affected.

Radiographic Findings. Saccular protrusion of the end of a long bone with multiple fine septae internally, and sharply demarcated, bulging, scalloped borders. It appears to begin in the cancellous bone and is surrounded by a thin identifiable cortex or periosteal new bone layer, which has a "blister of bone" appearance. In vertebrae the neural arch is usually the site of involvement.

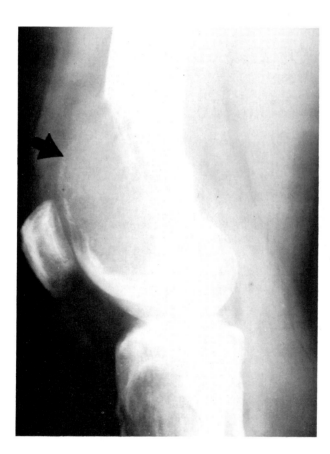

Figure 9–13 Aneurysmal bone cyst involving the distal metaphysis and epiphysis of the femur, a "blister of bone" appearance. Although this is called an aneurysmal bone cyst by many, it has also been called cystic giant cell tumor, especially with a history of injury. The thin bony roof of the lesion is noteworthy. (Courtesy of Colonel William L. Thompson, Armed Forces Institute of Pathology.)

The Benign Osteoblastoma (Giant Osteoid Osteoma, Osteogenic Fibroma) (Figure 9–14)

The nidus characteristic of osteoid osteoma is absent. Clinically and radiographically, the osteoblastoma is an entirely different type of lesion; despite its osteoid content and benign nature, it is an actively growing neoplasm.

Principal Sites of Involvement

In more than one-half of the cases, the tumor is situated in the *vertebral column*. The *neural arch* is the favorite region, and the pedicle in most instances is also invaded.

The second most frequent location (20 per cent) is long bone where the tumor has been identified as equally distributed between the ends and the shafts (Figure 9–14).

Many of the tumors involve small bones Most of the time the tumor appears to have an eccentric origin.

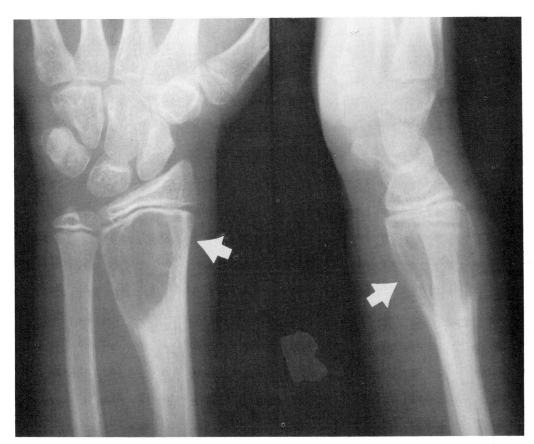

Figure 9–14 Antero-posterior and lateral views of the wrist showing a benign osteoblastoma (giant osteoid osteoma) in the distal shaft of the radius.

Radiographic Findings

Predominantly an osteolytic expanding process with evidence of cortical erosion, but there may be occasional bone production or calcification of varying degree within the tumor or around it.

A soft tissue mass arising from the eroded cortex is noted in about two-thirds of the cases.

In some cases a definite calcific shell of a characteristic nature sharply delimits the soft tissue mass. Usually an intact shell can be detected.

The tumor is usually well demarcated from the normal neighboring bone.

The tumors vary in size from approximately 2 by 1.5 cm. by 6 cm. to 10 by 6 by 6.5 cm., with an average of 2 by 3 cm.

RADIOLUCENT DISEASES OF BONE AFFECTING THE METAPHYSIS PRIMARILY WITHOUT MARGINAL SCLEROSIS

The diseases most frequently encountered in this category are:
1. Suppurative osteomyelitis
2. Nonsuppurative osteomyelitis
3. Sarcoid of bone
4. Giant cell tumor
5. Osteosarcoma
6. Metastatic tumor to bone (Chapter 7)
7. Radiation osteitis

Suppurative Osteomyelitis. The radiographic stages may be summarized as follows.

Radiographic Stages

No roentgen abnormalities usually occur until seven to ten days or longer after onset of infection.

Soft tissue swelling adjacent to the involved bone may be the earliest roentgen manifestation.

In untreated cases **small areas of rarefaction** may appear in the metaphyseal ends of the involved long bones.

The spread of the infection through the medullary bone and cortex causes **an elevation and reaction in the overlying periosteum.** Indeed, the appearance of new bone formation by such elevated periosteum may precede the roentgen observation of the lucency of the bone involved.

The **radiolucency spreads,** involving more and more of the shaft of the bone, but ordinarily **the epiphyseal plate is not crossed.** Arthritic involvement may occur if this barrier does break down.

Devitalization of the bone causes the formation of **sequestra** which can be recognized radiographically as dense osteosclerotic spicules of dead bone surrounded by a lucent zone of bone resorption.

Reactive new bone formation adjoining the destruction gives rise to the appearance of **involucra.**

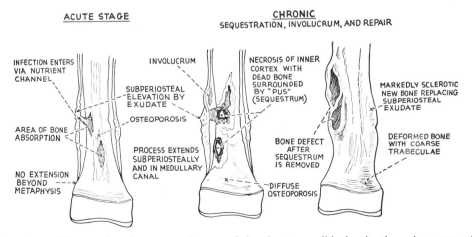

Figure 9–15 Diagram of a primary type of acute and chronic osteomyelitis showing the various stages of its development and pathogenesis.

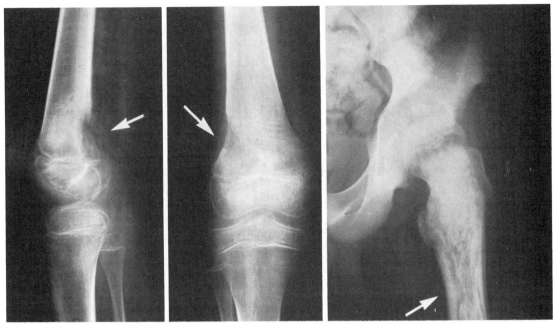

Figure 9–16 *A*. Acute osteomyelitis affecting the distal metaphysis of the left femur. *B*. A more advanced stage of osteomyelitis in the subchronic phase demonstrating advanced necrosis and sequestrum formation. Note that the destructive process stops at the epiphyseal line and does not cross into the epiphysis.

Nonsuppurative Osteomyelitis involves: tuberculosis of bone; mycotic infections of bone; fungus infections; syphilis of bone; brucella osteomyelitis; and possibly viral osteomyelitis.

Tuberculous Osteomyelitis may be classified into four types: (1) spine (Chapter 14); (2) osteitis and arthritis combined (Figure 9–17); (3) diaphyseal tuberculosis; and (4) tuberculoid reactions in bone.

Tuberculous Osteomyelitis and Arthritis. These usually coexist in long bones. The hip and knee are most commonly involved. Tuberculosis of the phalanges is shown in Figure 9–17.

RADIOGRAPHIC FINDINGS

Marked **radiolucency** and some evidence of **bone dissolution,** with minimal or **no sequestration.**

There is ordinarily **very little reactive bone formation** and **little or no periosteal reaction.**

Surrounding soft tissue atrophy results if the process is of long duration.

Diaphyseal Tuberculosis Without Adjoining Joint Involvement is rare, but extensive bone destruction with it is also rare, since this disorder heals more readily. The *greater trochanter* of the femur and the *diaphysis of the small bones of the hands* (spina ventosa) are sites of such involvement.

Tuberculoid Reactions in Bone Adjoining Tuberculous Arthritis. There is usually a disappearance of cancellous bone adjoining tuberculous arthritis.

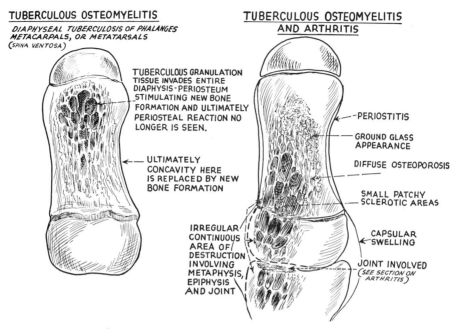

Figure 9–17   Tuberculous osteomyelitis and arthritis.

Nocardial Osteomyelitis produces lesions in bone which are radiographically identical to those of tuberculosis.

Fungus Infections of Bone.   These are usually secondary to involvement of the overlying or adjoining soft tissues, with the exception of coccidioidomycosis and blastomycosis. The latter are hematogenous in origin usually.

Actinomycosis affects the bones of the mandible, rib cage, and vertebrae especially, and is accompanied by draining sinuses. The granulomatous reaction is much like tuberculosis. Apart from *site* predilection, no special radiologic appearances can be attributed to these.

Blastomycosis Usually Produces a Slow Dissolution of Involved Bone and May Involve Peripheral Small Bones Especially (Figure 9–18). Occasionally a thick zone of sclerosis in the involved area may be identified surrounding the zone of bone dissolution.

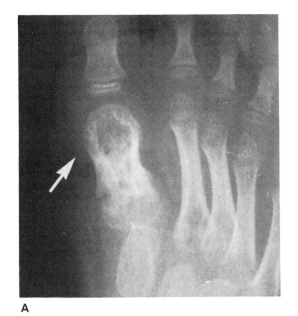

A

Figure 9–18   *A* and *B*. Blastomycosis of the great toe.

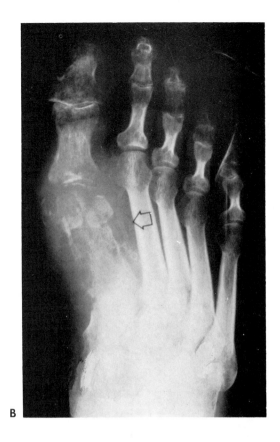

B

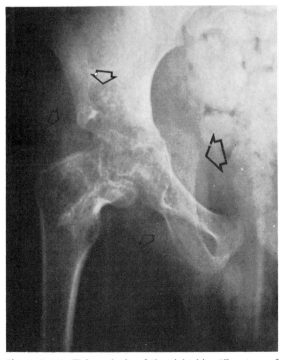

Figure 9–19   Tuberculosis of the right hip. (Courtesy of Dr. J. Johnston, Oakland, California.)

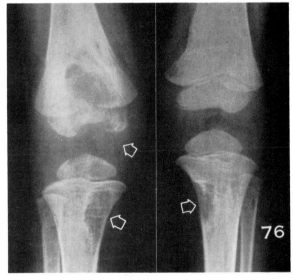

Figure 9–20   Tuberculosis of the knee. Tuberculosis of the phalanges is often referred to as "spinaventosa." (Courtesy of Dr. J. Johnston, Oakland, California.)

Sarcoid in Bone most frequently occurs in the small bones of the *hands and feet,* particularly the metacarpals, metatarsals, and phalanges. Any part of the reticuloendothelial system may be involved as well. The granulomatous process in the marrow of these small bones is destructive without inner or periosteal reaction.

Radiographic Findings

Small "pseudocystic" foci of lucency are especially observed in the hands and feet, because of destruction of the small trabeculae.

A coarse reticular trabecular pattern may also be observed (Figure 9–21).

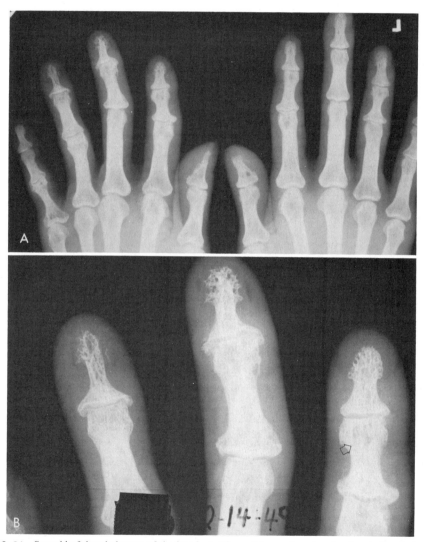

Figure 9–21   Sarcoid of the phalanges of the hand. *A.* View of the scattered and rather indiscriminate involvement of the ends of these short bones. *B.* Close-up view of several of the digits showing the cystic type resorption of the proximal and distal ends of the involved phalanges. Note also the frayed appearance of the phalangeal tufts.

The Giant Cell Tumor (Figure 9–22).   This lesion is usually situated in the end of some long tubular bone but may be situated in flat bones such as the ilium or scapula. The lower end of the femur, the upper end of the tibia, and the lower end of the radius are the three most common sites for the lesion. These account for 60 to 70 per cent of the localizations.

When there is a multiplicity of involvement, one must strongly suspect hyperparathyroidism, in which case *osteitis fibrosa cystica* may closely resemble the histologic appearance of the giant cell tumor.

Patient's age is usually following epiphyseal closure (greater than 20 years).

Radiographic Findings

The bone cortex in the affected region is thinned and expanded and has a large "soap bubble" appearance.

This is **very little periosteal new bone formation** over the thinned and expanded cortex.

A marginal zone of sclerosis is usually absent.

Unfortunately, the radiographic picture of fibrosarcoma can perfectly simulate that of a giant cell tumor.

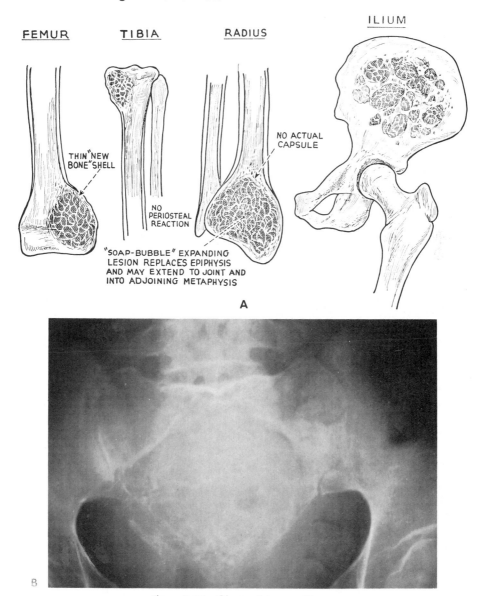

Figure 9–22   Giant cell tumor of bone.

Osteosarcoma.   Approximately three-quarters of osteosarcomas occur in the metaphyses of the lower femur or upper tibia in persons between 12 and 25 years of age.

Radiographic Findings.   Various types of osteosarcomas are illustrated in Figure 9–23. These include primary manifestations of:

Peripheral osteolysis with a break in the cortex and a soft tissue mass.

Central osteolysis with a break in the cortex and a soft tissue mass.

Combined sclerosis and osteolysis, a break in the cortex, and a soft tissue mass.

Osteosclerosis with a sunray-type reaction of the periosteum and a soft tissue mass.

A mosaic intermixture of sclerosis and radiolucency with periosteal layering and reactions which suggest malignant degeneration from an osteitis deformans (Paget's disease of bone). The latter occurs particularly in patients over 50 years of age.

In the periosteum, Codman's triangle (the zone of reactive bone formation adjoining the tumor periosteum) is very often identified, but this may also occur with inflammatory benign lesions.

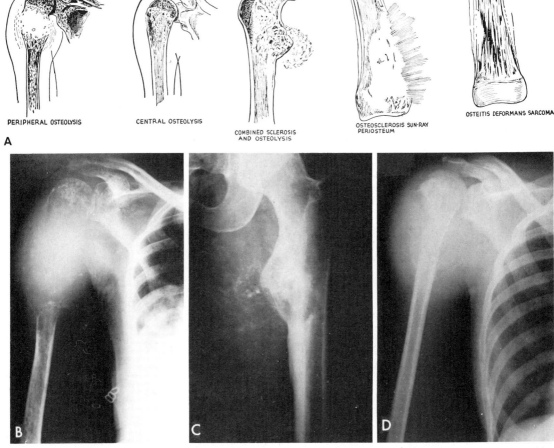

Figure 9–23   *A*. Sketches demonstrating peripheral osteolytic and central osteolytic types of osteosarcoma, combined sclerotic and osteolytic type, sclerotic sunray type, and type derived from osteitis deformans by malignant degeneration thereof. *B*. Radiograph demonstrating the osteolytic variety of osteosarcoma. *C*. Radiograph demonstrating the combined osteolytic and osteosclerotic type of osteosarcoma. *D*. Osteolytic variety of osteosarcoma, less advanced. (Sketches modified from Schinz-Case: Roentgen-Diagnostics.)

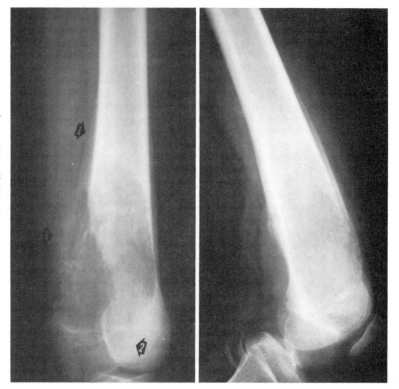

Figure 9-23 *Continued E.* Osteosarcoma of a lytic type involving the distal femur. Arrow 1 shows Codman's triangle as well as the lysis and some tendency to new bone formation with invasion of the adjoining soft tissues. Arrow 2 shows the marked lysis of the distal ends of the femur crossing into the epiphysis, with the layerlike periosteal reaction on the anterior aspect of the femur. Codman's triangle is shown on the posterior aspect. *Left,* oblique view; *right,* lateral view.

E

DIAPHYSEAL CORTICOPERIOSTEAL LESIONS

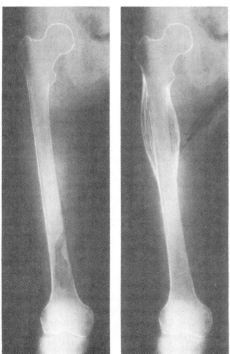

3. Neurofibromatosis
4. Traumatic periostitis and fractures
5. Pseudofractures (milkman's disease)
6. Osteosarcoma
7. Hemangioma
8. Osteomyelitis, secondary type
9. Fibrosarcoma

Figure 9-24 Diaphyseal corticoperiosteal radiolucent lesions. (Diagrammatic intensified radiographs.)

1. Osteomyelitis
2. Ewing's tumor and other round cell tumors

115

Osteomyelitis (see Figure 9–28)

Ewing's Tumor (Endothelioma)

General Comments. Ewing's tumor is one of the round cell tumors. *It is the third most common malignant primary bone tumor* and is surpassed only by plasma cell myeloma and osteosarcoma. Virtually all patients are seen *before the age of 30.*

Principal Sites. Most cases in younger persons begin in cylindrical bones, whereas the flat bones are more frequently involved in older patients. The tumor is situated most frequently in the femur and tibia but even the small bones of the feet, especially the os calcis, may be affected. Of the flat bones, those of the pelvic girdle are most commonly involved. Ribs and vertebrae may also, however, be affected.

Radiographic Findings (Figure 9–25)

(1) **A large soft tissue mass is usually associated.** (2) The **periosteum is elevated in layers,** producing the so-called "onion skin" appearance. (3) At the extremes of the periosteal elevation there is new bone formation **(Codman's triangle).** (4) The metaphysis is frequently involved and even the epiphysis may occasionally be the site of origin.

Sclerosis of the bone may at times be indicated by a streaky appearance of the involved areas, and it is accentuated by radiolucency (due to the osseous destruction) of the adjoining bone.

Unfortunately, only 25 per cent of Ewing's tumors present this classic radiographic appearance (Sherman and Soong).

Also, although a diagnosis may possess a high index of suspicion, **there is a close radiographical resemblance to osteomyelitis, eosinophilic granuloma, osteosarcoma, and reticulum cell sarcoma, and biopsy is therefore essential** for definitive diagnosis.

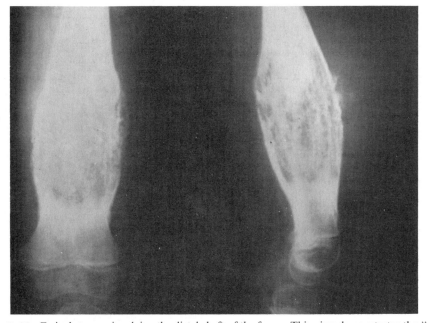

Figure 9–25 Ewing's tumor, involving the distal shaft of the femur. This view demonstrates the "onion peel" appearance of the entire destroyed portion of the distal shaft of the femur.

Neurofibroma (Figure 9–26)

General Comment.   Neurofibromas of bone are variable in appearance but are usually secondary to nerve involvement.

Radiographic Findings

The bone changes include: **scoliosis, bone atrophy, bone hypertrophy of individual bones, and skeletal anomalies. Many of the defects in the bone, but not all, apparently are the result of pressure from associated neurofibromas.**

At times only slight irregularity of bone contour is noted, with cystlike cavities adjoining.

Holt and Wright reported that 29 per cent of the total group of cases studied by them showed some form of skeletal defect, and these were classified as follows:

    a. Erosive defects.

    b. Scoliosis, with dysplasia of the vertebral body.

    c. Disorders of growth, including both over- and underdevelopment.

    d. Bowing and pseudoarthrosis of the lower legs.

    e. Intraosseous cystic lesions.

    f. Numerous congenital anomalies.

Hunt and Pugh have added the following:

    g. Defects of the posterior-superior orbital wall.

    h. Disorders of growth in bone associated with elephantoid hypertrophy of overlying soft tissues.

    i. Intrathoracic meningocele.

The latter authors indicated that sarcomatous degeneration of the neurofibromas occurred in 5 per cent of the patients.

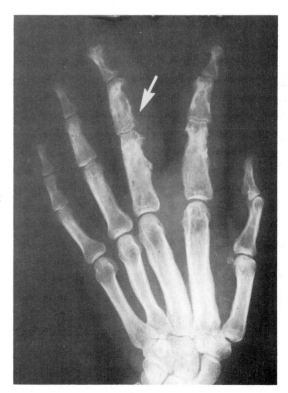

Figure 9–26   Neurofibromatosis affecting the right hand.

Hemangioma of Bone and Lymphangiomas of Bone (Figure 9–27)

General Comment. These lesions are usually located in the spine or skull, but other areas such as the extremities may also be involved.

Radiographic Findings

Vertebrae are involved in 10 to 30 per cent of cases, and a **characteristic vertical striated radiographic appearance may be noted** (Figure 9–28). Collapse of the involved vertebral body may result in pressure upon cord or nerve roots.

In the **extremities** there is often an **overgrowth** of the involved part. The lesion is usually corticoperiosteal with an expansion of the cortex and extension toward the medulla.

It has a multilocular appearance but the "bubbly" appearance is smaller and scattered, unlike the "soap bubble" appearance earlier described for the giant cell tumor and the aneurysmal bone cyst.

Also the lesions are usually in the diaphysis rather than in the epiphysis or metaphysis.

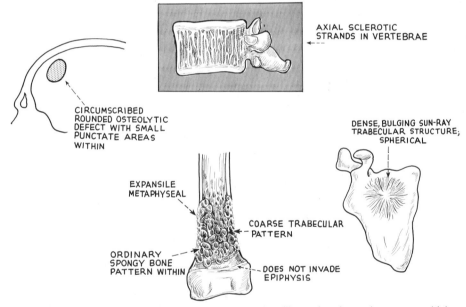

AXIAL SCLEROTIC
STRANDS IN VERTEBRAE

CIRCUMSCRIBED
ROUNDED OSTEOLYTIC
DEFECT WITH SMALL
PUNCTATE AREAS
WITHIN

DENSE, BULGING SUN-RAY
TRABECULAR STRUCTURE;
SPHERICAL

EXPANSILE
METAPHYSEAL

COARSE TRABECULAR
PATTERN

ORDINARY
SPONGY BONE
PATTERN WITHIN

DOES NOT INVADE
EPIPHYSIS

Figure 9–27 Hemangioma of bone: diagrammatic sketches illustrating the various types which may occur in different areas of the skeleton.

Osteomyelitis, Secondary Type (Figure 9–28)

General Comments. Osteomyelitis may involve bone by contiguous involvement from soft tissue infection. When this occurs there is usually an associated vascular deficiency such as occurs with peripheral arteriosclerosis or diabetes.

Most Frequent Sites are the feet. Usually the bones involved are the metaphysis and epiphysis of the distal aspects of the metatarsals or phalanges.

Radiographic Findings

The osteolytic process tends to extend irregularly in all directions from a cortical and periosteal site, but the area of maximum involvement is usually the site of soft tissue swelling.

The **periosteal reaction may be minimal.**
Very little if any sequestration is ever seen.
Very little sclerosis or evidence of new bone formation is obtained.

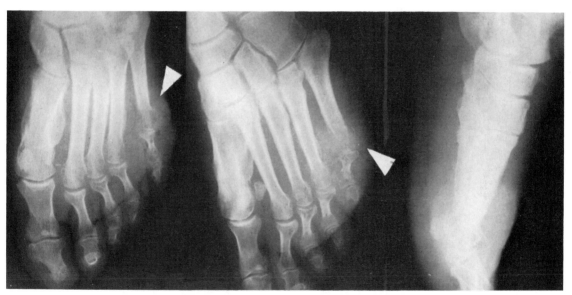

Figure 9–28   Osteomyelitis, secondary type.

Fibrosarcoma of Bone (Figure 9–28)

General Comment. Fibrosarcoma of bone is the least common of the primary malignant tumors with a probable predilection for persons in their second and third decades of life. There are two types: (1) a *medullary or endosteal variety* which arises centrally; and (2) *a periosteal type* arising in the periosteum. Both types are slow growing, and *they do not tend to metastasize until very late.* Recurrence following inadequate surgical removal is frequent.

Principal Sites are the condyle of the femur or an epicondyle of the humerus (Aegerter and Kirkpatrick). The jaw, usually the mandible, is also a frequent site of involvement.

Radiographic Findings

The periosteal variety usually appears as a **large soft tissue mass** which may **invade the underlying bone, causing lysis and radiolucency.**

The endosteal or central type fibrosarcoma destroys the trabeculae in the medullary portions of bone and later erodes the inner aspect of the surrounding cortex.

The **margins** of the tumor are **poorly defined** and usually there is **no overlying periosteal reaction,** until the entire cortex is destroyed.

Periosteal new bone may then be apparent but even it may shortly be destroyed as the tumor grows out into the adjoining soft tissues.

The primary radiographic appearance is that of radiolucency with destruction of bone and minimal or no periosteal reaction.

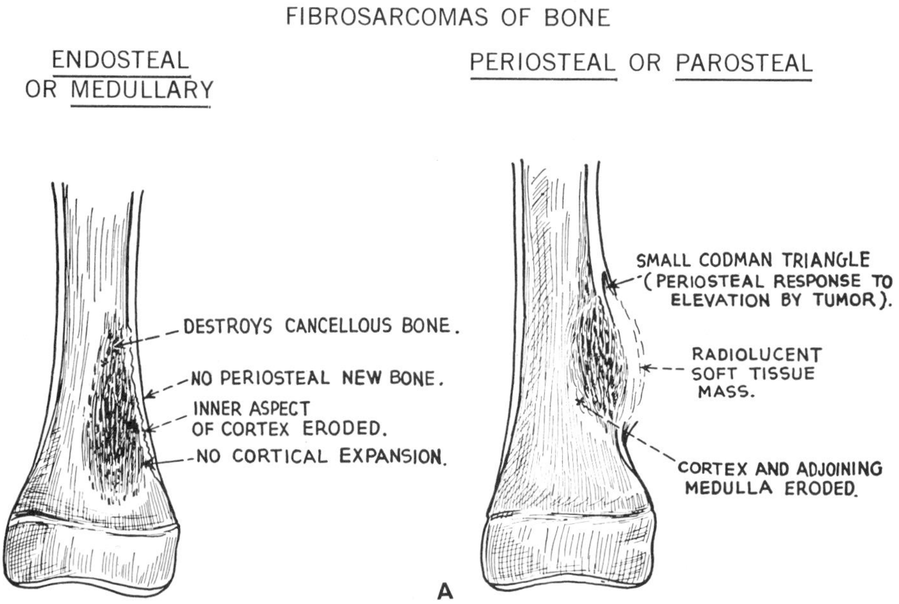

FIBROSARCOMAS OF BONE

ENDOSTEAL
OR MEDULLARY

PERIOSTEAL OR PAROSTEAL

DESTROYS CANCELLOUS BONE.

NO PERIOSTEAL NEW BONE.

INNER ASPECT
OF CORTEX ERODED.

NO CORTICAL EXPANSION.

SMALL CODMAN TRIANGLE
(PERIOSTEAL RESPONSE TO
ELEVATION BY TUMOR).

RADIOLUCENT
SOFT TISSUE
MASS.

CORTEX AND ADJOINING
MEDULLA ERODED.

A

B

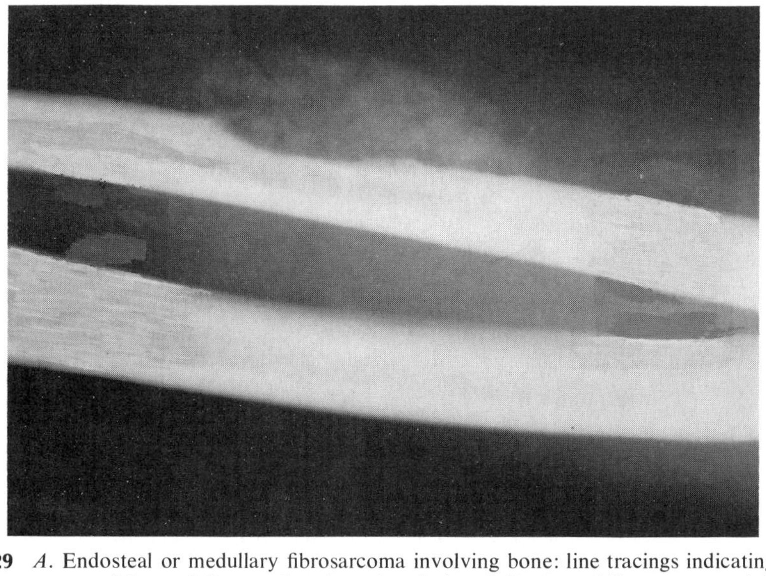

Figure 9–29 *A.* Endosteal or medullary fibrosarcoma involving bone: line tracings indicating the most frequent appearance of the medullary and periosteal varieties. *B.* Periosteal fibrosarcoma of the forearm involving the ulna.

Eosinophilic Granuloma of Bone

1. The sites of involvement by frequency can be inferred from a report by Ochsner. He reported 20 cases as follows: skull, six; ribs and spine, each three; mastoid, pelvis, femur, each two; mandible and humerus, each one.

2. The essential roentgenographic lesion is a localized area of rarefaction which occurs in the medullary portion of the bone; it may develop a scalloped defect in the inner cortical profile as it enlarges.

3. Pathologic fracture may supervene with a periosteal reaction.

4. There is usually no sclerotic zone otherwise.

5. In the spine a single vertebral body may collapse, producing a vertebra plana. This is not pathognomonic.

6. In the mandible there may be a cystlike area around a tooth producing a "floating tooth sign" similar to histiocytosis.

7. Ribs, pelvis, and long bones do not have specific lesions otherwise.

8. Epiphysis may be affected.

9. In the lung the lesion tends to be honeycombed.

10. Gastrointestinal tract lesions may also occur, especially polypoid lesions of the stomach (Rigler et al.; Ochsner).

Localization of Bone Neoplasms

From previous descriptions it is apparent that there are certain regions within the bone where tumors are most apt to occur, although there are exceptions. These are shown in Figure 9–30.

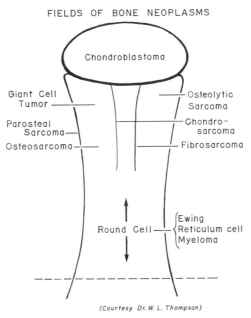

FIELDS OF BONE NEOPLASMS

Chondroblastoma

Giant Cell Tumor

Parosteal Sarcoma

Osteosarcoma

Osteolytic Sarcoma

Chondro-sarcoma

Fibrosarcoma

Round Cell — Ewing Reticulum cell Myeloma

(Courtesy Dr. W. L. Thompson)

Figure 9–30

Questions — Chapter 9

1. What basic classification have we employed involving radiolucent bone diseases affecting a single extremity from the radiologic standpoint?

2. Which are the most significant diseases affecting the epiphyses primarily?

3. What is the pathogenesis of osteochondrosis as presented in the femoral head?

4. What is meant by osteochondritis dissecans? Where is its most frequent site and where are some of the less frequent localizations of this disease process?

5. Describe the radiographic features of epiphyseal chondroblastoma.

6. Describe some of the clinical and radiographic features of neurotrophic osteopathy.

7. List the most important osteoporotic lesions affecting metaphyses primarily.

8. Indicate the pathogenesis and radiographic appearances of acute and chronic osteomyelitis.

9. Describe the radiographic features of a Brodie's abscess.

10. Describe some of the radiographic features of tuberculous osteomyelitis.

11. Describe the important radiographic features of enchondroma. What are some of the most frequent sites of involvement?

12. Describe the most frequently affected areas by a solitary bone cyst and the important radiographic features of this entity. What are the important differential diagnoses to be considered here?

13. Describe the important radiographic features of giant cell tumor.

14. Describe some of the important radiographic features of the nonosteogenic fibroma of Lichtenstein and Jaffe.

15. Describe the main radiographic features of osteosarcoma, indicating the several varieties of radiographic appearances which may occur.

16. List the most important disease entities affecting the diaphyses of bone predominantly.

17. List some of the important clinical and radiographic features of neurofibroma involving bone.

18. Describe the important radiographic features of hemangioma of bone, indicating its several appearances in the skull, vertebrae, long bones, and flat bones.

19. List those important disease entities that involve the periosteal zone primarily and the bone possibly secondarily.

20. Describe the important radiographic features of a secondary type osteomyelitis.

10

Bone Diseases of the Extremities Characterized by Increased Density, Expansion, or Enlargement

INTRODUCTION

Bone lesions may be arbitrarily categorized as sclerotic or radiolucent, with gradations between these poles (Figure 10–1). When the bone is not uniformly sclerotic or radiolucent, the alterations in density may be further subdivided as follows:

1. *Transverse* bands, usually at the *metaphyses;*

2. *Longitudinal reticular bands,* roughly parallel to the cortex, which may be asymmetrical and corticoperiosteal;

3. *Indiscriminate, patchy* foci of lucency or sclerosis: these may be localized to epiphyses, metaphyses, or diaphyses predominantly.

As always, neighboring soft tissues and joints must be carefully noted.

This proposed classification does not necessarily refer to any particular disease. The entire concept has evolved as a method of interrelating the pathologic entity with its radiographic counterpart, so that a system of thinking and analyzing may be developed.

As with the lucent disorders, these may be considered as (Figure 10–1):

1. Osteosclerosis affecting several extremities or disseminated.

2. Osteosclerosis, localized or regional.

OSTEOSCLEROTIC—HYPERTROPHIC BONE DISEASE
INVOLVING SEVERAL BONES

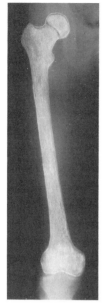
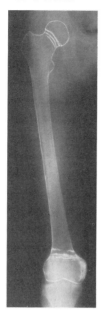
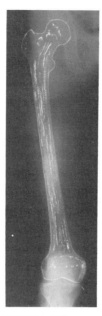
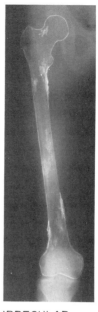
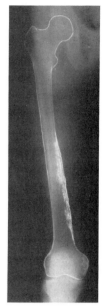

DIFFUSE   TRANSVERSE   FIBRILLAR   IRREGULAR   CORTICO-
                 BANDS   NETWORK   "PATCHY"   PERIOSTEAL
                                                                     INVOLVING
A   SEVERAL BONES

LOCALIZED TO ONE BONE OR REGION

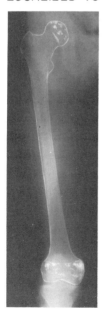
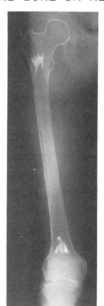
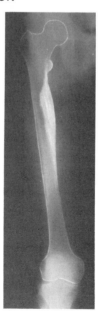
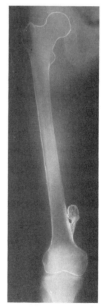

       LOCALIZED   LOCALIZED   LOCALIZED   OUTGROWTH OR
       EPIPHYSEAL   METAPHYSEAL   DIAPHYSEAL   OVERGROWTH
                                        PATCHY OR   (May be single or
B   SOLID   multiple)

Figure 10–1 General spectrum of osteosclerotic or hypertrophic bone diseases involving several bones or localized to one bone or region. (Intensified radiographs.)

OSTEOSCLEROSIS AFFECTING SEVERAL EXTREMITIES

Diffuse Osteosclerosis of Several Extremities

The following classification illustrated in Figure 10–2 shows this group of diseases conforming to three general categories:

DIFFUSE   FLASKLIKE   SHAFT ELLIPSOID

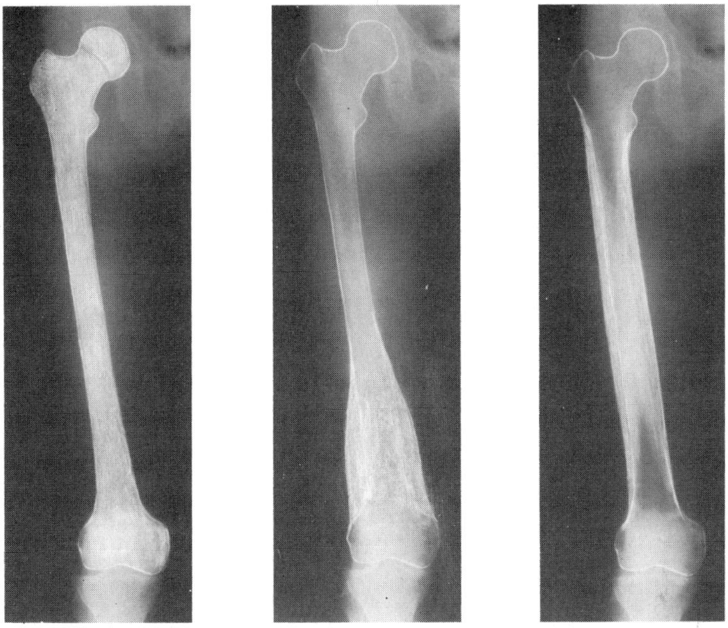

1. Fluorine poisoning
2. Mastocytosis (Urticaria pigmentosa)
3. Hypoparathyroidism
4. Hypervitaminosis A and D
5. Myelofibrosis Anemias, lymphomas
6. Carcinoid metastases or syndrome
7. Metastases — carcinoma prostate

} May be "reticulated" or "spotted" in appearance

1. Osteopetrosis
2. Pyle's disease

1. Engelmann's disease
2. Juvenile and tertiary syphilis

Figure 10–2 Osteosclerosis affecting several extremities of the diffuse osteosclerotic type: general categories. (Intensified radiographs.)

Marrow Disorders Related to Leukemias and Anemias
(see also Chapter 8)

General Comment. Osteomyelosclerosis may occur with any of the diseases which are accompanied by hypoplasia or aplasia of the bone marrow; hence, it is particularly related to the anemias, lymphomas, and leukemias.

Secondary myelosclerosis may also occur in association with, or from reaction to certain toxic agents, such as irradiation and industrial solvents.

Radiographic Findings

Diffuse bone sclerosis is the end stage of the metaplastic process.

Linear longitudinal streaking and mottling due to fibrosis may precede the diffuse sclerotic process.

At times there is an irregular coarsened and somewhat reticulated pattern in these disorders because the radiolucent aspect may have been uppermost.

Sclerosis of bone is present in more than one-half the cases and is of a diffuse rather than a localized variety. There is no expansion of the bone, as in osteopetrosis or Engelmann's disease, nor is there a tendency to thickening of the individual bony trabeculae, as in Paget's disease of bone. The ribs, pelvis, vertebrae, clavicles, and scapulae are most affected. Rarely is one able to detect changes in the skull, radius, ulna, tibia, or fibula, and no changes are ordinarily found in the hands or feet.

Splenomegaly and hepatomegaly are often associated, especially in severe cases.

In advanced sclerosis the trabecular pattern becomes irregular and indistinct, and the inner margin of the cortex blends with the spongiosa. When this occurs in vertebral bodies adjacent to end plates, it has been called the "rugger jersey" effect or "sandwich appearance." However, complete obliteration of the medullary space may occur in time in both vertebrae and long bones.

The proximal humerus and femur are especially involved—eventually, trabeculated bone may show a complete obliteration of the normal architecture. In the ribs the sclerosis leads to the striking appearance described as "jail bars" crossing the thorax.

DIFFERENTIAL DIAGNOSIS

Metastases from carcinoma of the prostate will be manifest as a diffuse sclerosis of all the bones of the skeleton. However, since this manifestation is more likely to take on the form of indiscriminate and irregular patchy sclerosis throughout the skeleton, this disorder is described elsewhere in this text.

Marble bone disease.

Engelmann's disease.

Paget's disease of bone.

OSTEOSCLEROSIS MANIFESTED CHIEFLY BY LONGITUDINAL CORTICOPERIOSTEAL THICKENING IN MULTIPLE BONES (Figure 10–3)

1. Melorheostosis leri
2. Juvenile or tertiary syphilis
3. Infantile cortical hyperostosis of Caffey-Silverman
4. Hypertrophic pulmonary osteoarthropathy
5. Chronic fungus osteomyelitis
6. Hypervitaminosis A
7. Acropachy (thyroid)
8. Venous stasis
9. Sclerosing sarcoma
10. Battered child syndrome
11. Obstructive jaundice

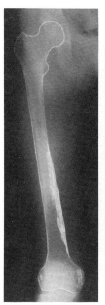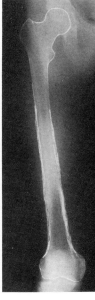

Figure 10–3 Intensified radiographs characterized chiefly by osteosclerosis of a longitudinal, cortical, or corticoperiosteal type in multiple bones or regions.

Infantile Cortical Hyperostosis of Caffey-Silverman (Figure 10–4).   Infantile cortical hyperostosis is a condition which appears in infants within the first five months of life and which ordinarily undergoes regression within twelve months following its initial appearance. It most frequently affects the mandible, clavicles, humeri, and ribs.

Radiographic Findings

There is dense periosteal thickening, hyperostosis of compact portions of bone, and sclerosis of spongy portions of the diaphysis, mandible, humeri, ribs, or other long bones which may be involved.

The major involvement is in the **diaphysis** of the bone.

Lamellated periosteal reaction occurs with an uneven outer border to the periosteal reaction.

Usually the disease is unilateral, but it may be bilateral.

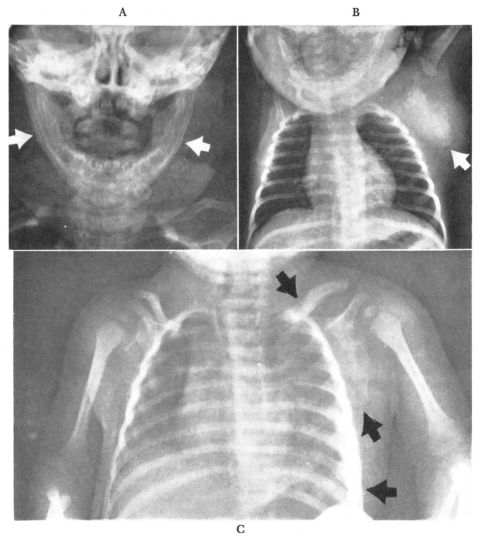

A

B

C

Figure 10–4   Infantile cortical hyperostosis. *A*. Mandible. *B*. Scapula. *C*. Scapula, approximately two months after *B*, showing considerable resolution of the process. At this later time, however, there is considerable involvement in the clavicle and ribs.

Syphilis of Bone (Figure 10–5).   This may be congenital or acquired.

Congenital Syphilis has been previously described as predominantly a metaphyseal osteochondritis and periostitis. The "saber shin" is a late manifestation (Figure 10–5; see also Chapter 8).

Acquired Syphilis of bone is a tertiary manifestation with involvement primarily of the walls of arterioles. Both long and flat bones may be involved. Necrotizing and proliferating responses in the involved sites coexist; thus, radiographically, *bone destruction and proliferation are usually found simultaneously.* There may be numerous jagged appearances with irregular subperiosteal new bone formation, imparting to the involved bone a combined lucent and sclerotic appearance. Since the sclerotic appearance may predominate, the description is placed in Chapter 10.

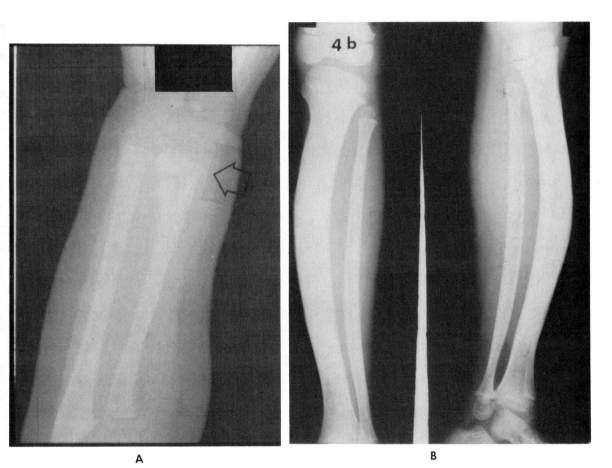

A   B

Figure 10–5   Congenital syphilis involving bone. *A.* Syphilitic osteochondritis involving the distal radius in an infant with evidence also of periostitis overlying the distal radius. *B.* Congenital syphilis in an older child showing the typical saber shin bowing of the tibia.

Hypertrophic Pulmonary Osteoarthropathy (Figure 10–6)

Clinical Features.   Pain and thickening of the long and short tubular bones, especially in the peripheral parts of the body. There may be clubbing of the digits. It is associated with chronic lung disease or carcinoma of the lung.

Radiographic Findings.   Thickening of the cortex of the long bones due to periosteal proliferation. The outermost margin of the bone is thickened and quite irregular. The ends of the bones are relatively free of involvement in comparison with the diaphyses. At the same time, the carpal and tarsal bones show a subcortical osteoporosis.

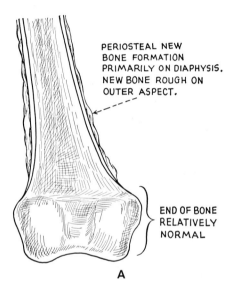

PERIOSTEAL NEW
BONE FORMATION
PRIMARILY ON DIAPHYSIS.
NEW BONE ROUGH ON
OUTER ASPECT.

END OF BONE
RELATIVELY
NORMAL

A

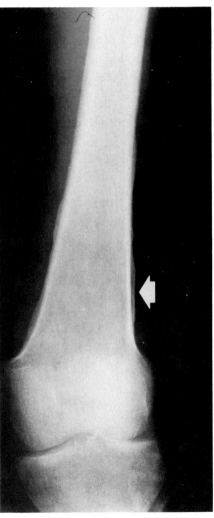

B

Figure 10–6 *A.* Diagrammatic illustration of radiographic findings in hypertrophic pulmonary osteoarthropathy. *B.* Hypertrophic pulmonary osteoarthropathy involving the distal shaft of the femur.

"Battered Child" Syndrome

Fractures or other manifestations of trauma are not infrequently discovered in infants incidental to some other examination. A history of trauma cannot always be obtained because of family concealment or because an older child may be responsible and the parents are unaware of the assault.

Infantile growth is rapid, and the periosteum is loosely applied and vascular. **Radiographically** the lesions tend to be multiple and superimposed on bones of normal density and architecture. Subperiosteal new bone beneath the elevated periosteum may involve an entire diaphysis (Figure 10–7). The metaphysis may be fragmented near the epiphyseal plate with or without gross epiphyseal displacement, especially around the elbows, knees, and ankles.

Subdural hematoma is often an associated abnormality.

The *differential diagnosis* must include: scurvy, congenital syphilis, infantile cortical hyperostosis, and malignant neoplasia. Usually the presence of an outright fracture of the diaphysis, the absence of bone destruction, and the absence of a radiolucent zone adjoining the zone of provisional calcification make the diagnosis evident (Caffey).

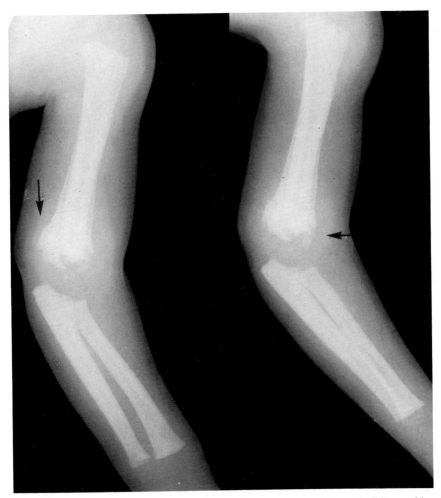

Figure 10–7 Radiographs of the arm and forearm of a child subjected to "battering" by an older sibling ("battered child syndrome"). (Courtesy of Dr. Joseph G. Gordon, Reynolds Memorial Hospital, Winston-Salem, N. C.)

OSTEOSCLEROSIS MANIFESTED PRINCIPALLY BY TRANSVERSE BANDS IN THE METAPHYSIS
(Figure 10–8)

1. HEAVY METAL POISONING

2. CRETINISM

4. DEBILITATING DISEASE WITH RECOVERY

5. HYPERVITAMINOSIS A (AND D)

6. LEUKEMIA

8. IDIOPATHIC HYPERCALCEMIA OF INFANCY
   (HYPERVITAMINOSIS D)

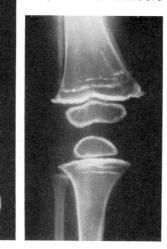
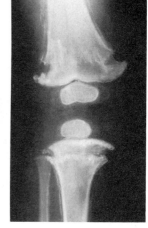

7. SCURVY   3. SYPHILIS
                         OSTEOPERIOSTITIS

Figure 10–8   Osteosclerosis manifested principally by transverse bands in the metaphyses: general categories. (Intensified radiographs.)

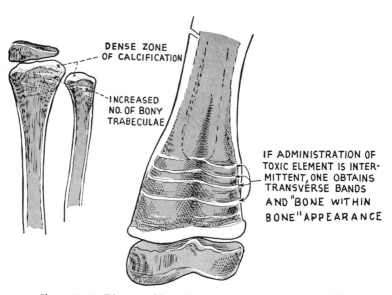

DENSE ZONE OF CALCIFICATION

INCREASED NO. OF BONY TRABECULAE

IF ADMINISTRATION OF TOXIC ELEMENT IS INTERMITTENT, ONE OBTAINS TRANSVERSE BANDS AND "BONE WITHIN BONE" APPEARANCE

Figure 10–9   Diagram of bone in heavy metal poisoning in a child.

Zone of Metaphyseal Sclerosis Following Treatment and Improvement in Severe Debilitating Disease (Figure 10–10). With systemic illness there may be a temporary cessation of osteoblastic activity at the zones of provisional ossification in metaphyses of long bones. Calcium deposition in the zones of provisional calcification continues. When systemic improvement ensues there is a temporary increase in osteoid deposition. The dense calcified cartilage is only partially resorbed. The new growth which bypasses these transverse calcified cartilaginous zones and transverse sclerotic lines which indicate temporary growth arrest are shown radiographically. Aggravated forms of these transverse growth arrest lines occur in the acute leukemias.

Transverse lines and bands of increased density in the metaphyses of growing bones are *usually found in children,* those apparently healthy as well as those chronically ill. When these lines occur late in the growth period, they may persist into adult life. The transverse lines are due to failure of normal resorption or removal of the calcified cartilage in the zone of provisional calcification. In the case of heavy metal poisoning, the heavy metal may be intermixed with the zone of provisional calcification.

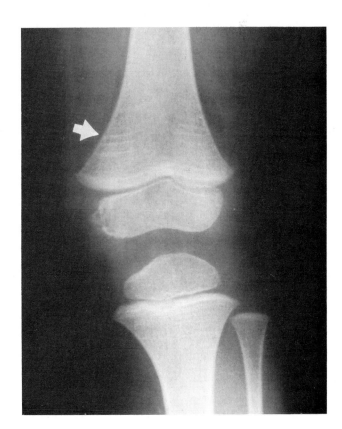

Figure 10–10 Transverse growth arrest lines around the knee.

MULTIPLE IRREGULAR AREAS OF OSTEOSCLEROSIS OF INDISCRIMINATE DISTRIBUTION (Figure 10–11)

IRREGULAR
"PATCHY"

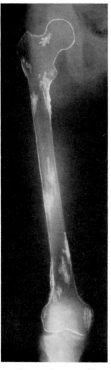

1. SCLEROTIC BONE ISLANDS

2. OSTEOPOIKILOSIS

3. PAGET'S DISEASE (OSTEITIS DEFORMANS)

4. OSTEOSCLEROTIC TUMOR METASTASES

5. OCCASIONAL MULTIPLE MYELOMA

6. MASTOCYTOSIS

7. LYTIC METASTASES FOLLOWING THERAPY (RADIATION, STEROIDS, CHEMOTHERAPY

8. OSTEOPATHIA STRIATA (VOORHOEVE)

9. OSTEOSCLEROSIS WITH PARATHYROID ADENOMA + CHRONIC RENAL FAILURE

Figure 10–11 General categories of bone diseases characterized by multiple irregular areas of osteosclerosis of indiscriminate distribution. (Intensified radiographs.)

Normal Variant Sclerotic Bone Islands (Figure 10–12). Normal sclerotic bone islands occur frequently in the metaphyses and epiphyses of long bones, in the innominate bone, and in the short bones of the hands and feet. The upper metaphysis of the femur, the head of the humerus, the heads of the metacarpals and metatarsals, and the iliac bones are most frequently involved. These small islands of compact bone measure 3 to 5 mm. in diameter. They may or may not be symmetrical. In "osteopoikilosis" they are multiple, bilateral, and quite symmetrical, affecting peripheral small bones especially.

In certain instances differentiation from slcerotic bone metastases, particularly in the large bones, and from sesamoid bones presents the most important diagnostic problems.

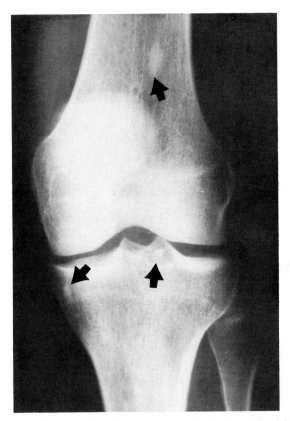

Figure 10–12 Antero-posterior view of the knee showing sclerotic bone island in the distal femur and proximal portion of the tibia.

Osteitis Deformans (Paget's Disease of Bone) (Figure 10–13)

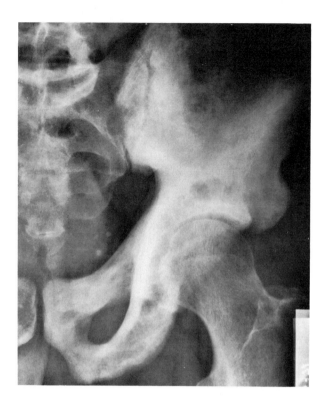

Figure 10–13 Radiograph illustrating the roentgen findings in Paget's disease of the hip. Note the coarsened and somewhat mosaic appearance of the ilium, ischium, and pubis, with a tendency toward thickening and a similar mosaic appearance of the trabecular pattern. This mosaic appearance corresponds with the pathologic appearance of the osseous matrix.

Clinical Features

Possibly up to 3 per cent of the population have this disease, but it is subclinical.

It may be monostotic or polyostotic.

Primary sites: spine, cranium, femora, pelvis, clavicles, ribs, tibiae, and sternum.

Laboratory Findings

Blood calcium, phosphorus, and urinary calcium are normal.

Alkaline phosphatase is markedly elevated.

Radiographic Findings

Bones are markedly thickened, widened and bent, with coarse trabecular pattern.

Early skull: circumscribed osteoporosis (called **osteoporosis circumscripta**).

Late skull: "cotton ball" appearance.

Vertebrae: "picture frame" appearance.

Facial bones: Leontiasis ossea.

Pelvis: "sheaves of grain" appearance of trabeculae.

Course. Progressive over years; 10 per cent develop *sarcoma*.

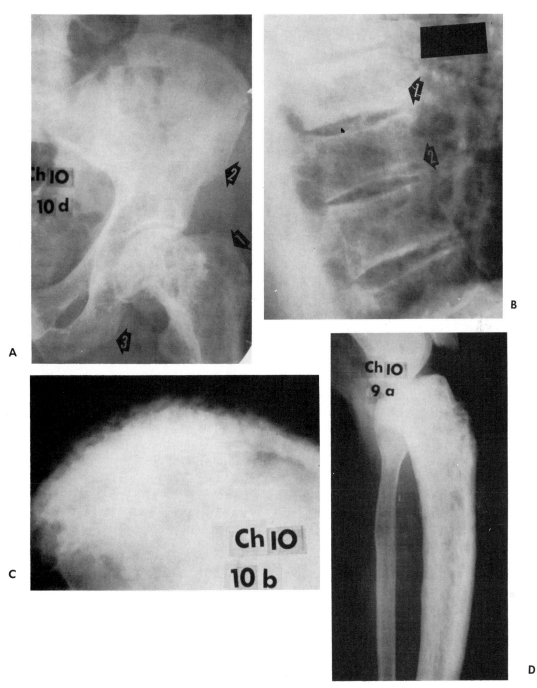

Figure 10–14 Paget's disease involving bone. *A.* Antero-posterior view of the hip in Paget's disease showing a coarsened trabecular pattern not only of the ilium but also of the adjoining portions of femur and ischium.

B. Lateral view of the thoracic vertebrae showing the boxlike, coarsened and thickened appearance of some of the vertebrae as well as a tendency to coarsened trabeculation without the boxlike appearance in others.

C. Closeup view of the "cotton ball" appearance of the bones of the calvarium, showing marked involvement of all the layers of the calvarium with thickening of the diploë and marked irregularity of both the inner and outer table. The outer table at times has a shell-like appearance.

D. Lateral view of the leg showing the bowed appearance of the shaft of the tibia with an irregular coarsened trabecular lytic process diffusely involving the entire shaft of the tibia.

Osteosclerotic Involvement from Tumor Metastases (Figure 10–15)

Most Frequent Origins of Tumors are the prostate, stomach, lung, pancreas, and, rarely, breast. Lymphomatous tumors should also be included here. Malignant carcinoid, urinary bladder carcinoma, and mucinous adenocarcinomas of the colon, when metastatic to bone, are also especially apt to produce sclerotic metastases (Greenfield).

Carcinoma of Prostate Metastases

These may produce a diffuse chalkiness of all bones.

The earliest metastases often appear on the inner aspect of the acetabulum, passing via valveless veins (Batson's plexus), also to the sacrum and other sites in the pelvis.

The appearance may closely resemble Paget's disease of bone but can usually be differentiated on the basis of the architectural pattern.

The high serum acid phosphatase level is almost pathognomonic. It may be related to release from the prostate by disruption of its capsule.

Metastatic Foci from Carcinoma of the Breast or Other Lytic Metastases Following a Favorable Therapeutic Response

Metastatic foci which have been treated by chemotherapy, hormonal treatment, or radiotherapy will frequently be replaced by sclerotic bone even when the primary lesion is not responsive to therapy. **Rarely the sclerosis is "ring-like" in appearance, surrounding the prior lytic foci in the bones.**

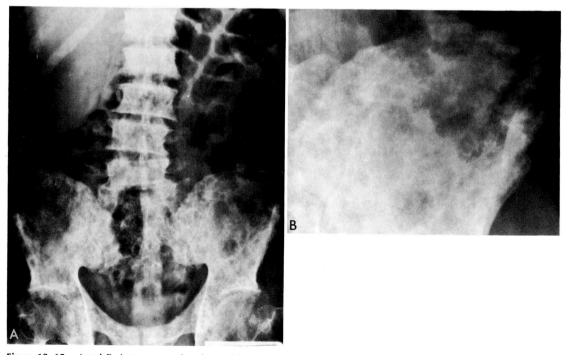

Figure 10–15 *A* and *B*. Antero-posterior views of the abdomen showing the lumbar spine and pelvis in a patient with widespread metastases from carcinoma of the prostate. In *A*, the entire lumbar spine and pelvis are shown. In *B*, a close-up view of the ilium is shown in better detail. Note the spotted lucency and marked dense sclerosis of the variety of tumor metastases.

Osteosclerosis with Parathyroid Adenoma and Chronic Renal Failure. Usually primary hyperparathyroidism due to parathyroid adenoma with resulting bone disease, as well as secondary hyperparathyroidism with bony manifestations, is ac-

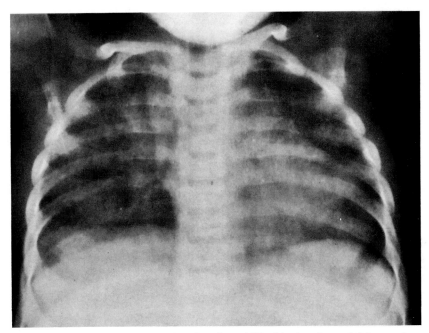

Figure 10–16 Antero-posterior view of the chest in a child with chronic renal failure and secondary hyperparathyroidism, which is responsible for the markedly osteosclerotic appearance of the bones of the thoracic cage. In contrast, there is a faintly frayed appearance of the metaphyseal zone in the right shoulder region at the epiphyseal plate zone between the humerus and its proximal epiphysis. The middle third of the clavicle is perhaps the best area to look for such zones of sclerosis.

companied by osteolytic radiolucencies. However, there are occasional cases of osteosclerosis reported. More frequently the bony appearance may be that of an admixture of sclerosis and lucency. The admixture of radiolucency and sclerosis often has an amorphous, homogeneous ground-glass appearance due to coarsened trabeculae and widening of the individual trabeculae.

In the thoracic and lumbar spine occasionally marked bone sclerosis affects the upper and lower thirds of the vertebral body, leaving a translucent band in the center of each vertebra (Kaye et al.; Beveridge et al.).

OSTEOSCLEROSIS OF A LOCALIZED OR REGIONAL TYPE

<table>
<tr><td align="center">EPIPHYSEAL</td><td align="center">DIAPHYSEAL
CORTICOPERIOSTEAL</td><td align="center">METAPHYSEAL
PATCHY OR SOLID</td></tr>
</table>

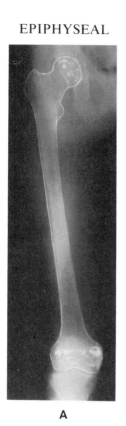 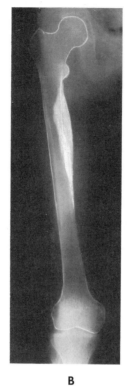 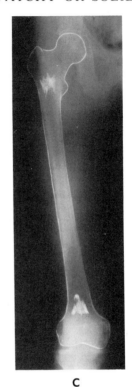

<table>
<tr><td align="center">A</td><td align="center">B</td><td align="center">C</td></tr>
</table>

1. Epiphyseal dysplasia	1. Osteoid osteoma	1. Bone infarcts
2. Hypothyroidism	2. Traumatic periostitis	2. Osteomyelitis of Garré
3. Congenital stippled epiphyses		3. Brodie's abscess (See Chapter 9)
4. Osteochondrosis		
5. Bone infarction (epiphyseal type)		

Figure 10–17   *A*. Osteosclerosis of a localized or regional type, predominantly epiphyseal. *B*. Osteosclerosis of a localized or regional type, predominantly corticoperiosteal or diaphyseal. *C*. Osteosclerosis predominantly metaphyseal, patchy, or solid. (Radiographs intensified.)

(Categories 1, 2, 3, and 4 have been previously considered.)

Bone Infarction (Figure 10–17)

Principal Sites in Bones.   Femur, humerus, tibia, and fibula.

Radiographic Appearance.   Wedge of sclerotic bone surrounded by a narrow dense line of demarcation. The base of the wedge runs along the scar of an old epiphyseal plate but at a slight distance from it. The sides are parallel to the cortex of the shaft but separated from it by a narrow band of normal bone. Ordinarily the cortex of the bone is not affected. Sometimes the lesion takes the shape of chains or clusters of dense rings.

The bone changes in **sickle cell anemia** are often related to hemorrhagic and infarcted areas, and may resemble the findings of bone infarction.

Osteoid Osteoma (Figure 10–18)

Clinical Features

Local tumefaction.
Extreme bone pain.
Peak incidence occurs in the second and third decades of life.
Males are affected more frequently than females.
Most frequent sites are the tibia, femur, fibula, humerus, vertebrae, and phalanges; rarely, the skull, ribs, and pelvis.
Osteoid osteoma in the femoral neck may produce a severe growth disturbance of the hip (Giustra and Feriberger).
Otherwise, when it is located near a joint it can produce both synovitis and proliferative arthritis.
When situated in a vertebra it often causes curvature of the spine—the result of muscle spasm rather than of bone deformity.
Gross Pathology. Eccentric marked cortical thickening extending inward toward cancellous structure of the bone, usually diaphyseal.

Radiographic Findings

1. Marked cortical thickening
2. Rarefied nidus with central sclerotic focus

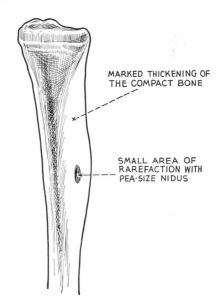

MARKED THICKENING OF THE COMPACT BONE

SMALL AREA OF RAREFACTION WITH PEA-SIZE NIDUS

Figure 10–18   Diagram of osteoid osteoma of tibia.

Osteomyelitis of Garré

Clinical Features

Usually affects males less than 30 years of age.
Usually a long bone is involved in its diaphysis.

Pathologic Features.   Devascularization of the cortex of the bone with scattered small areas of necrosis. No evidence of fistula formation or suppuration.

Radiographic Findings

Principal sites are the tibia, femur, fibula, ulna, and metatarsals.
Marked layering of the periosteum with subperiosteal calcification, and marked thickening of the associated cortex, with sclerotic encroachment on the medullary portion of the bone.
One may identify small disseminated areas of rarefaction and circumscribed areas of sequestration, but no extensive necrosis and sequestration are seen.

DISEASES OF BONE CHARACTERIZED BY OUTGROWTH OR OVERGROWTH OF BONE

Diseases of bone characterized by outgrowth or overgrowth may be subdivided into those involving a single bone and those involving several or many bones. The classification is rendered as follows:

1. Outgrowth or overgrowth of a single bone:
   a. Solitary osteochondroma.
   b. Osteoma (see Chapter 12).
   c. Osteochondromatosis or chondrocalcinosis of joints; perhaps a better term is synovial chondrometaplasia (see Chapter 11).
   d. Chondrosarcoma.
   e. Osteosarcoma, sclerotic type (see Chapter 9).
   f. Localized gigantism (see Chapter 7).
2. Overgrowth or outgrowth involving several or many bones.
   a. Hereditary multiple cartilaginous exostoses (multiple osteochondromas, diaphyseal aclasis).
   b. Pituitary gigantism.
   c. Acromegaly.
   d. Arachnoidactyly (Marfan's syndrome) (see Chapter 7).
   e. Engelmann's disease (see earlier in this chapter).
   f. "Erlenmeyer flask" type failure of bone modeling: Gaucher's disease; also marble bone disease or osteopetrosis (see Chapters 7 and 8).
   g. Pyle's disease (see Chapter 7).

Osteochondroma (Figure 10–19)

Clinical Features

Malignant transformation in 1 to 7 per cent of cases.
Maximum age incidence in first two decades.

Most Frequent Sites

At sites of tendon attachment.
Lower femur, upper tibia, upper femur, upper and lower humerus, lower tibia, and pelvis.

Radiographic Findings

Mushroom-shaped cancellous bony excrescence at sites mentioned above.
Hyaline cartilage cap is radiolucent and is not seen radiographically.
Cortex and medulla of host bone are continuous with tumor, but the compact bone is found only at the base of the lesion.

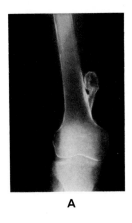

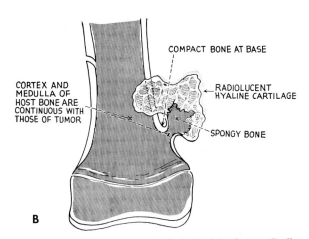

COMPACT BONE AT BASE

CORTEX AND
MEDULA OF
HOST BONE ARE
CONTINUOUS WITH
THOSE OF TUMOR

RADIOLUCENT
HYALINE CARTILAGE

SPONGY BONE

A   B

Figure 10–19 *A* and *B*. Radiograph and diagram of an osteochondroma of the distal shaft of the femur. (Radiograph intensified.)

Hereditary Multiple Cartilaginous Exostoses (Diaphyseal Aclasis). This condition is familial and hereditary in about 75 per cent of cases. Cartilaginous and bony exostoses similar in appearance to those described for osteochondroma may occur at any portion of the skeleton which has been preformed in cartilage, but the localizations are *particularly frequent in the metaphyseal portions of the long bones.*

The Most Frequent Sites are the upper shaft of the humerus, hands, knee, ankle, flat bones of the pelvis, scapula, ribs, and vertebrae. Malignant change is said to occur in about 5 per cent of the cases but otherwise the prognosis is usually considered favorable.

Differential Diagnosis. It is readily distinguished from chondrodysplasia (Ollier's disease), since in the latter condition an enchondromatosis appears first and the protuberant aspects of the disease come later.

Chondrosarcoma (Figure 10–20)

Clinical Features

Age incidence: primary type usually occurs prior to the third decade; secondary type occurs after the third decade.

Favored Sites

Fifty per cent of cases occur around knee.
Also occurs in proximal femur, pelvis, and humerus.

Radiographic Findings

Bone-destructive tumor mass with large, amorphous calcific foci which have a mulberry, peppery, or flocculent appearance in contrast to calcified osteoid matrix, which has a more patchy appearance. The calcium is sometimes described as "popcorn" type calcification.
Minimal periosteal reaction and Codman's triangle.
Osteolytic variety also occurs, with little or no sclerosis or calcification.

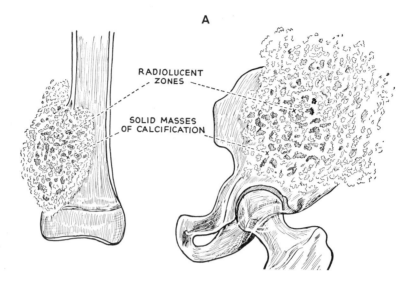

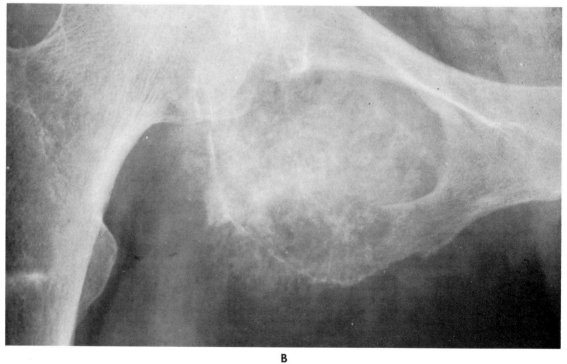

Figure 10–20 Chondrosarcoma. *A.* Diagrammatic illustration of radiographic findings. *B.* Chondrosarcoma involving the ischium and pubis, magnified view.

Generalized Pituitary Gigantism. Acromegaly (Figure 10–21 A, B)

Pathology

Ordinarily this disease is related to an eosinophilic adenoma of the anterior pituitary gland in the preadolescent period or is due to a hyperplasia of the eosinophilic cells of the anterior pituitary gland.

If overproduction of hormones persists into adult life, the typical clinical picture of acromegaly is produced, between 20 and 50 years of age most commonly.

Radiographic Findings in Acromegaly

Skull: bony tables markedly thickened; prominent bossae; mandible markedly thickened and increased in dimension with an obtuse angle between the ramus and the body. Sella turcica: thinning of the dorsum sellae and clinoid processes with evidence of intrasellar expanding lesions often present. Increased intracranial pressure may also coexist.

Hands: shafts of phalanges are markedly thickened with an increase in the tufted ends of the distal phalanges giving a "spade" appearance (Figure 10–28 A).

Heel: the soft tissues overlying the os calcis are increased in dimension to 23 mm. or more (Steinbach) (Figure 10–21 B). This sign is not pathognomonic of acromegaly since it may occur in hypothyroidism and in 1 to 2 per cent of nonedematous, nonacromegalic subjects even when the results are expressed in relation to body weight. All osseous trabeculations are markedly coarsened.

The product of the two greatest perpendicular diameters of the medial sesamoid bones of the first metacarpophalangeal joint (sesamoid index) (Figure 10–21 C) may also be used to identify acromegalics if it is greater than 29 for both men and women.

1. The heel-pad thickness sign is still a valuable diagnostic tool in acromegaly, provided that results are expressed in relation to body weight.

2. Gonticas et al. showed a normal range of 15 to 30 mm. for the thickness of the heel-pad, with a mean of 20.7 mm. (Steinbach and Russell had reported a range of 13 to 21 mm. with a mean of 17.8 mm.) There was, however, a good correlation of heel-pad thickness to body weight in kilograms. The larger heel-pads were invariably found in persons of greater than 70 kilos body weight. The heel-pad thickness in normal people was under 27 mm. in those who were 90 kilograms or less in weight.

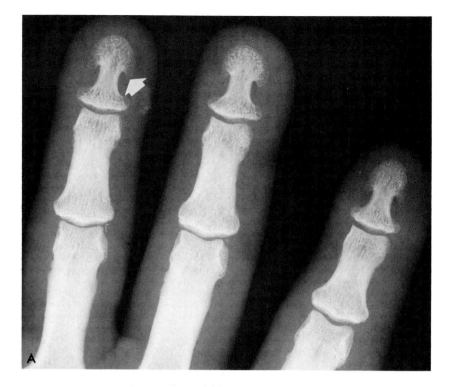

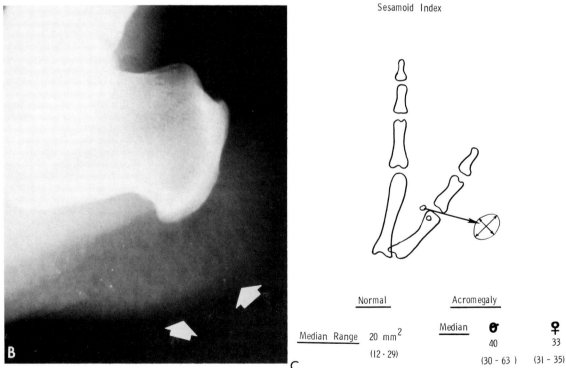

Sesamoid Index

		Normal		Acromegaly	
				Median	♂ ♀
Median	Range	20 mm^2			40 33
		(12 · 29)			(30 - 63) (31 - 35)

Figure 10–21 *A*. The phalanges in acromegaly. Note the typical "spade" appearance of the tufted ends of the distal phalanges with the overhanging broadened edges. Pituitary gigantism may produce a similar appearance when the individual attains adulthood.

B. Increased soft tissue width in lateral view of heel in acromegaly. The measured distance from the tuberosity of the os calcis to the adjoining skin surface usually exceeds 23 mm.

C. Method of computation of sesamoid index for diagnosis of acromegaly (Kleinberg et al.). Normally, median 20, range 12 to 29 in acromegalics. Male, median 40, range 30 to 63. Acromegalic women, median 33, range 31 to 35. The smaller indices are usually obtained from persons under 37 years age.

GENERAL CONCEPTS REGARDING TUMORS OF BONE

Introduction

The neoplasms of bone may be either benign or malignant.

Unfortunately, the line that separates malignant from benign tumors is not always distinct and every experienced pathologist has found that he must have all clinical and radiologic information at his disposal when he attempts to differentiate bone lesions of this or related types.

To understand the types of primary bone tumors, it is necessary to bear in mind a scheme of tissues that compose the skeleton; such a scheme may be given as follows:

I. *Osteogenic Series*
   A. Benign
      1. Osteoid osteoma
      2. Benign osteoblastoma
      3. Osteoma
      4. Osteochondroma
   B. Malignant
      1. Osteosarcoma
      2. Periosteal sarcoma
      3. Osteoclastoma (giant cell tumor)

II. *Chondrogenic Series*
   A. Benign
      1. Enchondroma
      2. Benign chondroblastoma
      3. Chondromyxoid fibroma
   B. Malignant
      1. Chondrosarcoma

III. *Collagenic Series*
   A. Benign
      1. Nonosteogenic fibroma
      2. Subperiosteal cortical defect
      3. Angioma
      4. Aneurysmal bone cyst
   B. Malignant
      1. Fibrosarcoma
      2. Angiosarcoma

IV. *Myelogenic Series*
   A. Malignant
      1. Plasma cell myeloma
      2. Ewing's tumor
      3. Reticulum cell sarcoma
      4. Hodgkin's disease

V. *Neurogenic Series*
   A. Benign
      1. Neurofibroma
   B. Malignant
      1. Neuroblastoma
   C. Tumors of sympathetic nerve origin, benign or malignant

Tumors Metastatic to Bone. The great majority of metastatic tumors in bone are of epithelial origin; however, a few sarcomas fall into this group. Ewing's tumor metastasizes to one or more bones in less than half the cases. It is usually encountered in children. Bone involvement may also be found in cases of leukemia, malignant lymphoma, and Hodgkin's disease.

Practically any tumor, with the exception of tumors of the central nervous system, may occasionally metastasize to bone. Cancers that frequently develop secondary deposits in bone are those which are primary in the *breast, prostate, thyroid, kidney,* and *lung.* Bone metastasis is also very common in *neuroblastoma.*

The thoracic vertebrae, ribs, sternum, and clavicles are most commonly involved in breast cancer, whereas lumbar and sacral vertebrae and the pelvic bones are the bones usually affected by a primary carcinoma of the prostate. Metastases in bones distal to the elbows and knees are unusual but do occur.

A primary carcinoma of the prostate, if it has grown out of the capsule of the prostate gland, will ordinarily produce an elevation of *acid phosphatase* in the blood serum. Almost any tumor, however, that destroys a considerable amount of bone and initiates osteoblastic reparative activity produces a rise in serum *alkaline phosphatase.* Elevated serum phosphatase levels may also occur with liver malfunction and disease.

Serum calcium levels may be altered in extensive skeletal metastases. High serum calcium levels may lead to metastatic calcification of soft tissues. Nephrocalcinosis may also result. Excessive osteoid production is usually induced by a malignant tumor, but irradiation and hormone therapy may also stimulate new bone formation. Sclerotic metastatic bony appearances may result in previously osteolytic areas as a result of such therapy.

The **most important functions of the radiologist** in respect to tumors of bone may be summarized as follows:

He should attempt to recognize the bone tumor type in collaboration with the pathologist.

He should attempt to label the tumor as either benign or malignant.

ROENTGEN CRITERIA FOR DIFFERENTIATION OF BENIGN FROM MALIGNANT BONE TUMOR PROCESSES

The most important are:
1. *Location*
2. *Architecture*
3. *Age of patient*

Location

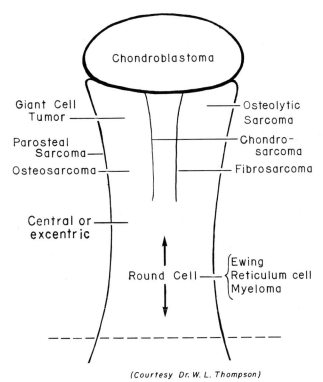

(Courtesy Dr. W. L. Thompson)

Figure 10–22 Location of bone neoplasms.

Architecture

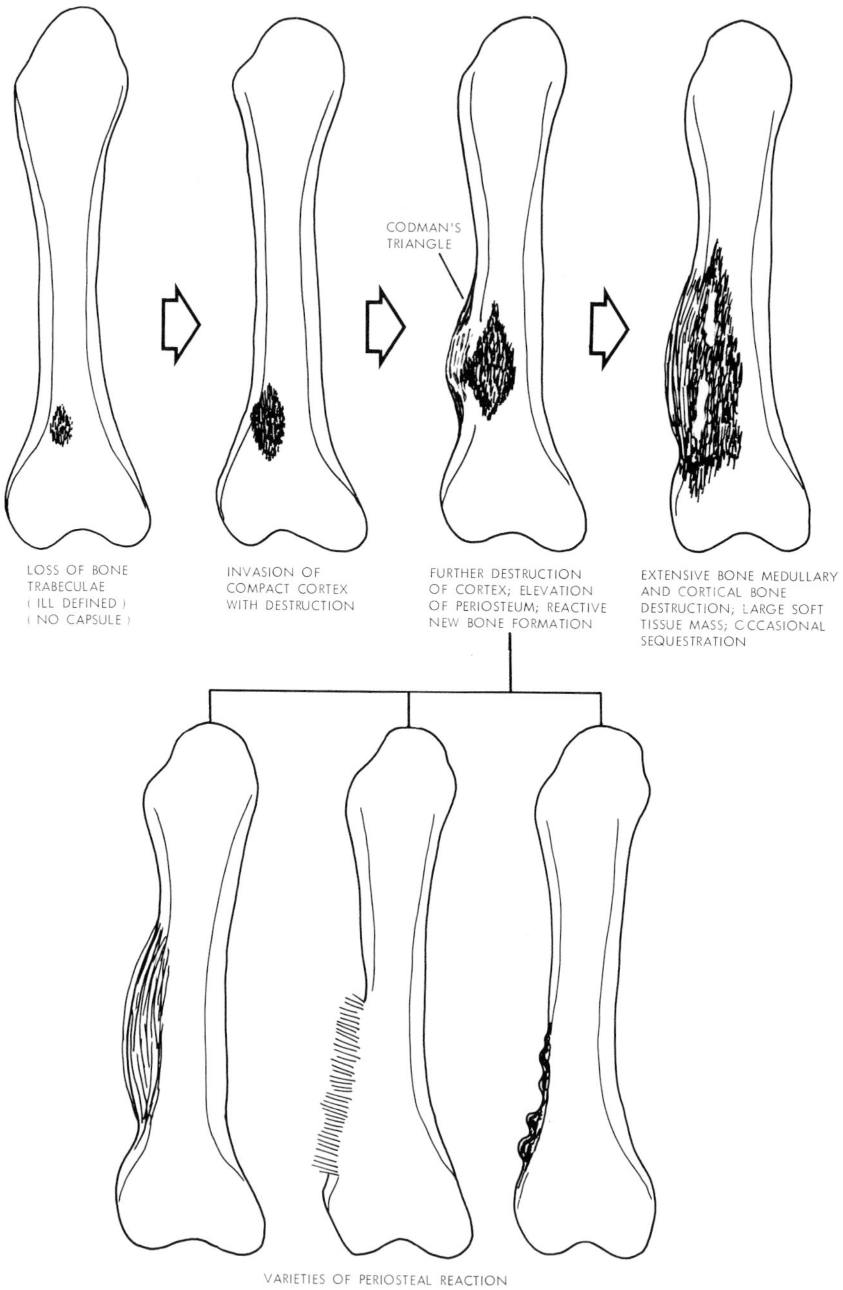

CODMAN'S
TRIANGLE

LOSS OF BONE
TRABECULAE
(ILL DEFINED)
(NO CAPSULE)

INVASION OF
COMPACT CORTEX
WITH DESTRUCTION

FURTHER DESTRUCTION
OF CORTEX; ELEVATION
OF PERIOSTEUM; REACTIVE
NEW BONE FORMATION

EXTENSIVE BONE MEDULLARY
AND CORTICAL BONE
DESTRUCTION; LARGE SOFT
TISSUE MASS; OCCASIONAL
SEQUESTRATION

VARIETIES OF PERIOSTEAL REACTION

Figure 10–23 Endosteal, cortical, and periosteal changes with a malignant tumor of bone.

Internal vs. External Architecture. The most characteristic features of both benign and malignant tumors are found in the intimate study of the architecture of the lesions. An architectural description may include the following:

1. Presence or absence of a discrete linear or sclerotic margin.

2. A close description of the "inside" pattern of the lesion. Is it trabecular? Is it irregular? Are there vertical strands? Are there small punctate areas of calcification, or is the intricate pattern more that of "popcorn" type calcification? Is there an "onion skin" layering?

3. Is there a periosteal reaction? If so, is this periosteal reaction vertically oriented ("sunray"), layered or "onion skin-like," or irregular or lacelike?

The importance of the *outer margin* in differentiating a benign from a malignant neoplasm is illustrated in Figure 10–24. It will be noted from this illustration that, generally, malignant lesions do not have a discrete outer margin—and this includes the giant cell tumor or osteoclastoma. The thickness or thinness of this sclerotic line or margin is also important. For example, the nonosteogenic fibroma, the fibrous dysplasia, the Brodie's abscess have all rather thick margins. By contrast, the bone cyst, the angioma, and epidermoidoma have a thin discrete margin.

The "Inside" or Trabecular Pattern or Calcium Deposition in a lesion is of importance in differential diagnosis as indicated here (Figure 10–24). In fibrous dysplasia or in a Brodie's abscess, even though there are small segments of bone contained within the lesion microscopically, this ordinarily cannot be differentiated radiologically. In a fibrosarcoma the lesion is ordinarily completely lytic with no demonstrable osseous or calcium deposition within the lesion proper. This is also true of a metastatic tumor usually, particularly of the osteolytic variety.

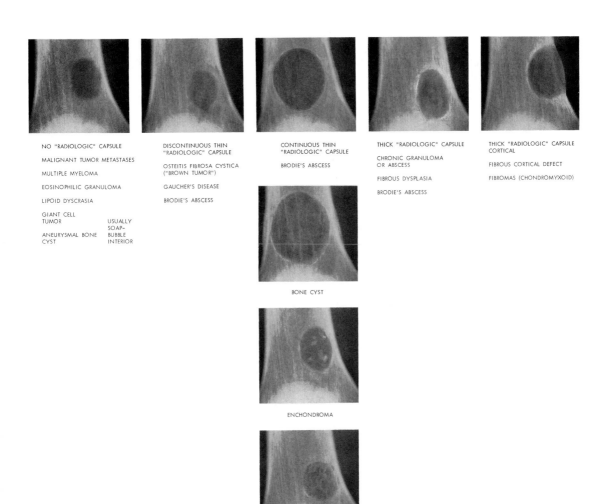

Figure 10–24 *A.* Importance of outer margin in differentiating a benign from a malignant bone tumor.

However, small septate trabecular patterns of an irregular type may be differentiated in such lesions as the chondromyxoid fibroma, the bone cyst, the giant cell tumor, the epidermoidoma, or the angiosarcoma. The inner pattern of the vertebral hemangioma is ordinarily vertically oriented, while the inner pattern of a reticulum cell sarcoma may well be coarse, irregular "woven" trabeculations. In contrast to these, the inner pattern of an enchondroma may have punctate small foci of calcified cartilage or calcification, and the chondrosarcoma contains large clumps of "mulberry" of "popcorn-like" calcification.

The importance of the type of *periosteal reaction* in respect to a bone lesion is indicated in Figure 10–23. In these diagrams the laminated periosteal elevation of congenital syphilis, rickets, and tuberculous osteitis is differentiated from the "onion skin" laminated periosteal elevation of a Ewing's tumor or reticulum cell sarcoma. The irregular proliferating or subperiosteal calcification of healing scurvy, chronic toxic proliferating periostitis, periostitis and osteitis secondary to chronic cellulitis, osteoperiosteal abscess, or periosteal neurofibroma are diagrammatically indicated. The "sunray" type periosteal reaction of sickle cell anemia and Mediterranean type anemias is indicated. Periosteal proliferation with new bone formation, such as is found in osteitis deformans, osteoid osteoma, the saber shin of juvenile syphilis, osteogenic sarcoma, and the osteomyelitis of Garré, is also diagrammatically indicated. It is a composite, therefore, of these major entities which helps to differentiate benign from malignant tumors and processes.

Another important feature in differentiation is the presence of a *break in the outer cortex of the bone*. Ordinarily when a break in the outer cortex of the bone occurs in the absence of pathologic fracture it spells malignant invasion of the cortex and the surrounding tissues. One must, however, be careful to determine that a pathologic fracture has not occurred which may make this kind of determination difficult.

And lastly, it is important to study the soft tissue surrounding the bone lesion very carefully. This helps to determine whether or not invasion has occurred. If invasion from the bone lesion has occurred, very often there is a notably increased density. On the other hand, inflammatory lesions may also produce soft tissue swelling and make this kind of differentiation difficult in itself.

Age

TABLE 10–1   AGES OF OCCURRENCE OF PRIMARY BONE TUMORS

0 to 10 Years	11 to 20 Years	21 to 30 Years	31 to 70 Years
Bone cysts	Osteogenic sarcoma	Giant cell tumors (sex incidence equal)	Multiple myeloma (sex incidence equal)
Neuroblastoma	Ewing's tumor		Lymphosarcoma and reticulum cell sarcoma
Ewing's tumor			Paget's sarcoma

Questions—Chapter 10

1. What is the general classification of the osteosclerotic and hypertrophic bone diseases of the extremities?

2. In the group of osteosclerotic diseases that are localized or regional, what are some of the main disease entities?

3. In the group of hypertrophic bone diseases representing a bone overgrowth, what are the main diseases represented?

4. Describe some of the radiographic features of marble bone disease.

5. What is the characteristic radiographic pattern of fluorine poisoning involving bone?

6. Describe the radiographic features of hypoparathyroidism and indicate how these differ from pseudohypoparathyroidism and pseudopseudohypoparathyroidism.

7. What are the main diseases characterized by transverse bands of osteosclerosis, particularly in the metaphyses?

8. Describe the main radiographic features of cretinism.

9. List the main disease entities in the osteosclerotic group that are manifested chiefly by longitudinal cortical sclerosis or corticoperiosteal thickening.

10. What are the main radiographic features of infantile cortical hyperostosis?

11. Describe the main radiographic features of juvenile and tertiary syphilis of bone.

12. Describe the main radiographic features of hypertrophic pulmonary osteoarthropathy.

13. Name the main osteosclerotic diseases that are characterized by multiple irregular osteosclerotic areas.

14. Describe the main radiographic features of osteitis deformans.

15. Describe the radiographic appearance of osteosclerotic tumor metastases and indicate the most frequent tumors of origin of such metastases.

16. What are the main radiographic features of bone infarction?

17. What are the main radiographic features of osteoid osteoma?

18. What are the main radiographic features of osteochondroma?

19. What are the main radiographic features of chondrosarcoma?

20. What is the order of frequency of the primary bone tumors?

21. Which are the bone tumors in which there is frequently multiple bone involvement?

22. Divide the various bone tumors in accordance with ages of occurrence of these primary tumors.

23. Classify the primary bone tumors in relation to the principal tissues of origin.

24. Indicate the sites of predilection of the following tumors: fibrous cortical defect; aneurysmal bone cyst; giant cell tumors; chondroblastoma; giant osteoid osteoma or osteoblastoma; osteosarcoma; reticulum cell sarcoma; osteochondroma; bone cyst; endothelioma; fibrosarcoma; multiple myeloma; and parosteal bone tumors.

25. Describe the radiographic features of the following diseases: multiple cartilaginous exostoses, pituitary gigantism, acromegaly, and localized gigantism.

26. Describe the most important features which differentiate a benign from a malignant bone tumor.

27. Describe the inner architectural pattern of such lesions as the vertebral hemangioma, enchondroma, chondrosarcoma, Brodie's abscess, and metastatic tumors. What is the most frequent inner architectural pattern of the giant cell tumor?

28. How would you differentiate a giant cell tumor from a benign bone cyst?

11

Radiology of Joints

ROUTINE USED IN RADIOGRAPHIC INTERPRETATION OF SYNOVIAL JOINT DISEASE

A guide for routine examination of the synovial joints is presented as follows:
1. The *alignment* of the bones on either side of the joint is noted and compared with the normal alignment.
2. The *capsular and pericapsular soft tissues* may show evidence of swelling or calcium deposition in the ligamentous structures.
3. The roughness or smoothness of the *subchondral bone* is noted, together with excrescences and any rarefaction or sclerosis in the adjoining cancellous bone.
4. The *width of the joint space* is estimated and at the same time an estimate is made of the condition of the joint cartilage. The joint space itself is examined for loose bodies.
5. The *status of the bony structures* on either side of the joint is examined, and both epiphyses and diaphyses are noted, as well as whether or not rarefaction is present.
6. Finally, *arthrography* with air or positive contrast media offers further elucidation of pathology. A bone survey or surveys of other parts of the body may also be of assistance.

As a result of this routine, a method of analysis of joint radiographs for evidence of joint disease can be devised and is described below.

CLASSIFICATION OF JOINT DISEASE FROM RADIOGRAPHIC STANDPOINT

1. Abnormalities of alignment (see Traumatic Disorders and other later categories).
2. Diseases characterized by capsular distension without bony involvement.
   a. Simple hydrarthrosis.
   b. Idiopathic capsulitis.
   c. Acute pyogenic infection (early).
   d. Rheumatic fever (periarticular arthrosis); migratory polyarthritis.

3. Diseases characterized by subchondral and capsular proliferative response. Capsular lipping, spurring, calcification, and ossification are seen in variable degrees.
    a. Traumatic arthritis.
    b. "Hypertrophic" arthritis (also called degenerative arthritis or osteoarthritis).
    c. Hemophilic arthritis.
    d. Neurotrophic arthropathy.
4. Diseases characterized by osteoporosis of neighboring bone and narrowing of the joint space with subchondral bone resorption.
    a. Tuberculous arthritis.
    b. Rheumatoid arthritis.
    c. Pyogenic arthritis (but with somewhat less surrounding osteoporosis).
5. Diseases characterized by periarticular bone resorption without significant adjoining osteoporosis.
    a. Gout.
    b. Sarcoid.
    c. The osteochondroses (see preceding chapters on bone).
    d. The primary tumors of joints (xanthoma, synovioma-sarcoma).
6. Diseases characterized by ankylosis. This is a nonspecific late change in any destructive joint disease.
    a. Late rheumatoid arthritis.
    b. Late post-traumatic arthritis.
    c. Late pyogenic arthritis.
    d. Late tuberculosis.
7. Diseases characterized by loose bodies ("joint mice") within the joint and articular irregularities.
    a. Osteochondritis dissecans.
    b. Chondromatosis of joints (chondrocalcinosis).
    c. Traumatic arthropathy (of the knee particularly, following meniscal injury).
    d. Neurotrophic arthropathy.
    In the case of the knee, special studies for demonstration of these loose bodies include arthrography and a special intercondyloid view of the knee joint through the flexed knee.
8. Diseases characterized by synovial, cartilaginous, capsular, pericapsular, bursal, or peritendinous calcification.
    a. Pseudogout.
    b. Peritendinitis calcarea.
    c. Pellegrini-Stieda disease (calcification of medial collateral ligament of the knee).
    d. Capsular fibrositis with calcification.

    In the above classification it is noteworthy that a disease of one etiology may appear under several categories of objective radiographic appearance. *It is incumbent upon the radiologist to be thoroughly familiar with the pathogenesis of the various arthropathies.* This will require a careful analysis of the patient's history, and reconstruction of joint appearances as they probably were, as well as what they are at present. In many instances previous films will not be available for sequential interpretation. Only a careful history will supply the necessary information.

DISEASES CHARACTERIZED BY CAPSULAR DISTENTION WITHOUT BONY INVOLVEMENT

1. Simple hydrarthrosis.
2. Idiopathic capsulitis.
3. Acute pyogenic infection (early).
4. Rheumatic fever (periarticular arthrosis).
5. Acute tenosynovitis.
6. Gastrointestinal disorders with arthralgia (such as Whipple's disease).

Simple Hydrarthrosis. Fluid accumulation within a joint from trauma, internal derangement, or mild degenerative change. The knee is frequently affected.

Idiopathic Capsulitis (Figure 11–1). Painful hip with marked disability in an infant with a mild systemic reaction. Usually a subsidence of this process ensues without sequelae after antibiotic therapy. No definite etiologic agent is isolated usually (Edwards).

Knee Joint Effusions are readily identified in lateral roentgenograms by the swelling of the suprapatellar pouch. Other signs described are anterior displacement of the patella, distention of the posterior capsule, and bulging of the infrapatellar ligament. A swelling of the suprapatellar bursa can also be demonstrated on frontal views by visualizing a semicircular lucency on each side of the distal femur at the level of the suprapatellar bursa (Harris and Hecht).

Acute Rheumatic Fever. In acute rheumatic fever there are very few radiographic manifestations.

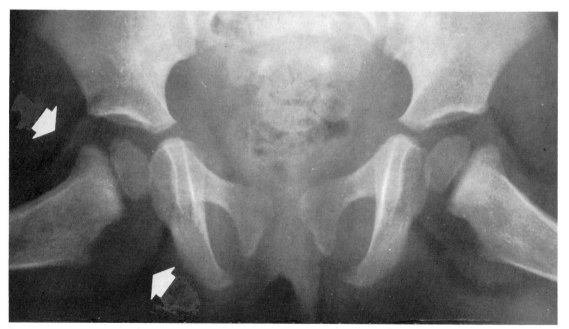

Figure 11–1 Idiopathic capsulitis of an infant. Painful hip with mild systemic reaction. No definite etiology known; the illness ordinarily subsides spontaneously or after antibiotic therapy. (Radiograph intensified.)

DISEASES CHARACTERIZED BY SUBCHONDRAL AND CAPSULAR PROLIFERATION IN ASSOCIATION WITH CARTILAGINOUS INJURY

1. Traumatic arthritis.
2. "Hypertrophic" arthritis (osteoarthritis).
3. Hemophilic arthritis.
4. Neurotrophic arthropathy.

Traumatic Arthritis (Figure 11–2)

Radiographic Findings (Figure 11–2 *A* and *B*)

Narrowed, irregular joint space due to cartilaginous thinning and fragmentation.

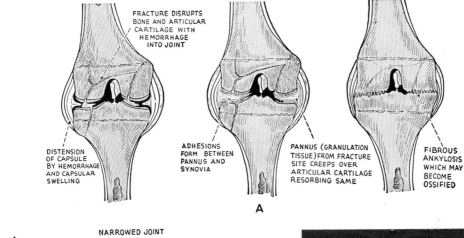

A

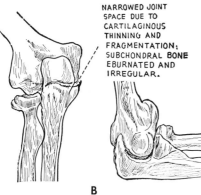

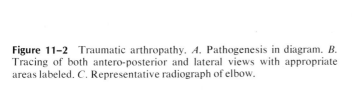

B

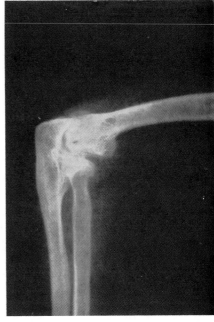

C

Figure 11–2 Traumatic arthropathy. *A.* Pathogenesis in diagram. *B.* Tracing of both antero-posterior and lateral views with appropriate areas labeled. *C.* Representative radiograph of elbow.

Subchondral bone is eburnated and irregular but is usually of normal or sclerotic density.

The joint, and even the extremity at the site of the joint abnormality, may be considerably deformed. Some joint motion is usually preserved, however, unless fibrous or ossific ankylosis has supervened.

Hypertrophic Arthritis (Figure 11–3)

Clinical Features

Weight-bearing joints are the ones most frequently involved (hips, knees, ankles, spine).

Distal interphalangeal joints of the fingers are frequently involved with associated soft tissue prominences known as Heberden's nodes.

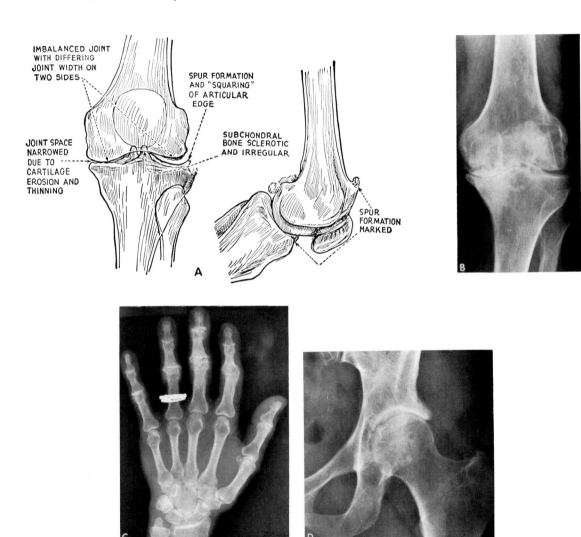

Figure 11–3 Hypertrophic arthritis. *A.* Pathogenesis in diagram. *B.* Antero-posterior view of the knee showing marked hypertrophic arthritis. *C.* Postero-anterior view of the hand showing marked hypertrophic arthritis affecting the small joints of the finger. The middle interphalangeal joints of the index, third, and fourth fingers are maximally involved. Note the good texture, however, of the surrounding bones. *D.* Minimal to moderate radiographic evidence of hypertrophic arthritis of the left hip. Notice the eburnation and sclerosis of the shelving portions of the bone, the narrowness of the joint space, and the asymmetry of the joint space with zones of lucency interspersed among those of sclerosis in the adjoining margin of the acetabulum.

Hemophilic Arthritis (Figure 11–4)

Joints affected especially are knees, hips, elbows, and ankles.

Stages in Pathogenesis (Figure 11–4)

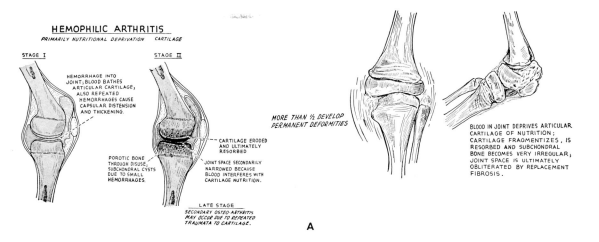

A

Radiologic Findings

Repeated hemorrhage causes a thickening of the capsule.

Deprivation of nutrition for the cartilage leads to erosion and thinning of the cartilage and narrowness of the joint space.

Subchondral bone cysts may develop.

Hypertrophic arthritis may also supervene.

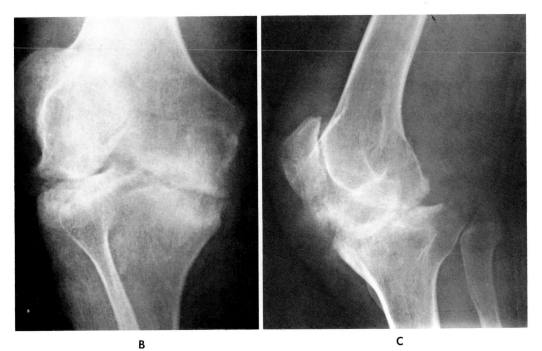

B   C

Figure 11–4 *A.* Stages in hemophilic arthritis. *B* and *C.* Hemophilic arthritis of the knee, antero-posterior and lateral views.

Neurogenic Arthropathy (Figure 11-5)

Hypertrophic Type

Approximately 90 per cent are related to tabes dorsalis, but only 5 to 10 per cent of tabetic patients develop these arthropathies; 10 per cent are associated with syringomyelia.

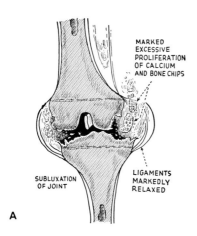

A

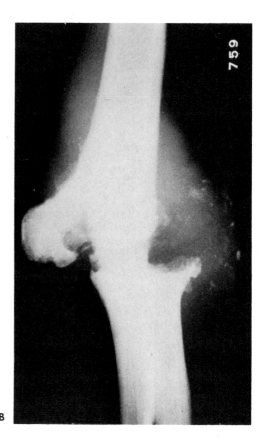

B

Figure 11-5 *A*. Pathogenesis of the hypertrophic type of neurogenic arthropathy. *B*. Charcot joint involving the elbow, antero-posterior view. Note the marked periarticular bony proliferation of the articular cartilaginous and osseous disruption, and the subluxation in the elbows. (Courtesy of Dr. James Johnston.)

Atrophic Type

This has been previously discussed in Chapter 9. A summary of the associated causes is given below.

1. Scleroderma, dermatomyositis
2. Raynaud's disease
3. Occlusive or traumatic vascular disease
4. Psoriasis
5. Leprosy
6. Tabes dorsalis
7. Syringomyelia
8. Burns, frostbite, electrical injuries
9. Diabetes

DISEASES CHARACTERIZED BY OSTEOPOROSIS OF THE NEIGHBORING BONES AND NARROWING OF THE JOINT SPACE WITH SUBCHONDRAL BONE RESORPTION

1. Tuberculous arthritis.
2. Rheumatoid arthritis and rheumatoidlike diseases.
   a. Psoriatic diseases
   b. Reiter's disease
   c. Sjögren's syndrome
   d. Colitic diseases
   e. Collagen diseases
3. Pyogenic arthritis (less surrounding osteoporosis than with the first two).

Tuberculous Arthritis (Figures 11–6 and 11–7)

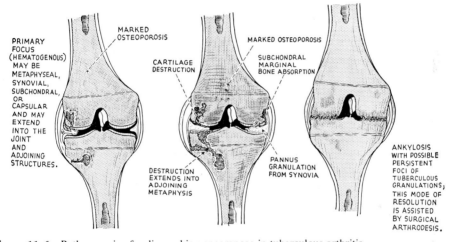

Figure 11–6 Pathogenesis of radiographic appearances in tuberculous arthritis.

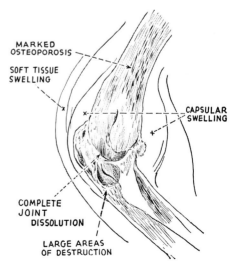

Figure 11–7 Line diagram and radiograph of the elbow in lateral view of a patient with tuberculous arthritis.

Clinical Features

Almost always hematogenous and at least 75 per cent are secondary to pulmonary tuberculosis in the first three decades of life.

Most frequent sites are the spine (one-third of cases); hip (one-sixth of cases); knee, elbow, wrist, and shoulder.

Rheumatoid Arthritis (Figure 11–8)

The essential lesion in this group of pathologic states is the "pannus."

This develops from a vascular synovial membrane and proceeds to grow over the avascular joint cartilage, depriving it of its proper nutrition.

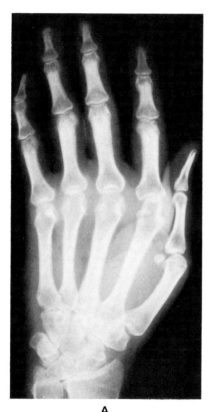

A

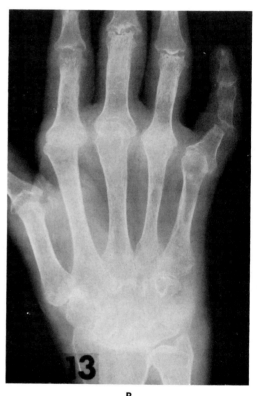

B

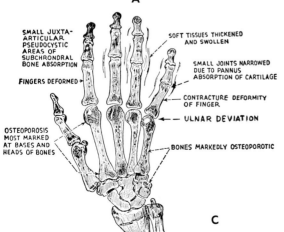

SMALL JUXTA-ARTICULAR PSEUDOCYSTIC AREAS OF SUBCHRONDRAL BONE ABSORPTION

FINGERS DEFORMED

SOFT TISSUES THICKENED AND SWOLLEN

SMALL JOINTS NARROWED DUE TO PANNUS ABSORPTION OF CARTILAGE

CONTRACTURE DEFORMITY OF FINGER

ULNAR DEVIATION

OSTEOPOROSIS MOST MARKED AT BASES AND HEADS OF BONES

BONES MARKEDLY OSTEOPOROTIC

C

Figure 11–8 Rheumatoid arthritis of the hand. *A.* Radiograph of early phase. *B.* Very late phase, approaching arthritis mutilans. *C.* Line diagram illustrating the major roentgen manifestations.

This granulation tissue resorbs the cartilage to the underlying subchondral bone and tends to resorb the bone as well, producing small pseudocystic areas.

Clinical Features

Any joint may be involved but especially the small joints of the hands and feet. Symmetrical involvement occurs in most instances.

The juvenile form of this disease is called Still's disease.

Radiographic Findings in Juvenile Rheumatoid Arthritis (Still's Disease)

1. Periarticular soft tissue swelling
2. Local osteoporosis
3. Periosteal thickening adjoining the joints involved
4. Cortical erosion
5. Destruction of joint cartilage and bone (late)
6. Growth disturbances (accelerated skeletal maturation, enlargement and ballooning of epiphyses, compression fractures of epiphyseal centers, decrease in width of shaft and osteoporosis)
7. Spondylitis is frequent, generally upper cervical, with ankylosis of apophyseal joints. Paraspinous ossification is rare as in sacroiliac involvement
8. Occasionally there are subluxations with an overgrowth of adjoining margins of the bone, resembling the overgrowth which occurs in the shelving portion of the acetabulum.

Rheumatoidlike Diseases

Psoriatic Arthritis

Roentgenologic Features

This condition resembles rheumatoid arthritis in the small joints of the hands and feet, but in this instance the earliest joints to be affected are the distal interphalangeal joints. Occasionally, there may also be involvement of the knees and other joints such as the ankles and wrists. The RA factor is usually absent.

The five roentgenological signs of greatest importance for recognition of psoriatic arthritis are:

1. Destructive arthritis, especially of the distal interphalangeal joints.
2. Bony ankylosis of the interphalangeal joints of the hands and feet.
3. Destruction of the interphalangeal joints of the hands and feet with abnormally wide joint spaces, and sharply demarcated adjacent bony surfaces.
4. Destruction of the interphalangeal joints of the great toe with bony proliferation at the base of the distal phalanx.
5. Resorption of the tips of the distal phalanges of the hands and feet.

Accessory Signs

1. Absence of osteoporosis.
2. Lack of ulnar deviation of the fourth and fifth fingers.
3. Lack of a positive RA factor in most instances.

In possibly as many as 10 per cent of patients, arthritis is present for a period varying from six months to as long as 25 years before the psoriasis is recognized dermatologically.

Sjögren's Syndrome. This syndrome may be defined as rheumatoid arthritis combined with keratoconjunctivitis sicca or xerostomia or both. In some patients there may be other associated phenomena, such as hepatomegaly, splenomegaly, congestive heart failure, leukopenia, and multiple serologic abnormalities including hyperglobulinemia.

Although the roentgenographic evidence of Sjögren's syndrome has generally been limited to its characteristic sialographic findings of ectasia and the well-known features of rheumatoid arthritis, there are some other notable roentgenographic manifestations. These include osteoarthritis in some patients with hand and wrist involvement, vascular calcification in some patients with involvement by rheumatoid arthritis of the ankles and feet, chondrocalcinosis, and occasionally osteoarthritis with involvement of the shoulder.

In the spine there are at times evidences of atlantoaxial separation, apophyseal joint destruction, osteoarthritis, sacroiliac arthritis, and rheumatoid arthritis of the hips (Silbiger and Peterson).

Pyogenic Arthritis (Figure 11–9)

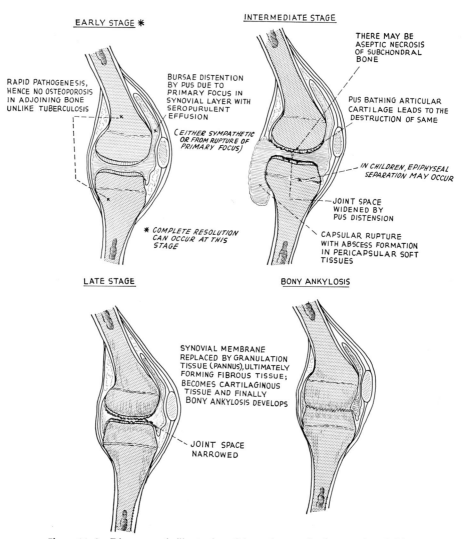

Figure 11–9   Diagrammatic illustration of the pathogenesis of pyogenic arthritis.

Arthritis with Ulcerative Colitis. This represents a form of arthritis which occurs in approximately 10 per cent of patients with ulcerative colitis in which the histologic lesion obtained in synovial biopsy resembles rheumatoid arthritis.

There is a close temporal relationship between the attacks of colitis and arthritis and the joint symptoms improve following surgical treatment for the colitis.

Usually the sedimentation erythrocyte agglutination test is negative in all patients by both agglutination and inhibition methods.

Reiter's Syndrome. This syndrome consists of urethritis, polyarthritis, and conjunctivitis.

The joints most frequently affected by rheumatoid arthritis in Reiter's syndrome are (1) the metatarsophalangeal; (2) the sacroiliac; (3) the proximal interphalangeal and the interphalangeal joint of the great toe; (4) the knee; and (5) the ankle. Many other joints are also affected but in a lesser frequency (Sholkoff et al.; Mason et al.). (6) The heel pad is often involved with bilateral calcaneal spurs, with a florid periostitis of the calcaneus.

Arthritis in the Collagen Diseases. Joint disease frequently constitutes an important aspect of several of the collagen diseases, including (1) 90 per cent of cases of lupus erythematosus; (2) serum sickness; (3) dermatomyositis; (4) erythema nodosum; (5) a small percentage of cases of scleroderma and polyarteritis nodosa.

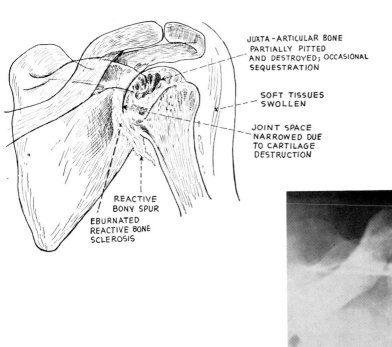

JUXTA-ARTICULAR BONE
PARTIALLY PITTED
AND DESTROYED; OCCASIONAL
SEQUESTRATION

SOFT TISSUES
SWOLLEN

JOINT SPACE
NARROWED DUE
TO CARTILAGE
DESTRUCTION

REACTIVE
BONY SPUR

EBURNATED
REACTIVE BONE
SCLEROSIS

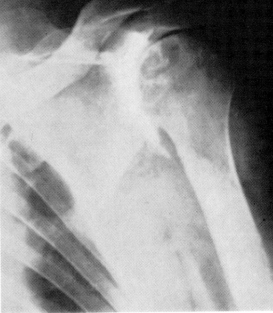

Figure 11–10 Pyogenic arthritis of the shoulder with line diagram of major roentgen findings.

DISEASES CHARACTERIZED BY PERIARTICULAR BONE ABSORPTION WITHOUT SIGNIFICANT ADJOINING OSTEOPOROSIS

1. Gout
2. Sarcoid
3. The osteochondroses (see bone section, Chapter 9)
4. The primary tumors of the joints (xanthoma, synovioma)
5. Tuberous sclerosis
6. Villonodular synovitis

Gout

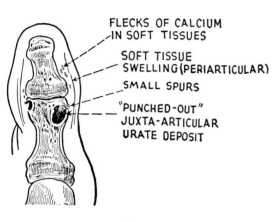

FLECKS OF CALCIUM IN SOFT TISSUES

SOFT TISSUE SWELLING (PERIARTICULAR)

SMALL SPURS

"PUNCHED-OUT" JUXTA-ARTICULAR URATE DEPOSIT

A

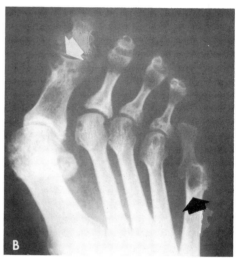

Figure 11–11   Gout. *A*. Tracing of a great toe affected by gouty arthritis. *B*. Radiograph demonstrating advanced gouty change.

Sodium biurate crystals may deposit anywhere within or outside a joint. Granulation tissue or pannus extends around the deposit, resorbing contiguous structures.

Sarcoid (Figure 11–12)

Roentgenologic Aspects

There are three types of bone manifestations:
(a) A reticular or honeycomb structure of the spongiosa. This is the most frequent bony manifestation.
(b) Round or ovoid, cystlike, punched-out lesions in the distal ends of the phalanges, with a thin sclerotic margin.
(c) A mutilating form, in which the cystlike areas coalesce, forming large areas of destruction (Greenfield et al.; Edeiken and Hodes).
Enlarged mediastinal lymph nodes are often associated.
Resembles rheumatoid arthritis (but with less osteoporosis) and tuberculosis cystica multiplex.

Villonodular Synovitis (Figure 11–13)

Synonyms are xanthoma, xanthogranuloma, giant cell tumor of tendon sheath, xanthomatous giant cell tumor, giant cell fibroangioma, and benign synovioma.

The cells contain hemosiderin pigment both within and outside the cells—hence the lesion has often been called a "pigmented tumor."

Localized Frontal or Parietal Bone Prominences

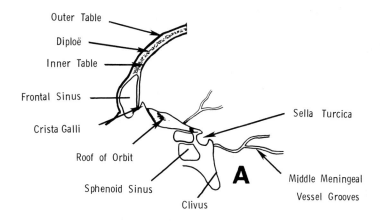

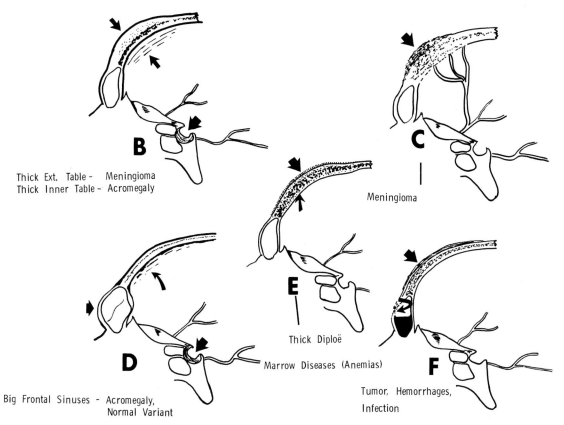

Figure 12–13 Varieties of prominence of the frontal bossae. *A.* Diagram of a frontal bone and normal anatomic parts. *B.* The thick external table as well as the internal table with erosion of the sella turcica such as might occur with either a meningioma or acromegaly. *C.* Illustrates what might occur with a meningioma. *D.* Possible results of a frontal sinus osteomyelitis. *E.* Prominence of the frontal bossae that may occur with marrow disorders such as anemia. *F.* Marked thickening of the periosteum with partial destruction of the inner or outer table (or both) resulting from hemorrhage, infection, or tumor.

Hair-on-end Pattern

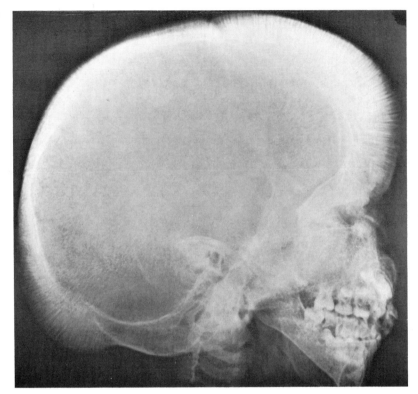

Figure 12–14 Lateral view of skull in thalassemia major, demonstrating "sun-ray" appearance just outside the external diploë.

1. Congenital hemolytic anemias (thalassemias, sickle cell disease, spherocytosis, and others)
2. Iron deficiency anemia
3. Metastases from neuroblastoma
4. Cyanotic congenital heart disease
5. Polycythemia vera in childhood

Localized Soft Tissue Prominences

1. Cephalohematoma
2. Encephalocele
3. Meningocele

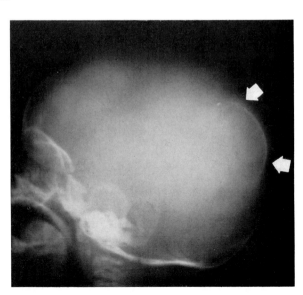

Figure 12–15 *B*. Calcified cephalohematoma in an infant.

Localized Depressions in the Calvarium or Base of the Skull

Depressed Skull Fracture (Figure 12–16)

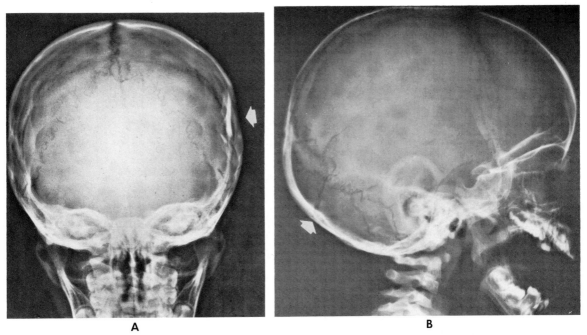

A   **B**

Figure 12–16 *A*. Lateral view of skull demonstrating a linear fracture of the occipital bone with no detectable depression of fragment. The appearance of the lambdoid suture for comparison is well demonstrated. *B*. Depressed fracture of the left parietal bone and adjoining squamous portion of temporal bone. A good tangential view is usually necessary to demonstrate the exact degree of depression.

Platybasia

DEFINITION. Flattening of the base of the skull with an increase in the basal angle. This may coexist with a basilar impression which is a separate entity and is an anomaly of the occipitocervical junction where the upper cervical segments and foramen magnum protrude into the cranial cavity. Klippel-Feil syndrome or Arnold-Chiari malformation may coexist also.

Platybasia may be congenital or acquired as the result of rickets, Paget's disease, hyperparathyroidism, osteomalacia, or osteogenesis imperfecta.

CLINICALLY there is a close resemblance to multiple sclerosis, spastic paralysis, syringomyelia, and adult Arnold-Chiari with adhesions.

Abnormalities of Density of the Bones of the Calvarium

Diffuse Radiolucency

1. Congenital disorders (cleidocranial dysostosis, osteogenesis imperfecta, and others)
2. Endocrine deficiencies (hypothyroidism)
3. Hyperparathyroidism
4. Neoplasms (neuroblastoma, lytic metastases)
5. Nonspecific radiolucencies

Hyperparathyroidism (See Chapter 8)

Neuroblastoma (Figure 12–17) (See Chapter 8)

DEFINITION.   Sympathicoblastoma originating in the cells of the sympathetic nervous system, most frequently in those from the adrenal gland.

RADIOGRAPHIC APPEARANCES (illustrated)

The tumor metastasizes widely to the skeleton, liver, and lymph nodes. In the skull metastases are most numerous adjoining sutures. The inner and outer tables of the skull become poorly defined, so that they virtually merge.

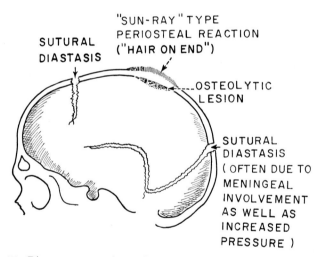

Figure 12–17   Diagram representing radiographic changes of the skull in neuroblastoma.

Demarcated Areas of Radiolucency in the Bones of the Calvarium

Fracture

CLASSIFICATION.   Linear, compound, comminuted, depressed.

RADIOGRAPHIC APPEARANCES

There is a jagged discontinuity in the bones of the calvarium—unlike sutures which appear serrated, and unlike vascular impressions which appear undulating. When a linear fracture has produced a separation of sutures, it is called "sutural diastasis." Multiple views of the skull including stereoscopic studies are necessary for greatest accuracy. At best, fractures of the base of the skull may be detected radiographically in only about 25 per cent of cases.

Depressed fractures have been discussed previously.

VALUE OF PLAIN FILMS FOR DETECTION OF FRACTURES OF THE SKULL

1. Roberts and Shopfner* have reported that only 8.6 per cent of 570 patients who had head trauma for which x-rays were obtained had demonstrable fractures. Most fractures were in the vault and were linear in type.
   a. There was no correlation with clinical symptoms or physical findings.
   b. The demonstration of the fracture affected the treatment in only 2 of the 49 cases, one a foreign body, and the other a depressed fracture.
2. Harwood-Nash et al.† reported an incidence of 26.6 per cent of skull fractures in 4465 children presenting with head trauma. The presence of the fracture was not correlated with clinical seriousness and did not alter the decision for medical care except in children with a depressed or compound fracture.
   a. The incidence of serious intracranial sequelae in head injuries regardless of the presence or absence of a skull fracture is 9 per cent, and the incidence of these sequelae in children without a fracture is 8 per cent.

---

*Roberts, F., and Shopfner, C. E.: Amer. J. Roentgenol., *114*:230, 1972.
†Harwood-Nash, D. C., Hendrick, E. B., and Hudson, A. R.: Radiology, *101*:151, 1971.

Wormian Bones.   They are found in:

1. Cleidocranial dysostosis
2. Osteogenesis imperfecta
3. Hypothyroidism
4. Progeria

Epidermoidoma (Figure 12–18)

DEFINITION.   A tumor formed from the inclusion of epidermal cells in the bones of the calvarium.

RADIOGRAPHIC APPEARANCES

Well-encapsulated zone of radiolucency with a well-defined scalloped sclerotic margin.

The tumor is usually situated in the diploë but involves both inner and outer table equally.

Unlike other lytic, well-encapsulated lesions of the calvarium, the central zones contain no trabeculae or foci of stippled calcification.

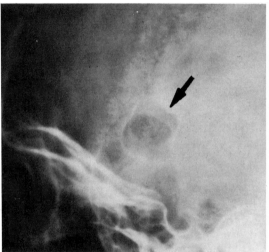

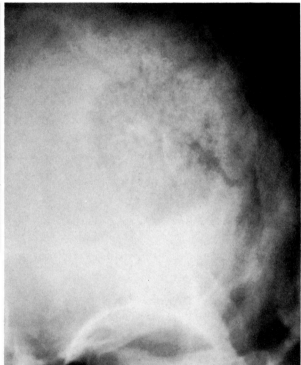

Figure 12–18   Epidermoidoma of the squama of the skull.

Figure 12–19   Hemangioma of the calvarium.

Hemangioma (Figure 12–19)

DEFINITION.   Blood vessel tumor of two types, cavernous or capillary. The lesion begins in the diploë and expands the inner and outer tables in fusiform fashion.

RADIOGRAPHIC APPEARANCES.   Two general types are recognized:

A lytic variety: sharply circumscribed with a thin sclerotic zone and an inner finely reticular bony structure.

A sclerotic variety: bony spiculation radiating from a central point, not perpendicular to the bony tables of the skull.

Multiple Areas of Demarcated Radiolucency

Foramina in the Base of the Skull (see preceding radiograph, page 179)

Normal lucencies of the cranial vault.
1. *Emissary veins* traverse small foramina, particularly in the parietal, temporal, and mastoid bones
2. *Parietal thinness*
3. *Parietal foramina* do not contain veins, and are similar to parietal thinness
4. *Pacchionian villi* (arachnoidal granulations)
5. *Venous diploë*
6. *Accentuated convolutional pattern*

Osteomyelitis of the Bones of the Calvarium

CLASSIFICATION. Pyogenic (acute or chronic); syphilitic; tuberculous; or fungal (actinomycosis, coccidioidomycosis; blastomycosis; or cryptococcosis, very rarely).

RADIOLOGIC APPEARANCES (Figure 12–20)

Early: Area of diminished density with ragged, irregular outline. There is a tendency for small areas to coalesce to form larger ones. **Late:** Sclerotic areas become intermixed with the lucencies. Actinomycotic involvement is characterized by a sclerotic response predominantly. Other lesions are difficult to distinguish one from the other radiologically.

Irregular areas of bone destruction giving the skull a moth-eaten appearance with small interspersed areas of sclerosis due to the contained sequestrae.

Chronic infections of the calvarium may be secondary to surgical craniotomy. A gradual lysis of bone at a surgical site is the diagnostic radiographic appearance.

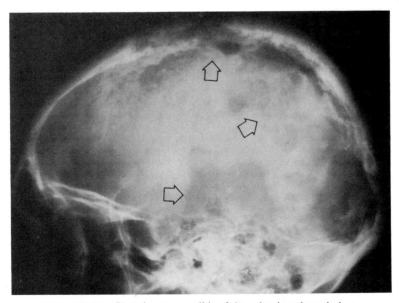

Figure 12–20 Chronic osteomyelitis of the calvarium, lateral view.

Fibrous Dysplasia (Figure 12–21)

RADIOGRAPHIC APPEARANCES.   An irregular radiolucency of the calvarium extending outward in projecting lobulations so that the affected bone appears scalloped and highly irregular in outline. The cortex appears to be eroded from within, while the periosteum attempts to compensate by laying down a thin shell of normal bone on the outer surface (Figure 12–21). There is usually a sclerotic zone surrounding the lytic zone within the calvarium, giving this lesion a thick outer margin.

In the skull the lesions are usually unilateral but may be bilateral.

In the paranasal sinuses, there may be an obliteration of the air space with diminution in the capacity of the adjoining orbits as the result of the marked thickening of the bony process.

The progress of the disease is variable and slow (Leeds and Seaman).

When facial bones are involved the process is called "leontiasis ossea."

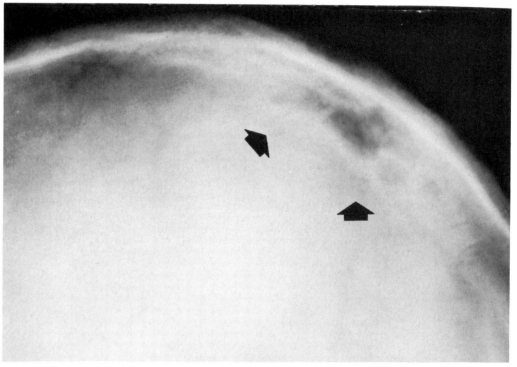

Figure 12–21   Close-up view of fibrous dysplasia of the calvarium. The relatively thick zone of sclerosis, coupled with the "shell of bone" appearance, is an important criterion for this diagnosis.

Paget's Disease of the Skull (Osteitis deformans) (Figure 12–22)

DEFINITION.   Acquired disorder of bone characterized by destruction and the formation of bizarre replacement bone which appears *expanded*, soft, poorly mineralized, and disorganized. It may be monostotic or polyostotic.

RADIOLOGIC ASPECTS

The skull is irregularly thickened, with scattered areas of involvement in the calvarium and facial bones. The outer table and diploë are most affected. There is a maplike or geographic resorption of the bone giving the appearance described as "osteoporosis circumscripta." Later the innner table may also be involved. Still later, there is a bizarre deposition of new bone in multiple, irregular patchy areas giving rise to the so-called "cotton ball" appearance. The tables and diploë ultimately become markedly thickened and the base of the skull may be so softened by the process that a basilar impression supervenes. The sella turcica may appear small. Sarcomatous degeneration may occur.

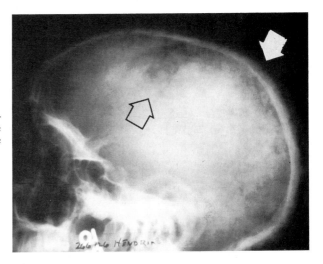

Figure 12–22 Paget's disease involving bone. Lateral view of the skull with late involvement of the skull showing the "cotton ball" type appearance of the bones of the calvarium.

Metastatic Malignancy to the Skull (Figure 12–23)

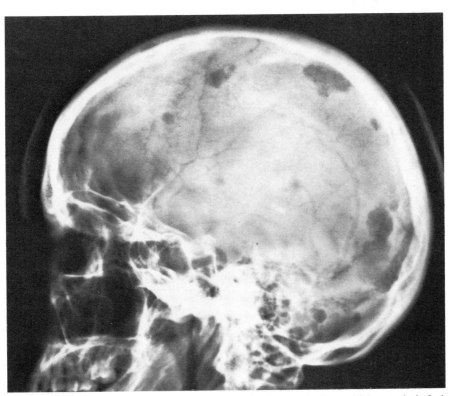

Figure 12–23 Metastatic tumors to the bones of the calvarium producing multiple osteolytic foci of a sharply circumscribed character in the bones of the calvarium.

Multiple Myeloma

PREFERENTIAL SITES.   Vertebral bodies, bones of the pelvis, shoulder girdle, skull.

RADIOGRAPHIC APPEARANCES (Figure 12–24)

No manifestations in approximately 25 per cent of cases.

Multiple areas of sharply defined bone destruction involving the vertebrae, pelvis, and especially, skull and shoulder girdle.

There is often an associated generalized osteoporosis.

When the cortex is completely destroyed, a soft tissue mass may be associated.

Occasionally, the process is not sharply defined and merely appears as multiple minute lytic foci throughout the bones, imparting an appearance closely resembling severe diffuse osteoporosis.

Pathologic fractures are frequent.

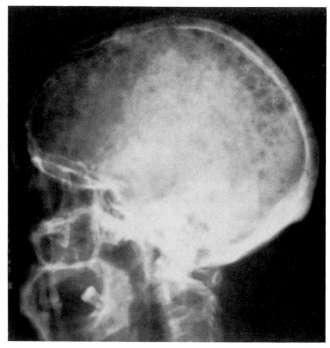

Figure 12–24   Lateral view of skull with advanced changes due to multiple myeloma.

Diseases of the Skull Manifest by Diffuse Increase in Radiopacity

Osteopetrosis (see Chapters 7 and 10)

Engelmann's Disease (see Chapters 7 and 10)

Metaphyseal Dysplasia (Pyle's disease; craniometaphyseal dysplasia)

Van Buchem's Disease

Fluorine Poisoning (see p. 125)

Marrow Disorders (see p. 125)

Diseases of the Skull Manifest by Multiple Demarcated Areas of Radiopacity

Osteitis Deformans of Paget's Disease. See previous description.

Osteoblastic Metastases. Prostatic carcinoma is the most common, but gastrointestinal tract, breast, and carcinoid metastases are often sclerotic. Metastatic lucent lesions often also become sclerotic after treatment (radiotherapy or chemotherapy).

Diseases of the Skull Manifest by Single or Confluent Demarcated Areas of Bony Sclerosis

Osteoma or Osteochondroma

Hyperostosis Frontalis Interna (Figure 12–25)

DEFINITION. This condition is characterized by marked hyperostotic change of the inner table of the frontal bone.

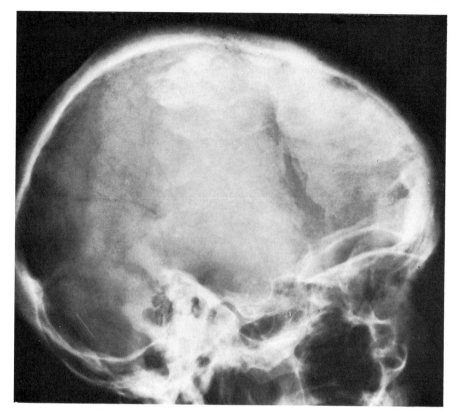

Figure 12–25   Hyperostosis frontalis interna, lateral view.

Meningioma

DEFINITION.   Meningiomas or fibroblastomas are tumors which arise from
the tissues surrounding the cerebrum, characterized by histological features of the
meningotheliomatous and psammomatous types. They are usually of either arachnoid or dural origin.

SITES OF ORIGIN (Figure 12–26).   The most frequent sites are parasagittal,
the petrous ridge, sphenoidal ridge, in the region of the olfactory groove, and over
the convexity of the cerebrum anterior to the fissure of Rolando. In general they
originate wherever arachnoid granulations are numerous and where the cerebral
veins enter the large venous sinuses.

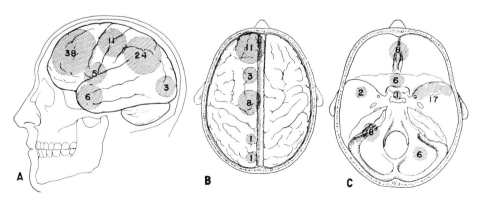

Figure 12–26   *A* to *C*. Diagrammatic sketch of the locations of intracranial meningiomas and the relative
frequency of each. (From Jacobson et al.: Radiology, *72*:358, 1959.)

RADIOGRAPHIC FINDINGS

Plain Films of the Skull

In parasagittal meningiomas: hypervascularity, hyperostosis, and calcification within the tumor, or a combination of these appearances.

Sphenoidal ridge and olfactory groove meningiomas: very marked hyperostosis and a very dense tumor mass. There may also be an associated enlargement of the sphenoidal fissure.

Jacobson et al. found that plain films of the skull were normal in only 22.5 per cent of the cases. The roentgenologic abnormalities most frequently encountered on the plain films of the skull were as follows: localized hyperostosis, 44.1 per cent; atrophy of the dorsum sellae, 29 per cent; localized increase in vascularity, 25.8 per cent; calcification, 20.4 per cent; significant pineal shift, 19.4 per cent; localized bone resorption, 16.1 per cent; and localized spiculation, 4.3 per cent.

Questions—Chapter 12

1. Describe the routine views of the skull and indicate the special significance and purpose of each of these views in respect to the roentgenology of the skull.

2. Describe a useful routine method for study of the radiographs of the skull.

3. Describe the growth and age changes of the skull in respect to the skull and facial proportions at birth, at six or seven years of age, at puberty, and after puberty.

4. Define the following terms: brachycephalic skull; dolichocephalic skull; turricephalic skull; plagiocephalic skull.

5. Describe a method of pineal localization.

6. Where is the habenula situated in the skull? What is its significance when calcified?

7. Describe the anatomy of the sella turcica.

8. What are the general causes for a small skull?

9. What are the general causes for an enlarged skull?

10. Define Arnold-Chiari malformation and indicate some of the lesions which are often associated.

11. Define "Dandy-Walker syndrome" and indicate the radiographic findings often found on plain films of the skull.

12. Define "cerebral aqueduct stenosis" and indicate radiographic findings which may be found on plain films early or late in life, and the significance of calcifications in the brain in respect to the above.

13. Define "Paget's disease of the skull" and describe the radiologic aspects of the skull appearances.

14. Define "meningocele" and "encephalocele" and indicate the radiographic findings often associated.

15. How does one demonstrate a depressed skull fracture most accurately and what is the significance of this finding?

16. Define "platybasia" and indicate the method you might employ in making the diagnosis roentgenologically.

17. What is the radiographic appearance of the skull in hyperparathyroidism?

18. Describe the radiographic appearances of the skull often associated with neuroblastoma.

19. What are the radiographic appearances of the bones of the calvarium associated with osteomyelitis affecting these bones?

20. Differentiate the radiographic appearance in the calvarium of epidermoidoma and hemangioma.

21. What are the most frequently encountered malignant lesions contiguous with the skull which may alter the roentgen appearance of the skull?

22. What foramina occur in the base of the skull in the middle fossa and how may they be detected?

23. What foramina occur in the posterior fossa of the skull and how may they be detected?

24. What foramina occur in the cranial vault and what is their radiographic appearance?

25. What is the clinical significance of an accentuated convolutional pattern? How does this appearance differ from lückenschädel?

26. Describe the radiographic appearance of a skull affected by fibrous dysplasia.

27. Classify the reticuloendothelioses. Which of these diseases are primary lipid disturbances and which are secondary?

28. How may metastatic malignancy to the skull alter the skull appearance roentgenologically?

29. Describe the radiographic appearance of multiple myelomas affecting the skull.

30. What are the most frequent sites of origin of meningioma and what are the radiographic findings in plain films of the skull?

31. Where do meningiomas originate which often do not alter the skull appearance?

13

Radiology of Special Areas of the Skull and Space-Occupying Lesions Within the Cranium

SELLA TURCICA

Plain Skull Film Changes in and Around the Sella Turcica and Their Significance

1. There are great variations in the normal size and configuration of the sella turcica (Weidner et al.). This must be evaluated in at least three views: lateral, P-A for floor of sella turcica, and A-P Towne's for dorsum sellae.

2. The double contoured appearance of the floor of the sella turcica is usually evidence of intrasellar tumor with asymmetrical expansion.

3. Intrasellar lesions causing enlargement of the sella are usually pituitary adenomas; less commonly they are craniopharyngiomas. Adenomas of the pituitary, usually arising from the anterior lobe of the pituitary, produce the following slight differences in appearance:

a. Chromophobe adenomas grow rapidly and become large with destruction and demineralization of the bony walls of the sella. There are no peripheral skeletal changes ordinarily.

b. Eosinophilic adenomas produce gigantism in the young and acromegaly in adults. They are slow-growing and the walls of the pituitary mold to conform to the configuration of a slow-growing tumor. They are well defined and the margins are well calcified usually.

c. Basophilic adenomas are tiny adenomas and rarely cause any enlargement of the sella; these patients usually have Cushing's syndrome and generalized osteoporosis. Rarely, predominantly basophilic adenomas are large expansile lesions.

d. Calcification in pituitary adenomas is rare, possibly 5 to 7 per cent (Deery).

e. Curvilinear calcification seen with chromophobe adenomas occurs in the capsule of the tumor or in the wall of the cyst. Calcification may occur in eosinophilic adenomas, called pituitary calculi.

4. Unilateral enlargement of the sella turcica may be secondary to intracavernous aneurysm of the internal carotid artery.

5. Enlargement of sella is also seen with hydrocephalus when the third ventricle enlarges and bulges into the sella.

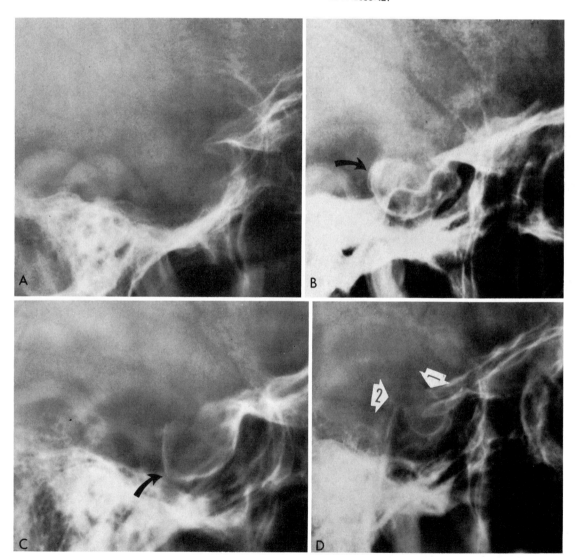

AS RESULT OF : 1. INCREASED INTRACRANIAL PRESSURE
2. INTRASELLAR EXPANDING LESION

EROSION OF POST. CLINOID PROCESSES
DUE TO :
1. INDIRECT PRESSURE AS IN
INCREASED INTRACRANIAL
PRESSURE, TUMORS,
HYDROCEPHALUS, ETC.
2. DIRECT PRESSURE FROM :
a. LOCAL TUMOR
b. ENLARGED 3rd. VENTRICLE

DORSUM
SELLA

SELLA TURCICA

SPHENOID AIR SINUS

BONE ABSORPTION OF FLOOR WITHOUT EXPANSION
OCCURS WITH SPHENOID SINUS MALIGNANCY.
THERE MAY BE ASSOCIATED BONY SCLEROSIS.

EROSION OF ANT. CLINOID PROCESSES
USUALLY UNAFFECTED BY INCREASED INTRA-
CRANIAL PRESSURE.

IF UNILATERAL EROSION (DETECTED BY
STEREO FILM IN CORONAL PLANE) IT IS
USUALLY DUE TO AN ANEURYSM OF
CAROTID ARTERY OR OPTIC NERVE TUMOR

SELLA TURCICA DECALCIFICATION
AND CIRCULAR EXPANSION DUE TO:
1. EXPANDING TUMOR WITHIN FOSSA
[MOST COMMON]   THERE MAY
ALSO BE A DOUBLE-CONTOURED
APPEARANCE OF THE FLOOR OF THE
SELLA
2. OCCASIONALLY OCCURS
WITH GENERALIZED INCREASED
INTRACRANIAL PRESSURE.

Figure 13–1 Diagram illustrating the changes in the sagittal contour of the sella turcica resulting from increased intracranial pressure or an intrasellar expanding lesion.

Figure 13–2 *A.* Lateral view of the sella turcica in a patient with a large pituitary adenoma. The posterior clinoids are completely eroded and there is considerable sclerosis and erosion of the floor of the sella turcica extending into the adjoining sphenoid sinus. *B.* Enlargement of the sella turcica caused by an aneurysm of the adjoining carotid artery siphon with some calcium deposit in the aneurysm (arrow). *C.* Marked thinning of the dorsum sellae and posterior clinoids with an increase in depth of the sella turcica posteriorly and some squaring off of its floor due to a Rathke pouch cyst adjoining (arrow). *D.* The sella turcica itself does not appear to be expanded or enlarged but note that the posterior clinoids are completely absent owing to erosion, and one of the anterior clinoids (arrow) is partially eroded and convex toward the eye. These findings indicate partial erosion of the anterior clinoids and considerable disappearance of the posterior clinoids, findings which were related to a chromophobe adenoma involving this area.

THE FACIAL BONES AND PARANASAL SINUSES

Normal Radiographic Anatomy

ROUTINE FOR STUDY OF PARANASAL SINUSES
I. CALDWELL'S VIEW

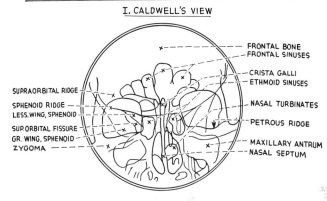

Figure 13–3

1. NOTE CLARITY AND INTEGRITY OF WALLS OF FRONTAL AND ETHMOID SINUSES.
2. NOTE FRONTAL BONE TEXTURE.
3. NOTE BONY NASAL SEPTUM AND ADJOINING TURBINATES; NOTE AERATION OF NASAL AIR PASSAGES.
4. NOTE ORBITS AND SPHENOIDAL MARKINGS THEREIN.
5. ONE CAN SEE MAXILLARY SINUSES ALSO, BUT NOT TO MAXIMUM ADVANTAGE.

II. WATERS' VIEW, MOUTH OPEN
(a) PATIENT UPRIGHT
(b) PATIENT RECUMBENT

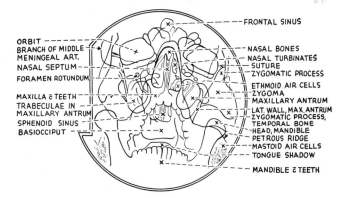

Figure 13–4

1. NOTE CLARITY OF MAXILLARY ANTRA, INTEGRITY OF ANTRAL WALLS, AND ADJOINING ZYGOMA.
2. NOTE SPHENOID SINUS.
3. OTHER SINUSES ARE ALSO SEEN, BUT NOT TO MAXIMUM ADVANTAGE.
4. NASAL BRIDGE AND SEPTUM.
5. FLUID LEVELS IN UPRIGHT FILM.

NOTE: *THIS VIEW WITH MOUTH OPEN, IN CONTRADISTINCTION TO THE ROUTINE WATERS' VIEW WITH THE MOUTH CLOSED, IS OUR INDIVIDUAL PREFERENCE, SINCE THE SPHENOID SINUS THEN COMES INTO VIEW.*

<u>III. LATERAL VIEW OF PARANASAL SINUSES</u>

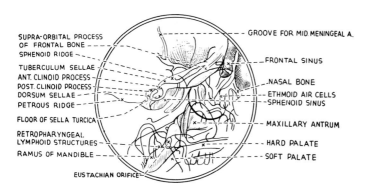

SUPRA-ORBITAL PROCESS OF FRONTAL BONE
SPHENOID RIDGE
TUBERCULUM SELLAE
ANT. CLINOID PROCESS
POST. CLINOID PROCESS
DORSUM SELLAE
PETROUS RIDGE
FLOOR OF SELLA TURCICA
RETROPHARYNGEAL LYMPHOID STRUCTURES
RAMUS OF MANDIBLE
EUSTACHIAN ORIFICE

GROOVE FOR MID. MENINGEAL A.
FRONTAL SINUS
NASAL BONE
ETHMOID AIR CELLS
SPHENOID SINUS
MAXILLARY ANTRUM
HARD PALATE
SOFT PALATE

1. NOTE FRONTAL, ETHMOID, SPHENOID AND MAXILLARY SINUSES.
2. NOTE POSTERIOR NASOPHARYNGEAL WALL.
3. NOTE SELLA TURCICA.
4. NOTE INTEGRITY OF SPHENOID RIDGE.
5. NASAL BONES MAY BE SEEN WITH BRIGHT LIGHT SOURCE.

Figure 13–5

Roentgen Pathology of the Maxilla and Paranasal Sinuses

Abnormal Alterations in Size

Congenital Occlusion of the Nares

Hypoplasia of the Facial Bones

1. Pierre Robin syndrome (congenital hypoplasia of mandible)
2. Mandibulofacial dysostosis (Treacher-Collins syndrome)

Acromegaly

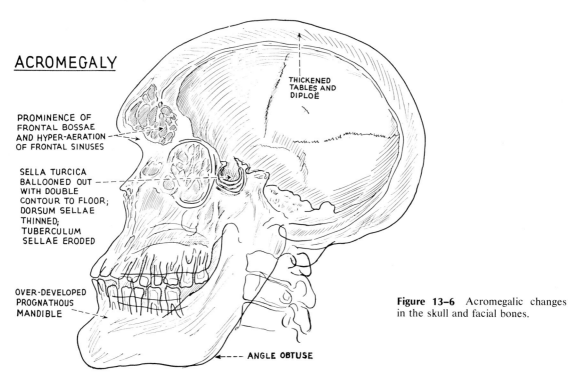

ACROMEGALY

THICKENED TABLES AND DIPLOË

PROMINENCE OF FRONTAL BOSSAE AND HYPER-AERATION OF FRONTAL SINUSES

SELLA TURCICA BALLOONED OUT WITH DOUBLE CONTOUR TO FLOOR; DORSUM SELLAE THINNED; TUBERCULUM SELLAE ERODED

OVER-DEVELOPED PROGNATHOUS MANDIBLE

ANGLE OBTUSE

Figure 13–6 Acromegalic changes in the skull and facial bones.

Changes in Density

Increased Density of the Paranasal Sinuses.   Representative lesions reflecting changes in aeration of the paranasal sinuses are shown in Figures 13–7 to 13–12. These include:

1. Acute and chronic sinusitis.
2. Thickening or edema of the mucous membrane of the paranasal sinuses.
3. Polypi.
4. Mucoceles.
5. Retention cysts.
6. Hemorrhage or blood clots in the sinuses.
7. Tumors, either primary or secondary to dental origin.
8. Malignant tumors originating in the epithelial lining of the paranasal sinuses (carcinomas). They may, however, on occasion be sarcomas or mixed tumors.
9. Foreign bodies in the sinuses.
10. Fibrous dysplasia (combined osteoblastic and osteolytic reaction).
11. Ossifying fibroma of the face—especially frontal bone, maxilla, mandible.

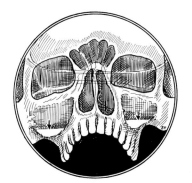

AIR-FLUID LEVEL
SINUSITIS HEMORRHAGE

Figure 13–7

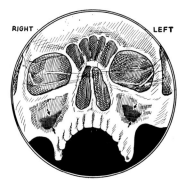

MUCOPERIOSTEAL THICKENING OF
MAXILLARY ANTRA; THE THICKENED
MUCOSAL LINE RUNS PARALLEL TO
THE ANTRAL WALL AND IS STRAIGHT;
ALLERGIC THICKENING IS OFTEN
SCALLOPED IN APPEARANCE.

Figure 13–8

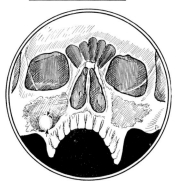

MAXILLARY ANTRAL
ALLERGIC POLYP

POLYPOID FILLING DEFECT IN
MAXILLARY ANTRUM, ALLERGIC
IN ORIGIN; MAY BE UNILATERAL
OR MULTIPLE; TURBINATES ARE
OFTEN SWOLLEN.

Figure 13–9

MUCOCELE OF LEFT FRONTAL SINUS

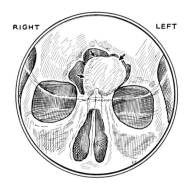

THERE IS A PRESSURE ATROPHY
OF SURROUNDING BONE CAUSED BY
A RADIOLUCENT, EXPANDING,
SHARPLY DEMARCATED LESION.

Figure 13–10

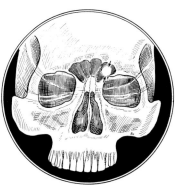

OSTEOMA-
FRONTAL SINUS

Figure 13–11

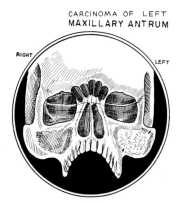

CARCINOMA OF LEFT
MAXILLARY ANTRUM

Figure 13–12

Diminished Density of the Bones of the Face

FRACTURES

Classification. Fractures are most readily classified by the major bones involved (mandible, maxilla, nose, zygoma, frontoethmoid, and mixed complex fractures).

Fractures of the Maxilla. Classification. LeFort's method of classification of fractures of the maxilla is shown in Figure 13–13.

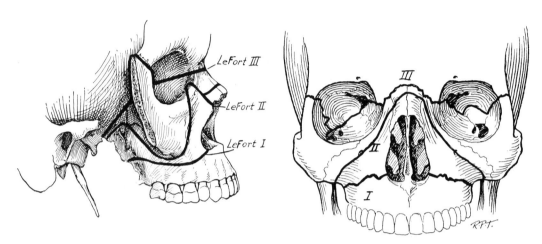

Figure 13–13 LeFort's method of classification of fractures of the maxilla. (From Kazanjian, V. H., and Converse, J. M.: *The Surgical Treatment of Facial Injuries,* 2nd Ed. Baltimore, The Williams and Wilkins Co., 1959.)

Fracture of the Orbit

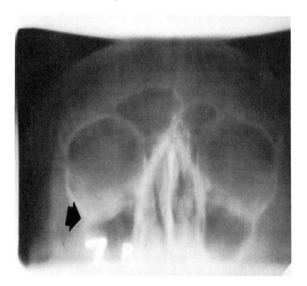

Figure 13–14 Body section radiograph at 7 cm. in Water's projection, demonstrating a definite depression of the infraorbital plate.

Radiographic Findings

The infraorbital foramen becomes cloudy.
Fragments may be identified in the maxillary sinus.
The floor of the orbit is broken into the maxillary sinus.
The maxillary sinus may be filled with orbital tissue (Figure 13–14).

OSTEOMYELITIS

CYSTS AND TUMORS

Tumors eroding the facial bones and paranasal sinuses by contiguous erosion from oral, nasal, or pituitary regions. These include carcinoma of the hard or soft palate, nasal tumors, and carcinoma or sarcoma of the paranasal sinuses. Likewise, tumors of the pituitary gland may erode downward into the sphenoid sinus.

Mixed tumors and plasma cell tumors. These are among the most frequent tumors involving the face and the adjoining bony structures.

ROENTGEN PATHOLOGY OF THE MANDIBLE

1. Decreased size
    a. Pierre-Robin syndrome (mandibular hypoplasia)
    b. Gargoylism ("amputated condyloid process")
2. Increased size
    a. Acromegaly
    b. Leontiasis ossea
    c. Fibrous dysplasia (cherubism)
3. Increased angle
    a. Acromegaly
    b. Progeria
4. Increased density
    a. Osteopetrosis (marble bone disease)
    b. Hyperphosphatasia
    c. Infantile cortical hyperostosis (Caffey-Silverman disease)
    c. Odontomas
5. Decreased density
    a. Fractures
    b. Abscesses and osteomyelitis (nonspecific; actinomycosis; periodontal)
    c. Periodontoclasia
    d. Epulis (giant cell tumor)
    e. Cysts and tumors
        (1) Fissural cyst
        (2) Odontogenic cysts
        (3) Ameloblastoma
        (4) Keratogenic (basal cell nevus syndrome)
        (5) Invasive tumors of gums
        (6) Histiocytic tumors
    f. Endocrine: hyperparathyroidism (loss of lamina dura)

RADIOLOGIC EVIDENCES OF INTRACRANIAL SPACE-OCCUPYING LESIONS

Introduction. Radiologic techniques have contributed significantly to the accurate localization and diagnosis of intracranial mass lesions. These methods, in the order of their complexity, include:

1. *Plain Films of the Skull,* including special coned-down and laminographic studies with the aid of polytomography, as described previously (see Figure 12–11).
2. *Radioisotopic Studies.* These include:
   a. *Cervicocranial scintiphotograms* in rapid sequence following the intravenous injection of a bolus of radionuclide.
   b. Rectilinear scans or scintiphotos of the head in frontal, lateral, and angled posterior projections.
3. *Angiograms of the Head,* which may be performed by:
   a. Four vessel arch and selective catheterization techniques.
   b. Percutaneous carotid angiograms of the neck.
   c. Percutaneous retrograde brachial angiograms—the left retrograde brachial being used for posterior fossa studies in lieu of a percutaneous left vertebral angiogram.
4. *Pneumograms of the Head.* These may be performed by:
   a. *Pneumoencephalography:* Withdrawal of fractions of cerebrospinal fluid via lumbar spinal puncture and replacement of the fluid with air or other suitable gaseous medium.
   b. *Ventriculography:* The instillation of the gaseous medium into the ventricles of the brain directly by puncture of the posterior parietal lobe of the brain through a small trephine opening in the parietal bone.
5. *Cisternomyelograms with Pantopaque:* In this technique, a small quantity of the Pantopaque is introduced into the lumbar region and carefully manipulated into each cerebellopontine angle under fluoroscopic control, and control of the patient's head.
6. *Ventriculograms with Pantopaque.*
7. *Dural Sinus Venograms,* where obstruction of a venous sinus is suspected.
8. *Instillation of Sterile Micropaque Barium into Known Abscess and Neoplastic Cavities,* in order to study the sequential diminution or enlargement of such cavities under treatment.
9. *Radioisotopic Myelocisternoencephalo Photograms:* In this technique the radioactive medium in high specific activity is injected into the lumbar region and is followed several hours later to the basal cisterns of the head; after 24 hours it is followed over the convexity of the brain. Abnormally, the radioactivated cerebrospinal fluid appears in the ventricles of the brain in certain cases of low pressure hydrocephalus.

The discussion of all these methods is outside the scope of this text except for the plain films of the skull, and it too must be outlined only in introductory fashion.

Abnormal Calcium Deposits. Abnormal calcification within the skull may be said to be either (a) non-neoplastic or (b) neoplastic in origin.

NON-NEOPLASTIC CALCIFICATION. This may be outlined as follows:
1. Congenital and neonatal
    a. Tuberous sclerosis
    b. Infantile hemiplegias
2. Parasitic diseases
    a. Toxoplasmosis
    b. Torulosis
    c. Cysticercosis
    d. Echinococcosis
    e. Trichinosis
3. Inflammatory processes
    a. Tuberculous meningitis
    b. Encephalitis
    c. Brain abscess
    d. Tuberculoma
    e. Luetic gumma
4. Vascular lesions
    a. Arteriosclerosis
    b. Angiomas
    c. Sturge-Weber syndrome
    d. Aneurysms (circle of Willis; vein of Galen)
    e. Endarteritis calcificans cerebri
    f. Cerebral hemorrhages
    g. Subdural hematoma
5. Endocrine disorders
   Parathyroid insufficiency
6. X-ray injury
   Necrosis of the brain following roentgen radiation

NEOPLASTIC CALCIFICATION
Pathologic Tumoral Calcifications. Calcification in intracranial neoplasms was reported in 13 per cent of 1557 tumors (Martin) and occurs far more frequently in the supratentorial lesions than in infratentorial ones. It occurs primarily in the walls of blood vessels or within the tumor areas of ischemic or hemorrhagic degeneration and necrosis. It occurs also in the walls of cysts or cystic neoplasms.

The tumors which are most frequently calcified are:
1. Gliomas
    a. Oligodendroglioma
    b. Astrocytoma
    c. Pinealoma
    d. Ependymoma
    e. Spongioblastoma polare
    f. Medulloblastoma
    g. Glioblastoma multiforme
2. Meningiomas

3. Congenital tumors
   a. Craniopharyngioma
   b. Chordoma
   c. Epidermoid
   d. Lipoma
4. Chromophobe pituitary adenoma
5. Choroid plexus papilloma

Parasellar or Intrasellar Calcification.   Calcification in or adjoining the sella turcica tends to fall into the following categories:

Flocculent (as in a craniopharyngioma — see section on brain) within the hypophyseal fossa.

Circumlinear in the arc of a circle or ellipse (also seen with craniopharyngiomas as well as with adjoining aneurysms).

Tubular, as with calcification in the carotid arteries in their cavernous portions.

Mulberry-type calcification posterior to the dorsum sellae, as seen with chronic granuloma or gliomas.

These pathological types of calcification must be differentiated from the normal calcification of the petroclinoid ligament.

Questions — Chapter 13

1. What is the range of normal measurement for the sella turcica by Camp's method?
2. Describe the changes which occur in and about the sella turcica in relation to intrasellar expanding lesions.
3. Describe the changes which occur in and about the sella turcica due to extrasellar intracranial expanding lesions.
4. Describe the changes which occur in and about the sella turcica in relation to destructive diseases of the sphenoid bone.
5. Which views are obtained routinely in the radiographic study of the face?
6. Which views are obtained routinely for radiographic examination of the mandible?
7. Which radiographic views are considered routine in examination of the paranasal sinuses?
8. Describe the skull in acromegaly.
9. List five general causes for increased density of the paranasal sinuses. How may they be recognized radiographically?
10. Indicate the LeFort classification for fracture of the maxilla.
11. Why is it important to recognize fractures of the zygoma?
12. Describe the radiographic appearances of the "blow-out fracture" of the orbit. What bone or bones are especially fractured in this region?
13. Describe at least four standard positions for radiography of the mastoid and temporal bone.
14. What is the significance of increase in opacity of the mastoid air cells with no loss of bone integrity?
15. What is the significance of increased radiopacity of the mastoid with destruction of mastoid air cells?
16. Describe the radiographic appearances of a cholesteatoma involving the mastoid region.
17. What are the most frequent tumors in the vicinity of the apex of the petrous bone? How do they manifest themselves radiographically?
18. What are the radiographic findings with optic nerve glioma?
19. Indicate the routine and special procedures utilized for diagnosis and localization of intracranial mass lesions.

20. List the changes in the skull indicative of increased intracranial pressure.

21. Describe the changes in the sella turcica related to increased intracranial pressure.

22. List the areas of physiologic calcification within the cranium and indicate which of these are significant in respect to the localization of mass lesions within the cranial cavity.

23. What are some of the causes of non-neoplastic calcification in the cranial cavity? Describe some of their appearances.

24. Which are the most frequent calcifying tumors found within the cranial cavity?

25. Describe various alterations in size and contour of the posterior fossa in respect to: (1) Arnold-Chiari malformation; (2) Dandy-Walker syndrome; (3) cerebral aqueduct stenosis; (4) medulloblastoma of the posterior fossa in a child.

14

The Radiology of the Vertebral Column

NORMAL ANATOMY OF THE CERVICAL SPINE

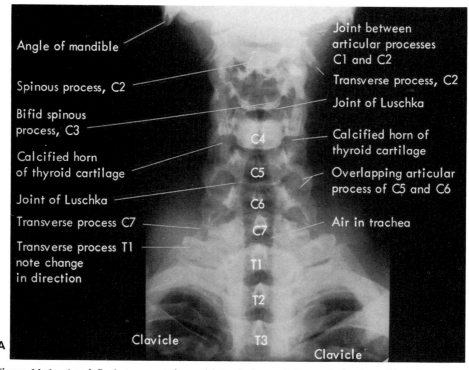

Figure 14–1 *A* and *B*. Antero-posterior and lateral views of the cervical spine with major anatomic parts labeled. Lateral view (xeroradiograph) permits a better detailed delineation of some of the anatomic structures partially hidden on conventional views of the cervical spine.

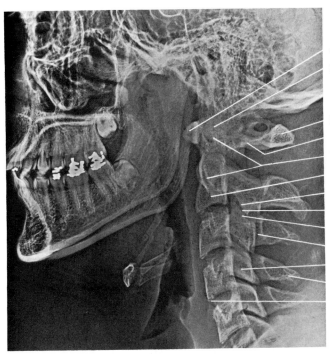

ANTERIOR TUBERCLE, CI
DENS (ODONTOID PROCESS)

POSTERIOR TUBERCLE, CI
POSTERIOR ARCH, CI
TRANSVERSE PROCESSES, CI−C2
BODY, C2
INFERIOR ARTICULAR PROCESS, C3
APOPHYSEAL JOINT
SUPERIOR ARTICULAR PROCESS, C4
LAMINAE, C3
ARTICULAR PILLAR
SPINOUS PROCESS, C4
INTERVERTEBRAL SPACE

B

Figure 14–1 (*Continued*)

(*Illustration continued on the following page*)

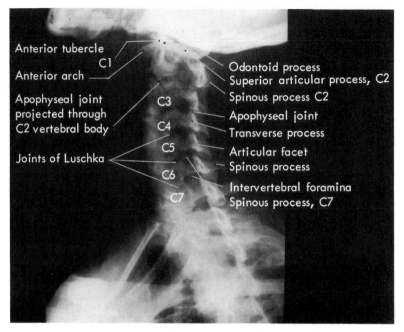

C

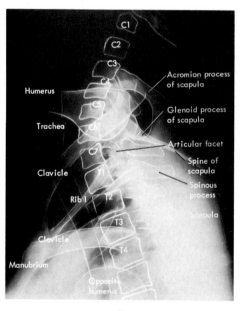

D

Figure 14–1 (*Continued*)   *C.* Oblique view of the cervical spine with major anatomic parts labeled.
D. Lateral (slightly oblique) view of upper two thoracic segments (Twining position).

Normal Sagittal Measurements

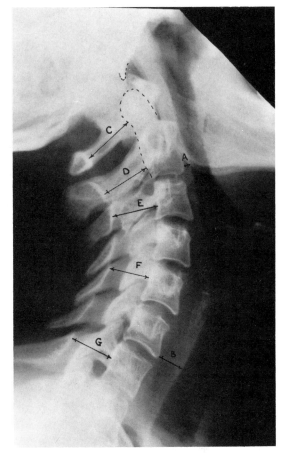

Figure 14–2 Normal lateral view of neck indicating regions evaluated. *A.* Retropharyngeal space, second cervical vertebra. *B.* Retrotracheal space, sixth cervical vertebra. *C* to *G.* Cervical spinal canal. *C,* first cervical vertebra; *D,* second cervical vertebra; *E,* third cervical vertebra; *F,* fifth cervical vertebra; *G,* seventh cervical vertebra. (From Wholey, M. H., Brewer, A. J., and Baker, H. L., Jr.: Radiology *71*: 350, 1958.)

NORMAL SAGITTAL MEASUREMENTS*

Region Evaluated	Normal Sagittal Measurements for Children 15 Years and Under (120 cases)		Normal Sagittal Measurements for Adults (480 cases)	
	AVERAGE (MM.)	RANGE (MM.)	AVERAGE (MM.)	RANGE (MM.)
Retropharyngeal space	3.5	2–7	3.4	1–7
Retrotracheal space	7.9	5–14	14.0	9–22
Cervical spinal canal:				
At first cervical vertebra	21.9	18–27	21.4	16–30
At second cervical vertebra	20.9	18–25	19.2	16–28
At third cervical vertebra	17.4	14–21	19.1	14–25
At fifth cervical vertebra	16.5	14–21	18.5	14–25
At seventh cervical vertebra	16.0	15–20	17.5	13–24

*From Wholey, M. H., Brewer, A. J., and Baker, H. L., Jr.: Radiology, *71*:350, 1958.

NORMAL ANATOMY OF THE THORACIC SPINE

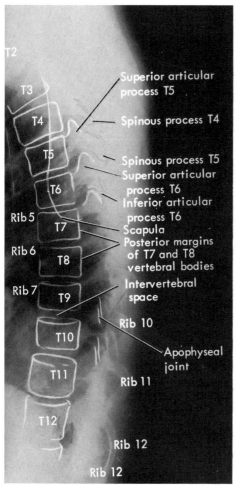

Figure 14-3   Lateral view of thoracic spine; labeled tracing on radiograph.

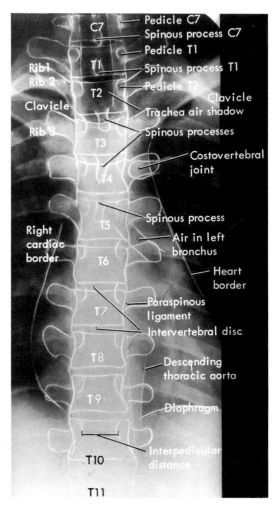

Figure 14-4   Antero-posterior view of the thoracic spine: labeled tracing on radiograph.

NORMAL ANATOMY OF THE LUMBOSACRAL SPINE

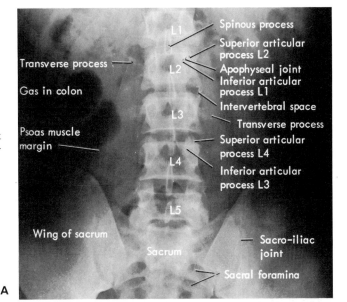

Figure 14–5 *A* and *B*. Antero-posterior and right antero-posterior oblique views of the lumbosacral spine: labeled radiographs.
  C. Lateral radiograph of lumbar spine.

A

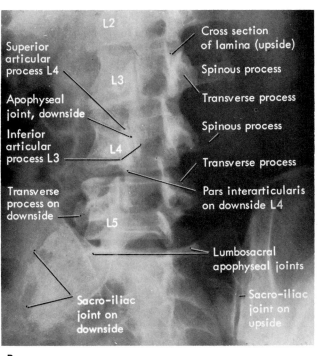

B

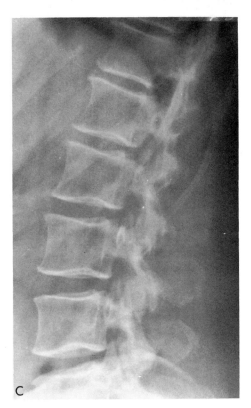

C

Illustration continued on the following page

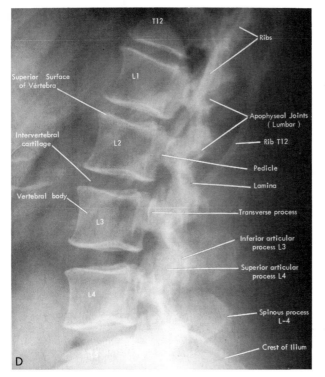

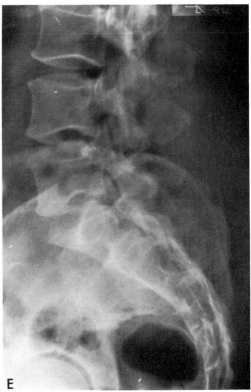

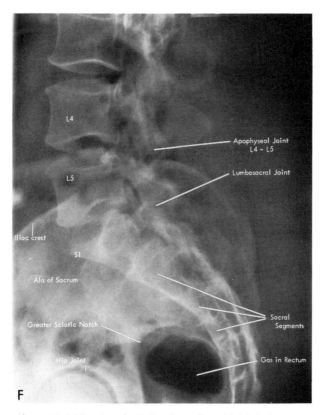

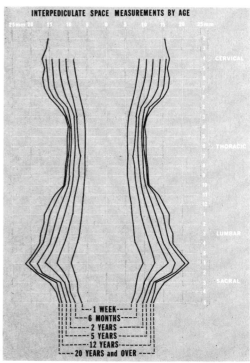

Figure 14–5 (*Continued*) *D*. Lumbar spine with labeled anatomic parts superimposed. *E*. Lateral radiograph of lumbosacral spine. *F*. Lumbosacral spine with anatomic parts labeled.

Figure 14–6 Chart for determination of interpedicular distances of the spine.

CLASSIFICATION OF ABNORMALITIES OF THE SPINE FROM THE RADIOGRAPHIC STANDPOINT

The spine is analyzed in relation to the usual classification of radiographic pathology, namely, abnormalities of *number, size, and shape* of the individual vertebral segments, *contour* of the spine generally, *density, architecture,* and *function* (study of the spine in motion).

In addition special consideration must be given to the following: *Joint abnormalities of the spine*—the intervertebral disks and true synovial joints are considered separately; and *special contrast studies* of the subarachnoid space (*myelography*).

Abnormalities in Number of Vertebral Segments

Failure of development

Fusion of elements

1. Klippel-Feil deformity—a synostosis of two or more of the cervical segments with varying degrees of partial fusion and malformation giving rise to associated hemivertebrae and irregularities in the laminae and spinous processes.
2. Block vertebrae—a fusion of two or more vertebrae.
3. The occipital vertebra—anomalies of fusion of the occipital bone and C-1 vertebra.
4. Atlantoaxial fusion—an assimilation of the atlas and axis.
5. Lumbarization and sacralization—when the fifth lumbar vertebra is completely assimilated in the sacrum it may be called "sacralization"; when the first sacral segment is integrated into the lumbar spine so that there are functionally six lumbar segments the condition is called "lumbarization."

Supernumerary elements

"BLOCK" VERTEBRAE

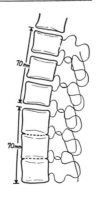

USUALLY HEIGHT OF
"BLOCK" VERTEBRAE =
HEIGHT OF CORRESPONDING
VERTEBRAE + INTERSPACES

Figure 14–7   Block vertebrae.

Abnormalities of Shape and Size

1. Congenital absence of the dens
2. Congenital absence of pedicles and articular facets
3. Clefts in vertebrae
   a. Coronal cleft
   b. Sagittal cleft
   c. Cleft spinous processes
      (1) With meningocele or myelomeningocele
      (2) Failure of fusion of neural arches in cleidocranial dysostosis
4. Increase in size (acromegaly, Paget's disease, fluorosis)
5. Platyspondyly (hypothyroidism, mucopolysaccharidoses)
6. Vertebra plana—Calvé's disease (eosinophilic granuloma, pathologic compression)
7. Biconcave vertebrae ("fishlike" vertebrae, osteoporosis, osteomalacia)
8. End-plate indentations
   a. Anterior: osteochondroses, epiphysitis
   b. Central ovoid: Schmorl's nodes
   c. Central "squared": sickle cell anemia, thalassemia
   d. Posterior: cretinism
   e. Entire: Scheuermann's disease (juvenile kyphosis)
9. Vertebral body indentations
   a. Anterior: aneurysm or pulsating masses
   b. Posterior: neurofibromatosis, intraspinous masses
10. Wedged vertebrae
    a. Trauma
    b. Infection
    c. Metastatic disease
    d. Hemivertebrae
11. Tonguelike anterior appearance
    a. Beaking of mucopolysaccharidoses
12. Butterfly vertebrae due to anomalous development

Some Abnormalities in Size and Shape

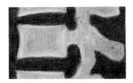

NORMAL

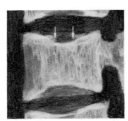

STEP-LIKE INDENTATION
END PLATES
(SICKLE CELL ANEMIA)

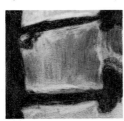

EPIPHYSITIS
SCHEUERMANN'S DISEASE

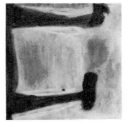

INCREASE HEIGHT
(ACROMEGALY)

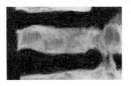

FLATTENED OSTEO-
CHONDRODYSTROPHY

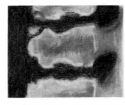

EPIPHYSITIS ADVANCED
WEDGED AND
UNDULATING END-PLATES
(ADVANCED
SCHEUERMANN'S DISEASE)

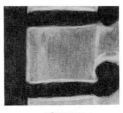

SQUARED
(TURNER'S SYNDROME)

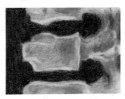

PERSISTANT EPIPHYSIS
INCREASED INTERSPACES
(CRETINISM
HYPOTHYROIDISM)

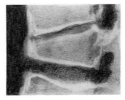

VERTEBRA PLANA
RETICULOENDOTHELIOSIS
EOSINOPHILIC GRANULOMA

Figure 14–8

Abnormalities of Radiodensity and Architecture

1. Homogeneously lucent
   a. Osteogenesis imperfecta
   b. Hypophosphatasia
   c. Primary hyperparathyroidism
   d. Cushing's syndrome
   e. Osteoporosis
   f. Osteomalacia
   g. Rickets (hypovitaminosis D)
   h. Multiple myeloma
   i. Ewing's sarcoma (occasionally, entire spine, but usually localized)
   j. Sickle cell anemia
   k. Thalassemia
2. Homogeneously sclerotic
   a. Osteopetrosis
   b. Ivory vertebrae
   c. Fluoride poisoning
   d. Myelosclerotic anemia

    e. Urticaria pigmentosa (mastocytosis)

    f. Idiopathic hypercalcemia of infancy

    g. Acquired hemolytic anemia

    h. Lymphoma

3. Spotted lucency

    a. Osteomyelitis

          Syphilitic

          Pyogenic

          Fungal

    b. Metastatic neoplasia and multiple myeloma

    c. Chordomas

    d. Sacrococcygeal teratoma

    e. Giant cell tumor

    f. Benign chondroblastoma

    g. Aneurysmal bone cyst

    h. Cystic angiomatosis

    i. Benign osteoblastoma (giant osteoid osteoma)

    j. Vertebral epiphysitis (Scheuermann's disease)

    k. Traumatic changes in the spine—Special considerations in each region of the spine

    l. Spondylolysis; spondylolisthesis; pseudospondylolisthesis; reverse spondylolisthesis

    m. Reticuloendothelioses, such as eosinophilic granuloma

4. Spotted sclerosis

    a. Osteopoikilosis

    b. Congenital stippled epiphysis

    c. Tuberous sclerosis

    d. Sclerotic bone islands

    e. Neoplastic metastatic disease

    f. Spinal lymphomas

    g. Osteoid osteoma

    h. Urticaria pigmentosa (mastocytosis)

5. Vertical irregular lucency and sclerosis

    a. Hemangioma

    b. Osteopathia striata (Voorhoeve's disease)

    c. Sickle cell disease

6. Boxlike sclerosis

    a. Paget's disease (osteitis deformans)

    b. Idiopathic hypercalcemia of infancy

7. Indiscriminate lucency and sclerosis

    a. Fibrous dysplasia

    b. Metastatic neoplasia:

          Malignant lymphomas

    c. Radiation effects on vertebrae

8. Spur formations with or without paraspinous ligamentous calcification

    a. Spondylosis deformans

    b. Syphilitic spondylitis

    c. Rheumatoid spondylitis

    d. Ankylosing spondylitis

    e. Ochronosis

Some Abnormalities in Architecture

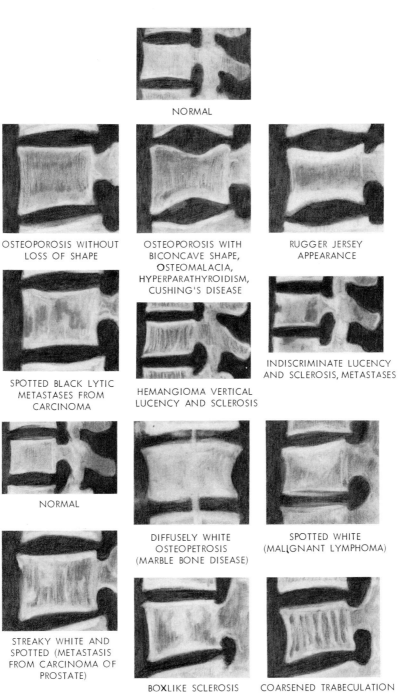

Figure 14–9   General categories of roentgen changes in the architecture of vertebrae.

Abnormalities of Contour and Alignment of the Spine as a Whole

The Normal Curvature of the Spine. These curves are illustrated in Figure 14–10. The major change with age occurs in the cervicothoracic junction when the child begins to lift its head and to assume the erect posture.

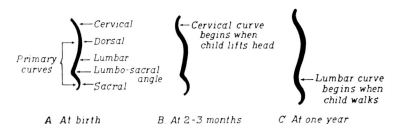

CHANGES IN SPINAL CURVATURE WITH AGE

Primary curves
— Cervical
— Dorsal
— Lumbar
— Lumbo-sacral angle
— Sacral

— Cervical curve begins when child lifts head

— Lumbar curve begins when child walks

A At birth   B At 2-3 months   C At one year

Figure 14–10 Changes in spinal curvature with age. (From Meschan, I., and Farrer-Meschan, R. M. F.: Radiology, *70*:637–648, 1958.)

Definition of Terms

Scoliosis: lateral curvature and usually an associated rotation of several vertebrae in the longitudinal axis.
Lordosis: increased concavity in the spine on the posterior aspect.
Kyphosis: angulation of the spine on its posterior aspect.

Disease Entities with Kyphosis or Scoliosis

1. Congenital torticollis
2. Morquio's disease
3. Hurler's disease

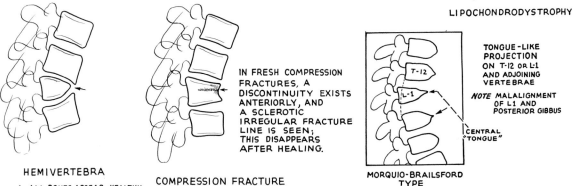

LIPOCHONDRODYSTROPHY

HEMIVERTEBRA

1. ALL *BONES APPEAR HEALTHY.*
2. *ANTERIOR HALF OF VERTEBRA IS ABSENT, NOT COMPRESSED.*
3. *ADJACENT VERTEBRAE ARE EXPANDED TO FIT DEFORMITY.*
4. *NO BULGING ANTERIORLY.*
5. *OTHER DEVELOPMENTAL ABNORMALITIES (RIB) MAY BE PRESENT.*
6. *INTERSPACES ARE WELL PRESERVED.*

COMPRESSION FRACTURE

IN FRESH COMPRESSION FRACTURES, A DISCONTINUITY EXISTS ANTERIORLY, AND A SCLEROTIC IRREGULAR FRACTURE LINE IS SEEN; THIS DISAPPEARS AFTER HEALING.

MORQUIO-BRAILSFORD TYPE

T-12
L-1
CENTRAL "TONGUE"

TONGUE-LIKE PROJECTION ON T-12 OR L-1 AND ADJOINING VERTEBRAE

NOTE MALALIGNMENT OF L1 AND POSTERIOR GIBBUS

Figure 14–11 Various types of wedged vertebral bodies.

4. Arthrogryposis multiplex congenita
5. Mongolism
6. Turner's syndrome
7. Fractures and dislocation
8. Juvenile kyphosis (osteochondrosis; Scheuermann's disease)

Abnormalities of Vertebral Alignment – One Vertebra with Another

1. Hemivertebrae
2. Atlantoaxial subluxation
3. Trauma
4. Spondylolisthesis
5. Pseudospondylolisthesis
6. Reverse spondylolisthesis

A Radiographic Analysis of Spondylolisthesis

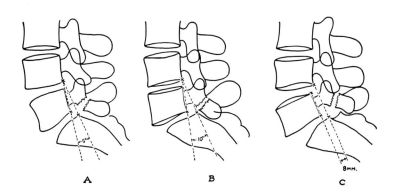

A RADIOGRAPHIC ANALYSIS OF SPONDYLOLISTHESIS

TRACINGS OF RADIOGRAPHS OF SUBJECTS WITH SPONDYLOLISTHESIS.
THE LINES EITHER INTERSECT ABOVE THE FIFTH LUMBAR VERTEBRA
AND FORM AN ANGLE EXCEEDING 2° (A and B) OR REMAIN PARALLEL,
BUT ARE MORE THAN 3 MM. APART (C).

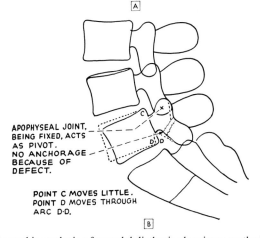

APOPHYSEAL JOINT, BEING FIXED, ACTS AS PIVOT. NO ANCHORAGE BECAUSE OF DEFECT.

POINT C MOVES LITTLE.
POINT D MOVES THROUGH ARC D·D.

Figure 14–12 *A.* Radiographic analysis of spondylolisthesis showing a method of lining and detection. *B.* Diagram illustrating the usual mechanism of spondylolisthesis.

Joint Abnormalities of the Spine

1. Anatomic considerations
2. Disease entities
    a. Atlantoaxial fusion
    b. Alkaptonuria and ochronosis
    c. Ankylosing spondylitis
    d. Rheumatoid arthritis
        (1) Juvenile
        (2) Adult
        (3) Reiter's syndrome
    e. Ulcerative colitic arthritis
    f. Neuropathic arthropathy of the spine
    g. Paraplegic neuroarthropathy
    h. Traumatic arthropathy
    i. Intervertebral disk alterations
        (1) Injuries
        (2) Infections
        (3) Herniations
        (4) "Vacuum" phenomenon
    j. Hypervitaminosis A

Anatomic Considerations

The joints of the spine fall into two categories: (1) synovial joints or diarthroses, and (2) amphiarthroses.

The synovial joints may be found in the following sites:

1. Atlantoaxial joint.
2. Synovial joint between the occipital condyle and C-1.
3. Intervertebral joints between the articular processes of the vertebrae.
4. The costotransverse and costovertebral synovial joints: joints between the ribs and the transverse processes and vertebral bodies respectively.
5. The sacroiliac joints—synovial joints between the wings of the sacrum and the iliac bones.

The amphiarthrodial joints are the fibrocartilaginous junctions between the intervertebral disks and the vertebral endplates.

Ankylosing Spondylitis vs. Rheumatoid Arthritis of the Spine (Figure 14-13)

Definition. Ankylosing spondylitis and rheumatoid arthritis resemble one another closely but have been separated from one another on the following differential points:

1. There is a difference in incidence in males and females.

2. There is an absence of streptococcal and sheep red cell agglutinins in ankylosing spondylitis.

3. Subcutaneous nodules are absent in pure ankylosing spondylitis.

4. Severe osteoporotic changes in peripheral joints occur with rheumatoid arthritis, whereas this does not ordinarily occur with ankylosing spondylitis with peripheral joint involvement.

5. Calcification of the paraspinal ligaments is frequent in ankylosing spondylitis but is not present with rheumatoid arthritis.

6. Sacroiliac and spinal changes are predominant with ankylosing spondylitis while these are rare in rheumatoid arthritis. The cervical spine, however, is involved frequently with rheumatoid arthritis.

Radiographic Manifestations

The paraspinous ligaments become thinly calcified and ultimately produce the so-called "bamboo" appearance. There is gradual loss of definition of the subarticular bone to the point of complete obliteration of the intervertebral joint.

The sacroiliac joints are involved very early in ankylosing spondylitis, perhaps in 98 per cent of cases (Forester). There are stages of involvement of the sacroiliac joints: (1) cloudy opacities in the para-articular bones; (2) spotted osteoporosis of the subchondral bone; (3) ultimate blurred obliteration of the joint space itself with complete ankylosis.

Ankylosing spondylitis is primarily a disease involving the synovial joints and intervertebral joints and affects the bones immediately adjoining these joint areas. Rheumatoid arthritis, on the other hand, may affect the bones of the vertebral bodies away from the joint.

The intervertebral disks may appear either wide or narrowed.

The joints between the ribs and the dorsal vertebrae are also involved, ultimately leading to a fixation of the thoracic cage and respiratory difficulties.

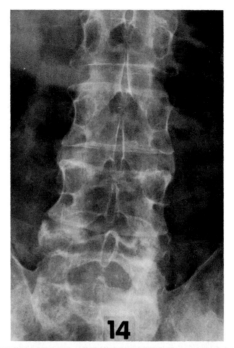

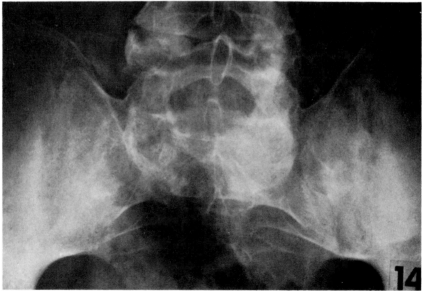

Figure 14–13   Ankylosing spondylitis. *A*. Paraspinous ligamentous calcification and ankylosis of synovial joints. *B*. Advanced sacroiliac arthritis.

Juvenile Rheumatoid Arthritis

Definition. Rheumatoid arthritis in the very young. The joints most commonly affected are hand, wrist, foot, ankle, knee, and temporomandibular joints. The cervical spine, however, is involved in about 13 per cent of the cases (Epstein, 1969).

Radiographic Manifestations

Early: no radiologic changes are apparent in the spine.

Late: x-ray findings are similar to those previously described for ankylosing spondylarthritis. Decalcification of the vertebral body may take place. The intervertebral disks even appear to expand. Certain parts of vertebral bodies are especially prone to osteoporosis, especially at the atlantoaxial junction where subluxation may result.

Later in life, ankylosis of the apophyseal joints of the upper cervical vertebrae may occur. The antero-posterior diameter of the vertebrae may appear diminished and the entire process tends to simulate a block vertebra.

Reiter's Syndrome

Definition. Disease of unknown etiology consisting of: (1) arthritis resembling rheumatoid arthritis; (2) conjunctivitis; (3) urethritis. (4) Involvement of the spine and sacroiliac joints is very infrequent (Hollander et al.). (5) In cases reported by Good (1962) Reiter's syndrome appeared to be closely associated with ankylosing spondylitis and clearly separable from rheumatoid arthritis involving the spine.

Spondylosis Deformans

Definition. Degenerative condition usually beginning in early middle age and characterized by spur formations along the margins of vertebral bodies with paraspinous ligamentous calcifications. Spurs may protrude into the spinal canal and the intervertebral foramina, producing pressure upon adjoining nerve structures.

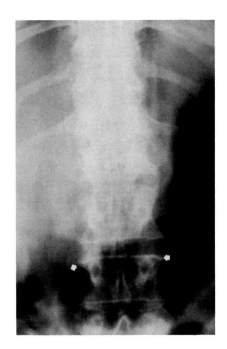

Figure 14–14 Antero-posterior view of lower thoracic and lumbar spine in deforming spondylosis. Note the lipping of the vertebrae (arrows) and the partial bridging of adjoining interspaces.

Intervertebral Disk Alterations

Disk Injuries. Disk injury may produce degeneration, fragmentation, and ultimately protrusion or herniation of the injured disk.

RADIOGRAPHIC MANIFESTATIONS

Narrowness of the interspace.
Degenerate lipping of adjoining vertebral bodies and end-plates.
Undulation and irregularity of the end-plates of adjoining vertebral bodies.
Degenerative calcification of portions or all of the intervertebral disks.
Protrusion posteriorly toward the spinal canal, best demonstrated by myelography.
"Vacuum phenomenon" in intervertebral disks, defined as radiolucent streaks in the intervertebral space presumably representing gas in the intervertebral disk region.

Disk Infections. In view of the fact that the intervertebral disk is avascular, direct infection of the intervertebral disk is rare. However, extension from an adjoining inflammatory process may occur. Thus, tuberculosis and other infectious processes may result in destructive changes in intervertebral disks. These have been previously described.

Intervertebral disk calcification, although very rare in children, has been reported by a number of investigators (Weens, Melnick, and Silverman). These calcifications may occur at any age, appear most frequently in the cervical spine, and do, on occasion, disappear over a period of several months.

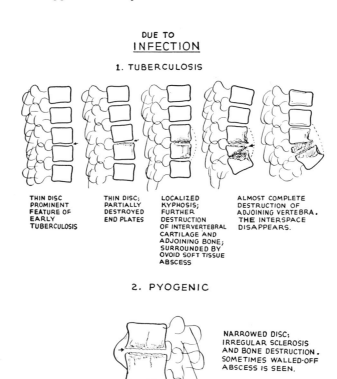

DUE TO
INFECTION

1. TUBERCULOSIS

THIN DISC PROMINENT FEATURE OF EARLY TUBERCULOSIS

THIN DISC; PARTIALLY DESTROYED END PLATES

LOCALIZED KYPHOSIS; FURTHER DESTRUCTION OF INTERVERTEBRAL CARTILAGE AND ADJOINING BONE; SURROUNDED BY OVOID SOFT TISSUE ABSCESS

ALMOST COMPLETE DESTRUCTION OF ADJOINING VERTEBRA. THE INTERSPACE DISAPPEARS.

2. PYOGENIC

NARROWED DISC; IRREGULAR SCLEROSIS AND BONE DESTRUCTION. SOMETIMES WALLED-OFF ABSCESS IS SEEN.

Figure 14–15 Diagram illustrating tuberculous and pyogenic spondylitis.

GENERAL COMMENTS CONCERNING MYELOGRAPHY

Definition. Examination of the subarachnoid space of the spinal column by the injection of a suitable contrast material into this space. This contrast material may be gaseous or a positive contrast material such as Pantopaque.

Myelography is Particularly Helpful in:

1. Demonstrating an operable lesion when the clinical and laboratory data are inconclusive.
2. Confirming or excluding an intraspinal lesion when all other methods have failed to establish a diagnosis.
3. Establishing the extent of a known lesion and possibly in giving some indication of its general pathologic nature.
4. Excluding multiple lesions, since approximately 4 per cent of spinal neoplasms are multiple.
5. Localizing the level of the lesion accurately prior to operation.
6. Determining the cause of recurrent symptoms in the patient with a previous laminectomy.
7. Medicolegal circumstances in which myelography may help to establish the presence or absence of a lesion, although a negative myelogram is not conclusive.

Questions — Chapter 14

1. Indicate some of the abnormalities in number of vertebral segments.
2. What is meant by the term block vertebrae?
3. What is meant by the term occipital vertebra?
4. What is meant by the terms lumbarization and sacralization?
5. What is the clinical importance of congenital absence of the dens?
6. What is the clinical significance of cleft spinous processes?
7. What is the clinical significance of a meningocele and how would you recognize this radiologically? Where are meningoceles most frequently situated?
8. What categories of abnormalities of radiodensity and architecture do we recognize?
9. Name some of the disease entities which are responsible for the homogeneously sclerotic appearance of vertebrae.
10. Name some of the disease entities which are characterized by a spotted radiolucency of vertebrae.
11. Describe some of the differential features between tuberculous and nontuberculous involvement of vertebrae.
12. Define "vertebral epiphysitis." Is this truly an inflammatory process? What is the pathogenesis of lesions and what is their ultimate radiographic appearance?
13. Describe some of the traumatic changes in the spine. What are the most frequent appearances in the cervical region, the thoracic region, and the lumbosacral region?
14. Define the following terms; spondylolysis; spondylolisthesis.
15. Indicate five or six disease entities characterized by spotted osteosclerosis of vertebrae.
16. Describe some of the radiographic appearances of urticaria pigmentosa as it affects the spine.
17. What is the most frequent lesion of vertebral bodies which is characterized by vertical irregular radiolucency and sclerosis?
18. What is the most frequent disease affecting vertebrae which is characterized by boxlike sclerosis or a "picture frame" appearance?
19. What differential features in respect to spur formation can you enumerate in respect

to the following: spondylosis deformans; syphilitic spondylitis; ankylosing spondylitis; rheumatoid spondylitis?

20. Define the following terms: (1) scoliosis; (2) lordosis; (3) kyphosis; (4) gibbus; (5) primary curvature in scoliosis; (6) secondary curvature in scoliosis.

21. Describe the deformity in Klippel-Feil deformity.

22. What is meant by "hemivertebrae"?

23. What is meant by atlantoaxial subluxation and what are some of its causes?

24. What types of joints are found in the spine? Which of these are synovial joints?

25. Describe the differences which are generally recognized between ankylosing spondylitis and rheumatoid arthritis as it affects the spine in both the juvenile and adult.

26. What is the radiographic appearance when the intervertebral disk is injured?

27. What is the radiographic appearance when infection involves the intervertebral disk? Name some agents which are responsible for this.

28. What is meant by the term "herniated disks"? Where is it found most frequently? How is it best demonstrated radiologically?

29. Relate some of the indications for myelography.

30. How would you distinguish between intramedullary, extramedullary, and intradural or extradural lesions of the spine?

31. List some lesions (approximately ten) which can be identified by myelography.

15

Introduction to Roentgenologic
Analysis of the Chest

INTRODUCTION

Basic Anatomy Review

Upper Air Passages, Larynx (see Chapter 14)

Bronchial Distribution of the Lung. The bronchial distribution of the lung is illustrated in Figure 15–2 in frontal, lateral, and oblique projections.

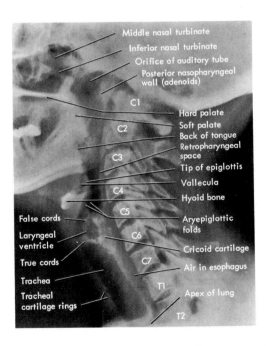
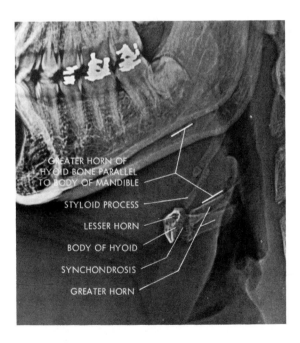

Figure 15–1 *A*. Lateral view of upper air passages and soft tissues of the neck, labeled. *B*. Further xeroradiographic study of the soft tissues of the upper neck to demonstrate the parallelism of the greater horn of the hyoid bone with the inferior margin of the body of the mandible. Other portions of the hyoid bone are also labeled.

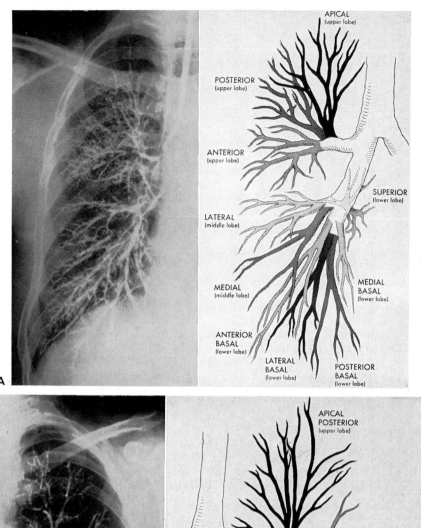

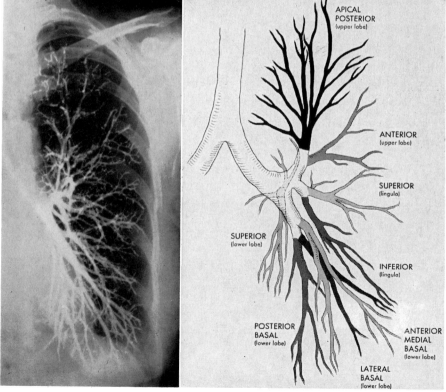

Figure 15–2 The normal human bronchial tree. *A*. Right postero-anterior projection. *B*. Left postero-anterior projection. (From Lehman, J. S., and Crellin, J. A.: Medical Radiography and Photography *31*, 1955.)

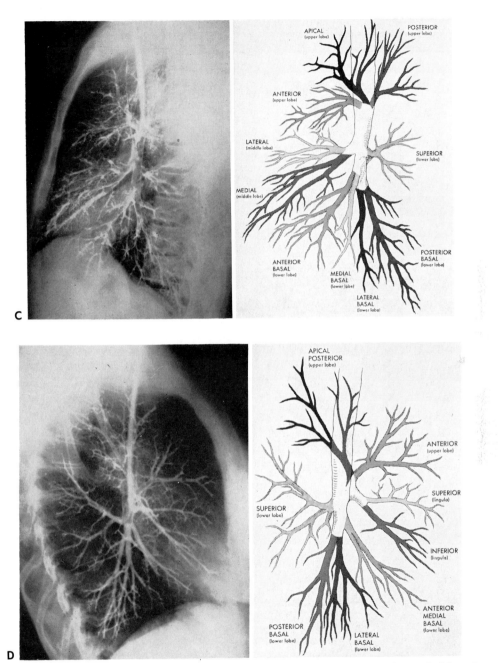

Figure 15–2 (*Continued*)   The normal human bronchial tree. *C*. Right lateral projection. *D*. Left lateral projection. (From Lehman, J. S., and Crellin, J. A.: Medical Radiography and Photography *31*, 1955.)

The Primary Lung Lobule and the Acinus. The *primary lobule* of Miller comprises a 1 to 1.5 mm. diameter air space supplied by each alveolar duct, its various vessels, atria, and alveoli.

The *acinus* represents that portion of the lung parenchyma distal to one terminal bronchiole—i.e., all of the respiratory bronchioles, alveolar ducts, and alveoli supplied by this terminal bronchiole. It measures approximately 5 to 7 mm. in diameter and contains approximately 18 last order respiratory bronchioles. Each alveolar duct in turn supplies a family of approximately 20 to 25 alveoli. A *secondary lobule* (Reid and Simon) consists of a cluster of 3 to 5 terminal bronchioles forming the millimeter pattern of branching at the end of a bronchial pathway, together with the respiratory tissue which they supply. Each secondary lobule measures 1 to 1.5 cm. in diameter (Fig. 15–3).

The acinus and secondary lobule are visible radiographically when filled with water density material.

The *alveolar pores* (pores of Kohn) are openings in the alveolar wall about 10 to 15 μ in diameter allowing "collateral air drift" into an adjoining air space or acinus.

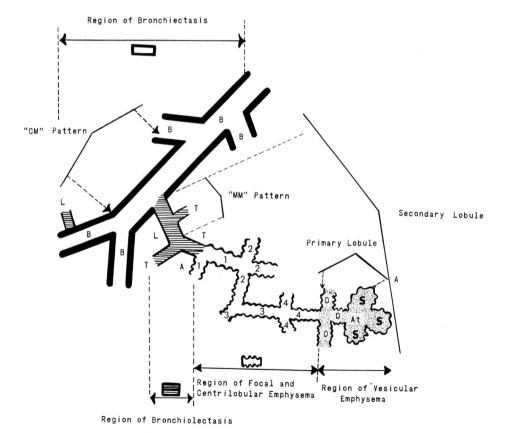

Figure 15–3   The "secondary lobule" (diagram).

The Pulmonary Vascular System

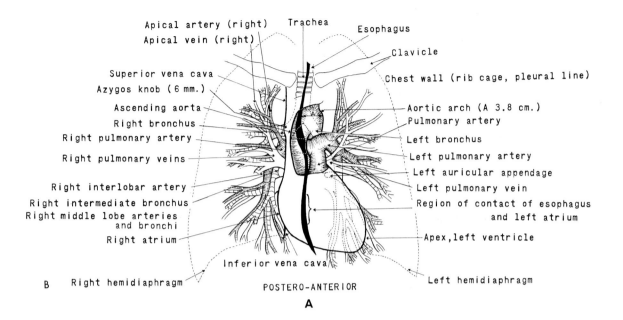

A

Apical artery (right)
Apical vein (right)
Trachea
Esophagus
Clavicle
Chest wall (rib cage, pleural line)
Superior vena cava
Azygos knob (6 mm.)
Ascending aorta
Right bronchus
Right pulmonary artery
Right pulmonary veins
Right interlobar artery
Right intermediate bronchus
Right middle lobe arteries
    and bronchi
Right atrium
Aortic arch (A 3.8 cm.)
Pulmonary artery
Left bronchus
Left pulmonary artery
Left auricular appendage
Left pulmonary vein
Region of contact of esophagus
    and left atrium
Apex, left ventricle
Inferior vena cava
B   Right hemidiaphragm
POSTERO-ANTERIOR
Left hemidiaphragm

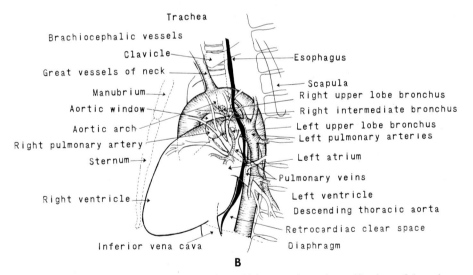

B

LATERAL VIEW OF CHEST

Trachea
Brachiocephalic vessels
Clavicle
Great vessels of neck
Manubrium
Aortic window
Aortic arch
Right pulmonary artery
Sternum
Right ventricle
Inferior vena cava
Esophagus
Scapula
Right upper lobe bronchus
Right intermediate bronchus
Left upper lobe bronchus
Left pulmonary arteries
Left atrium
Pulmonary veins
Left ventricle
Descending thoracic aorta
Retrocardiac clear space
Diaphragm

Figure 15–4 *A* and *B*. Relationships of tracheobronchial tree to the main ramifications of the pulmonary artery.

Postero-anterior View

Important facets with respect to the pulmonary vascular system are summarized as follows (Figure 15–4):

1. The main pulmonary artery forms a segment of the left border of the heart, and at the level of the carina and slightly to the left of the midline it bifurcates into right and left branches.

2. The left branch extends obliquely upward toward the left pulmonary apex, whereas the right branch is almost horizontal in position and *always relatively lower than the left pulmonary artery.*

3. The left hilus is higher than the right in 97 per cent of normal subjects.

4. The superior branch of the right pulmonary artery curves *anteriorly* over the upper lobe bronchus and divides into three branches. *It can usually be identified just anterior and to the left of the bronchus of the upper lobe. The vein is usually identified lateral to the bronchus* in a similar position in the upper lobe so that venous and arterial patterns can be readily distinguished.

5. The interlobar artery, which is a continuation of the pulmonary artery, passes in front of the intermediate bronchus and on the lateral aspect of this bronchus, descending into the major fissure. It supplies one branch to the middle lobe, one to the superior segment of the lower lobe, and four which accompany the similar basilar bronchi of the lower lobe.

6. The left pulmonary artery is more difficult to follow into the periphery of the lung. It is on a more posterior plane than the right. The upper of its two divisions sends two or more branches to the apical posterior segments and one to the anterior segment of the upper lobe. The other ramifications, all similar in distribution to comparable bronchi, are difficult to identify.

The spatial distribution of pulmonary veins is quite variable but the prevailing patterns comprise *two large veins on each side which enter the mediastinum at a level below the pulmonary arteries and anterior to them.* On the left side, superior and inferior pulmonary veins drain the upper and lower lobes respectively.

Identification of pulmonary arteries and veins as well as trachea and bronchi is of importance in the lateral projection also and is indicated in Figure 15–4 B.

Lateral View

TRACHEA. The region of first reference is the trachea. Both upper lobe bronchi course horizontally for a short distance from their origins in the main stem bronchi with the right upper lobe bronchus originating superior to the left upper lobe bronchus. The lumina of these structures are visible in the lateral view.

THE RIGHT PULMONARY ARTERY lies anterior to the tracheobronchial air column. The left pulmonary artery is somewhat superior to the right pulmonary artery and posterior to the tracheobronchial air shadow.

THE PULMONARY VEINS are quite variable. In most people they drain into the left atrium bilaterally through two main trunks. They tend to be confluent near their entry into the left atrium, contributing to the hilar shadow.

On the right side, the superior pulmonary vein enters the left atrium below the right pulmonary artery. This, unfortunately, is highly variable and slight degrees of rotation will cause even greater variability in appearance. The inferior pulmonary vein is inferior and posterior to the ipsilateral superior vein.

The upper lobe veins on the left converge anterior and inferior to the left upper lobe bronchus to form the superior pulmonary vein. The superior pulmonary vein and the immediately adjacent left atrium lie anterior to the left lower lobe bronchus.

The left inferior pulmonary vein usually enters the left atrium inferiorly and posterior to the superior vein. Often the veins on the left form a common trunk prior to draining into the left atrium.

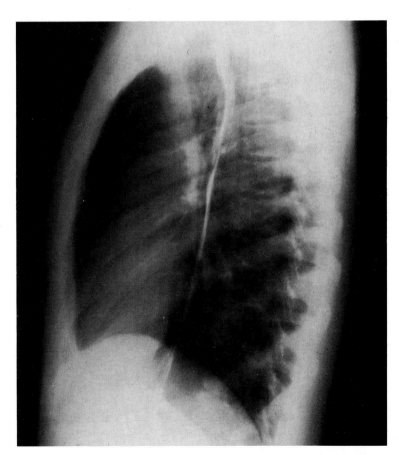

Figure 15-5 Normal lateral radiograph of the chest.

The Pleura and Interlobar Fissures (Figure 15–6)

Ordinarily, the pleura is not visualized unless it contains excessive fluid or foreign tissue such as inflammation or neoplasm. When the pleural shadow can be identified it is usually indicative of an active or previous abnormality.

The interlobar fissures may frequently be identified on normal routine radiographs of the chest and impart valuable information in respect to the volume of the enclosed lobe. Identification of the interlobar fissure between the right upper and middle lobe in frontal perspective and the major and minor fissures in the lateral views is especially frequent.

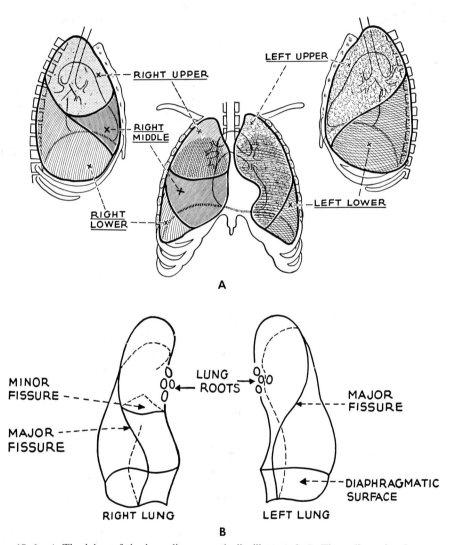

Figure 15–6   *A.* The lobes of the lung diagrammatically illustrated. *B.* Three-dimensional concept of interlobar fissures.

Heart and Mediastinum. The radiology of the heart and mediastinum is presented in subsequent chapters (Chapters 21, 22, and 23) for convenience in description. The heart, mediastinum, and lungs together form an integral, inseparable unit.

RADIOLOGIC METHODS OF EXAMINATION OF THE CHEST

1. Chest fluoroscopy
2. Postero-anterior and lateral films of the chest
3. Special film studies, including:
     a. Lateral decubitus films (patient on side, horizontal x-ray beam. Useful for demonstrating small pleural effusions)
     b. Right or left (or both) postero-anterior oblique films of the chest
     c. Apical lordotic projection (especially useful for demonstration of the lung apices and anterior mediastinum on tangent)
     d. Body section studies (tomography)
     e. Bucky films and air gap studies
     f. Esophagrams
     g. Angiocardiograms
     h. Diagnostic pneumothroax and pneumopericardium
     i. Bronchial brushing
     j. Lymphangiography
     k. Bronchography

METHODS OF STUDYING RADIOGRAPHS OF THE CHEST

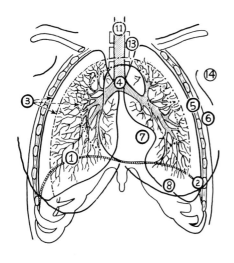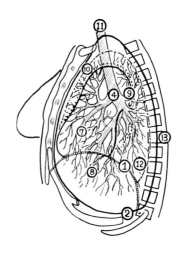

1. DIAPHRAGM	5. RIBS AND PLEURA	9. HILI ON LATERAL VIEW
2. COSTOPHRENIC SINUSES	*6. THORACIC WALL	10. ANT. MEDIASTINUM
3. ZONES OF LUNG FIELDS	7. HEART	11. TRACHEA IN NECK
4. TRACHEA IN THORAX AND HILI	8. UNDER DIAPHRAGM	12. POST. MEDIASTINUM
		13. VERTEBRA
		*14. SOFT TISSUES OF CHEST WALL AND AXILLA

Figure 15–7

1. Localize the abnormal shadow with respect to the chest wall, pleura, lung parenchyma, or mediastinum. If localized in the lung, determine the exact lobe or segment involved if possible.
2. Study the level of the diaphragm on each side, noting its general contour and position and any abnormalities contiguous with it.
3. Study the costophrenic and cardiophrenic sinuses in relation to their clarity and sharpness for indication of pleural disease.
4. Survey the lung fields. First compare the two sides in relation to one another. Secondly, divide the lung fields into three zones. The innermost zone contains hilar blood vessels of large caliber, the intermediate or middle zone contains the medium-sized blood vessels, the outer zone contains the very small blood vessels, usually so small that only minimal detection is obtained in the usual radiographs. When any shadows which are extraordinary in any respect appear, therefore, in each of these zones, they immediately attract attention from the standpoint of abnormal pathology.
5. Note the lung apices, particularly, and take care to look "under the bones" so that no actual pulmonary markings of unusual character are overlooked.
6. Study the hilar blood vessels and mediastinum. The position of the trachea and its major ramifications are noted. The trachea is ordinarily located near the midline. A further analysis of the mediastinum will follow in later chapters; here, it is enough to say that a study of the mediastinum cannot be separated from a study of the respiratory system.

   The major hilar blood vessels should be traced so that arteries and veins are distinguished, especially in the lung apices and the lung bases. Is there a "deflection" or "cephalization-of-flow" phenomenon in the upright position so that venous distention is noted? Is there an accentuation of the interstitial pattern? Is there arterial distention?
7. Study the thoracic cage, tracing each rib carefully. The widths and symmetry of the intercostal spaces are evaluated simultaneously. The clavicle, scapulae, and visible bony structures of the neck are noted. Although the skeletal structures of the dorsal spine are not seen adequately for careful diagnosis, it can be noted whether or not there is a scoliosis or other significant spine deformity which may affect the radiographic diagnosis of chest lesions. Is there a sternal depression or deformity, pectus excavatum, or pectus carinatum?
8. Study the soft tissue structures of the thoracic cage (Figure 15–7). Identify the breasts, nipples, areoli, the muscular shadows, particularly the pectoralis major and minor, and the sternocleidomastoids, which very often cast a significant soft tissue shadow across the medial aspect of the lung apices. A tegmental shadow, ordinarily seen above the superior border of the clavicle, must be identified and distinguished from the abnormal.
9. Any unusual pleural shadows are identified. The pleura does not ordinarily cast a significant visible shadow, except occasionally the posterior mediastinal (paraesophageal) stripe to a minimal degree in the costophrenic sinuses and overlying the lung apices. In the region of the lung apices small blebs may occur normally. They are without pathologic significance and must be identified and distinguished from a pathologic process.
10. Identify structures underlying the diaphrgam. A postero-anterior erect chest film offers a very good opportunity for visualizing free air under the diaphragm. Dense areas of calcification such as may occur with calcified cysts of the liver are also identified. The distance of the stomach (fundal air bubble or Magenglase) from the left hemidiaphragm is noted. Is there a filling defect in the fundus? Is the spleen enlarged?

11. In the lateral projection of the chest it is particularly important to identify the *mediastinal shadow* and to form in the mind's eye a concept of the normal in this regard. Identify the left and right pulmonary artery, the trachea, and the bifurcations. We find the lateral projection extremely valuable in detecting abnormal lymphadenopathy or tumor masses in the central mediastinum.

12. In the lateral view identify the *anterior mediastinal clear space* which is just anterior to the cardiac silhouette and underlies the sternal shadow. On occasion the lateral view will be the only projection in which the clear space is obliterated to indicate the presence of a space-occupying lesion in the anterior superior mediastinum.

13. In the lateral projection, the pleural reflection over the internal mammary vessels is studied. Metastases will at times produce detectable masses in this location.

14. In the oblique projections, further care must be exercised to carefully identify the trachea and bronchial structures which can be seen to excellent advantage. The oblique views are also particularly valuable in analysis of the cardiac silhouette, especially when barium delineates the esophagus. This will be described in Chapters 21 and 22.

15. Study the clear pneumonic space in the posterior mediastinum and identify the relationship it has with a posterior margin of the left ventricle and the reflection of the inferior vena cava especially.

16. Study the dorsal spine.

GENERAL CONCEPTS OF RADIOGRAPHIC PATHOLOGY OF LUNG PARENCHYMA

The usual initial approach of the radiologist to the examination of the chest is objective. An effort is made to classify the visualized abnormalities by their radiographic appearances.

Chest lesions are described as radiopaque or radiolucent. The radiopaque lesions may be (1) diffuse in appearance; (2) segmental; (3) nodular; (4) linear; or (5) reticular or reticulonodular.

Diffuse, ill-defined shadows are usually irregular in shape, vary in size from 5 to 10 mm. in diameter (when they have a mulberry appearance) and merge imperceptibly with the surrounding lung. The mulberry pattern usually denotes an *acinar* water density (secondary lobule).

The *segmental shadows* are closely related to the diffuse shadows, except that they are more sharply demarcated, roughly triangular in outline, and denote disease limited to a segment of the lung. These shadows of increased density result from the following:

1. Blockage of a peripheral bronchus;
2. Obstruction of a blood supply to a segment;
3. Compression of a lung segment by an adjoining pathologic process.

An abscess may supervene in any instance.

Nodular shadows are characterized by a clearly demarcated circumscribed outline. These vary from multiple small nodular shadows throughout both lung fields to a single shadow which may achieve a much larger size. The nodular shadows may be solid in density or may show variations in density because of calcific deposits or even air. They may demonstrate a fluid level if abscess formation occurs, and in this instance the walls of the cavity may be thin and uniform or wide and irregular. Each has its separate significance.

Linear (or reticular) shadows may be caused by an increase in size or density of the normal vascular, lymphatic, interstitial, or bronchial markings.

Linear and reticular markings are increased at the site of any area of chronic inflammation or malignant tumor formation—for example, in basal bronchiectasis or pulmonary carcinoma.

The venous vascular markings are increased in congestive heart failure. (An effort is made to distinguish distended veins in their appropriate areas in the lungs.)

Compression of the lung may cause a linear density (atelectasis, or a platelike atelectasis described by Fleischner).

Old organized infarcts may also produce linear shadows.

Chronicity is characterized by clear delimitation of outline, linear streaking in association with a mass and calcification.

Radiolucent abnormalities of the chest may be seen over large areas of parenchyma because of the breakdown of interalveolar septa in emphysema. They may be seen where the pleural cavity contains air, and they may be bilateral, unilateral, or localized to a small area. Small circumscribed areas of radiolucency are seen with pulmonary cysts, or supernatant air in a pulmonary abscess, in which case communication with a bronchus may be postulated.

Calcification in structures due to chronicity of disease, or secondarily to degeneration in tissues, is recognized in the lungs or elsewhere. It is important to note whether the calcification is peripheral to the density or central. Each has its separate pathologic significance.

After these objective classifications are carried out, the radiologist next attempts to reconstruct the pathophysiology of the disease process.

Thereafter, the patient's history and other laboratory evidences are studied, and the diagnosis is thus synthesized.

Questions—Chapter 15

1. Name the important anatomic parts of the upper air passages and larynx.

2. Describe the usual bronchial distribution of the lung, naming the major ramifications.

3. What is meant by the term "primary lung lobule"? What is meant by the term "secondary lobule"?

4. Describe in detail the pulmonary vascular system as it relates to the radiologic depiction. What is the relationship of the left and right pulmonary artery? What is the relationship of the pulmonary veins to the arteries? What is the relative importance of the bronchial arteries?

5. Describe the pleural and interlobar fissures and their approximate positions in the chest.

6. Enumerate the segments of the lungs and indicate their anatomic derivation.

7. What is meant by the term "tenting" and "scalloping" of the diaphragm?

8. What are three fundamental principles which apply to the radiographic examination of the mediastinum?

9. What is meant by the term "lung hilus" and what are the structures that occupy this area?

10. What bony structures compose the thoracic cage?

11. What are the important radiographic methods of examination of the chest?

12. Describe in detail a routine that is useful for studying radiographs of the chest in both the frontal and lateral perspective.

13. What part does bronchography play in the examination of the chest?

14. In the general concepts of the radiographic pathology of lung parenchyma, what are the major subdivisions?

15. Describe the embryologic development of the so-called "azygos" lobe.

16

Radiology of the Diaphragm, Pleura, Thoracic Cage, and Upper Air Passages

THE DIAPHRAGM

Methods of Study

Fluoroscopy for degree and manner of movement.

Films of the chest in full inspiration and expiration to detect extent of excursion Free air under the diaphragm may be detected if the patient is in the erect position.

Pneumoperitoneum may be employed to outline the inferior margin of the diaphragm if it is considered sufficiently important on any clinical basis.

Diaphragm: Abnormalities in Function

Immobility or Fixation

1. From phrenic paralysis or palsy
2. From inflammation
   a. Pleurisy with or without effusion
   b. Subdiaphragmatic abscess, usually accompanied by elevation of diaphragm, pleural effusion, segmental atelectasis, and free air under the diaphragm, all of which are cardinal signs of subdiaphragmatic abscess. Of the cardinal signs of subdiaphragmatic abscess, free air under the diaphragm is the most absolute
3. From pulmonary emphysema: the diaphragm is low and flat because of the persistent expanded state of the lungs

Paradoxical Movement: Upward movement on inspiration, downward movement on expiration.

1. From phrenic paralysis
2. From pneumothorax under tension

Diaphragm: Abnormalities in Position

Bilateral Elevation of the Diaphragm.   Found with:
1. Obesity
2. Abdominal masses
3. Ascites
4. Large liver
5. Pregnancy

Unilateral Elevation of the Diaphragm.   Found with:
1. Decrease in size of hemithorax
2. Weakness or palsy of half of diaphragm
3. Eventration of diaphragm
4. Gastric or colonic distention
5. Liver or splenic enlargement
6. Inflammation, fluid, or abscess under half of diaphragm
7. Interposition of colon
8. Diaphragmatic tumor

Small differences may be of no significance

Bilateral Low Position of the Diaphragm.   Found with:
1. Chronic pulmonary emphysema (with diminished respiratory excursion, "teardrop"-shaped heart, flared ribs, prominent pulmonary arteries, increased radiability of the anterior mediastinum)
2. Bilateral pneumothorax
3. Asthenic build

Unilateral Low Position of the Diaphragm as in check-valve obstruction of a bronchus by a foreign body.

General Comment.   In this instance it must be established that the opposite side is not elevated. This usually suggests unilateral check-valve type obstruction which may be due to either a foreign body or a neoplasm.

Radiologic Aspects

1. The additional film in full expiration will determine that the low position of the diaphragm persists in both phases of respiration.
2. During fluoroscopy, a sway of the mediastinum may be observed so that it moves toward the side which is obstructed in full inspiration, and away from the side which is obstructed in full expiration.

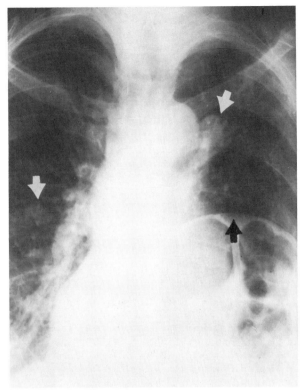

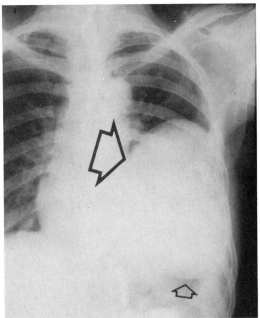

Figure 16–2 Leiomyoma of the diaphragm.

Figure 16–1 Marked elevation of the left hemidiaphragm with gas-containing loops of the colon and stomach projected beneath this. In this patient there were tumorlets of the lung as demonstrated by the arrows.

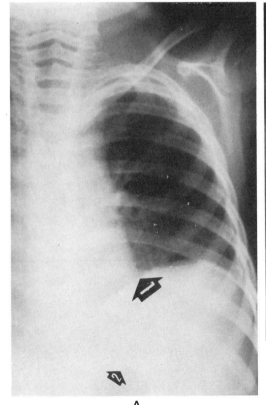

A

B

Figure 16–3 *A* and *B*. Infrapulmonary effusion simulating a tumor of the diaphragm, but in the lateral decubitus the free flow of the fluid from beneath the lung along the lateral chest wall establishes the diagnosis.

Diaphragm: Changes in Shape

Changes in diaphragmatic contour are somewhat difficult to interpret in view of the normal variations such as "scalloping" or "tenting." On the other hand, a local bulge or elevation of the diaphgram may be caused by:

1. Tumor within the diaphragm
2. Pleural tumor
3. Infrapulmonary encapsulated fluid (Figure 16–3B)
4. Subdiaphragmatic cyst, tumor, or encapsulation of fluid
5. Tumor of an enlarged organ beneath the diaphragm, raising it locally, such as occurs with the liver.

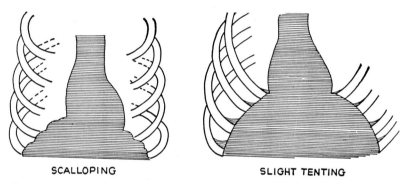

SCALLOPING   SLIGHT TENTING

Figure 16–4   Diagrammatic illustration of tenting and scalloping of the diaphragm.

Diaphragm: Abnormalities in Size and Integrity

Methods of Radiographic Recognition

1. An abdominal organ in the chest may be recognized either by its gas content or by introducing barium in the gastrointestinal tract (Chapters 27 through 30).
2. Increased intra-abdominal pressure can be shown by the Valsalva and Mueller tests with patient in the prone position.
3. Pneumoperitoneum—care must be exercised since pneumothorax may result, necessitating immediate withdrawal of air.
4. Liver or pancreas radioisotopic scans or scintiphotos may be superimposed over a chest radiograph.

Classification of Diaphragmatic Hernias

1. Traumatic through tear in the diaphragm
2. Through esophageal hiatus
3. Through foramen of Morgagni anteriorly
4. Through pleuroperitoneal hiatus (foramen of Bochdalek) posteriorly

Classification of Hernias Through Esophageal Hiatus (Chapter 27)

1. Congenital shortening of the esophagus. These are rare.
2. Paraesophageal hernia.
3. A sliding hernia with a tendency for the herniated portion of the stomach to move in and out through the esophageal hiatus with

changes in position caused by slight changes of pressure differential between the thorax and the abdomen.

Herniations Through the Foramina of Morgagni

General Comment. Only the omentum may be herniated without containing any incarcerated loops of bowel.

Radiologic Aspects

1. Stomach appears in a high transverse position with the distal body of the stomach drawn upward toward the region of the foramina of Morgagni and the transverse colon also drawn upward in an inverted "V" configuration. It may be necessary to fill both the stomach and the colon with barium for accurate demonstration.
2. On other occasions the loops of bowel, particularly the transverse colon and the distal body of the stomach, may be included in the hernia sac.

Hernias Through the Foramina of Bochdalek

General Comment

1. They usually occur early in infancy and childhood and most frequently contain bowel but at times contain other intra-abdominal organs such as the liver.
2. These hernias are found more frequently to the right of the midline, but occasionally to the left.
3. When the liver is included in the hernia on the right, the appearance may resemble a dense consolidation. A shift of the mediastinum away from the side of the hernia is common.

Diaphragm: Abnormalities in Density

Two Types:

1. Dissection of gas, producing an extrapleural emphysema of the diaphragm, often in association with perforations of the esophagus, tracheobronchial tree, or lower gastrointestinal tract (Figure 16–6)
2. Calcium density of the diaphragm, usually in association with a calcified pleural plaque.

Radiologic Aspects. Free air in the interstitial tissues of the diaphragm must be distinguished from free air in the peritoneal space. This can be done by altering the position of the patient and obtaining various views which might cause the air to rise to the uppermost level. If confined to the diaphgram, the free air will not be seen in the abdomen under these diverse conditions.

Diaphragm: Abnormality in Number; Accessory Diaphragm

An accessory diaphragm is a rare anomaly which is caused by the location of a second leaf of the diaphragm in the right chest cavity separating all or part of the right lower lobe from the remaining lung.

Radiologic Aspects. In this condition the right hemidiaphragm appears elevated and the oblique fissure accentuated and thickened (Nigogosyan and Ozarda).

THE PLEURA

Radiographic Classification of Pleural Disease

Abnormalities of Configuration and Size

Circumscribed widening of the pleural space may occur from pneumothorax, hydrothorax, granuloma, empyema, fibrosis, or neoplasm.

Abnormalities of Density

1. Diminished density may be caused by pneumothorax, either loculated or diffuse.
2. Water density caused by pleural effusion, free or encapsulated.
3. Calcification of the pleura, either in plaques or diffusely.
4. Thickened bands due to fibrous adhesions.
5. Nodulations of the pleura projected within a pneumothorax and indicative of primary pleural tumors, tumor metastases, granulomas, or pseudotumors (fibrin bodies).

Pneumothorax

General Comment.   Pneumothorax refers to air in the thoracic cage separating the parietal and visceral pleura. It may be generalized or sharply localized. It may be combined with either free-flowing fluid, adhesive fibrous bands, or loculations between the parietal and visceral pleura.

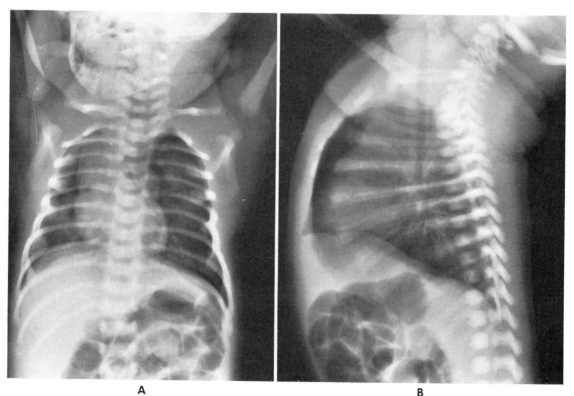

A   B

Figure 16–5   *A* and *B*. Infantile pneumothorax (*A*) and pneumomediastinum in postero-anterior and lateral projections.

When there is a communication between the lung or the bronchus and the pleural space, causing air to enter the pleura freely during inspiration, the check-valve mechanism which increases the tension in the pleural space causes a marked shift of the mediastinum toward the opposite side, and a tension pneumothorax is produced.

COMPARISON OF PNEUMOMEDIASTINUM AND PNEUMOTHORAX

	Pneumothorax	Pneumomediastinum
A-P view	Air lateral or inferior to the lung	Air is usually central, with or without a demarcating mediastinal pleura outlining a raised thymus
Lateral view	Anterior or subpulmonary air in some cases	The thymus is outlined or raised in about two-thirds of the cases
Oblique views	Lateral or subpulmonary air may be seen	The mediastinal pleura and thymus are usually outlined
Shift of air accumulation with change of position of the patient from supine to prone	Air shifts readily to an uppermost position	No shift of air
Mediastinal displacement	Common	Rare
Subcutaneous emphysema	Not present	It occurs but is uncommon

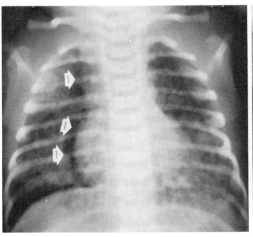 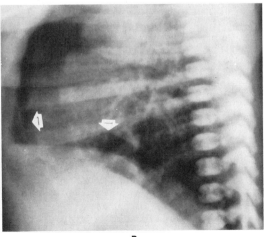

| A | B |

Figure 16–6 Pneumomediastinum and extrapleural sign in a newborn infant following aspiration of meconium. *A.* Postero-anterior view. *B.* Lateral view. Arrows point to the pneumomediastinum and the extrapleural accumulations of air.

Pleural Effusion

General Comment

Effusions are described as either generalized and free in the pleural cavity, or circumscribed and encapsulated.

Circumscribed effusions may be further subclassified in relation to their situation as: diaphragmatic (infrapulmonary), costal, interlobar, or paramediastinal.

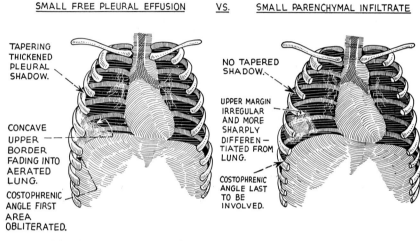

Figure 16–7 Differences in the radiographic appearance between small free pleural effusion and small parenchymal infiltrate at a lung base.

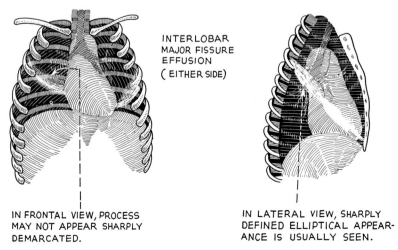

Figure 16–8 Interlobar circumscribed pleural disease in frontal and lateral perspectives.

In either case, whether the process is generalized or circumscribed, it may be unilateral or bilateral.

In the case of massive pleural effusion there is usually evidence of increased volume within the thorax, producing a spreading of the ribs and an increase in the width of the interspaces.

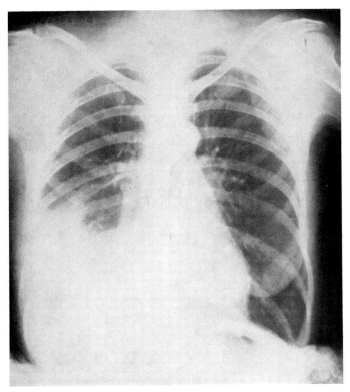

Figure 16–9   Radiograph demonstrating a small free pleural effusion in the right costophrenic sinus extending into the major interlobar fissure on the right.

An infrapulmonary effusion in the postero-anterior upright film study resembles (in radiographic appearance) an apparently elevated leaf of the diaphragm, with a contour similar to the diaphragmatic shadow and just as sharply outlined. On the left side, however, the gastric bubble will lie at a considerable distance from the superior margin of such a shadow (Figure 16–3).

Pleural Plaques and Adhesions

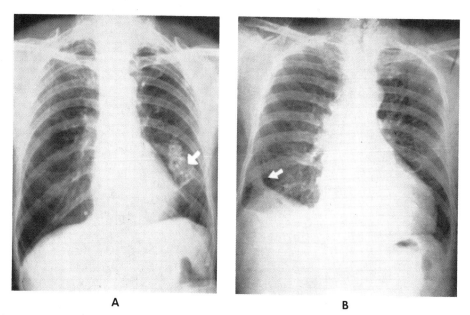

A

B

Figure 16–10 *A.* Radiograph demonstrating the appearance of calcified pleura adjoining the left heart as seen radiographically en face. *B.* Radiograph demonstrating a broad pleural adhesion between the right lower thoracic cage and the right hemidiaphragm.

Homogeneous, amorphous calcific pleural plaques are best demonstrated in tangent, and are continuous with the adjoining pleura. *En face,* the localized pleural disease may appear within the lung. In tangent, the obtuse contiguity with the pleura is demonstrated.

Tumors of the Pleura

Pathologic Classification

1. Primary
   a. Benign: fibroma, angioma, chondroma
   b. Malignant: (1) mesothelioma arising from the mesothelial layer; (2) mesothelioma arising from the stroma
2. Metastatic tumors of the pleura—usually a manifestation of lymphangitic spread of carcinoma, malignant lymphoma, or sarcoma throughout the pleural space

Radiologic Aspects of Malignant Pleural Mesothelioma (Heller et al.)

1. Pleural effusion
2. Irregularly thickened pleura
3. Mass lesions that may appear pulmonary rather than pleural

ROENTGEN SIGNS RELATED TO THE THORACIC CAGE

Symmetrical Changes Are Widening, Narrowness, Lengthening as in:

1. Pulmonary emphysema
2. Morquio's disease
3. Achondroplasia
4. Rickets
5. "Hourglass chest"
6. "Barrel chest"
7. "Flail chest"
8. Jeune's syndrome (asphyxiating thoracic dystrophy)

Asymmetrical Changes

1. Thoracoplasty
2. Crushing injuries to one side of the chest

Bony Abnormalities

1. Sternum:
   - a. Pectus excavatum (depressed sternum)
   - b. Pectus carinatum ("beaking" of sternum; "pigeon breast")
   - c. Sternal clefts or notches
2. Ribs:
   - a. Rib notching—superiorly, inferiorly, or both
   - b. Hypoplasia or aplasia
   - c. Supernumerary; diminished number; or "ectopic"
   - d. "Baseball bat" or "cricket bat" shape in chondrodystrophies or achondroplasias
   - e. Expansile lesions of ribs
   - f. Extrapleural sign
3. Spine (Chapter 14)
4. Pectoral girdle

Abnormalities of the Diaphragm Reflected in the Thorax

Abnormalities of the Soft Tissues of the Thoracic Cage

1. Atrophic or absent musculature
2. Breasts
3. Skin and subcutaneous tissues (tumors, gas)

Pleural Abnormalities Extending to the Thoracic Cage

Symmetrical Changes of Ribs and Thoracic Cage

"Barrel chest." The ribs are horizontal with an anterior bowing of the sternum, kyphosis of the thoracic spine, and flattening of the diaphragm. Typically described in patients with emphysema, emphysematous alterations follow acute exanthemas, pertussis, and cystic fibrosis of the pancreas. Air trapped in the lungs produces a hyperlucency of the lungs beneath the sternum anterior to the mediastinum.

"Hourglass chest." Narrowness at the mid-thorax with paralytic involvement.

Flail chest. Temporary abnormality during healing of multiple rib fractures combined with paradoxical respiration.

Rachitic chest. In rickets and scurvy, the costochondral junctions become expanded (beaded).

Achondroplastic chest. In achondroplasia the thorax is small because of *undergrowth of the ribs and sternum.* The scapulae and clavicles are unduly prominent and widely spaced in relation to the thoracic wall.

The chest in Morquio's disease. Short, deep thorax with the ribs expanded near their sternal junctions. They diminish in diameter near their necks, resembling a baseball or cricket bat.

Bony Abnormalities

Ribs

Rib Notching

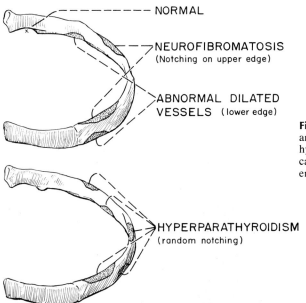

NORMAL

NEUROFIBROMATOSIS
(Notching on upper edge)

ABNORMAL DILATED
VESSELS (lower edge)

HYPERPARATHYROIDISM
(random notching)

Figure 16–11 Diagrammatic illustration of rib appearances in neurofibromatosis compared with those in hyperparathyroidism. Also shown are rib notchings caused by abnormal dilated vessels accompanying such entities as coarctation of the aorta.

Coarctation of the aorta is the most frequent cause in ribs three to nine on their inferior margins, and is produced by the pulsations from the dilated numerous collaterals around the coarctation site. The internal mammary and intercostal arteries are most frequently involved.

Superior rib notching or thinning, also affecting ribs three to nine, is most commonly the result of chronic paralytic poliomyelitis and is thought to be due to pressure by the scapulae (Bernstein).

Rheumatoid arthritis and scleroderma are also associated with superior rib erosion and distal clavicle resorption (Keats).

Expansile Lesions of the Ribs

1. Fibrous dysplasia
2. Aneurysmal bone cyst
3. Multiple myeloma
4. Histiocytosis-X
5. Chondromyxoid fibroma
6. Chondrosarcoma

Destructive Lesion with Extrapleural Sign

1. Tuberculosis, mycosis (actinomycosis, nocardiosis, blastomycosis)
2. Multiple myeloma
3. Metastatic tumor (usually intrinsic and not associated with extrapleural sign)

Miscellaneous Alteration of the Pectoral Girdle

1. Resorption or "pencilling" of distal clavicle or medial clavicular end
   a. Rheumatoid arthritis
   b. Hyperparathyroidism
2. Thickening of clavicle
   a. Infantile cortical hyperostosis (Caffey-Silverman disease)
   b. Healed fracture

Soft Tissues of the Thorax

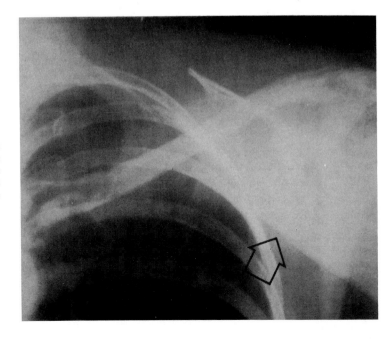

Figure 16–12 Closeup view of the axilla in a patient who has had a radical mastectomy. Complete absence of the pectoral muscles produces an oblique line across the left of the axilla.

RESPIRATORY DISTRESS IN INFANCY AND CHILDHOOD

Newborn and Young Infant

Many diverse causes must be considered:
1. *Extrapulmonary diseases* such as congenital heart disease, noninfectious enterocolitis, intestinal atresia, subdural hematoma, liver disease, adrenal disease, and anoxia and shock from any cause in the ante- through the postpartum period
2. *Palsies or paralysis* of the larynx or chest musculature
3. *Injuries* to the respiratory center of the brain
4. Primary respiratory distress may be from many causes, such as:
    a. *Neonatal atelectasis* (Chapter 17)
    b. *Transient tachypnea* of the newborn (wet lung syndrome)
    c. *Aspiration pneumonitis* (Chapter 17)
    d. *Hyaline membrane disease* and bronchopulmonary dysplasia (Chapter 17)
    e. *Congenital pneumonitis*
    f. *Pulmonary hemorrhage*
    g. *Pulmonary dysmaturity* (Wilson-Mikity syndrome) (Chapter 17)
    h. *Pulmonary lymphangiectasia* (Singleton and Wagner)
    i. *Congenital lobar emphysema* (Chapter 20)
    j. *Pneumothorax and pneumomediastinum*
5. Metabolic abnormalities (hypocalcemia; hypoglycemia)
    These entities, by their objective appearances, belong in subsequent chapters.

Older Infants and Children

Somewhat similar considerations are operative here, although causes may be different. Apart from the extrapulmonary causes, they may be divided into:
1. Upper tract obstruction, and
2. Lower tract ventilatory interference.

Upper Tract Obstruction

Clinical Manifestation: Suprasternal retraction; inspiratory stridor.

Radiographic Appearances

1. Epiglottitis (Figure 16–13)
2. Infantile croup (Figure 16–14)
3. Tracheomalacia and laryngomalacia
4. Tracheobronchomegaly (Mounier-Kuhn syndrome)
5. Bulbar and pseudobulbar palsy (infectious, toxic, or central nervous system origin)

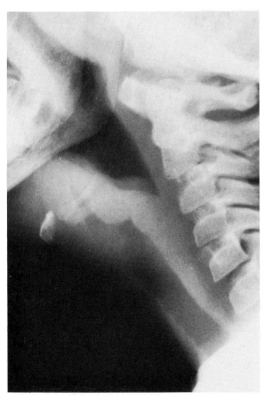

Figure 16–13 Soft tissue lateral film of the neck demonstrating the massively swollen aryepiglottic folds with epiglottitis. (Courtesy of Dr. J. S. Dunbar, Montreal, Canada.)

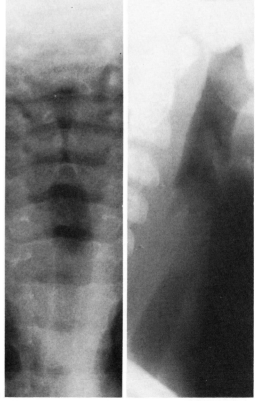

A   B

Figure 16–14 *A* and *B*. Radiographic appearance of croup. The walls of the conus elasticus of the trachea in the subglottic region show convexity medially instead of concavity medially. A secondary collapse of the trachea may appear particularly during inspiration but ordinarily disappears during expiration. (Courtesy of Dr. J. S. Dunbar, Montreal, Canada.)

Lower Tract Obstruction

Clinical Manifestation: Chest is hyperinflated. There is no retraction in the subcostal and intercostal regions, and expiration is prolonged and wheezy.

Radiographic Appearances

1. Masses in the oro- or nasopharynx, such as thyroglossal duct cysts and hemangiofibromas
2. Foreign body aspiration (Chapter 17)
3. Tracheo-esophageal fistula (Chapter 27)
4. Emphysema and asthma (Chapter 20)
5. Cystic fibrosis of the pancreas (mucoviscidosis) (Chapter 17)
6. Mediastinal lymph node enlargement from any cause, including pertussis, the acute exanthemas, or lymphomas (Chapter 21)

Questions—Chapter 16

1. What are the radiologic methods of study of the diaphragm?
2. What is the general classification of abnormalities of the diaphragm from the radiographic standpoint?
3. What are the cardinal radiographic signs of subdiaphragmatic abscess?
4. What are the cardinal roentgen signs of chronic obstructive pulmonary emphysema?
5. What is meant by "paradoxical movement of the diaphragm"?
6. Indicate at least four conditions in which there is a unilateral elevation of the diaphragm.
7. Indicate at least some conditions associated with bilateral low position of the diaphragm.
8. What is meant by "check-valve obstruction of a bronchus" and how would you demonstrate this radiologically?
9. What is meant by the terms "scalloping" and "tenting" of the diaphragm?
10. What is meant by infrapulmonary encapsulation of fluid?
11. Give a clinical classification of a diaphragmatic hernia.
12. Give a classification of those hernias that are found through the esophageal hiatus of the diaphragm.
13. What is the radiographic technique for examination of the pleura?
14. What is a radiographic classification of pleural disease?
15. How does one recognize circumscribed pleural disease radiographically?
16. What are the radiographic features of pneumothorax and what is the importance of the expiratory-phase film in its study?
17. What are the radiographic characteristics of a small free pleural effusion compared to a small parenchymal infiltrate?
18. What are the radiographic characteristics of massive effusions as compared to a parenchymal pneumonia or a massive atelectasis?
19. What are the various appearances of encapsulated intralobar effusion?
20. Describe the radiographic appearance of a calcified pleura.
21. Describe the radiographic appearance of a free pleural effusion.
22. Describe the radiographic appearance of marked fibrous thickening of the pleura, such as may occur in the upper thoracic cage. What are the concomitant findings in relation to the mediastinal structures?
23. Describe the radiologic aspects of tumors of the pleura. What special diagnostic technique is available to us for demonstration of small nodulations of the pleura?
24. What is meant by the following terms: pectus excavatum; pectus carinatum; barrel chest; hourglass chest; flail chest; rachitic chest; achondroplastic chest?
25. Describe the ribs in Morquio's disease.

26. Indicate some of the causes of pathologic rib notches. In what particular cardiac condition are they of special significance and how does one recognize this radiographically?

27. Indicate the clinical entities responsible for resorption of the distal ends of the clavicle.

28. Indicate which abnormal soft tissues of the thoracic cage may be recognized radiologically.

29. List the common primary causes for respiratory distress in the newborn and very young infant.

30. What are some of the causes of upper tract obstruction in older infants and children?

31. Describe the radiographic appearances in epiglottitis, infantile croup, and tracheomalacia. How would you go about making an appropriate radiographic study to make these diagnoses?

17

Diffuse, Poorly Defined, Homogeneous Shadows of the Lung Parenchyma

GENERAL OUTLINE

Poorly Defined, Diffuse, Homogeneous Densities of the Lung Parenchyma

1. Those which are lobar or segmental in distribution, moderately sharply demarcated, and roughly triangular or polygonal in shape.
2. Those which are scattered, poorly defined, irregular, and often acinar in distribution.
3. Those which tend to occur in apices or subapical regions.
4. Those occurring in any situation in the lung parenchyma.
5. Those with a tendency to basilar distribution.
6. Those with a tendency to migrate from one area to another.
7. Those with a tendency to involve the inner two-thirds of the lungs or the hilar lymph nodes.
8. Those with a tendency to pneumatocele formation, suppuration or abscess formation.
9. Those with a tendency to a miliary pattern.
10. Those with a strong tendency to interstitial involvement along with acinar involvement.

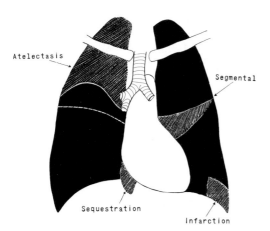

Figure 17–1 Diagram illustrating various entities that may produce lobar or segmental homogeneous but moderately sharply demarcated shadows.

THOSE WHICH ARE LOBAR OR SEGMENTAL IN DISTRIBUTION, MODERATELY SHARPLY DEMARCATED, AND ROUGHLY TRIANGULAR OR POLYGONAL IN SHAPE

1. Atelectasis
2. Lobar or confluent pneumonia
3. Pulmonary infarction
4. Pulmonary sequestration (Chapter 18)
5. In adults: Hemophilus influenza pneumonia
6. Pulmonary hypogenesis (Chapter 16)
7. Pseudolymphoma

Atelectasis

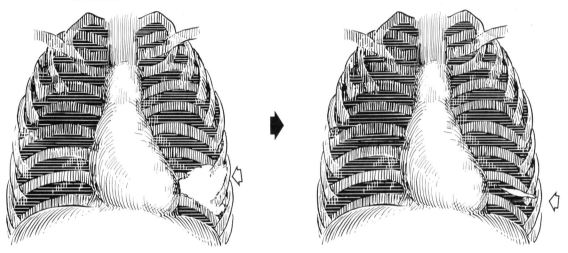

SCARRING FROM INFARCTION OR INFECTION

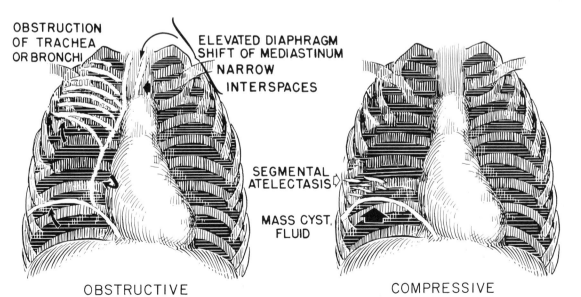

Figure 17–2 Line diagrams demonstrating the various different kinds of pulmonary atelectasis.

ADVANCED COLLAPSE LEFT LOWER LOBE

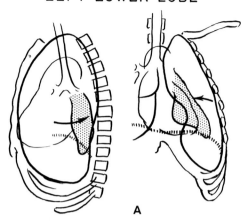

Figure 17–3 Changes with lobar atelectasis. *A.* Findings with collapse of the left lower lobe, shown diagrammatically. *B.* Diagram of roentgen findings with advanced collapse of the left upper lobe.

A

Collapse of Left Lower Lobe

a. Reduction in size and number of visible vascular structures may be minimal or not apparent.

b. The anterior segmental artery of the upper lobe is deflected and runs horizontally or downward.

c. The hilus may be slightly depressed or in a normal position but appears reduced in size.

ADVANCED COLLAPSE LEFT UPPER LOBE

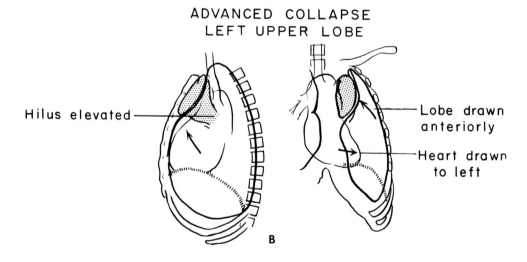

Hilus elevated

Lobe drawn anteriorly

Heart drawn to left

B

Left Upper Lobe Collapse

a. Slight elevation of left hilus.

b. Fanning out and reduction in the number of the visible vessels.

c. Reduced caliber and absence of the lingular branches.

d. In lateral view an anterior mass may be identifiable

Collapsed right middle lobe or lingula of left upper lobe produces the "silhouette sign" (Figure 17–6). This sign, originally described by Robins and Hale in 1944, and later by Felson and Felson, refers to obliteration of portions of the outline of the heart, aorta, and diaphragm by disease in the lungs in contact with these structures.

ADVANCED COLLAPSE
RIGHT UPPER LOBE

ADVANCED COLLAPSE
RIGHT LOWER LOBE

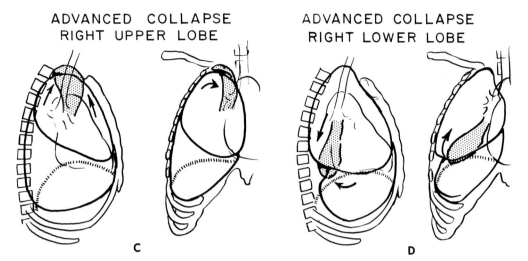

C

D

Figure 17–3 *Continued*   *C*. Roentgen findings with advanced collapse of the right upper lobe. Note that the lobe collapses posteriorly, cephalad, and centrally. *D*. Advanced collapse of the right lower lobe. The right lower lobe collapses posteriorly, cephalad, and centrally.

ADVANCED COLLAPSE
RIGHT MIDDLE LOBE

RIGHT MIDDLE AND
LOWER LOBE

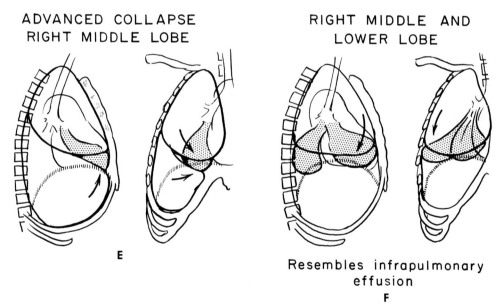

E

Resembles infrapulmonary
effusion

F

E. Roentgen findings with advanced collapse of the right middle lobe. Note that the right middle lobe collapses cephalad and medially. Usually this collapse produces a "silhouette" sign in which the right cardiac margin can no longer be distinguished in frontal perspective. *F*. Roentgen findings with combined collapse of the right middle and lower lobes. Note that this resembles an infrapulmonary effusion. (Modified from Krause and Lubert, Amer. J. Roentgenol., *79*:258–268, 1958.)

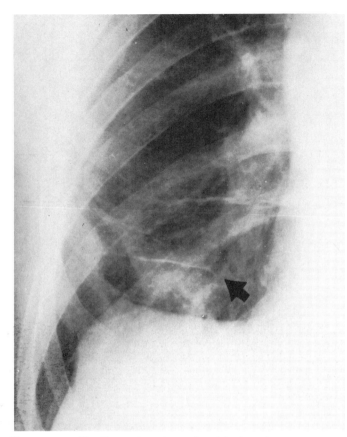

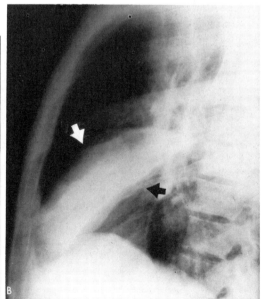

Figure 17–5   Confluent pneumonia involving the right middle lobe (arrow 1) and the right lower lobe (arrow 2), for comparison with Figure 17–6.

Figure 17–4   Platelike atelectasis at the right lung base; many such shadows have their origin, however, in pulmonary infarction.

Confluent Pneumonia (Figure 17–5)

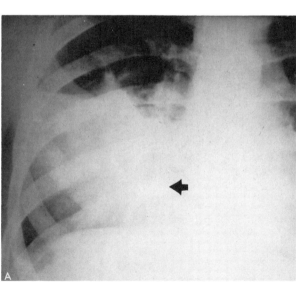

Figure 17–6   *A* and *B*. "Silhouette sign." Lobar consolidation with some atelectasis in the right middle lobe demonstrating the loss of definition of the right cardiac margin (black arrow in *A*).

Confluent Pneumonia (Figures 17–5, 17–6C)

Homogeneous area of increased density, usually in a dependent portion of the lung, involving a lobe or a section of a lobe, irrespective of anatomic segments.

The margin between involved and uninvolved lung is ordinarily sharply demarcated.

There is no diminution in volume as with atelectasis.

Very often there is contiguous involvement of the pleura, and a pleural effusion may accompany the alveolar involvement.

If the basilar lobe is involved, the costophrenic sinus is the last to be involved, unlike an uncomplicated case of pleural effusion, in which the costophrenic sinus is involved first.

During resolution, the confluent shadow becomes less homogeneous and more "weblike" and radiolucent until normal radiolucency supervenes.

Incomplete resolution may occur and fibrosis may develop, chiefly in the peribronchial and subpleural regions of the lungs.

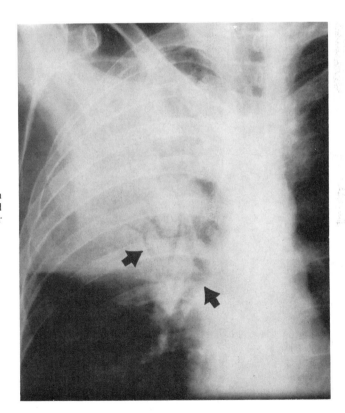

Figure 17–6 *Continued   C.* "Air bronchogram sign" of pulmonary consolidation. (Intensified for photographic purposes.) Patient with lobar consolidation due to lobar pneumonia.

DIFFERENTIATION OF MASSIVE DENSE SHADOWS IN THE CHEST

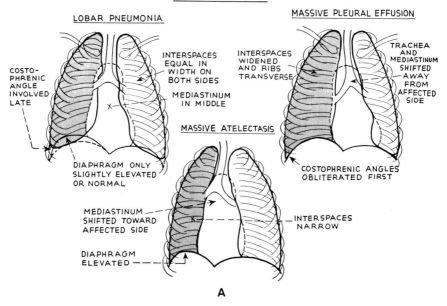

LOBAR PNEUMONIA

MASSIVE PLEURAL EFFUSION

INTERSPACES EQUAL IN WIDTH ON BOTH SIDES

MEDIASTINUM IN MIDDLE

COSTO-PHRENIC ANGLE INVOLVED LATE

DIAPHRAGM ONLY SLIGHTLY ELEVATED OR NORMAL

INTERSPACES WIDENED AND RIBS TRANSVERSE

TRACHEA AND MEDIASTINUM SHIFTED AWAY FROM AFFECTED SIDE

COSTOPHRENIC ANGLES OBLITERATED FIRST

MASSIVE ATELECTASIS

MEDIASTINUM SHIFTED TOWARD AFFECTED SIDE

INTERSPACES NARROW

DIAPHRAGM ELEVATED

A

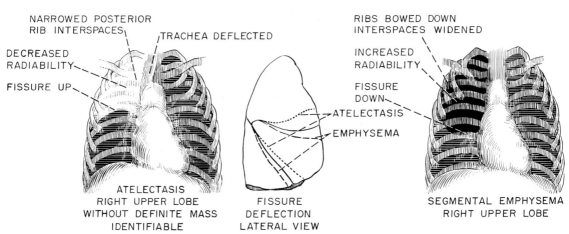

NARROWED POSTERIOR RIB INTERSPACES

TRACHEA DEFLECTED

DECREASED RADIABILITY

FISSURE UP

ATELECTASIS RIGHT UPPER LOBE WITHOUT DEFINITE MASS IDENTIFIABLE

FISSURE DEFLECTION LATERAL VIEW

ATELECTASIS

EMPHYSEMA

RIBS BOWED DOWN INTERSPACES WIDENED

INCREASED RADIABILITY

FISSURE DOWN

SEGMENTAL EMPHYSEMA RIGHT UPPER LOBE

B

Figure 17–7   *A*. Characteristics of a massive pleural effusion as compared with parenchymal lobar pneumonia and massive atelectasis. *B*. Differences in roentgen signs for lobar atelectasis and lobar emphysema.

Pulmonary Infarction (Figure 17–8)

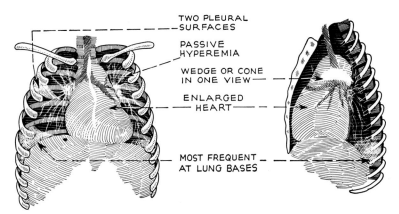

TWO PLEURAL SURFACES

PASSIVE HYPEREMIA

WEDGE OR CONE IN ONE VIEW

ENLARGED HEART

MOST FREQUENT AT LUNG BASES

Figure 17–8 Diagram illustrating roentgen findings with pulmonary infarction.

The majority of pulmonary thromboembolic episodes are not associated with detectable changes on plain chest radiographs. When present, radiographic findings include:

1. Ischemia of the lung peripheral to the embolus, resulting in a hyperlucent area with diminished or absent vascularization.
2. Dilatation of the hilar arteries as the result of vasospasm of the peripheral arteries and mechanical obstruction.
3. Impaired ventilation of the lung due to broncho-constriction, chest pain, and bronchial edema.
   a. Obstructive emphysema or atelectasis may follow ("line shadow" in 20 per cent).
4. With infarction, necrosis of alveolar walls and extravasation of blood into alveolar spaces results.
   a. A homogeneous, poorly outlined density resembling pneumonia is seen, as early as 10 to 12 hours, or as late as one week.
   b. The size and shape will depend upon the projection in relation to the obstructed area.
   c. Cavitation may occur if the necrotic process is extended.
5. Elevation of the diaphragm is frequent (30 per cent of cases).
6. Small pleural effusions are also common (at least 46 per cent of cases).
7. Pulmonary hypertension and cor pulmonale may supervene.
8. Acute pulmonary edema may accompany pulmonary embolization.
9. The diagnosis may be assisted materially by pulmonary angiography.
10. If infected emboli have given rise to the pulmonary ischemia and infarction, abscess formation after several days or even weeks may result.
11. The time of resolution varies greatly. It may occur within 7 to 10 days or less, sometimes without any residual finding, but it may be much longer, averaging as long as 20 days according to Fleischner, or even up to five weeks.

POORLY DEFINED, HOMOGENEOUS, IRREGULARLY SCATTERED DENSITIES OF THE LUNG

Bronchopneumonias

This group of diseases includes many different respiratory viruses (Fraser and Paré) and microbial infections.

Radiologic Appearances

Highly variable, including acinar, segmental, and even lobar consolidation.

There may be diffuse or local accentuation of lung markings due to interstitial and peribronchial inflammation.

There may be a widespread, reticular pattern with hilar lymph node enlargement, as in measles (rubeola).

Segmental pneumonia and atelectasis are also often present.

The lower lobes may be predominantly affected.

Pleural effusion is rare.

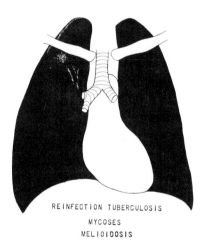

SCATTERED, POORLY DEFINED, IRREGULAR

OFTEN ACINAR

OFTEN APICAL OR SUBAPICAL

1. Pulmonary tuberculosis (reinfection type)
2. Mycotic infections of the lung
3. Pseudomonas
4. Pseudomallei (melioidosis)

REINFECTION TUBERCULOSIS

MYCOSES

MELIOIDOSIS

Figure 17–9   Differential diagnosis of apical or subapical chronic infectious acinarlike shadows.

Pulmonary Tuberculosis (All Types)

General Principles

The radiographic manifestations of tuberculosis are protean, although a general pattern in relation to the pathogenesis may be recognized. It is convenient to describe all forms of tuberculosis at this time, with the recognition that tuberculosis may enter any of our chapters or sections on pulmonary disease.

The outright diagnosis of pulmonary tuberculosis on radiographic grounds must never be made. Bacteriologic proof is required for a positive diagnosis.

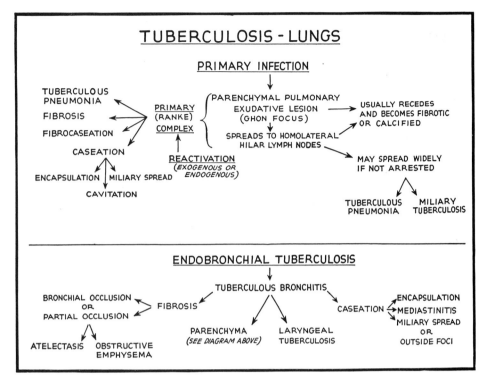

Figure 17–10   Diagram demonstrating the various possible sequential occurrences in association with tuberculosis of the lungs.

Primary Infection.   The primary lesion usually occurs in the peripheral interstitial tissues of the lung and may be barely detectable in infancy and childhood (Ghon focus). There occurs a focus of pneumonic consolidation a few millimeters in diameter, usually under the pleura of the lung peripherally or near the hilus. This lesion may undergo fibrosis and ultimately calcify, or it may be the source of a widespread dissemination of the disease. Usually the infection spreads to the homolateral hilar lymph nodes, where it may once again undergo fibrosis and calcification (forming the Ranke complex) (Figure 17–11), or it may be arrested and may undergo fibrocaseation and ulceration.

PRIMARY PULMONARY TUBERCULOSIS
VARIOUS APPEARANCES

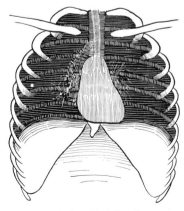

HILAR LYMPH NODES, GHON'S FOCUS; OCCASIONAL CALCIFICATION.

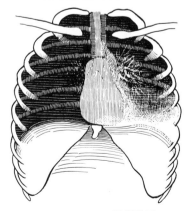

HILAR LYMPH NODES, ATELECTASIS AND EFFUSION.

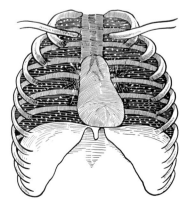

MILIARY HEMATOGENOUS

Figure 17–11   Examples of primary pulmonary tuberculosis in diagram.

Adult Reinfection Type. The primary complex may remain dormant, or in adult life, reinfection may occur by either an exogenous or endogenous source of tubercle bacilli. Reactivation in the adult gives rise to a new exudative response which *usually lies in the apical or subapical region.* This may undergo fibrosis, fibrocaseation, or outright caseation with ulceration—cavitation. Occasionally, an acute exudative pneumonia may be part of any of these various phases.

RADIOLOGIC FEATURES (Figure 17–12)

In its exudative phase when subapical or apical, it will appear as an ill-defined homogeneous shadow of increased density.

In its proliferative phase it may be characterized as a nodule, particularly if it has undergone scar formation, fibrosis, or calcification.

In its cavitary phase it may also appear somewhat nodular but less well-defined, with a reactive zone around it.

At times when the interstitial tissues are affected mostly, it may appear reticular or reticulonodular.

It may involve the pleura or the pericardium, or extend itself outside the chest.

It may disseminate through almost any modality—the bloodstream, the lymphatics, by extension over surfaces, direct extension, or migration of endothelial cells which contain the bacilli. Dissemination through the lymphatics is probably most common, and tuberculosis is typically a lymphogenous disease.

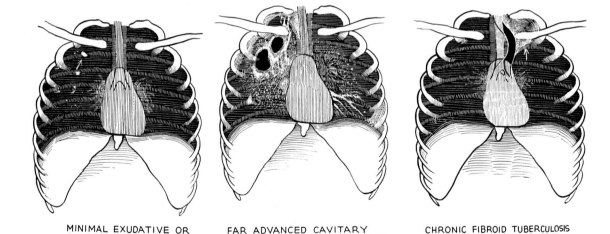

MINIMAL EXUDATIVE OR PROLIFERATIVE AREA.　　FAR ADVANCED CAVITARY WITH PERIBRONCHIAL TUBERCLES IN OPPOSING LUNG BASE; EFFUSION　　CHRONIC FIBROID TUBERCULOSIS

Figure 17–12　Radiographic appearances in diagram of pulmonary tuberculosis in adults.

Atypical Tuberculosis (anonymous tuberculosis, chromogenic tuberculosis, unclassified tuberculosis). This has been differentiated as a result of newer cultural techniques, sensitivity studies, and special differentiation methods.

Roentgen Appearances

1. Thin-walled cavities, often with a lack of pericavitary inflammation
2. Lack of hilar elevation
3. Little evidence of bronchogenic spread
4. Little pleural reaction

Mycotic Infections of the Lungs

General Considerations.   The radiologic aspects of mycotic infections of the lungs are generally nonspecific and resemble tuberculosis in its many manifestations. There are, however, some salient outstanding characteristics in respect to one or another of these, but demonstration of the causative organism is the ultimate proof.

Fungus infections may occur as a serious complication in compromised hosts (i.e., debilitating diseases; chemotherapy; diabetes; and others).

Actinomycosis

RADIOGRAPHIC APPEARANCES

1. Pleural disease (empyema or pleural thickening)
2. Chest wall involvement (soft tissue swelling, rib periostitis, rib destruction, vertebral destruction)
3. Mass lesion
4. Chronic alveolar infiltrate
5. Cavitation
6. Transgression of an interlobar fissure
7. Pulmonary fibrosis
8. Esophagopleural and bronchopleural fistula
9. Pulmonary osteoarthropathy

Nocardiosis.   This is often classified with actinomycosis. The appearances simulate those of tuberculosis, lung abscesses, single or multiple, and empyema. Unlike the situation in actinomycosis, when fistulae occur they are usually quite superficial.

Blastomycosis.   Pulmonary blastomycosis may appear as multiple nodules or abscesses or areas of pneumonic consolidation. It may simulate bronchogenic carcinoma at times. Nodular or caseous masses in the lungs and hilar nodes may resemble tuberculosis closely. In general, there is a greater predilection for the skin, the lungs, and the bones than with the other mycotic infections.

Histoplasmosis

RADIOGRAPHIC APPEARANCES (Figure 17–13)

Round shadow complexes measuring 1/2 to 3 cm. in diameter associated with large, hilar lymph nodes. Calcific centers may or may not be present. This stage may be followed by soft infiltrations in the surrounding tissue and usually these are ill-defined and homogeneous, whereas the former are nodular.

Ill-defined, homogeneous infiltrations in the lungs that have a macular appearance.

A true miliary dissemination over both lungs may occur and after two to four years, calcifications are found in this distribution.

In some cases only enlargement of hilar and mediastinal lymph nodes occurs.

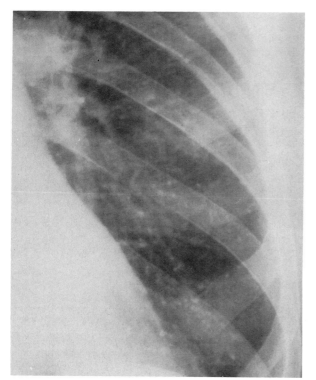

Figure 17–13   Histoplasmosis. Calcified nodules due to old histoplasmosis.

Figure 17–14   P-A view of the chest in a patient with coccidioidomycosis. Note the thin-walled cavity. (Courtesy of the Armed Forces Institute of Pathology, Washington, D.C.)

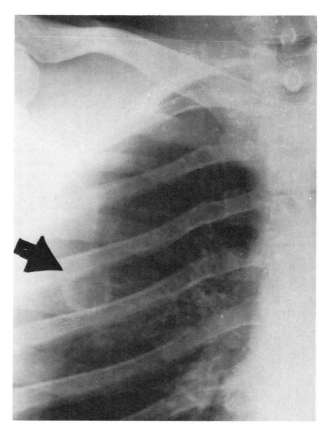

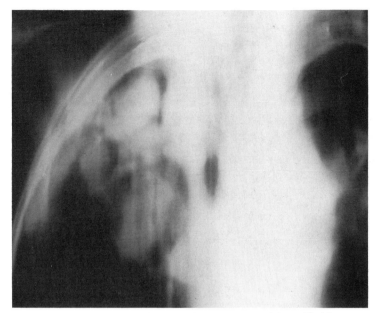

Figure 17–15 Aspergillosis showing the fungus ball appearance and intensified by a tomogram of the right upper lobe.

Coccidioidomycosis. The *roentgen findings* are rather variable and include:

1. Pneumonitis
2. Pleural effusion with hilar and mediastinal lymphadenopathy
3. Thin-walled cavity in the lung field
4. Granuloma without cavitation
5. In approximately 20 per cent of cases, the roentgenographic appearance is identical to that of tuberculosis

OTHER PNEUMONIAS WITH A PREDILECTION FOR BASILAR DISTRIBUTION

TENDENCY TO BASILAR DISTRIBUTION

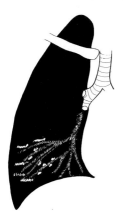

Bronchiectasis
Hypostatic pneumonia
Mucoviscidosis
Aspiration pneumonia
Bacterioides

Figure 17–16   Differential diagnosis of pneumonias with a predilection for basilar distribution.

Mucoviscidosis (Figure 17–17) (with cystic fibrosis of the pancreas)

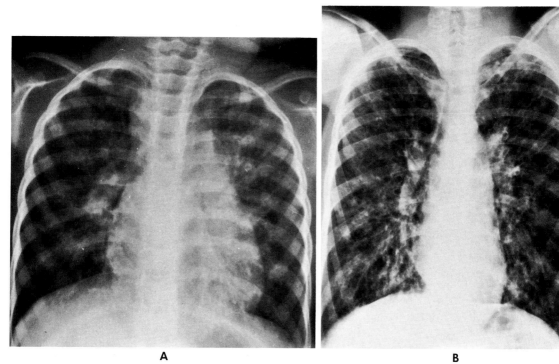

A   B

Figure 17–17   *A.* Mucoviscidosis in the lung of a child. Note the marked increase in the interstitial pattern and the prominence of the right pulmonary artery, which suggests that pulmonary hypertension is already present.

B. Postero-anterior view of the chest in an adult with mucoviscidosis of the lung. Note the marked increase in the interstitial pattern and the areas of lucency that suggest associated chronic obstructive pulmonary disease and probably associated chronic bronchitis and pneumonitis. Bronchiectasis is often present as well. (A lateral view of this same patient is shown in Figure 19–6.)

Radiographic Appearances

Patchy ill-defined areas of increased density, especially in the lung bases
Segmental foci of atelectasis

Alveolar Proteinosis — Roentgenographic Appearances

1. Bat wing appearance closely resembling pulmonary edema

2. On close inspection, however, the appearance suggests acinar involvement with mottled or granular densities creating a rosette appearance. These are aggregates of alveolar densities.

3. Lobar consolidation

4. Nodular lesions

5. There may be clearing peripherally or (more rarely) centrally, with a variety of patterns created.

6. No lymph node enlargement is noted.

7. There may be hyperinflated and atelectatic areas as well (Prager; Ramirez).

THOSE PNEUMONIC LESIONS WITH A TENDENCY TO PNEUMATOCELE FORMATION, SUPPURATION, OR ABSCESS FORMATION AND PLEURAL INVOLVEMENT

1. Staphylococcus pneumonias
2. Klebsiella and Aerobacter (Friedländer's) pneumonia
3. In infants: Hemophilus influenzae pneumonia
4. Bacteroides pneumonias (see previously)
5. Tuberculosis (see previously)
6. Wegener's necrotizing granuloma
7. Wilson-Mikity syndrome
8. Pulmonary hematoma

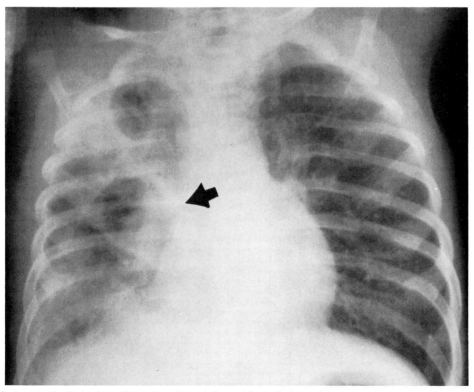

Figure 17–20   P-A view of the chest in an infant with staphylococcic pneumonia. Note the following combination of findings: (1) unilaterality; (2) pleural involvement; (3) pulmonary consolidation; (4) pneumatocele formation. The arrow points to a large pneumatocele adjoining the right side of the mediastinum.

THOSE LESIONS OF THE LUNG PARENCHYMA WITH A TENDENCY TO DISTRIBUTE THEMSELVES IN A MILIARY PATTERN

1. Infectious granulomas, such as tuberculosis and the mycoses (see previously)
2. Varicella pneumonia
3. Cytomegalovirus pneumonia
4. Ornithosis
5. Chemical pneumonitis
6. Renal transplantation pneumonia
7. Loeffler's pneumonia (rarely)

LUNG LESIONS WITH A TENDENCY TO INTERSTITIAL INVOLVEMENT AS WELL AS ACINAR INVOLVEMENT

1. Interstitial edema (see previous description with alveolar edema)
2. Atypical viral pneumonia and mycoplasma pneumonia (see previous discussion)
3. Reticuloendothelioses (mostly interstitial—see Chapter 19)
4. Goodpasture's syndrome (pulmonary-renal syndrome)
5. Wilson-Mikity syndrome (pulmonary dysmaturity)
6. Pulmonary hemosiderosis
7. Pulmonary hemorrhages in infants
8. Hyaline membrane disease of the newborn (respiratory distress syndrome)
9. Bronchopulmonary dysplasia
10. Rheumatoid pneumonia (mostly interstitial—Chapter 19)
11. Scleroderma (mostly interstitial—Chapter 19)
12. Dermatomyositis (mostly interstitial—Chapter 19)
13. Chronic fibroid tuberculosis (see previous discussion)
14. Transient tachypnea of the newborn (Chapter 19)

Pulmonary-Renal Syndrome (Goodpasture's syndrome) (Figure 17–47). Repeated episodes of pulmonary hemorrhage, iron-deficiency anemia, and glomerular disease of the kidneys.

Radiographic Manifestations

Patchy air-space consolidations of irregular shape.
Air bronchograms.
In a few days, the fluffy areas become reticular and interstitial.
After 10 or 12 days the chest may return to normal, but with repeated episodes the involved patchy areas may become fibrotic.
Pulmonary hypertension and cor pulmonale may ensue (Benoit et al.).

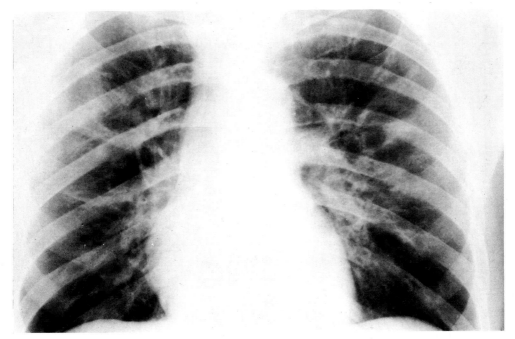

Figure 17–21   P-A film of the chest in Goodpasture's syndrome.

Wilson-Mikity Syndrome (pulmonary dysmaturity) (Figure 17–23).   Although respiratory disturbance may be noted in the neonatal period, the clinical respiratory embarrassment is most manifest several weeks after birth. About one-half die, and the others improve slowly after a period of six months to a year.

Radiographic Appearances

Diffuse linear and reticular areas of density with interspersed "cystlike" areas of lucency.

Resembles "bronchopulmonary dysplasia."

In the "intermediate stage" the pattern may consist of coarse streaks radiating from the hilus, most commonly into the upper lobe, with air-trapping and emphysema in the lower lobes.

No residual pathologic or radiologic findings in those infants who survive and recover after 4 to 11 months of age.

Hyaline Membrane Disease of the Newborn (Respiratory Distress Syndrome) (Figure 17–22).   Ninety per cent of cases are premature infants in the newborn period, and about one-half die within the first 24 hours of life.

Radiographic Appearances

The lungs are diffusely granular in appearance, with scattered air-filled alveolar ducts giving rise to "bubbles" of air in the homogeneous ground glass and granular appearance.

If the infant survives, there may be a gradual development of interstitial fibrosis (bronchopulmonary dysplasia).

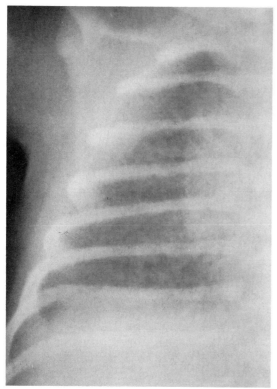

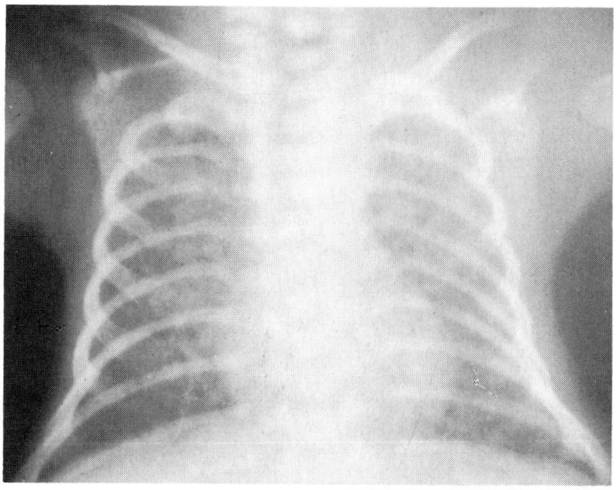

Figure 17–23 Postero-anterior view of the chest in an infant with Wilson-Mikity syndrome.

Figure 17–22 Magnified view of the right lung in a newborn infant with a respiratory distress syndrome (hyaline membrane disease).

Bronchopulmonary Dysplasia (Oxygen toxicity in infants)

Pathology. In infants who have survived after hyaline membrane disease treated with oxygen, four stages have been described (Northway), including:
1. Patchy infiltrate with segmental atelectasis, "granular" appearance of lungs, scattered "background of aeration."
2. Necrosis and repair; coalescence of emphysema; focal thickening of capillaries.
3. Atelectasis and emphysema with a "spongy" appearance of the lung.
4. Large emphysematous areas with interspersed hypertrophied peribronchial muscle and fibrosis.

Similar Fibroplastic Proliferation and change has been described in adults with other agents, especially "free radical producers" (Meschan et al.).

Radiographic Appearances

Complete opacification of the lung with interspersed cystlike lucencies. Later, it simulates a sponge or swiss cheese.

Affects the peripheral zones especially and is **not** associated with pleural effusion (dry lung).

Transient Tachypnea of the Newborn

Roentgenographic findings include prominent vascular markings, hyperaeration, fluid in the costophrenic sulci, Kerley lines, and widened interlobar fissures.

NEOPLASMS OF THE LUNG, BRONCHI, AND MEDIASTINUM

Although neoplasms may have an ill-defined, homogeneous appearance, it is probable that other appearances are more frequently encountered. Hence, lung neoplasia is discussed in this text with those diseases which tend to produce mass nodular shadows in the lung parenchyma. *It should be stated, however, that in any pneumonic process of an ill-defined type that persists for a period longer than three months, in a person past the age of 40, the possibility of bronchogenic carcinoma or lung neoplasm must be suspected and excluded by every available means.*

Questions – Chapter 17

1. Which parenchymal lung disease entities are represented by poorly defined, homogeneous densities of the lungs, tending to be lobar or segmental in distribution, moderately sharply demarcated, and roughly triangular or polygonal in shape?

2. Which of these poorly defined, homogeneous densities tend to be scattered and irregular in distribution everywhere but primarily in the lung apices or in subapical regions?

3. Which of the poorly defined, parenchymal lung diseases tend to have a basilar distribution?

4. Which of the poorly defined, homogeneous densities of the lung tend to be confined to the inner two-thirds of the lung?

5. Which of the poorly defined, homogeneous densities of the lung tend to be widely disseminated, especially in the outer zones of the lung, and have a strong tendency to pneumatocele formation, suppuration, or abscess formation?

6. Which of the poorly defined, homogeneous densities of the lung tend to have a rather miliary pattern?

7. Which of the poorly defined, homogeneous parenchymal diseases of the lung tend to have with them a considerable interstitial involvement as well as the acinar involvement?

8. What are the cardinal roentgen signs of atelectasis?

9. What is meant by the "air bronchogram sign"?

10. What are the most prevalent roentgen findings in relation to bronchial adenoma?

11. What are the main radiographic features of lobar (Diplococcus) pneumonia?

12. What are the main roentgen features of a pulmonary infarction?

13. What is the sequential appearance of a pulmonary infarction in a small area of the lung?

14. What is the most definitive single radiographic investigative technique in the diagnosis and evaluation of thromboembolic disease?

15. What are the different radiographic types of pulmonary tuberculosis?

16. What are the main groups of mycotic infections of the lungs?

17. What are some of the main roentgen features of pulmonary actinomycosis?

18. What are the main radiologic features of blastomycosis?

19. What different types of pulmonary histoplasmosis do we recognize? How do they manifest themselves radiographically?

20. What are the main radiographic features in coccidioidomycosis?

21. What are the main roentgen features in aspergillosis as it affects the lung?

22. What are the main radiographic features of viral bronchopneumonias? Which of these is most prevalent?

23. List the collagen diseases as they affect the lung and indicate some features which might help differentiate one type from another.

24. What is meant by the respiratory distress syndrome or hyaline membrane disease of the newborn?

25. What is meant by "bronchopulmonary dysplasia" of the infant?

26. Indicate some of the special roentgen features of mucoviscidosis.

27. Indicate some of the different types of aspiration pneumonia. How may they be classified? What are the different types of lipoid pneumonia? What are the main roentgen features of these several types of aspiration pneumonia?

28. What is meant by "Loeffler's syndrome" and what are its main roentgen features?

29. Indicate the different morphologic types of pulmonary edema and tell how they are usually manifest radiographically.

30. Indicate the main roentgen features of alveolar proteinosis.

1. What are the main roentgen features of most of the acute exanthemas of childhood, especially measles and whooping cough?

32. What are the main radiographic features of staphylococcus pneumonia in the infant?

33. What are the main radiographic features of staphylococcus pneumonia in adults?

34. What are the main radiographic features of klebsiella and aerobacter pneumonias (Friedländer's pneumonias)?

35. What are the main roentgen features of chemical pneumonitis?

36. What are the main roentgen features of renal transplantation pneumonia?

37. What are the main roentgen features of the pulmonary renal syndrome (Goodpasture's syndrome)?

38. What is meant by "pulmonary dysmaturity" or the "Wilson-Mikity syndrome"?

39. What are the main radiologic features in pulmonary hemosiderosis? What other disease entity does this resemble closely?

40. What are the main radiologic features of bronchopulmonary dysplasia "as it may be applied to adults"?

41. As a general rule, how does the concept of bronchogenic carcinoma or lung neoplasm fit into the category of poorly defined, homogeneous densities of the lung?

18

Radiology of Nodular Lesions of the Lung Parenchyma

DEFINITION AND CLASSIFICATION

A "nodular lesion" of the lung parenchyma by our definition refers to those solid or partially solid lesions which tend to be clearly demarcated in the lung, as opposed to the poorly defined, homogeneous, and diffuse shadows previously discussed in Chapter 17, the linear and reticular shadows described in Chapter 19, and the lucent, largely air-containing lesions in Chapter 20.

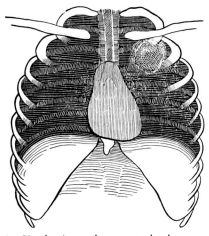

1. Single, irregular mass shadows:
   a. 5 mm. to 3 cm. in diameter
   b. greater than 3 cm. in diameter

A

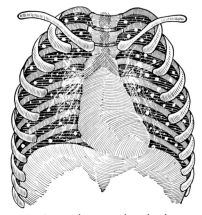

2. Coarsely granular shadows

B

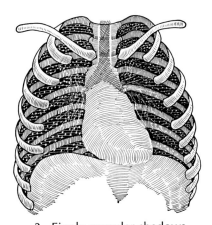

3. Finely granular shadows

C

Figure 18–1 General classification of nodular lesions of lung parenchyma. *A*. Single irregular mass shadows. *B*. Multiple coarse nodular shadows. *C*. Finely nodular shadows. *Note:* Single irregular mass shadows less than 3 cm. in diameter are not alluded to here. These so-called "coin lesions" usually represent granuloma, early malignancy, hamartomas, adenomas, exudate, or blood vessels in cross section.

SINGLE IRREGULAR MASS SHADOWS 3 CM. OR LESS IN DIAMETER (Figure 18–2)

Classification

1. Granulomas
2. Hamartomas
3. Exudative lesions
4. Blood vessels in cross section
5. Neoplasms

The contents may be either calcified or necrotic and hence cavitated. If cavitary, the inner wall may be shaggy and thick or thin and regular. There may or may not be a reactive zone around the lesion.

In the erect position, a fluid level may be present.

The 3 cm. size limitation is arbitrary, and these lesions are often called "coin lesions" of the lung. Actually, they are not strictly coin-shaped, but rather small spherules.

From the foregoing, it is most apparent that body section radiography is essential to help distinguish the architecture and hence the probable pathology of the lesion.

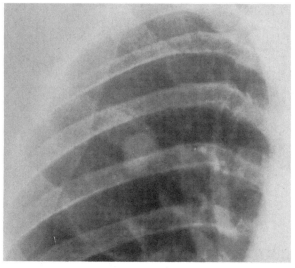 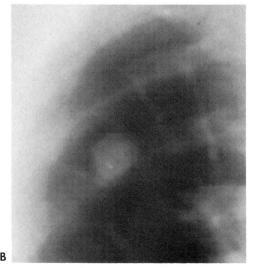

A   B

Figure 18–2 *A.* Nodule in the right upper lobe. *B.* Polytomogram of this nodule showing a small nidus of calcification within the nodule not otherwise demonstrable, establishing that this lesion is a benign lesion caused by a granuloma.

SINGLE IRREGULAR MASS LESIONS IN THE LUNG PARENCHYMA GREATER THAN 3 CM. IN DIAMETER

The radiographic appearances of single mass shadows greater than 3 centimeters in diameter may be classified as follows:

1. Sharply demarcated
   a. Fluid-filled lung cyst (see Chapter 20)
   b. Tumors of pleura, thoracic cage, or lung (previously considered)
   c. Hamartoma (flat on one side in tangential view)
   d. Lipoid pneumonia (occasionally; more frequently irregular)
   e. Granuloma
2. Irregular with "fuzzy" outline representing zone of peripheral inflammation or infiltration
   a. Abscess, granuloma (lipoid, infections; see Chapter 17)
   b. Infarct (Chapter 17)
   c. Arteriovenous aneurysm
   d. Bronchial adenoma (including bronchiolar or alveolar carcinoma)
   e. Bronchogenic carcinoma
   f. Lipoid pneumonia
3. Containing air or fluid
   a. With thick shaggy walls
      (1) Abscess
      (2) Carcinoma
      (3) Tuberculosis
   b. With thin walls
      (1) Lung cyst
      (2) Mycotic cavities
      (3) Tuberculosis (caseous)
      (4) Pulmonary hematoma
   c. With cavity disproportionately small in relation to the wall or surrounding consolidation, with possible irregular projections into the cavity
      (1) Bronchogenic carcinoma
4. Associated with calcium
   a. Hamartoma
   b. Conglomerate granulomas
      (1) Histoplasmoma—the target calcification appearance

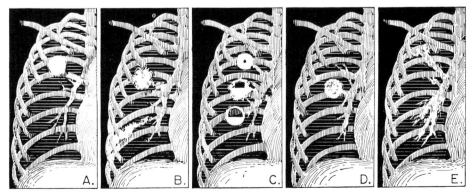

Figure 18–3 Categories of appearance of single irregular mass shadows. *A.* Sharply demarcated, solid. *B.* Irregular, fuzzy outline, but solid. *C.* Containing air or fluid. *D.* Associated with calcium. *E.* Associated with linear extension to the hilus. (For pathological entities, see outline.)

(2) Tuberculoma with multiple foci of calcification
(3) Solitary metastasis from osteogenic sarcoma which may at times contain bone
5. Associated with linear extension to the hilus
   a. Arteriovenous aneurysm
   b. Pulmonary carcinoma
   c. "Dunham's fan" in tuberculosis
   d. "Sequestration" of the lung

Sharply Demarcated Lesions

Hamartoma (Figure 18–4)

Definition. An overdevelopment of some tissue element which belongs normally at the site where it is found. Thus, a hamartoma of the lung consists of an overgrowth of such tissue as cartilage, fibrous tissue, smooth muscle tissue, or blood vessels.

Radiographic Features

Sharply defined, rounded shadow of an intermediate soft tissue density, varying in diameter from 2.5 to 9 cm. with no other associated findings.

Punctate areas of calcium deposit are contained within the sharply demarcated mass in about 50 per cent of cases. This calcium may have a "popcorn" configuration.

Body section radiography is indicated in all such cases.

Occasional umbilication.

May enlarge slowly.

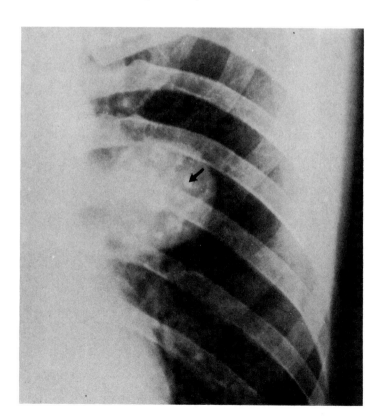

Figure 18–4 Hamartoma of the lung. P-A radiograph demonstrating such a tumor. The arrow points to calcium contained within the tumor mass and resembling "popcorn" calcification.

Irregular Outline With or Without Cavitation

Lung Abscess (Figure 18–5)

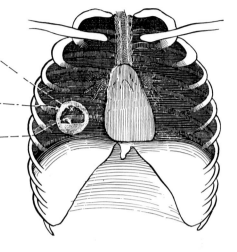

SINGLE-CHAMBERED OR
MULTICHAMBERED CAVITY
(*MAY BE FILLED WITH FLUID AND
NOT BE SEEN*)

INFLAMMATORY OR
GRANULOMATOUS WALL;
OR WALL OF ATELECTATIC
TISSUE

AIR-MENISCUS LEVEL

*USUALLY SITUATED NEAR
PLEURAL SURFACE (75%)
MAY RUPTURE INTO PLEURA
AND FORM BRONCHOPLEURAL
FISTULA*

Figure 18–5 Diagram of radiographic appearances in association with lung abscess.

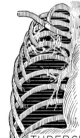

1. More apt to be irregular
2. Less fluid levels
3. More apt to be in lobe apices or subapices

TUBERCULOSIS

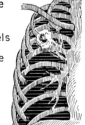

1. Shaggy
2. Tumefaction within cavity
3. Satellite metastatic nodes

BRONCHOGENIC CARCINOMA

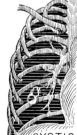

1. Thin-walled
2. May be multiple
3. May be associated emphysema

CYSTIC DISEASE

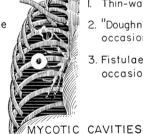

1. Thin-walled
2. "Doughnut" occasionally
3. Fistulae occasionally

MYCOTIC CAVITIES

Figure 18–6 Differential diagnosis of cavitary lesions.

1. Basilar often
2. Peribronchial beading
3. Segmental atelectasis

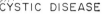

BRONCHIECTASIS

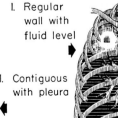

1. Regular wall with fluid level
1. Contiguous with pleura

EMPYEMA

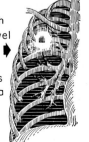

LUNG ABSCESS

Arteriovenous Aneurysm or Pulmonary Angioma of the Lung
(Figures 18–7, 18–8)

Telangiectasis elsewhere (in over 50 per cent of the cases) (Rendu-Osler-Weber's disease).

Radiographic Features

Strandlike vascular bands can often be traced to and from the lesion which is usually found in middle and lower lobes.

On fluoroscopy, the lesion pulsates; it decreases in size with straining against a closed glottis (Valsalva test); it increases in size with inspiration against a closed glottis (Müller test).

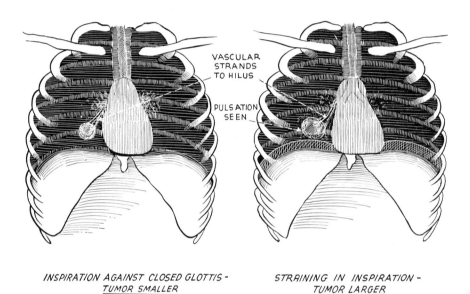

INSPIRATION AGAINST CLOSED GLOTTIS –
TUMOR SMALLER

STRAINING IN INSPIRATION –
TUMOR LARGER

Figure 18–7   Diagrammatic appearances of arteriovenous aneurysm (angioma) of the lung.

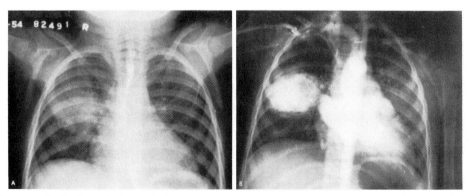

Figure 18–8   Radiograph demonstrating the appearance of an arteriovenous malformation of the lung.

Bronchial Adenoma. The average bronchial adenoma ranges in size from 1 to 10 cm. in diameter (with an average of about 4 cm.); it is sharply circumscribed, slightly lobulated, and is ordinarily detected by the adjoining abnormalities of the lung rather than by the nodulation itself. It is probable that only about one in four of these may be detected by its nodular appearance. It appears in three histologic forms: (1) the carcinoid type; (2) the cylindroma type; (3) the mixed tumor type comparable with tumors of the salivary glands.

Clinical Manifestations

Cough, pain, hemoptysis, and repeated pneumonia in a 20 to 40 year old person, usually female. After bronchial occlusion, pneumonia and bronchiectasis follow.

The "carcinoid syndrome" appears in association with a carcinoid neoplasm that is more invasive and more active physiologically than the usual bronchial adenoma.

Roentgenologic Presentations

1. No radiographic pattern is diagnostic.
2. A hilar mass alone or in combination with a parenchymal infiltration is the most common appearance.
3. Atelectasis.
4. Pleural effusion or a negative chest film is rare.
5. Tomography and bronchography may demonstrate intrabronchial tumors or obstructions in a high percentage of cases, but differentiation from other bronchial neoplasms is usually not possible.
6. Metastases to bone do occur and are usually lytic in variety.
7. Bronchial adenomas may be malignant pulmonary neoplasms whose radiographic presentation is indistinguishable from that of bronchogenic carcinoma (Giustra and Stassa).

Primary Malignant Tumors of the Lung. Bronchogenic carcinoma is by far the most frequent primary malignant tumor of the lung. More rarely, carcinomas arise from alveolar epithelium.

VARIOUS APPEARANCES OF PRIMARY BRONCHOGENIC CARCINOMA

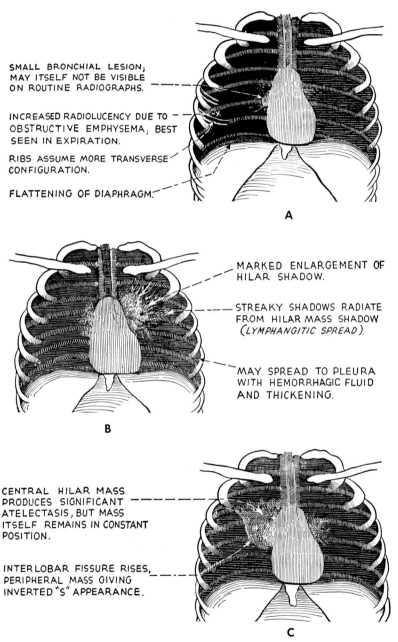

SMALL BRONCHIAL LESION; MAY ITSELF NOT BE VISIBLE ON ROUTINE RADIOGRAPHS.

INCREASED RADIOLUCENCY DUE TO OBSTRUCTIVE EMPHYSEMA; BEST SEEN IN EXPIRATION.

RIBS ASSUME MORE TRANSVERSE CONFIGURATION.

FLATTENING OF DIAPHRAGM.

A

MARKED ENLARGEMENT OF HILAR SHADOW.

STREAKY SHADOWS RADIATE FROM HILAR MASS SHADOW (*LYMPHANGITIC SPREAD*).

MAY SPREAD TO PLEURA WITH HEMORRHAGIC FLUID AND THICKENING.

B

CENTRAL HILAR MASS PRODUCES SIGNIFICANT ATELECTASIS, BUT MASS ITSELF REMAINS IN CONSTANT POSITION.

INTERLOBAR FISSURE RISES, PERIPHERAL MASS GIVING INVERTED "S" APPEARANCE.

C

Figure 18–9 *A.* Central type of bronchogenic carcinoma diagrammatically illustrated showing the check valve type of hyperlucency which may result with relatively small lesions. *B.* Diagram illustrating the central type of bronchogenic carcinoma associated with a marked enlargement of hilar nodal shadow with streaky shadows radiating from this hilar mass shadow due to retrograde lymphangitic spread. *C.* The central type of bronchogenic carcinoma in association with atelectasis, giving rise to the so-called inverted S appearance.

BRONCHOGENIC CARCINOMA (Continued)

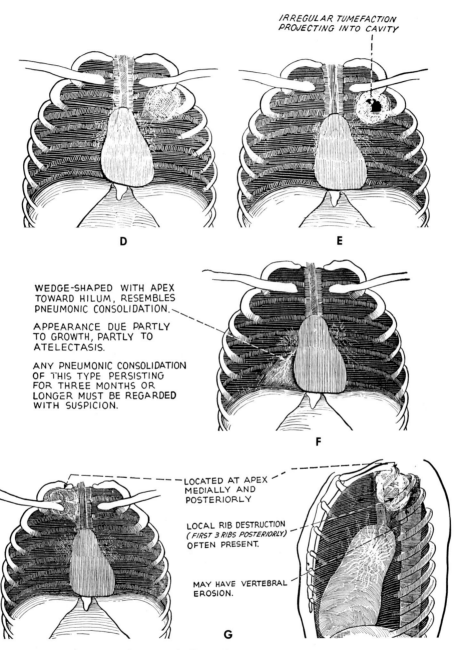

IRREGULAR TUMEFACTION
PROJECTING INTO CAVITY

D   **E**

WEDGE-SHAPED WITH APEX
TOWARD HILUM, RESEMBLES
PNEUMONIC CONSOLIDATION.

APPEARANCE DUE PARTLY
TO GROWTH, PARTLY TO
ATELECTASIS.

ANY PNEUMONIC CONSOLIDATION
OF THIS TYPE PERSISTING
FOR THREE MONTHS OR
LONGER MUST BE REGARDED
WITH SUSPICION.

F

LOCATED AT APEX
MEDIALLY AND
POSTERIORLY

LOCAL RIB DESTRUCTION
(FIRST 3 RIBS POSTERIORLY)
OFTEN PRESENT.

MAY HAVE VERTEBRAL
EROSION.

G

Figure 18–9 *Continued   D*. Diagrammatic illustration demonstrating the radiographic appearances of the peripheral type of bronchogenic carcinoma. *E*. Diagram representing the most frequent appearance of the pneumonic type of bronchogenic carcinoma. *F*. Diagram illustrating the radiographic appearances in association with the posterior sulcus apical type of bronchogenic carcinoma (Pancoast's tumor). *G*. Lymphangitic type. A similar appearance may be seen with metastatic malignancy from stomach, breast, pancreas, lung, lymphomas and leukemias, and prostate.

SUMMARY OF RADIOGRAPHIC FEATURES OF BRONCHOGENIC CARCINOMA

1. Elevated or depressed hilus
2. Obtuse arteriovenous angle
3. Increased space between esophagus and tracheobronchial tree (lateral projection) when esophagrams are available. Normal space is only 2 to 3 mm.; when greater than 5 mm. a solid mass interposed in this area must be suspected
4. Obliteration of the anterior mediastinal clear space
5. Obliteration of the paramediastinal radiolucent line
6. Double-contoured appearance of the aortic knob
7. Disproportionate elevation of the diaphragm with symptoms of recurrent laryngeal palsy
8. Segmental atelectasis or emphysema with air-trapping
9. Accentuated interlobar fissure with adjoining mass lesion
10. Mass lesion with Kerley's "B" lines (suggesting lymphangitic tumor spread)
11. Morton's S curve (see Figure 18–9C)
12. Eccentric cavitation
13. Persisting bronchopneumonia
14. Associated chronic lung diseases

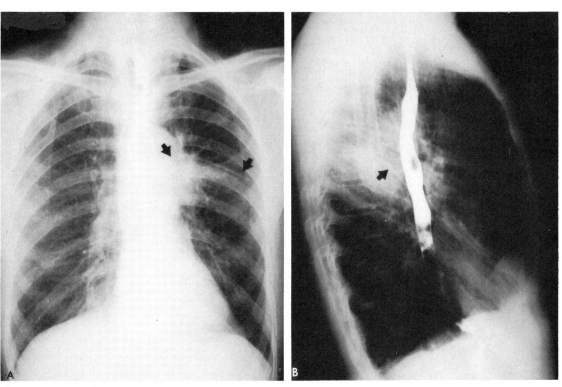

Figure 18–10 *A* and *B*. Mass shadow in the left hilus, coupled with extension to the adjoining interlobar fissure producing an accentuated appearance of this fissure. This mass also tends to produce a somewhat double-contoured appearance in the region of the aortic knob.

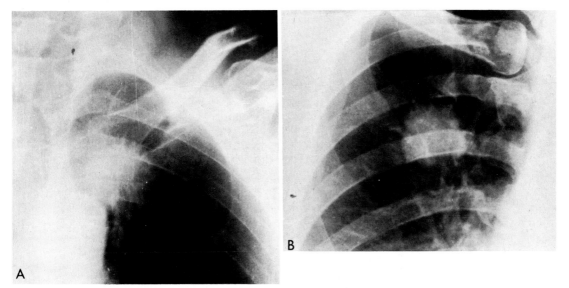

Figure 18–11 *A.* Squamous cell carcinoma of the left upper lobe forming in an old scar and hence called "scar carcinoma." *B.* Carcinoma of the right upper lobe having a stellate radiation around a relatively discrete nodule.

Carcinoma of Alveolar Origin (Bronchiolar Carcinoma)

1. No radiographic finding is pathognomonic.
2. Four major patterns, however, may be seen:
    a. Nodular
    b. Coalescent
    c. Infiltrative
    d. Mixed
3. The nodules may be single or multiple; small, medium, or large.
    a. They are usually fluffy with irregular and spiky margins. Some, however, tend to be regular and well-defined.
    b. "Coalescent" indicates grouping of the nodules.
    c. The infiltrative lesions are usually homogeneous with poorly defined transitions to normal lung. Kerley's "B" lines may be seen.
    d. "Mixed" patterns are composed of mixed nodules and infiltration.
4. Pleural effusion is not uncommon and may be extensive.
5. Metastases occur in 50 per cent of the cases.

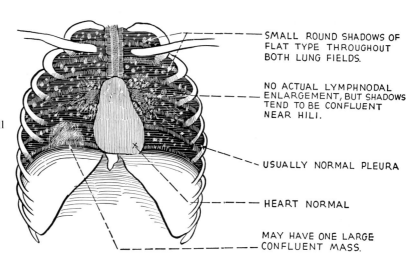

Figure 18–12 Alveolar cell (bronchiolar) carcinoma.

SMALL ROUND SHADOWS OF FLAT TYPE THROUGHOUT BOTH LUNG FIELDS.

NO ACTUAL LYMPHNODAL ENLARGEMENT, BUT SHADOWS TEND TO BE CONFLUENT NEAR HILI.

USUALLY NORMAL PLEURA

HEART NORMAL

MAY HAVE ONE LARGE CONFLUENT MASS.

Lipoid Pneumonia and Granuloma

Lipoid and Cholesterol Pneumonitis

Classification

1. Cholesterol pneumonitis — endogenous
    a. Obstructive
    b. Nonobstructive
2. Exogenous (chronic aspiration of oily substances)

Radiographic Manifestations of Cholesterol Pneumonitis

1. Endogenous types
    a. Confused with tumor, lung abscess, or infarct
    b. May be extensive and lobar, with collapse
    c. May be segmental, usually peripheral near the pleura, or along a fissure
    d. Occasional enlargement of mediastinal lymph nodes
    e. Rarely, cavities 1 to 1.5 cm. in diameter
2. Exogenous type (due to chronic aspiration of oily substances)
    a. Alveolar consolidation, with homogeneous consolidation of one or more segments, usually in lower lobes, depending on gravity
    b. May be several centimeters in diameter
    c. May have fairly well circumscribed margins simulating peripheral bronchogenic carcinoma
    d. Usually no calcification or cavitation radiographically
    e. The granulomas may resemble tuberculosis or sarcoid

TABLE 18–1   DISTINGUISHING FEATURES OF SOLITARY PULMONARY LESIONS

Characteristic	Favors Benign Lesion	Favors Malignant Lesion
Roentgenologic findings:		
Size	Less than 1 cm.	More than 4 cm.
Shape	Regular	Irregular
Margin	Smooth and round	Notched or indefinite — Rigler's notch sign
Calcification		
"Popcorn" type	Hamartoma probable	Absent
Laminated type	Granuloma probable	Absent
Central type	Granuloma probable	Absent
Marginal flaky type	May be granuloma	May be malignancy
Cavitation		
Smooth internally	Benign abscess or cyst	Usually absent
Rough internally	Less likely to be benign	Eccentric, usually present
Incidence	Granulomas — approximately 40 per cent Adenomas — 2 to 4 per cent Hamartomas — 7 per cent	Approximately 30 per cent

Pulmonary Sequestration

Definition. Separation of a segment or group of segments of lung from normal continuity with the rest of the bronchial tree whose blood supply comes from a systemic artery.

Types. Intralobar and extralobar.

General Comments Regarding Intralobar Sequestration. This is a nonfunctioning portion of lung within the visceral pleura of a pulmonary lobe. Its blood supply comes directly from the aorta or one of its branches, such as the descending thoracic aorta, abdominal aorta, intercostal artery, or aberrant vessels, while the pulmonary veins drain the blood from the lesion.

In about two-thirds of the cases, the lesion occupies the position of the posterior basilar segment of the left lung. In the remainder it is in a similar position on the right.

Ordinarily, there is no communication with a bronchus unless infection has supervened and produced drainage into a bronchial branch.

Radiographic Manifestations of Intralobar Sequestration

Homogeneous mass of water density in the left or right lower lobe.

In the presence of superimposed infection and communication with a bronchus, it may contain an air-fluid level or be surrounded by infected lung.

It requires angiographic demonstration of the blood supply for definitive diagnosis. The anomalous vessel extends like a "finger" medially toward the aorta.

Extralobar Sequestration

Differences from intralobar sequestration:

It is an accessory lung bud enclosed in its own pleural envelope.

It is said to be related to the left hemidiaphragm in 90 per cent of cases, either above or below it.

It drains via a systemic vein (azygos or gastrointestinal), but is supplied arterially directly from the aorta or one of its branches.

Occurs in neonates, and is associated with other congenital anomalies.

Radiographic Appearances of Extralobar Sequestration

Homogeneous mass of water density contiguous with the diaphragm, most frequently on the left.

Best demonstrated by angiography, otherwise accurate diagnosis is possible only by surgical exposure and excision.

Pulmonary Hematoma

Etiology. Penetrating or nonpenetrating chest injury.

Roentgen Appearance. Single or multiple spherical densities sometimes sharply demarcated, occasionally spindle-shaped.

Associated Findings. In the sequence of radiologic changes, a central area of radiolucency may develop (cavitation).

Ultimate Course. Usually resolves spontaneously (Williams).

MULTIPLE COARSELY NODULAR LESIONS IN LUNG PARENCHYMA (Figure 18–13)

Definition

This group of diseases comprises those containing multiple small nodulations of the lung of a clearly demarcated nature, generally with a diameter greater than approximately 5 mm., but less than 3 cm.

GROSS DIFFERENTIATION OF VARIOUS PARENCHYMAL SHADOWS

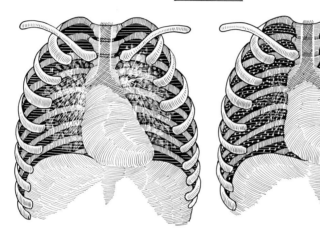

FLUFFY, DIFFUSE, HOMOGENEOUS SHADOWS
SLIGHTLY NODULAR (*PULMONARY EDEMA*)

FINELY GRANULAR SHADOWS

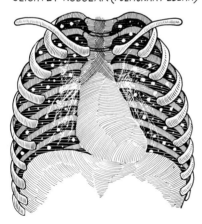

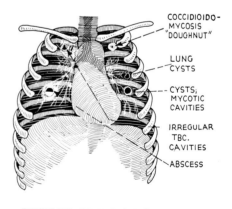

COCCIDIOIDO-
MYCOSIS
"DOUGHNUT"

LUNG
CYSTS

CYSTS;
MYCOTIC
CAVITIES

IRREGULAR
TBC.
CAVITIES

ABSCESS

COARSELY GRANULAR SHADOWS

SPHERICAL, DEMARCATED
MASS SHADOWS
(*MAY BE SOLID OR CAVITARY,
INCREASED RADIOLUCENCY
SHARPLY DEMARCATED.*)

Figure 18–13   Different appearances of the coarsely nodular lesions of the lung parenchyma.

Size and Shape (Figure 18–14)

1. Round or sharply circumscribed
2. Irregular
   a. Malignant lymphomas
   b. Necrotizing granulomatous processes

Location

1. Upper lobe: mycotic infections, tuberculosis
2. Uniform distribution: hematogenous spread
3. Lower lobes:
   a. Hematogenous spread of any lesion
   b. Autoimmunologic disorders such as rheumatoid arthritis, periarteritis nodosa, and disseminated lupus erythematosus. Rheumatoid nodules tend to be subpleural while lesions of periarteritis nodosa are more central in location.

Presence or Absence of Calcification

1. "Target" calcification: mycosis such as histoplasmosis
2. Peripheral calcification: other granulomata
3. Calcification (even ossification) may occur in metastatic neoplastic processes but is very rare in primary neoplasms
4. Pulmonary alveolar microlithiasis: small, "sandlike" calcifications with uniform distribution
5. Pneumoconioses
6. Pleural calcification
   a. Asbestosis
   b. Talc or mica inhalation
7. Parasitic parenchymal calcifications (rare). Curvilinear.
8. Multiple hamartomas: "popcorn" type calcification
9. Metastatic calcification: systemic or metabolic processes such as chronic mitral stenosis, renal failure, hypo- or hyperparathyroidism, and primary myeloid metaplasia

Presence or Absence of Cavitation

1. Very thin walls
   a. Mycoses
   b. Lung cysts
   c. Hematomas
2. Irregular, shaggy inner walls
   a. Neoplasms
   b. Tuberculosis
   c. Pyogenic abscesses (occasionally)
   d. Pulmonary metastases (occasionally). Melanoma, mucinous adenocarcinoma
   e. Necrotizing granulomatous processes (Wegener's, for example)
3. Nodule on inner wall
   a. Neoplasms
   b. Fungus ball

Edge Pattern and Internal Architecture

1. Irregular or "fuzzy" external edge: most likely inflammatory but may often be neoplastic
2. Sharply circumscribed
   a. Metastases (sarcomas, clear cell renal carcinomas, seminomas)
3. Coarsely nodular lesions: often metastases from gastrointestinal tract or lymphosarcoma
4. Lymphangitic metastases: linear, radiating from hilus
   a. Lymphomas
   b. Breast
   c. Lung
   d. Pancreatic carcinoma
5. Feeding artery or vein suggests arteriovenous malformation. These may change in size with Valsalva or Mueller maneuvers. Forty to sixty per cent have hereditary hemorrhagic telangiectasias.

Associated Findings in Hili, Bones, and Pleura: separately considered.

Metastatic Tumors of the Lung

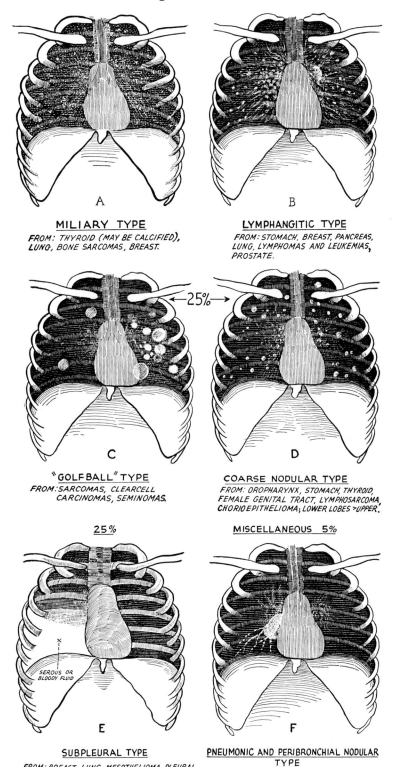

A

MILIARY TYPE
*FROM: THYROID (MAY BE CALCIFIED),
LUNG, BONE SARCOMAS, BREAST.*

B

LYMPHANGITIC TYPE
*FROM: STOMACH, BREAST, PANCREAS,
LUNG, LYMPHOMAS AND LEUKEMIAS,
PROSTATE.*

←25%→

C

"GOLFBALL" TYPE
*FROM: SARCOMAS, CLEARCELL
CARCINOMAS, SEMINOMAS.*

D

COARSE NODULAR TYPE
*FROM: OROPHARYNX, STOMACH, THYROID,
FEMALE GENITAL TRACT, LYMPHOSARCOMA,
CHORIOEPITHELIOMA; LOWER LOBES >UPPER.*

25%

MISCELLANEOUS   5%

*SEROUS OR
BLOODY FLUID*

E

SUBPLEURAL TYPE
*FROM: BREAST, LUNG; MESOTHELIOMA PLEURAL
LESIONS USUALLY TOO SMALL TO BE SEEN
(SEEN ONLY IN 3%).*

F

**PNEUMONIC AND PERIBRONCHIAL NODULAR
TYPE**
FROM: ESOPHAGUS, LUNG, BREAST.

Figure 18–14 *A* through *F*. Diagrams illustrating the various roentgen appearances of metastatic tumors of the lung.

Pneumoconioses

We may place the pneumoconioses in this category of nodular lesions of the lung parenchyma, realizing that the range of appearances with pneumoconioses includes the following:

Intensification of the pulmonary linear markings.

Diffuse and symmetrical stippling or nodulation throughout the lung fields.

Widening and increased density of the hilar shadows.

Diffuse, discrete small nodules throughout the lungs, 3 to 5 mm. in diameter.

Conglomerate masses superimposed on the above.

Cavitation within a conglomerate mass with or without a fluid level within the cavity.

The so-called "eggshell" calcification involving hilar and perihilar lymph nodes.

Pleural thickening and fibrosis.

Areas of calcification of various types in the pleura.

In acute beryllium pneumonitis (Figure 18–15), the chest film may show woolly, patchy densities throughout both lung fields, and these may undergo resolution in the acute phase of the disease.

Asbestosis is one of the chief causative agents of calcification of pleural plaques.

It is important to recognize that there is no special correlation between radiographic appearances and the clinical aspects of the case.

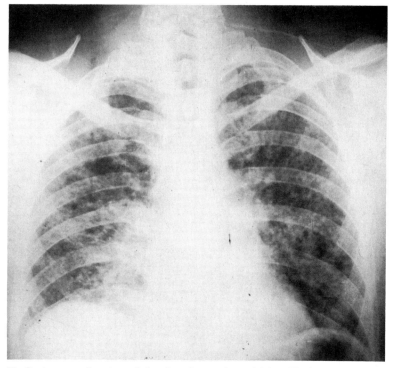

Figure 18–15 Postero-anterior view of the chest in a patient with berylliosis. (Courtesy of the Armed Forces Institute of Pathology. Washington. D.C.)

TABLE 18-2 CLASSIFICATION OF PNEUMOCONIOSES IN RELATION TO THE REACTIONS INDUCED (Adapted from Shanks and Kerley)

A. Dusts which induce fibroplastic tissue reactions:
   1. Free silica producing silicosis.
   2. Certain silicates such as asbestos, china clay, talc, mica, and sillimanite (silicatosis).
   3. Silica mixed with coal dust (anthracosilicosis).
B. Dusts merely stored in the lungs (no tissue reaction);
   1. Ferric oxide (siderosis); tin (stannosis); barium (baritosis).
   2. Ferric oxide mixed with a silver (argyrosiderosis).
C. Dusts of doubtful activity:
   1. Aluminum.
   2. Graphite.
D. Inorganic dusts causing a chemical pneumonitis:
   1. Beryllium.
   2. Manganese.
   3. Vanadium.
   4. Osmium.
   5. Platinum.
E. Organic dusts causing fibrosis or allergic reactions:
   1. Bagasse sugar cane dust (bagassosis).
   2. Cotton or linen dust (byssinosis).
   3. Wheat dust ("thresher's disease").
   4. Diatomite.
   5. Farmer's lung (possibly due to sensitization to mold) (Mindell).
F. Carcinogenic dusts:
   1. Arsenic.
   2. Radioactive dusts.
   3. Asbestos (?) (Freundlich and Greening).
G. Gases or fumes which produce a chemical pneumonitis or fibrosis (pneumoatmosis):
   1. Nitrous fumes (silo-filler's disease).
   2. Sulfuric fumes.
   3. Chlorine compound fumes.
   4. Acetone.
   5. Acrolein.
   6. Ammonia.
   7. Carbon tetrachloride.
   8. Cadmium fumes.
   9. Insecticides (peritachlorophenol).
  10. Isoamyl acetate (banana oil).
  11. Refrigerants (methyl chloride or methyl bromide).

LUNG DISEASE CHARACTERIZED BY FINELY GRANULAR SHADOWS

More than 80 conditions are characterized by the presence of disseminated miliary lesions in the lungs (Felson).

Those most frequently encountered are:

1. *Acute: changes demonstrated in less than two weeks*
   a. Primary atypical and other interstitial pneumonia (see Chapter 19)
   b. Influenzal pneumonia
   c. Bronchiolitis fibrosa obliterans (see Chapter 19)
2. *Subacute: changes apparent in two to eight weeks*
   a. Miliary tuberculosis and mycosis
   b. Miliary carcinosis
   c. The pneumoconioses
   d. Allergic pneumonias and "collagen diseases"
3. *Chronic: no changes observed within eight weeks*
   a. Pneumoconiosis
   b. Alveolar carcinoma of the lung
   c. Pulmonary arteriolar endarteritis
   d. Sarcoidosis
   e. Lipoid dyscrasias
   f. Pulmonary amyloidosis
   g. Arrested mycoses

Further differentiation of these various lesions is possible by utilizing specific clinical, laboratory, and other roentgenographic aids.

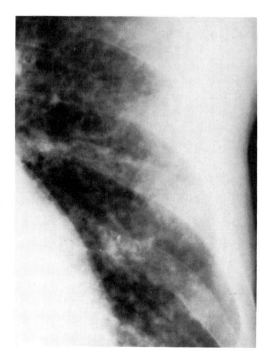

Figure 18–16 Postero-anterior close-up view of the lung fields in a patient with miliary tuberculosis to demonstrate the roentgen appearance of finely granular shadows.

Questions — Chapter 18

1. What is the general classification of nodular lesions of the lung parenchyma?

2. What is meant by "coin lesions" of the lung and what general pathologic conditions usually produce this radiographic appearance?

3. What are the various categories of radiographic appearance of single irregular mass shadows?

4. What are the main entities that must be considered among the sharply demarcated single mass shadows greater than 3 cm. in diameter?

5. What are the main clinical entities that must be considered among the single mass shadows which have an irregular ill-defined outline?

6. What are the main entities that produce single irregular mass shadows but contain air or fluid?

7. What single mass shadows which are ordinarily quite sharply demarcated are associated with calcium deposits?

8. What single mass shadows in the lung parenchyma are usually associated with linear extension to the hilus?

9. What are the main radiographic features of a lung abscess?

10. Indicate some of the differential diagnostic radiographic features of various cavitary lesions.

11. Describe the various categories of radiographic appearances of primary bronchogenic carcinoma.

12. Describe the radiographic features of the alveolar cell or bronchiolar-type carcinoma.

13. Describe the main radiographic features of hamartomas of the lung.

14. Describe the main radiographic features of arteriovenous aneurysm or angioma of the lung.

15. Describe the radiographic appearances and classification of bronchopulmonary sequestration.

16. Describe the roentgen features of pulmonary hematomas.

17. What differential features are recognized for various multiple parenchymal nodular shadows?

18. Which metastatic neoplastic processes in lung tend usually to be rather irregular in shape rather than typically round or sharply circumscribed?

19. Is it possible to differentiate between the various autoimmunologic disorders ("collagen diseases") of the lung?

20. How may the presence or absence of calcification within multiple lesions in the lung help in determining the cause?

21. Which metabolic processes or systemic diseases, other than infectious granulomas or neoplasms, may appear as metastatic calcific foci in the lung?

22. How may the presence or absence of cavitation and its characteristics help in the differentiation of multiple neoplastic processes? Which metastatic neoplasms of the lung are apt to cavitate?

23. Which of the pneumoconioses is characterized by calcification of the pleura?

24. What are some of the pneumoconioses which induce a fibroplastic tissue reaction?

25. Which of the inhaled dusts do not produce a serious tissue reaction?

26. Which of the inhaled substances produce a chemical pneumonitis?

27. Which inhaled organic dust causes fibrosis or allergic reactions?

28. Which of the inhaled dusts may be carcinogenic?

29. Which of the gases or fumes may produce a chemical pneumonitis?

30. What is a general classification for the lung diseases characterized by fine granular shadows?

31. What are the most frequently encountered lung diseases characterized by fine granular shadows?

19

Radiology of Lesions of the Lungs Characterized by Increase in Linear Markings

ANATOMICAL ENTITIES IN THE CHEST RESPONSIBLE FOR LINEAR OR RETICULAR MARKINGS OF THE LUNG

1. Pulmonary arteries
2. Pulmonary veins
3. Accentuation of the bronchial pattern
4. Other linear shadows projected in the interstitium of the lung
    a. Septate or accentuated lymphatic lines
    b. Line shadows caused by pleura
    c. Fleischner's linear or platelike atelectasis
    d. Lines resulting from infarction, segmental collapse, and lung scarring
    e. Line shadows radiating out of infectious granulomas, tumors, or pneumoconiosis lesions
    f. Weblike shadows and honeycombing
    g. Bandlike shadows

Postero-anterior View

Blood Flow in Upper and Lower Lungs (Figure 15–4)

Normally, *in the erect position* the blood flow in the lung bases is approximately three times the flow in the upper lung fields. In minimal passive hyperemia, one of the earliest manifestations of venous distension and passive hyperemia of the lungs is a "cephalization" of the flow pattern in the upper lobes so that the ratio of upper to lower begins to approach 1:1 rather than the 1:3 in the erect position.

When the *flow of blood is impeded on its return from the lungs* (Figure 15–4), both the arteries and the veins in the lower lung appear constricted, while the upper lobe arteries and veins become dilated. Early mitral stenosis is especially responsible for this appearance.

When there is an *increased pre- or postcapillary resistance in the lungs*, the veins of the lower lung fields appear constricted, while the upper lobe veins appear slightly dilated. The central pulmonary arteries appear enlarged, and there is a rapid tapering of the more peripheral and midzone arteries, the arteries of the outer zone appearing constricted. This is found with pulmonary arterial and venous hypertension.

When there is *increased pulmonary blood flow* (as with some of the congenital heart diseases especially), the pulmonary arteries and veins appear distended in all areas.

When there is a *diminished flow in the main pulmonary arteries,* such as may occur with infundibular stenosis, all of the vessels both centrally and peripherally appear small. At times, especially with congenital lesions such as pulmonic valvular stenosis, the main pulmonary artery dilates, yet the peripheral flow is diminished and the peripheral vessels are small, as with infundibular stenosis. This is possibly due to the "jet" of blood through the isolated stenotic valve.

With *increased peripheral resistance* there is a marked dilatation of the main pulmonary artery, but the peripheral branches are constricted. There is a reduced venous return to the heart via the pulmonary veins, and they become narrowed.

Interalveolar Interstitium

Ordinarily, the interalveolar septa are microscopic in size and are not visible radiographically. When they become thickened by edema fluid, fibrosis, or tumor cell infiltration, they may become visible radiographically.

Some of these interstitial accentuated lines are caused by the dilated intercommunicating lymphatics; when centrally situated these have been called Kerley's "A" lines and when peripherally situated, particularly at the lung bases, they have been called Kerley's "B" lines. *These have not been found unless the pulmonary capillary pressure is 18 mm. of mercury or more and the pulmonary arterial diastolic pressure is greater than 25 mm. of mercury.*

As edematous fluid accumulates in interstitial tissues, a perivascular haziness causes the involved vessels to become indistinct in outline. The central lung zones become slightly increased in density. The accumulation of fluid in the subpleural fibrous tissues causes an accentuation and thickening of the interlobar fissures, which become more readily visible radiographically.

ACCENTUATION OF THE PULMONARY ARTERIES

Classification

Barely Perceptible Dilatation of Arteries, occasionally in association with poorly defined homogeneous shadows of increased density, as in bronchopneumonia (see Chapter 17) (Figure 19–1).

Diffusely Dilated Pulmonary Arteries with increased pulmonary arterial flow, as in congenital heart disease in left-to-right shunts (see Chapter 23).

Centrally Enlarged Pulmonary Arteries, With a Rapid Tapering of the pulmonary arteries toward the midzones of the lung, as in pulmonary hypertension.

Pulmonary Hypertension

The central engorgement and rapid tapering of pulmonary arteries is seen in five differing *physiologic* circumstances.

Hyperdynamic. When the left-to-right shunt approaches a 3:1 ratio, vasoconstriction of the peripheral pulmonary arteries results.

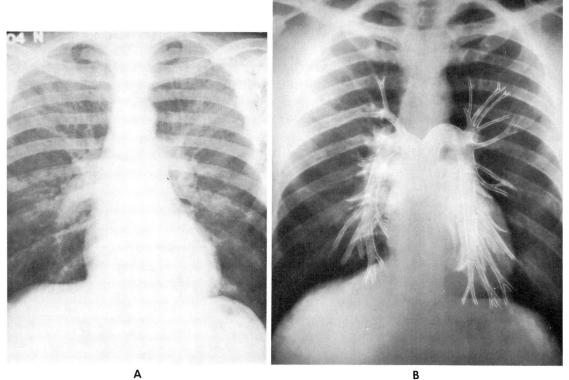

A   **B**

Figure 19–1 *A*. Distension of the arterial components of the lung fields. There is also a prominence of the pulmonary arteries. *B*. Diagrammatic representation of active hyperemia of the lungs.

Vasoconstrictive. Obstruction to venous return at the left atrial level (mitral stenosis, atrial myxoma, cor triatriatum) causes a rise in venous pressure. As this becomes chronic, the main pulmonary arteries dilate, but beyond the third division the arteries are narrow, tortuous, and irregular in contrast to the hyperdynamic type. In some instances, the lower lobe veins appear to contract, whereas the upper lobe veins dilate.

Obliterative (Figure 19–2)

In chronic obstructive pulmonary disease (emphysema) there is an obliteration of the interalveolar septa, with loss of capillaries peripherally. This diminution in the capillary bed results in a pulmonary hypertension.

In pulmonary fibrosis, pneumoconiosis, and rarely, sarcoidosis, there is an increased resistance to flow in the pulmonary arteriolar and capillary bed, and pulmonary hypertension results.

In scleroderma, periarteritis nodosa and rheumatoid disease, intimal thickening and sclerosis lead to increased peripheral resistance and pulmonary hypertension.

Thromboembolic disease, with emboli lodging in the large or small pulmonary arteries, may cause infarction, and this also results in pulmonary hypertension (Goodwin et al.). Pulmonary angiography is especially important in the demonstration of this type of pulmonary artery disease.

When a major pulmonary artery is obstructed, a somewhat different radiographic picture results, described as the "pruned tree" appearance (Figure 19–3).

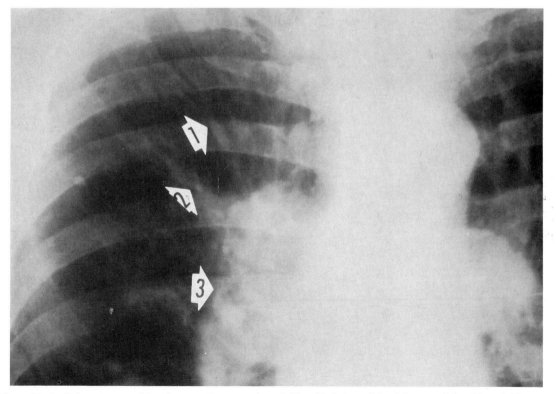

Figure 19–2 Pulmonary arterial and venous hypertension. *A*. Magnified view of the right upper lobe: (1) probable artery distended with rapid tapering, indicating arterial hypertension; (2) a distended vein; (3) the markedly distended right pulmonary artery.

High Altitude Pulmonary Hypertension. Chronic oxygen lack in individuals who live in high altitudes may have a direct constrictive effect on the arterial tree and produce the so-called "high altitude pulmonary hypertension."

Primary Idiopathic Hypertension. This occurs primarily in women under 40 years of age or in children in whom the fetal histologic structure of the muscular arterial media persists beyond the age at which involution to the adult form normally occurs.

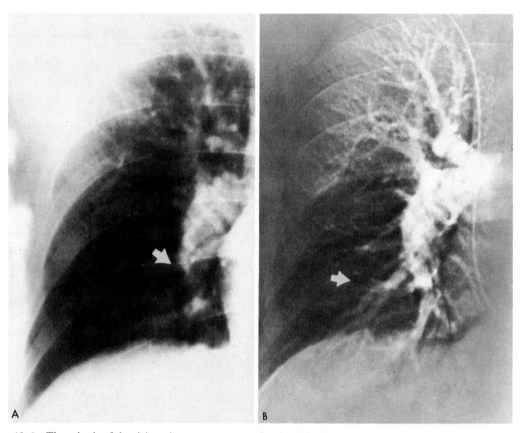

Figure 19–3 Thrombosis of the right pulmonary artery. *A.* On the plain film study, the pulmonary artery shows a sharp margination near the second order branches, with only faint vascularity peripheral to this region. *B.* The injection of contrast material into the pulmonary artery shows the "pruned tree" appearance of the thrombosed artery, whereas there is a normal arborization in the right upper lobe. This appearance has been intensified by subtraction (see text for this special technique).

ABNORMALITY OF THE PULMONARY VEINS

1. **Increase in size of the pulmonary veins**
    a. Left-to-right intracardiac shunts (septal defects)
    b. Extracardiac shunts
        (1) Patent ductus arteriosus
        (2) Aortic-pulmonary window
        (3) Anomalous pulmonary venous return
2. **Decrease in size of pulmonary veins**
    a. With decrease in pulmonary arterial circulation
        (1) Congenital heart lesions (i.e., pulmonic stenosis; tetralogy of Fallot)
        (2) Thrombosis of the main pulmonary artery
    b. With postcapillary hypertension
        (1) Acquired mitral valvular disease
        (2) Left ventricular failure
        (3) Cor triatriatum
        (4) Left atrial myxoma
        (5) Primary pulmonary venous obstruction
        (6) Total anomalous pulmonary venous return below the diaphragm
3. **Diffuse increase followed by a decrease in the size of the pulmonary veins. Left heart failure**
    a. Sequence of events
4. **Anomalous pulmonary veins**
    a. Total and partial anomalous pulmonary venous return
    b. Scimitar syndrome
5. **The pulmonary varicosity**
    a. Part of a generalized pulmonary venous engorgement
    b. Solitary pulmonary varix

Postulate by Simon (1958): Increase in pulmonary venous pressure above a critical level results in venous vasoconstriction. Since hydrostatic pressure is higher in the lower lobes than in the upper when a person is erect (12–15 mm. Hg. in adults), venous vasoconstriction occurs first in the lower lobes, and pulmonary perfusion increases in the upper lobes. As the venous hypertension persists, the constriction of upper lobe veins also occurs, and pulmonary arterial hypertension supervenes. This postulate has not been proved but serves to explain the radiographic manifestations of both mitral valvular disease and left heart failure.

Diffuse Increase Followed by a Decrease in the Size of the Pulmonary Veins. Left Heart Failure

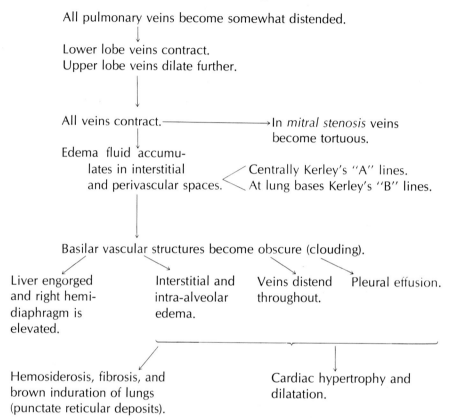

SEQUENCE OF PULMONARY VENOUS CHANGES WITH LEFT HEART FAILURE

All pulmonary veins become somewhat distended.

Lower lobe veins contract.
Upper lobe veins dilate further.

All veins contract. ──────────→ In *mitral stenosis* veins become tortuous.

Edema fluid accumulates in interstitial and perivascular spaces.
⟨ Centrally Kerley's "A" lines.
At lung bases Kerley's "B" lines.

Basilar vascular structures become obscure (clouding).

Liver engorged and right hemidiaphragm is elevated.

Interstitial and intra-alveolar edema.

Veins distend throughout.

Pleural effusion.

Hemosiderosis, fibrosis, and brown induration of lungs (punctate reticular deposits).

Cardiac hypertrophy and dilatation.

Bone formation with mitral stenosis: 2 to 5 mm. calcific deposits in the midlung zones (3 to 13 per cent of cases) (Kerley; Galloway et al.).

ACCENTUATION OF THE BRONCHIAL PATTERN

General Comment. The trachea and major central bronchi produce tubular air-containing shadows with minimal but visible wall thickness, at least to the level of the intermediate bronchus on the right and the left lower lobe bronchus on the left. Beyond the hilar regions and these defined areas, the bronchial shadows are blended into the air space shadows so that they are normally invisible. When seen, they represent either:

1. An air bronchogram—consolidated lung around the visualized bronchus (pneumonia) (Chapter 17).
2. Chronically inflamed bronchi, or those which have elements of both muscular hypertrophy, glandular hyperplasia, and inflammation, as in asthma, coupled with bronchitis (Robbins; Hodson and Trickey).
3. Thickened bronchial walls due to peribronchial fibrosis, particularly when this is coupled with bronchial dilatation, as in bronchiectasis.
   a. When bronchiectatic segments become filled with retained secretions, they produce fingerlike shadows (the "gloved finger" shadow of Simon).
   b. Atelectasis and pneumonitis are frequently associated with bronchiectasis, which add to the tubular or fingerlike appearance.
4. Mucoid impactions.
   a. May be central or
   b. Peripheral, as in mucoviscidosis and asthma.

The above roentgen signs are found in multiple disease categories, which are described in the following paragraphs.

Bronchiectasis

Definition. Abnormal and irreversible dilatation of the bronchi and bronchioles caused by a chronic necrotizing infection.

Major Lobes Involved. It is bilateral in about 50 per cent of cases, and is usually found in the basal segments of the lower lobes. When the lingula or middle lobes are affected, usually the adjoining segments of the lower lobes are also involved.

Radiographic Findings (Figure 19–4)

Peribronchial fibrosis, retained secretions produce accentuated linear markings.

There is atelectasis and reduction of volume in the affected area of lung.

Cystic spaces (up to 2 cm. in diameter), which adjoin the accentuated markings and areas of atelectasis, impart a beaded appearance to the involved lung. This may progress to outright "honeycombing" and emphysema.

Compensatory overinflation of the adjoining lung may occur.

Occasionally, there may be adjoining pleural thickening.

Bronchography is essential for a more detailed description of findings prior to treatment.

The "dirty" chest appearance of Simon usually indicates mucous gland hypertrophy, and may be associated with bronchitis.

Emphysema (see Chapter 20) accompanies bronchitis in at least 15 per cent of patients who seek medical assistance for this disorder (Simon, G., 1959).

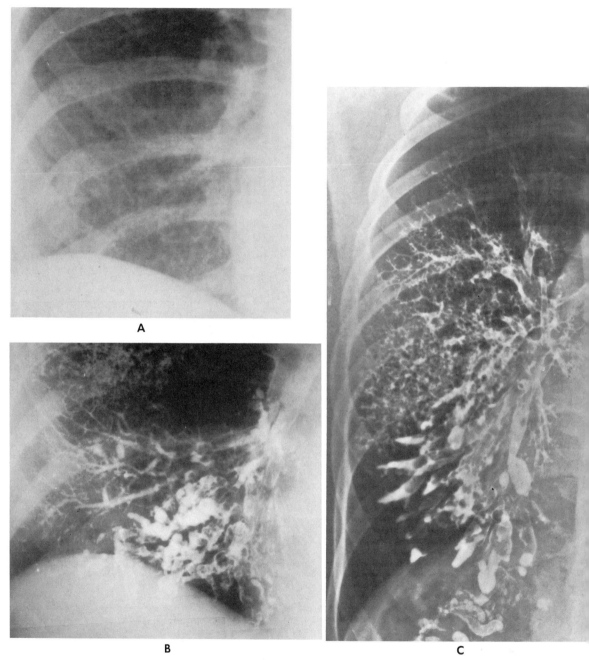

Figure 19–4   Bronchiectasis, plain films, and bronchograms, all magnified. *A*. Postero-anterior view at the right lung base demonstrates the increased interstitial pattern with a lucent and higher density of reticulonodularity on the plain film. *B* and *C*. Bronchograms. Note the counterpart of the sacculation as demonstrated by the bronchogram on the films without the additional opaque contrast.

Mucoid Impaction (Figure 19–5)

Definition.   Plugging with inspissated mucus of one or more bronchi distal to a major lobar bronchus.

Sites of Occurrence.   Predominantly in the upper lobe, although it may occur in any lobe, or even in multiple sites in the lung (Urschel et al.).

Precursory Diseases.   Asthma and bronchitis usually. Mucoviscidosis.

Radiographic Appearances

The plugs may be seen as Y- or V-shaped densities in a second order bronchus.

May appear round, oval, or elliptical and may simulate a tumor.

The distal lung is usually not atelectatic.

When the plug is removed or expectorated, there remains a central area of bronchiectasis.

May be associated with cavitation.

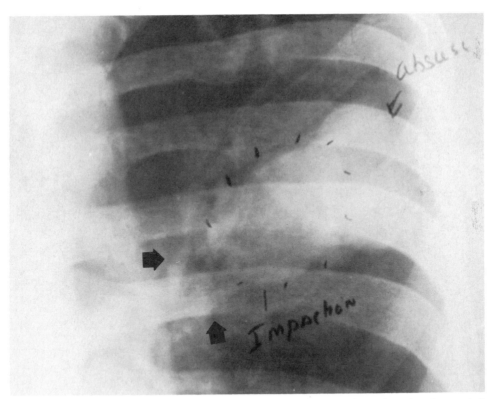

Figure 19–5   Mucous plug impaction of the left upper lobe. The arrows point to the rather characteristic V appearance with the impaction shown peripherally and the abscess most peripherally. (Film obtained courtesy of Dr. Alvin Sears, Dallas, Texas.)

Mucoviscidosis (Cystic Fibrosis) (Figure 19–6)

Radiographic Appearances

Accentuation of an irregular type of the linear markings throughout the lungs.

Thickened bronchial walls which give rise to numerous "parallel line shadows."

Large or small areas of atelectasis.

Recurrent pneumonitis.

Interspersed nodular, fingerlike shadows (Waring et al.), thought to represent peripheral mucoid bronchial impactions.

Late in the disease: Numerous strandlike shadows suggesting fibrosis, and cystlike radiolucencies due to a superimposed emphysema (Figure 19–6).

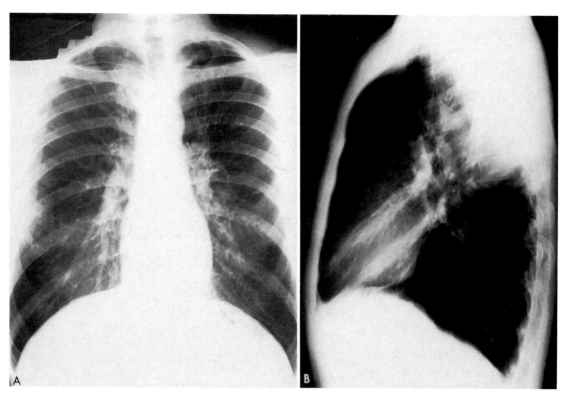

Figure 19–6   Mucoviscidosis in an adult.

OTHER LINEAR SHADOWS PROJECTED IN THE INTERSTITIUM OF THE LUNG

Classification

1. "Septate" or accentuated lymphatic lines.
2. Line shadows caused by pleura.
3. Fleischner's "linear or platelike atelectasis."
4. Line shadows resulting from infarctions, segmental collapse, and lung scarring.
5. Line shadows radiating out of infectious granulomas, tumors, or pneumoconiosis deposits.
6. Weblike shadows and honeycombing.
7. Bandlike shadows.

Septate or Accentuated Lymphatic Lines

(Kerley's "A" and "B" lines)

Pathogenesis

1. Pulmonary edema
2. Pulmonary venous hypertension
3. Mitral valvular disease
4. Lymphangitic carcinomatosis; lymphomas
5. Hemosiderosis and other disease entities where depositions occur in the interlobular septa

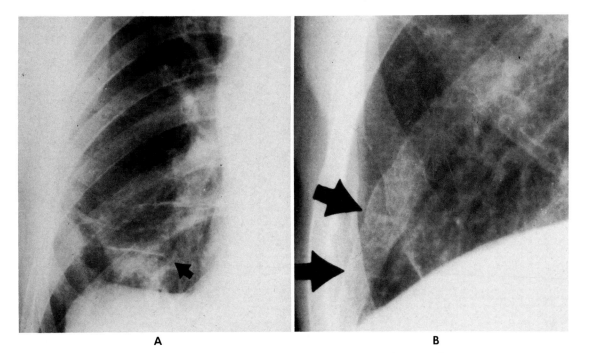

A   B

Figure 19–7   *A*. Platelike (segmental) atelectasis. *B*. Kerley's "B" lines.

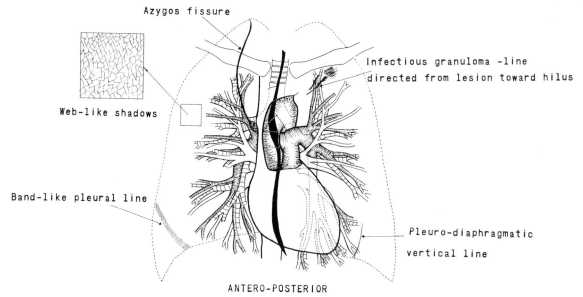

Figure 19–8 Other linear lung shadows.

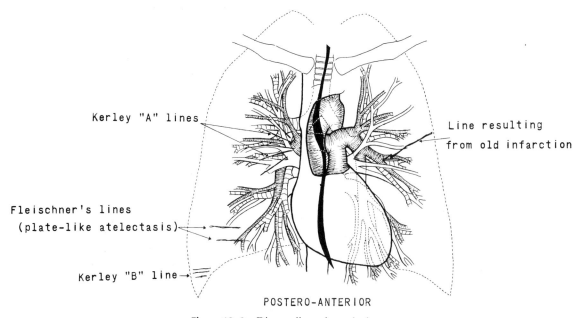

Figure 19–9 Diverse linear lung shadows.

Figure 19–10 Reticulonodular disease of the lung, such as may occur with histiocytosis.

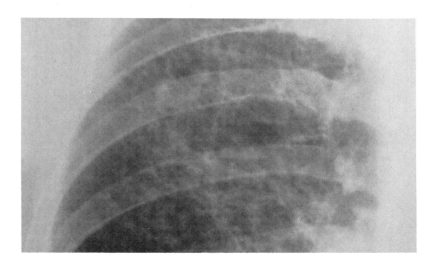

Line Shadows Caused by Pleura

General Types

1. Horizontal or oblique fissures (Chapter 16).
2. Accessory fissures (Chapter 16).
3. Azygos fissure (Chapter 16).
4. Pleurodiaphragmatic vertical lines: These are at times referred to as "adhesions" but probably represent indentations of the pleura toward a scar in the lung parenchyma.
5. Vertical mediastinal pleural lines (especially with herniated lung across the midline).

Fleischner's Linear or Platelike Atelectasis

Definition. Linear shadows of increased density at the lung bases in a roughly horizontal plane, from 1 to 3 mm. in thickness and several centimeters in length. These lines can usually be shown to extend to the pleura.

Pathogenesis. Diminished diaphragmatic excursion, as in splinting of the diaphragm following abdominal surgery. Usually there is an exudate within the collapsed alveoli and in the interalveolar septa. It is thought that small airway obstruction is usually associated with stagnant secretions as well.

This is usually a temporary process, disappearing with good ventilatory measures.

Lines Resulting from Infarctions, Segmental Collapse, and Lung Scarring

Definition. Linear shadows, usually arising from segmental or subsegmental atelectasis, or scars resulting from healed infectious granulomas or infarcts.

At times, these cannot be traced to a truly segmental origin (Reid) and may be caused by thrombosed pulmonary veins. These latter lines are more apt to be obliquely, rather than horizontally, oriented.

Line Shadows Radiating Out of Infectious Granulomas, Tumors, or Pneumoconiosis Lesions

Line shadows are frequently found which radiate away from a nodular lesion of the parenchyma toward the lung hilus. They are at times caused by an admixture of tubercles, fibrous tissue, and thickened lymphatics, as in cases of healed tuberculosis; or they may be related to a "tumor track" from a malignant neoplasm of the lung to the lung hilus (Marmorshtain).

Similar line shadows may at times be identified as radiating from a nodular lesion toward the pleura and may be related to "indrawn pleura" or subsegmental atelectasis (Simon, G., 1971).

Rigler observed the latter sign in 20 of 25 cases of alveolar cell carcinoma.

Weblike Shadows and Honeycombing

Definition. These linear shadows form a network resembling a spider's web which may have small or large interstices. Honeycombing is a term widely used to represent a coarse reticular pattern, which suggests a cellular appearance or "honeycomb." Unfortunately, this term has also been widely used to suggest interlacing areas of fibrosis or interstitial involvement of the lung by the reticuloendothelial diseases.

Pathogenesis. Interstitial replacement in the lung gives rise to this pattern in its varying degrees. Thus, this may occur with asbestosis, interstitial fibrosis, interstitial pneumonias or rheumatoid lung.

The term honeycomb was originally used to describe the late changes of histiocytosis X in the lung, when the air-containing spaces are 5 to 10 mm. in diameter and are separated by a coarse network. This pattern, however, may also be seen with tuberous sclerosis, tuberculosis, bronchiectasis, and chronic fungal infections.

In the case of Hamman-Rich disease, the "cysts" tend to be somewhat smaller (up to 3 mm. in diameter), more closely resembling the picture described for bronchopulmonary dysplasia (Chapter 17).

Bandlike Shadows

Wide bandlike shadows are seen particularly with the broad adhesions between lung parenchyma and pleura (Chapter 16).

A bandlike curvilinear appearance is seen with the "scimitar" syndrome.

GENERAL COMMENTS RELATED TO FIBROTIC DISEASE OF THE LUNG

Fibrotic disease of the lung may occur in a wide variety of situations and from many causes.

Thus, it may be interstitial, peribronchial, perivascular, perialveolar, or pleural in origin.

It may occur with Boeck's sarcoidosis, lipoid storage diseases, collagen diseases, chronic beryllium poisoning, asbestosis, other pneumoconioses, postradiation, with idiopathic pulmonary hemosiderosis, and with idiopathic progressive interstitial fibrosis (Hamman-Rich syndrome, Ceelen-Gellerstedt syndrome) (Fleischner and Reiner).

From the physiological point of view, when the fibrosis involves the interstitium of the alveolar walls an alveolar-capillary block syndrome may develop.

When there is a perivascular fibrosis and interference with proper flow of blood through the lungs, a pulmonary hypertension may result with secondary cor pulmonale.

Most Common Diseases Responsible for Accentuated Interstitial Markings in the Lung

1. Histiocytosis X
2. Sarcoid
3. Scleroderma rheumatoid arthritis (i.e., autoimmune [collagen] diseases)
4. Idiopathic interstitial fibrosis
5. Tuberous sclerosis
6. Bronchiolar dilatation with muscular hyperplasia
7. Pneumoconiosis
8. Hemosiderosis
9. Mucoviscidosis
10. Lymphangitic carcinomatosis
11. Interstitial pneumonias
    a. Usual or classical interstitial pneumonia (UIP)
    b. Bronchiolitis obliterans and diffuse alveolar damage (BIP)
    c. Desquamative interstitial pneumonia (DIP)
    d. Lymphoid interstitial pneumonia (LIP)
    e. Giant cell interstitial pneumonia (GIP)

The common characteristic of all these is the so-called honeycomb appearance.

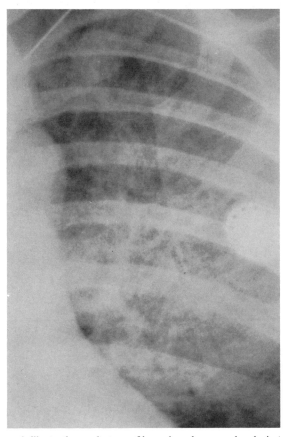

Figure 19–11   Radiograph illustrating end stage of bronchopulmonary dysplasia (oxygen toxicity) in the adult.

Questions — Chapter 19

1. What are the anatomical entities in the chest responsible for linear or reticular markings of the lung?

2. Draw a diagram showing the usual orientation of the apical arteries and veins as well as the main pulmonary arteries and lower pulmonary veins as they drain into the left atrium. Indicate the etiology of the so-called "azygos" fissure.

3. Where is the azygos "knob" usually found and what is its maximum normal measurement?

4. Where does the right pulmonary artery lie in respect to the tracheobronchial air column in the lateral view? The left pulmonary artery?

5. Where do the pulmonary veins lie in the lateral view?

6. What is the physiologic significance of pulmonary arteries which are centrally enlarged and taper rapidly toward the midzone of the lung?

7. Indicate some of the causes of increase in size of the pulmonary veins.

8. Indicate some of the causes of a decrease in size of the pulmonary veins.

9. Indicate causes of a diffuse increase followed by a decrease in the size of some pulmonary veins, and describe the sequence of events in such clinical entities.

10. What is the sequence of pulmonary venous changes with left heart failure?

11. What is meant by the "scimitar syndrome" and what are its roentgenographic manifestations?

12. What is meant by the term air bronchogram and what is its pathologic and roentgenologic significance?

13. What are the radiographic findings usually associated with bronchiectasis in plain films as well as bronchograms?

14. What is the roentgenologic appearance often associated with mucoviscidosis?

15. Indicate some of the line shadows on a chest film which are caused by pleura.

16. What are some of the other line shadows on the chest apart from accentuated lymphatics and pleural lines?

17. What does the term honeycombing usually signify and what is its pathological parallel?

18. What is a bandlike shadow usually caused by?

19. Indicate some of the disease entities characterized by pulmonary fibrosis.

20. What is meant by the term platelike atelectasis?

21. What are the most common diseases responsible for interstitial fibrosis in the lungs?

22. What is meant by the term muscular sclerosis of the lungs? What are other synonyms for this condition? Describe the roentgenologic aspects of these.

Radiology of Lung Lesions Characterized by Increased Radiolucency in the Lung Fields — Either Localized or Generalized

CLASSIFICATION OF ROENTGEN SIGNS

A. Extrapulmonary
  1. Chest Wall Lucency (Chapter 16)
      a. Interstitial emphysema
      b. Neuromuscular atrophy or paralysis
      c. Congenital absence of muscle groups
      d. Surgical resections (radical mastectomy)
  2. Pleural Space Lucencies (Chapter 16)
      a. Pneumothorax
      b. Bronchopleural fistula
          (1) Empyema
  3. Mediastinal Lucency (Chapter 21)
      a. Paramediastinal emphysema
      b. Pneumopericardium
      c. Bronchogenic cyst
  4. Gas-Containing Organs in Abdomen Normally, Herniating into Chest (Chapters 16, 24, 28, 29, 30)
B. Pulmonary
  1. Generalized
      a. More air than is normally present
          (1) Acute bronchiolitis in infants
          (2) Generalized air-trapping with asthma
      b. Loss of interalveolar septa in interstitium
          (1) Chronic obstructive pulmonary disease
      c. Diminished blood flow and pulmonary vascularity
          (1) Congenital heart disease (Chapter 23)
          (2) Pulmonary hypertension (Chapter 19)
  2. Localized to One Area — One Lung or Less. This sign is further studied in relation to the marginal architecture and the inside pattern.

a. No marginal wall; adjoining lung relatively normal
- (1) Lobar emphysema
- (2) Check-valve obstruction of a bronchus (foreign body; congenital left upper lobe stenosis; bronchial adenoma) (Chapter 17)
- (3) Pulmonary artery thrombosis (Chapter 19)
- (4) Unilateral hyperlucency of lung
  - (a) Swyer-James or MacLeod's syndrome
  - (b) Unequal aeration of lung in certain congenital heart lesions such as patent ductus arteriosus

b. No wall; adjoining lung abnormal
- (1) Localized emphysema, with "pseudocysts" or bullae
- (2) Pneumoconiosis (Chapter 18)
- (3) Sarcoidosis (Chapter 21)

c. Thin wall; inside-content air only
- (1) Cyst
- (2) Blebs (protruding from pleural surface)
- (3) Bullae, contained within the lung
- (4) Thin-walled cavities, especially from fungus infections; occasionally other infections
- (5) Pneumatoceles

d. Thick wall; inside-content air, fluid, or solid substance (necrosis; fungus ball)
(When both air and fluid are present, there is a fluid level in the erect position or with the horizontal x-ray beam projection.)
- (1) Abscesses (Chapter 18)
- (2) Cavitary infarcts (Chapter 17)
- (3) Cavitary neoplasms, primary or metastatic (Chapter 18)
- (4) Arteritis (Wegener's necrotizing granuloma) (Chapter 17)
- (5) Hydatid cysts; air crescent in wall
- (6) Fungus ball in a cavity (mycelia; aspergillosis; moniliasis) (Chapter 17)

3. *Multiple Circumscribed Areas: Cavities, Blebs, Bullae*
   a. "Honeycombing" (Chapter 19)

DISCUSSION OF ABOVE ENTITIES, ESPECIALLY AS PERTAINS TO RADIOLOGY

Generalized—Pulmonary—More Air Than Normal

Acute Bronchiolitis in Infants and in Adults with Bronchial Asthma

Roentgenologic Features

General overinflation of lungs may be the only finding (Koch; Engle). Widespread miliary nodulations may be present.

Chronic Obstructive Pulmonary Disease (Figure 20–1)

Definition.   Anatomic alteration of the lung characterized by an abnormal enlargement of the air spaces distal to the terminal, nonrespiratory bronchioles, *accompanied by destructive changes of an irreversible type in the alveolar walls.*

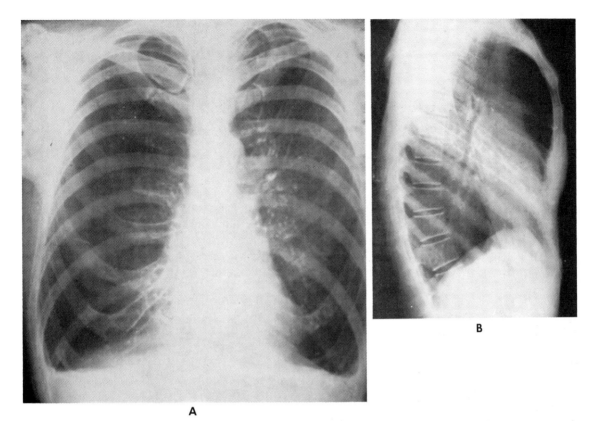

Figure 20–1   *A*. Extensive chronic obstructive pulmonary disease with pseudocystic change. *B*. Lateral radiograph of the chest demonstrating pulmonary emphysema. Note the increased radiolucency in the anterior mediastinal clear space, the heart and aorta being displaced backward. When this occurs in children, it is sometimes referred to as the "trapped air syndrome."

Radiologic Findings

1. Overinflation with hyperlucency of the lungs
2. Increased lung markings of interstitial type
3. Anterior mediastinal clear space measures 2.5 cm. or more to the anterior margin of the ascending aorta
4. Trapped air syndrome, with a "sway" of the mediastinum in expiration
5. Bullae, 1 to 2 cm. or greater in diameter
6. Cor pulmonale with evidence of right ventricular hypertrophy
7. Pulmonary artery hypertension with dilated main pulmonary arteries, and rapid tapering of midzone arteries
8. "Hanging drop" type of heart
9. Low flat diaphragm
10. Intercostal lung bulging in oblique views especially
11. Increased transverse diameter of the chest, the ribs assuming a transverse horizontal configuration which gives the chest a "squared" appearance
12. Diminished mobility of the diaphragm with full inspiration and expiration—2 to 3 cm. or less instead of 5 to 10 cm.—and a diaphragmatic lag in forced expiration, further suggesting air-trapping

The Radiographic Manifestations of Alpha-1 Antitrypsin Deficiency (Bett).

In alpha-1 antitrypsin deficiency the roentgenographic appearance of the chest is basically that of severe emphysema.

The symptoms are those of chronic obstructive pulmonary disease and usually the entity is found in a young female who has a long history of chronic bronchitis, asthma, or smoking, or who has a family history of emphysema.

PULMONARY LUCENCY LOCALIZED TO ONE AREA—NO MARGINAL WALL

Infantile Lobar Emphysema (Figure 20–2)

General Comments

In most infants it is manifest at birth, but may occur somewhat later.

It most frequently affects the left upper lobe, but may affect the right upper and middle lobes also. The lower lobes are seldom involved.

This diagnosis is extremely important to make, since progression and even death may supervene without appropriate therapeutic intervention.

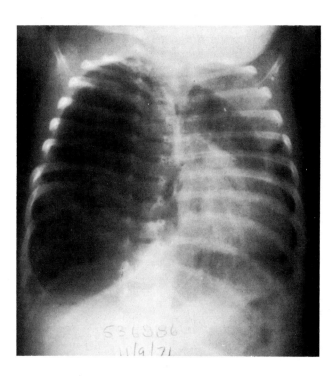

Figure 20–2   Lobar emphysema, infantile.

Congenital cardiac anomalies are associated in about 50 per cent of cases (Reid et al., Staple et al.).

Roentgenologic Features

Marked increase in volume of the affected lobe, even to the extent of depressing the ipsilateral hemidiaphragm and displacing the mediastinum to the opposite side.

The affected lobe is hyperlucent, but it contains discernible vascular markings which are widely separated, thus differing from a cyst or pneumothorax.

Mediastinal swing between inspiration and expiration.

Idiopathic Unilateral Hyperlucent Lung (Unilateral Lobar Emphysema) (Figure 20–3)

General Comments (Swyer-James or MacLeod's syndrome)

Etiology is unknown, but it may be related to a childhood infection or pneumonia.

Roentgenologic Features

Marked hyperlucency of one lung with diminutive pulmonary vasculature. Although the hilar vasculature is present, the vessels are very small in size.

Air-trapping during expiration, with a swing of the mediastinum toward the normal side in expiration, is always present.

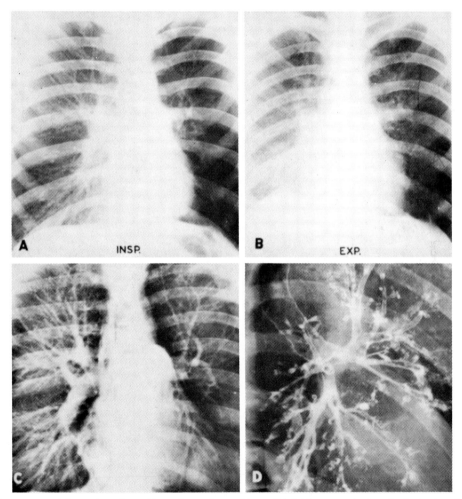

Figure 20–3 Idiopathic unilateral hyperlucent lung with small left hilus. *A* and *B*. Inspiration and expiration films. There is hyperlucency of the left lung which persists on expiration. The heart shifts toward the left on inspiration, and the left hemidiaphragm shows poor excursion. *C*. The pulmonary angiogram shows marked decrease in the size of the left main pulmonary artery and its branches, with compensatory increase on the right. *D*. The bronchogram shows a peculiar diffuse form of bronchiectasis with absence of "alveolar" filling. This suggests the presence of a peripheral form of obstructive emphysema. (From Margolin, H. N., Rosenberg, L. S., Felson, B., and Baum, G.: Amer. J. Roentgenol., *82*:63, 1959.)

PULMONARY LOCALIZED LUCENCY—THIN-WALLED, INSIDE-CONTENT AIR ONLY

Cysts of the Lung

Classification

1. Solitary lung cysts
    a. Developmental
    b. Infectious
    c. Neoplastic
2. Multiple lung cysts
    a. Apical
        (1) Blebs and bullae
    b. Basal in lung
        (1) Cystic bronchiectasis (Chapter 19)
    c. Indiscriminate in distribution
        (1) Pneumatocele formation, especially in staphylococcus aureus pneumonia in infants
        (2) With late tuberculosis or other chronic pneumonitides

Roentgenologic Features (Figure 20–4)

The appearance of the cyst is very much the same irrespective of its cause, except for adjoining appearances in the lung. Thus, there may be opacities in adjoining lung or pleura in some infectious or neoplastic processes. The appearance of unilateral pleural effusion and adjoining pneumonia in an infant suggests staphylococcus pneumonia. A prior injury to the lung (homogeneous density due to hematoma) may, in several days, demonstrate a pneumatocele.

A cyst usually appears spherical or ellipsoid radiographically in all projections. It may contain fluid, in which case a fluid level may be presented in the erect position if free air is also contained within the cyst. Air may enter a cyst by communication with a bronchus.

Occasionally, an encapsulated pneumothorax will simulate the appearance of a cyst, requiring body section radiographs and oblique and stereoscopic views to establish the differentiation.

If infection supervenes, a cyst wall becomes thicker, loses its clear demarcation from adjoining pulmonary tissues, and acquires the appearance of an abscess.

Dissecting communication with a bronchus may produce a crescentic air shadow, as occasionally seen in hydatid disease (Figure 20–4).

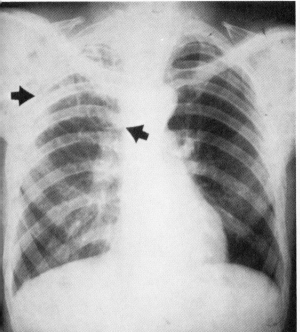

A

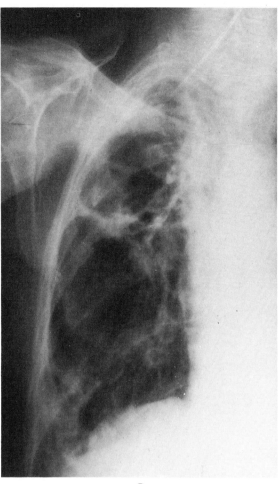

B

Figure 20-4 *A.* Radiograph demonstrating cystic lung disease in the right upper lobe such as might be related to congenital cyst formation. *B.* Cavitation throughout the right lung in far advanced pulmonary tuberculosis.

PULMONARY LUCENCY — LOCALIZED — SINGLE OR MULTIPLE — THICK-WALLED, CONTENT AIR, FLUID OR SOLID MEDIUM (See Chapter 18)

Questions — Chapter 20

1. In an infant with acute bronchiolitis, what roentgen signs could be expected?

2. What are the roentgen signs attributed to chronic obstructive pulmonary disease? What is their relative accuracy in predicting morphologic change? How does this correlate with the clinical diagnosis of emphysema?

3. In those localized pulmonary lesions characterized by increased radiolucency, what disease entities should be borne in mind when a specific marginal wall or cyst cannot be seen?

4. What are the roentgen signs of lobar emphysema in infants? Why is it important to make this diagnosis promptly?

5. What is unilateral hyperlucency of the lung? How is it characterized radiographically?

6. How would you define a "cyst" of the lung? bleb? bulla? What differential features are there among certain thin-walled cavities such as fungus infection, congenital cysts, cysts from chronic obstructive pulmonary disease, pneumatoceles following staphylococcal pneumonia, cavitary infarction, cavitary neoplasia, either primary or secondary, Wegener's necrotizing granuloma, and cavities characterized by a fungus ball?

7. What are the roentgenologic features of chronic bronchitis?

21

Radiology of the Mediastinum, Excluding the Heart

BASIC ANATOMY

Mediastinal Boundaries

The mediastinum is that compartment of the thoracic cage which is bounded laterally by the parietal pleural reflections along the medial aspects of both lungs, by the thoracic inlet superiorly, the diaphragm inferiorly, the sternum anteriorly, and the anterior surfaces of the thoracic vertebral bodies posteriorly.

Arbitrary Compartments of the Mediastinum

For descriptive purposes the mediastinum is divided into four compartments.

The Superior Mediastinum, bounded superiorly by the thoracic inlet and inferiorly by a line drawn from the manubriosternal angle to the intervertebral disk between T-4 and T-5 vertebrae.

The Inferior Mediastinum below this imaginary line is further subdivided into three compartments or subdivisions:

1. An anterior mediastinum bounded anteriorly by the sternum and other tissues beneath the sternum, and posteriorly by the pericardium covering the heart and major vessels anteriorly.

2. A middle mediastinum, which contains the heart, the aorta, the origin of the great vessels to the upper extremities and neck, the pulmonary arteries, superior and inferior vena cavae, and the vessels of the root of the lung.

3. The posterior mediastinum, which is bounded anteriorly by the heart and posteriorly by the thoracic spine.

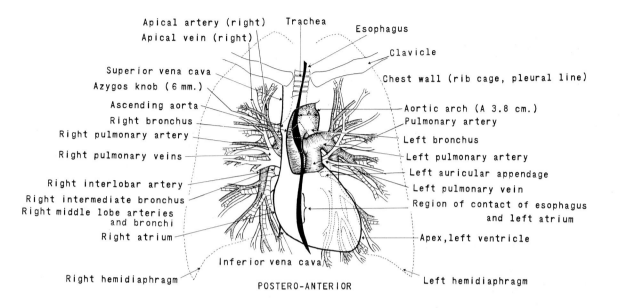

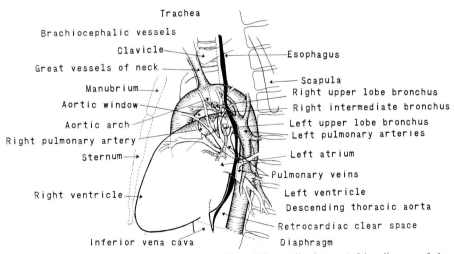

Figure 21–1 *A*. Line diagram of chest showing a frontal view of the mediastinum. *B*. Line diagram of chest showing a left lateral view.

Basic Anatomic Structures Contained in the Mediastinum

In frontal perspective (Figure 21–1) the *trachea, left and right main bronchi,* and *pulmonary arteries* are readily identified. *The pulmonary veins* are faintly seen. The *azygos vein* produces an ovoid shadow in the right tracheobronchial angle and is important to identify. It is considered enlarged when its measurements exceed 6 to 10 mm. in the erect position or 14 mm. in the recumbent position (Felson, 1968; Keats et al.; Doyle et al.).

The *arch of the aorta* and *descending thoracic aorta* produce a definite line along the left lateral aspect of the thoracic spine. With clear definition, paraspinal lines can be distinguished on either side of the thoracic spine (Figure 21–3), closely applied to the thoracic spine and representative of the *paravertebral mediastinal pleura,* which is applied to the paraspinous ligamentous tissue on either side. With body section radiographs an *anterior mediastinal line* can usually be seen, projected into the trachea; this represents the confluence of the pleura anteriorly (Figure 21–2). Similarly, a *posterior mediastinal line* can be demonstrated, especially with body section radiography, representing the confluence of the esophagus and pleura and called the *superior and inferior esophageal-pleural stripe* or the posteromedial pleural stripe.

In the lateral view (Figure 21–1 B), the *manubrium and sternum* are clearly defined. Beneath the sternum, a soft tissue space is identified where the costal and mediastinal pleurae are contiguous with each other. The pleura at the level of the manubrium passes backwards over the superior mediastinum from the sternum to

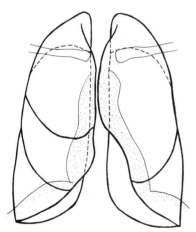

Figure 21–2 Line diagram showing the boundaries of the anterior and posterior mediastinal pleura.

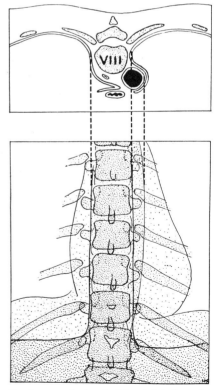

Figure 21–3 *Upper:* cross section through the posterior mediastinum at the level of the eighth thoracic vertebra. *Lower:* diagram taken from a roentgenogram depicting the posterior portions of the visceral or parietal pleura as lines along the vertebral column. Dotted lines indicate anatomical substrates of pleural lines and aortic lines in cross section. (From Lachman, E.: Anat. Rec., *83:*521, 1942.)

the vertebral column and is reflected over the apex of lung tissue protruding slightly above the first rib laterally but no higher than the first rib posteriorly. The anterior margins of the two pleurae converge behind the sternoclavicular joints and come into apposition with each other at the lower border of the manubrium. The anterior margins remain in apposition to approximately the fourth costal cartilages. The left pleura at this level turns away from the median plane as much as 2 to 3 cm. and finally reconverges with the right pleura at the level of the xyphoid process.

The costal surface of the lung and pleura lies in close relationship with the ribs, intercostal muscles, and innominate veins. The fat and remains of the *thymus* (in the adult) lie beneath the manubrium and anterior to the innominate veins. Somewhat laterally, beneath the costal cartilages, the *internal mammary vessels* descend deeply to the pectoralis muscles. In the lateral view, the thymus in the adult cannot be identified unless enlarged or unless it is the site of tumor formation. Lymph nodes are not detected unless enlarged abnormally.

In the *superior aspect of the anterior mediastinum,* the right and left lung projected over one another create a *clear space* in the adult, which should not ordinarily measure more than 2.5 cm. in maximum antero-posterior measurement. (Air-trapping as defined in Chapter 20 will increase this measurement.)

In the middle of the superior mediastinum, at the level of the first costal cartilage, the *innominate veins* and *innominate artery lie anterior to the trachea.*

The *trachea* lies just to the right of the midline at this level, while the *esophagus,* more posteriorly is in the midline closely applied to the thoracic vertebra (usually the third thoracic vertebra at this level).

At the inferior margin of the superior mediastinum (fourth thoracic level), the pericardium comes into intimate contact with the substernal connective tissue and fat, separating the right and left pleural sacs. The internal mammary vessels lie immediately anterior to the pericardium at this level, just anterior to the pleural margins.

Enlargement of the internal mammary vessels, as in coarctation of the aorta, enlargement of the lymph nodes and lymphatics (which course along the internal mammary vessels), or infiltration by any neoplasia or fluid may sometimes be recognized beneath the sternum in the lateral view.

Also at the inferior boundary of the superior mediastinum (fourth thoracic level) is the arch of the aorta, located approximately in the midline and traversing toward the left posteriorly, while the superior vena cava lies just to the right of the midline, both structures situated anterior to the trachea. The esophagus, posteriorly, is closely applied to the fourth thoracic vertebra, with the *thoracic duct* on its left.

Occasionally, the *esophagus* may be seen on radiographs when it contains air in sufficient quantity, but otherwise it requires barium esophagrams for delineation.

In infancy and early childhood, the thymus gland extends into the anterior mediastinum, producing a distinct shadow in lateral and frontal projections.

The inferior mediastinum is divided into anterior, middle, and posterior subdivisions. The anterior subdivision at this level may at times be demonstrated in a lateral view, employing a horizontal x-ray beam, with the patient lying supine. Normally, the pericardium is in close contact with the posterior soft tissues adjoining the sternum.

The middle mediastinum is largely occupied by heart and pericardium, with the right ventricle lying anteriorly. The major vessels (ascending aorta, superior vena cava, main and branching right and left pulmonary artery, and inferior vena cava inferiorly) occupy this subdivision also. The left atrium forms a posterior chamber for the cardiac silhouette.

The *posterior subdivision of the inferior mediastinum* extends between the posterior aspect of the pericardium and the spine, to the level of the fourth thoracic vertebra.

A transverse section at the level of the interspace between the seventh and eighth thoracic vertebrae is very helpful in visualizing the structures in this region. The pleura and lung, applied closely to the lateral aspects of the spine, form a *"thoracic gutter,"* which extends to a level beyond the posterior line of the spinal canal. Thus, in a straight lateral view, much lung is obscured by the thoracic spine. The pulmonary veins enter the left atrium at the anterior margin of the posterior mediastinum. The esophagus, situated just to the right of the midline behind the left atrium, and the descending thoracic aorta, placed just to the left, are in close approximation to each other. The azygos vein lies immediately posterior to the esophagus at this level. The left and right bronchi lie at the same level along the anterior margin of the esophagus, with the left bronchus slightly posterior and to the right.

The space between the right and left pleura at this level is slightly less than the width of a vertebral body (2 cm. or less)—just sufficient to allow easy visibility for the paraspinous ligamentous silhouette.

The posterior mediastinum also contains the vagus nerves (closely applied to the esophagus on either side); the thoracic duct; the superior hemiazygos vein just posterior to the thoracic aorta; the sympathetic chain; and numerous paravertebral lymph nodes.

Esophagrams show the following important indentations (Figure 21–1):

1. Indentation to the left and slightly posteriorly at the level of the aortic arch.
2. Slight indentation anteriorly by the left main bronchus and close to the bifurcation of the trachea.
3. A minimal impression at the level of the left atrium.

MEDIASTINAL LYMPH NODES

The lymph nodes of the mediastinum are numerous and are liberally distributed along the internal mammary vessels, in juxtavertebral loci, and in foci adjoining the diaphragm anteriorly and laterally to the pericardial sac (Figure 21–4). They are nestled among the large vessels, both arteries and veins, and are found adjacent to the lower esophagus and descending aorta, and at bifurcations of the trachea and bronchi in both hili and the lungs.

Although normally not visible, they take on great significance in inflammatory and neoplastic disease.

The right paratracheal lymph node chain represents a principal drainage area for the entire right lung and a major portion of the left. Thus, the careful analysis and identification of each shadow of this region on the chest radiograph is imperative.

The lymphatic drainage of the esophagus also takes on great significance, since it usually occurs in longitudinal pathways in submucous and muscular lymphatic networks, extending from the internal jugular chains through the paratracheal nodal groups and the posterior mediastinal nodes, into the nodes of the cardia and lesser curvature of the stomach. Careful observation of metastases from neoplasms of the esophagus corroborate the early spread of these lesions to subdiaphragmatic sites.

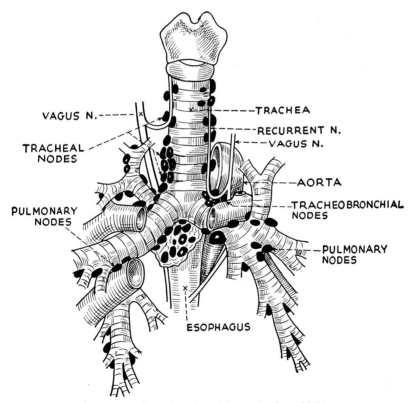

Figure 21–4 Lymph nodes of the tracheobronchial tree.

RADIOLOGIC TECHNIQUES OF EXAMINATION OF THE MEDIASTINUM

1. Postero-anterior and lateral chest roentgenograms in maximal inspiration, moderately overpenetrated, and with barium in the esophagus (using high kilovoltage, short exposure time, and a Bucky grid)
2. Fluoroscopic examination may be used to evaluate the following, especially:
   a. Pulsation—intrinsic or by impact
   b. Abnormal response to positive intrathoracic pressure
   c. Relationship of the movement of the mass lesion to structures within the chest: diaphragm, tracheobronchial tree, esophagus, heart, and major vessels
   d. The relationship of the cardiopericardial shadow to the epicardial fat (especially to exclude pericardial effusions)
3. Body section radiography. This is especially useful in:
   a. Determining the relationship of the abnormality to a specific anatomic structure
   b. Studying the relationship of the abnormality to the vascular structures of the mediastinum
   c. Studying the nature of calcification in the lesion, if it is present
   d. Studying the nature of fat within the lesion, if it is present
4. Angiography. This is especially useful in:
   a. Determining the relationship of the abnormality to opacified vascular structures such as the heart, aorta, major vessels arising from the aorta including the internal mammary (Boijsen and Reuter), and pulmonary arteries and veins
   b. Studying the great veins leading into the heart (venacavography)
   c. Studying the azygos venous system (azygography). This may be done by intraosseous injection of the contrast agent or by selective catheterization
5. Bronchography may indicate widening, narrowness, or filling defects in the air passages
6. Myelograms may demonstrate the status of the subarachnoid space and indicate whether the mediastinal lesion is related to the spine or spinal cord
7. Pneumomediastinography (Sumerling and Irvine). In this technique, the gas is introduced into the fascial planes of the mediastinum by a number of differing routes. Tomography coupled with this technique is especially helpful in certain cases. This method is useful for:
   a. Ascertaining the exact relationship of a lesion to the adjoining structures
   b. Helping to determine resectability of a lesion in the mediastinum, or of bronchogenic carcinoma
8. Diagnostic pneumothorax and pneumoperitoneum may be used to localize the suspected lesion in relation to these potential spaces; they are especially helpful in studying herniations from the abdomen into the thoracic cage. These procedures must be performed with great care, in order to avoid a tension pneumothorax and its deleterious symptoms
9. Radioisotopic techniques:
   a. Blood pool scans
   b. Radioisotopic angiograms
   c. Study of pericardial effusions
   d. Localization of some tumors: thymoma, thyroid, and occasionally, lymph node enlargements

CATEGORIZATION OF ROENTGEN SIGNS IN RESPECT TO MEDIASTINAL LESIONS

The Anatomic Position of the lesion is carefully defined.

The more cephalad an upper mediastinal mass lesion appears while still remaining visible in the lung, the more posterior it lies.

Contiguity of the lesion to bone may cause bone erosion (spine; sternum; ribs).

Lesions which erode or destroy bone are arterial aneurysms, tumors of peripheral nerves, tumors of sympathetic ganglia, and lesions of cartilage and bone.

Localization charts are shown in Figure 21–5. Lesions projecting into the mediastinum from the abdomen are hiatal hernias, foramen of Morgagni hernias, thoracic diverticula, and pseudocysts of the pancreas.

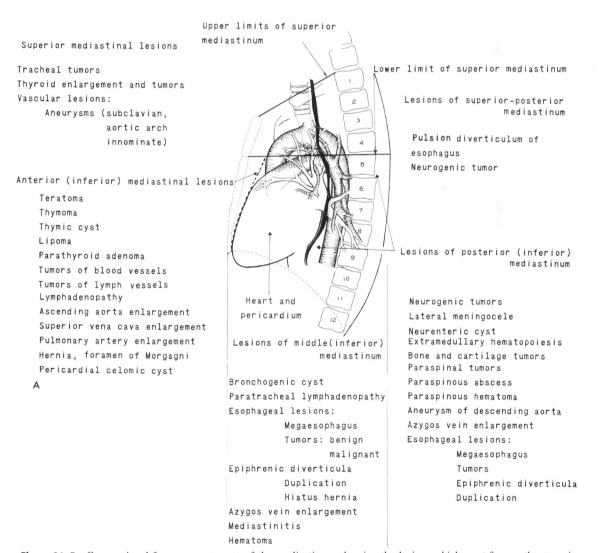

MOST FREQUENT SITES FOR MEDIASTINAL LESIONS *

Upper limits of superior mediastinum

Superior mediastinal lesions

Tracheal tumors
Thyroid enlargement and tumors
Vascular lesions:
    Aneurysms (subclavian,
           aortic arch
           innominate)

Lower limit of superior mediastinum

Lesions of superior-posterior mediastinum

Pulsion diverticulum of esophagus
Neurogenic tumor

Anterior (inferior) mediastinal lesions

Teratoma
Thymoma
Thymic cyst
Lipoma
Parathyroid adenoma
Tumors of blood vessels
Tumors of lymph vessels
Lymphadenopathy
Ascending aorta enlargement
Superior vena cava enlargement
Pulmonary artery enlargement
Hernia, foramen of Morgagni
Pericardial celomic cyst

A

Heart and pericardium

Lesions of posterior (inferior) mediastinum

Neurogenic tumors
Lateral meningocele
Neurenteric cyst
Extramedullary hematopoiesis
Bone and cartilage tumors
Paraspinal tumors
Paraspinous abscess
Paraspinous hematoma
Aneurysm of descending aorta
Azygos vein enlargement
Esophageal lesions:
    Megaesophagus
    Tumors
    Epiphrenic diverticula
    Duplication

Lesions of middle (inferior) mediastinum

Bronchogenic cyst
Paratracheal lymphadenopathy
Esophageal lesions:
    Megaesophagus
    Tumors: benign
           malignant
Epiphrenic diverticula
    Duplication
    Hiatus hernia
Azygos vein enlargement
Mediastinitis
Hematoma

Figure 21–5   Conventional four compartments of the mediastinum showing the lesions which most frequently occur in each of the main subdivisions. (Modified from Leigh, T., and Weens, H.: Seminars in Roentgenology, *4*:59–73, 1969.)

The Outer Margin of the Lesion is carefully described to determine its site of origin (Figure 21–6).

Sharp margination favors a mediastinal lesion rather than a lesion in the lung.

Acute angulation at a margin favors intrapleural or intrapulmonary disease, whereas an obtuse margin which tapers toward the chest wall favors an extrapleural source (extrapleural sign).

If the margin of the lesion blends imperceptibly into the adjoining vascular system, it is likely that the origin of the mass is in fact the vascular system.

The Density and Internal Architecture of the Lesion Are Defined

Fat: This is not readily detected in chest lesions, but if seen it points toward lipomas, teratomas, excess fat following steroid therapy, fat pads, or omental hernia.

Calcification:

Circumlinear, with a fine line: probable cyst.
Laminated: probable aneurysm.
Annular or stippled: thyroid carcinoma or neurosarcoma.
Formed bone or tooth: teratoma.
Concentric small speckled calcification: probable phleboliths in hemangioma.
"Popcorn"-like conglomerations: chondroma or hamartoma.

Gas: Hernia, esophageal origin, mediastinal abscess, or communicating duplication cyst; megaesophagus.

The Shape of the Lesion is Carefully Defined

Multiple Lobulations: lymph nodes enlarged from lymphoma or granuloma.
Teardrop: pedunculated lesion, with the upper end of the teardrop pointing to the site of origin, often a bronchogenic cyst.
Fusiform and Elongated: megaesophagus.
"Sail-shadow":   thymus.

The Size of the Lesion is not in itself very helpful, since mediastinal lesions vary so greatly in size.

Function Studies

Fluoroscopy, with the Aid of Esophagrams may help determine whether the lesion moves with respiration, the tracheobronchial tree, the esophagus, the diaphragm, or the heart and major vessels. Unfortunately, the evaluation of pulsations in or contiguous to the mass may not be helpful, since aneurysms may not pulsate if full of clot, and masses may appear to pulsate only because of close contact with a pulsatile structure.

Careful study of the esophagus may reveal its involvement by such lesions as diverticula, megaesophagus, leiomyomas, and duplication.

Response to Treatment.   *Steroid test:* Shrinkage of mediastinal lymph nodes in sarcoid, or the thymus in thymic hyperplasia.

Changes in Respect to Time.   Some mediastinal lesions such as pericardial or bronchogenic cysts may remain quiescent for many years; malignant tumors tend to increase in size in relatively short intervals of time, while inflammatory lesions may recede with time, or undergo organization or calcification.

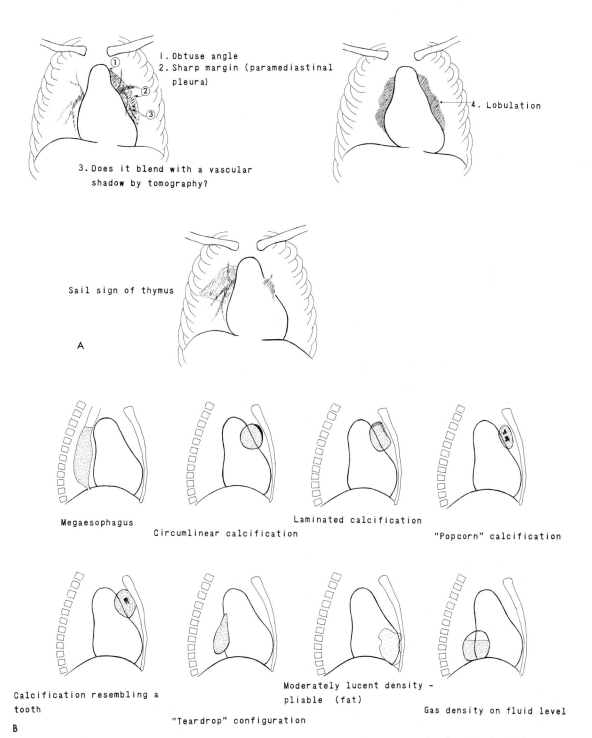

Figure 21–6 Diagrams illustrating some of the roentgen signs of abnormality in respect to mediastinal lesions.

EXAMPLES OF SOME MEDIASTINAL LESIONS AND THEIR RADIOGRAPHIC APPEARANCES

Superior Mediastinal Lesions

Thyroid Enlargement and Tumors

Roentgenologic Aspects

The trachea and esophagus appear to be deviated and compressed.

The substernal portion moves upward with swallowing, coughing, and sniffing.

Calcification may be identified in the lesion of an amorphous type.

The detection of radioactive iodine uptake over the mass may be further corroborative evidence of the intrathoracic goiter.

Vascular Lesions: Aneurysms (See Chapter 22)

Anterior (Inferior) Mediastinal Lesions

Teratomas (Figure 21–7)

Roentgenologic Aspects

They usually contain opacities that vary from linear calcifications in a capsule to skeletal parts such as teeth, mandible, or a bone.

At times, teratomas contain fatty or radiolucent material.

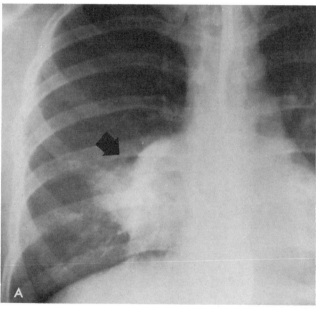
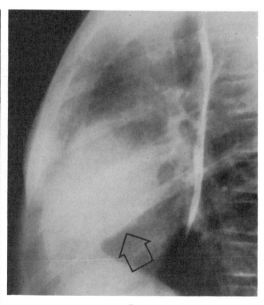

Figure 21–7 Dermoid of the mediastinum. *A.* Postero-anterior view. *B.* Right lateral projection. These are usually anteriorly situated tumors.

Thymomas and Thymic Cysts

Roentgenologic Aspects

The small tumors are usually less than 6 cm. in diameter, are round, and situated adjacent to and just superior to the aortic arch in the midline.

The larger tumors assume a pattern not unlike a large thymus in normal children, and usually they exceed 6 cm. and tend to grow inferiorly.

10 to 12 per cent of all thymomas show calcification, usually linear, suggesting the lining of a cystic cavity.

Some cases show a "mottled" calcification. This usually indicates a histologically malignant tumor.

Pericardial Cysts and Diverticula (Figure 21–8)

Roentgenologic Features

These are usually sharply circumscribed, rounded, or oval-shaped masses of water density in the right cardiophrenic angle anteriorly. Usually, they appear to be resting upon the diaphragm.

At times, they assume a teardrop configuration, particularly in the lateral view.

They must be differentiated from omental herniations through the foramina of Morgagni and normal epicardial fat pads in these situations.

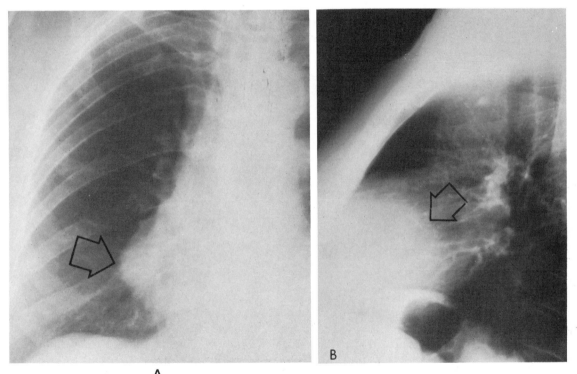

A

Figure 21–8   Pericardial cyst. *A.* Postero-anterior view of the chest. *B.* Right lateral view of the chest. The pericardial cyst is usually situated in the right cardiophrenic angle anteriorly as indicated here, but it may, on rare occasions, also be situated on the left.

Lymphadenopathy

Roentgenologic Aspects

The borders are usually smooth, rounded, and lobulated, sometimes symmetrically enlarged on either side of the mediastinum.

They are usually of homogeneous density.

They may compress or displace surrounding structures.

They may be differentiated from adjoining vascular structures by the compressibility of vascular structures with positive pressure chest x-ray studies. Also, the "epicardial fat line" surrounding the heart is often obliterated by enlarged lymph nodes in the lung hilus.

Middle (Inferior) Mediastinal Lesions

Bronchogenic Cysts

Roentgenologic Aspects

Bronchogenic cysts are usually seen as smoothly outlined masses within the mediastinum, adjoining the bifurcation of the trachea and extending below this level (in "tear drop" fashion).

The cyst may actually elevate and flatten the interbronchial angle.

They may communicate with the trachea or one of the bronchi and a fluid level will then be demonstrated within the cyst. Otherwise they are sharply circumscribed, homogeneous masses of water density.

Sarcoid

Roentgenologic Aspects

Most common lymph nodes are tracheobronchial.

The involvement tends to be symmetrical.

Pulmonary parenchymal, bone, skin, eye, and salivary gland lesions are often associated.

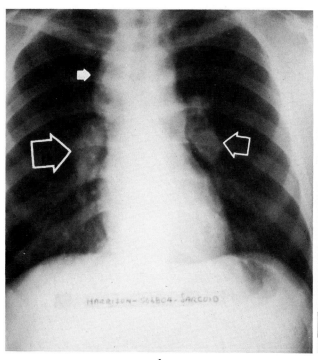
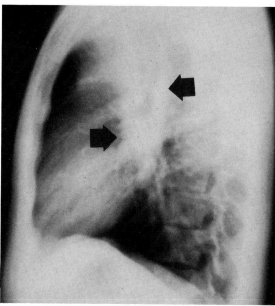

A   B

Figure 21–9 *A* and *B*. Mediastinal sarcoid occupying the midmediastinum. Postero-anterior and lateral projections.

Malignant Lymphoma

Roentgenologic Aspects

Most common lymph node involvement is paratracheal.

Any lymph nodes or lymphatics in the chest may be involved.

The lesions are more asymmetrical than those that occur with sarcoid.

The borders of the lesions are lobulated and smooth.

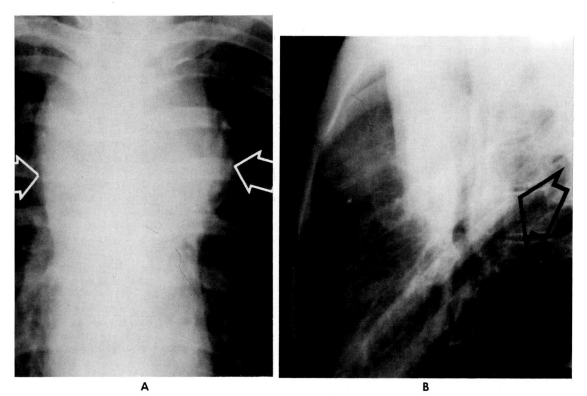

A   **B**

Figure 21–10   *A* and *B*. Examples of malignant lymphoma occupying the midmediastinum.

Acute Mediastinitis (Figure 21–11)

INFLAMMATORY AFFECTIONS OF MEDIASTINUM

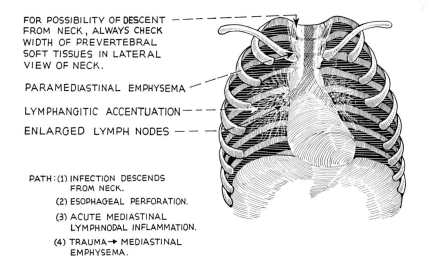

FOR POSSIBILITY OF DESCENT
FROM NECK, ALWAYS CHECK
WIDTH OF PREVERTEBRAL
SOFT TISSUES IN LATERAL
VIEW OF NECK.

PARAMEDIASTINAL EMPHYSEMA

LYMPHANGITIC ACCENTUATION

ENLARGED LYMPH NODES

PATH: (1) INFECTION DESCENDS
        FROM NECK.
     (2) ESOPHAGEAL PERFORATION.
     (3) ACUTE MEDIASTINAL
        LYMPHNODAL INFLAMMATION.
     (4) TRAUMA → MEDIASTINAL
        EMPHYSEMA.

Figure 21–11   Diagram illustrating the radiographic appearances in association with inflammatory infections of the mediastinum.

Chronic Mediastinitis

General Comments. These lesions are usually granulomatous or fibrotic. Granulomatous mediastinitis may be caused by any of the infectious granulomas, such as histoplasmosis, tuberculosis, or other mycoses. Sarcoidosis and silicosis have also been associated with granulomatous mediastinitis.

Roentgenologic Aspects

The most common manifestation is a general widening of the mediastinum with scalloped, lobulated margins, somewhat more marked on the right.

Obstruction of the superior vena cava may be present.

Adjoining mediastinal structures are obscured frequently by this inflammatory process.

Posterior (Inferior) Mediastinal Lesions

Neurogenic Tumors (Figure 21–12)

Roentgenologic Aspects

The neurofibromas, neurilemmomas, and schwannomas, or those neurogenic tumors having origin in the peripheral nerves, are usually the ones which cause bony deformity (Leigh).

The neurofibromas tend to have a narrowed mediastinal base as seen in a frontal projection.

The ganglioneuromas originating from sympathetic ganglia tend to have a broader mediastinal base and may contain calcification.

The angle between the tumor and the mediastinum tends to be obtuse in the ganlioneuroma and acute in the neurofibroma.

Aortography may be necessary to distinguish these lesions from aneurysms.

Myelography may also be helpful in determining whether or not a "dumbbell" type tumor of the spinal canal is present.

Neuroblastoma

Roentgenologic Aspects

This is a highly invasive tumor usually found in the posterior mediastinum and quite aggressive in its growth.

Usually there is a paravertebral widening.

Pheochromocytomas and Paragangliomas

Roentgenologic Aspects

The majority of these tumors originate from the adrenal medulla or the retroperitoneal region, but they can occur in the thoracic area, particularly in the posterior mediastinum.

They may occur from multiple sites of origin.

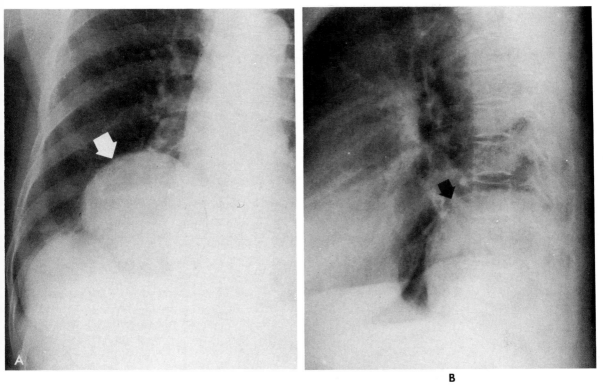

Figure 21–12 *A* and *B*. P-A and lateral films of the chest demonstrating a neurofibroma affecting the posterior inferior mediastinum. Although these films were not obtained for bone detail, the erosion of the intervertebral foramina in the lower thoracic region is quite readily demonstrated.

WIDENING OF THE PARAVERTEBRAL FASCIAL PLANES

1. Tuberculosis of the spine
2. Hematoma secondary to fracture of the spine
3. Neoplasms of the spine
4. Spinal osteomyelitis
5. Posterior mediastinal lymphomatous masses
6. Extramedullary hematopoiesis

Esophageal Lesions (also see Chapter 27)

General Comment. Esophageal lesions which may appear as mediastinal tumors include (1) megaesophagus; (2) tumors, especially of the intramural type; (3) epiphrenic diverticula; (4) duplication; (5) hiatus hernia.

Questions – Chapter 21

1. Define the four classically recognized arbitrary compartments of the mediastinum.

2. Which are the most frequent pathologic lesions found in the superior compartment?

3. Which are the most frequent lesions found in the anterior subdivision of the inferior compartment?

4. Which are the most frequent lesions found in the middle subdivision of the inferior compartment?

5. Which are the most frequent lesions found in the posterior subdivision of the inferior compartment?

6. What is meant by the "anterior mediastinal clear space"?

7. What is the importance of the measurement of the anterior mediastinal clear space in respect to "air-trapping"?

8. Where do the internal mammary vessels and lymph nodes lie and what is their radiologic significance?

9. Where anatomically does the ascending part of the arch of the aorta lie? Where does the transverse part of the arch of the aorta lie?

10. Where does the descending thoracic aorta lie? What is the significance of these anatomic positions and relationships?

11. In what compartment does the esophagus lie and what is its significance from the standpoint of a study of mediastinal lesions?

12. Where does the thymus gland lie in infants and in adults and what is its significance radiologically?

13. What is meant by the "thoracic gutter"? Where is it seen on a lateral roentgenogram of the chest?

14. Where does the esophagus lie in respect to the left atrium and what is the radiologic significance of this?

15. Where does the esophagus lie in respect to the descending thoracic aorta and what is its radiologic significance?

16. Where do the right and left bronchi lie in respect to the esophagus? Indicate this radiologic significance.

17. What are the normal indentations on the esophagus in frontal perspective? in lateral perspective? and what is the significance of a careful study of these impressions and indentations?

18. What is the relationship of the upper level of the manubrium to the apex of the lung? Why is it important to know the relationship of the apex of the lung to the thoracic inlet, and what is this relationship?

19. Describe the anatomy of the mediastinal lymph nodes and indicate the pathologic and radiologic significance of these.

20. Describe briefly the lymphatic drainage of the esophagus. What is the pathologic and radiologic significance of this?

21. Indicate the basic radiologic techniques for examination of the mediastinum.

22. What is the importance of body section radiography as a supplement to the basic radiologic technique for examination of the mediastinum?

23. What is the importance of angiography in the investigation of mediastinal lesions?

24. What is the importance of myelography in the examination of mediastinal lesions?

25. Categorize the important roentgen signs in respect to mediastinal lesions.

26. Which are the lesions which frequently erode or destroy bone in the mediastinum?

27. Which lesions in the mediastinum are commonly located around the base of the heart?

28. Which lesions in the mediastinum may be projected from the abdomen?

29. What is the importance of a careful study of the outer margins of lesions of the mediastinum?

30. What is the importance of study of internal density and architecture of the lesions? What radiolucent shadows can be identified and what is their significance?

31. What calcific shadows can be identified within mediastinal lesions and what is their significance?

32. What is the importance of fluoroscopy with esophagrams in respect to mediastinal lesions?

33. Why is it important in respect to mediastinal lesions to know about any other disease in the patient?

34. If there is abdominal involvement such as hepatosplenomegaly, what mediastinal disease processes would be considered likely?

35. Which lesions of the mediastinum may be accompanied by pleural fluid?

36. Describe the roentgen appearances of a thymoma. Where is it most frequently situated and what disease processes may be associated with it?

37. Describe the roentgen appearance of a nonpenetrating injury of the thorax producing a disrupted aortic wall.

38. Describe the roentgen appearance of acute mediastinitis, chronic mediastinitis.

39. Describe the most frequent sites for hyperparathyroid adenoma. What systemic manifestations would assist in recognition of this tumor?

40. What is the most frequent roentgen appearance of heterotopic substernal thyroid? What adjunctive tests are most helpful?

41. What adjunctive symptoms are frequently present with pheochromocytomas and paraganglionomas? How may these lesions be investigated other than by the radiologic techniques described?

42. How may one distinguish bone erosion occurring in the region of the spine by aneurysms from that which is produced by a neurofibroma?

22

Roentgenology of the Heart (Exclusive of Congenital Heart Disease)

RADIOLOGIC METHODS USED IN THE ROENTGEN CARDIAC EXAMINATION

1. **The Postero-anterior (P-A) Teleroentgenogram of the Chest** (six foot target-to-film distance), preferably with barium outlining the esophagus (Figure 21–1A)
2. **The Left and Right Anterior Oblique Films of the Chest,** also with barium outlining the esophagus and usually following fluoroscopy (Figures 22–1 and 22–2)
3. **A Lateral Film of the Chest with Esophagram** (Figure 21–1B).
4. **A P-A Teleroentgenogram of the Chest in the Recumbent Position** for comparison with the erect film, if pericardial fluid is suspected. Other special procedures are listed below.
5. **Fluoroscopy.** Fluoroscopy with image amplification should accompany the film studies. The following routine is recommended.
   a. *The heart and mediastinal structures are studied in the frontal* and *both oblique projections* (and lateral, if necessary).
   b. *A barium swallow should always be part of the fluoroscopic and radiographic study of the heart,* with good delineation of the esophagus in all projections. Since the esophagus is so closely applied to the descending aorta on the one hand and the posterior cardiac structures on the other, changes in the course of the esophagus become of considerable value in the interpretation of cardiovascular and aortic anatomy.
   c. The patient is then lowered into a recumbent position and a study of the mediastinum is repeated as described earlier in the frontal and oblique projections, noting carefully the changes which occur with change in body position.

Specialized Cardiovascular Investigations

Additional procedures are available which may supplement the information obtained by routine studies described previously. These include
1. Venous angiocardiography.
2. Selective angiocardiography.
3. Cardiac catheterization. This is followed by injection of the radiopaque substance directly into the desired area or chamber.
4. Aortography by catheterization technique.
5. Coronary angiography.
6. Cavography.
7. Transosseous venography.
8. Lymphangiography.

NORMAL ANATOMY*

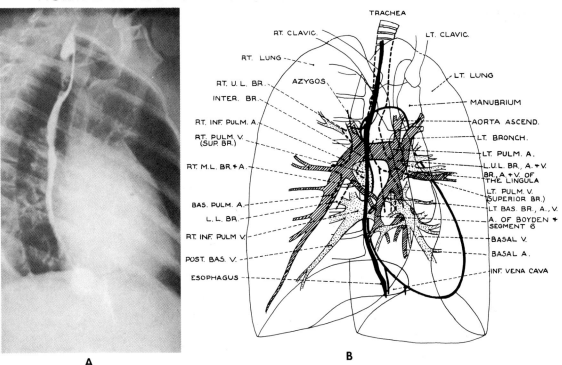

Figure 22–1   Cardiac esophagram: right anterior oblique projection. *A.* Radiograph. *B.* Labeled tracing of *A.*

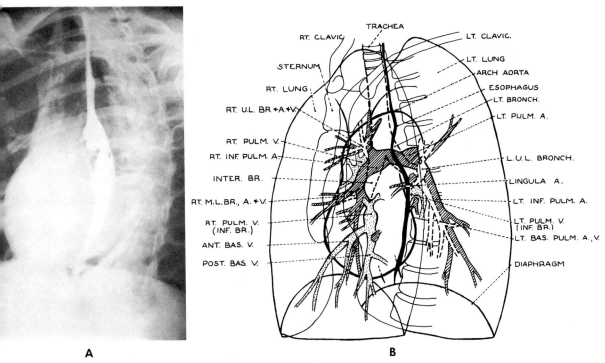

Figure 22–2   Cardiac esophagram: left anterior oblique projection. *A.* Radiograph. *B.* Labeled tracing of *A.*

*For postero-anterior and lateral projections, see Figure 21–1A and B.

Projection of Cardiac Valves in Routine Position in Radiography

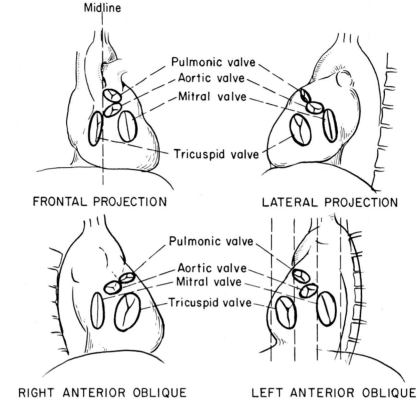

FRONTAL PROJECTION

LATERAL PROJECTION

RIGHT ANTERIOR OBLIQUE

LEFT ANTERIOR OBLIQUE

Figure 22–3   Projection of cardiac valve in the routine position used in radiography of the heart.

Determination of Relative Cardiac Volume (Amundsen)

The physical factors employed are (1) a target-to-film distance on frontal view of 2 meters, and (2) a target-to-film distance on lateral view of 1.5 meters.

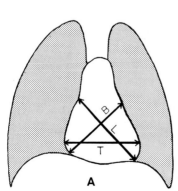

A

Figure 22–4 *A.* Usual measurements employed in calculating relative cardiac volume. *B.* Lateral view of the normal heart showing the method of obtaining D, the greatest antero-posterior measurement of the heart in calculation of relative heart volume.

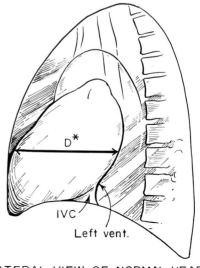

LATERAL VIEW OF NORMAL HEART

B

Basic Formula.   Volume $= K \times L \times B \times D$ (Figures 22–4 and 22–5), where $K =$ 0.42 (standard deviation 7.4 per cent) — based on 45 cases, comparing calculated value with autopsy-determined value.

Relative heart volume is defined as the volume per square meter of surface area using the DuBois nomograms for calculation of surface area from body height and weight. Thus, the formula for *relative heart volume* is:

$$\frac{0.42 \times L \times B \times D}{\text{Body Surface Area in square meters}}$$

A difference of 90 ml. per square meter or more between two successive examinations of the same patient indicates a significant change in relative heart volume.

Relative Heart Volume Determination (Amundsen)

Predicted Heart Volume (PHV) $= 0.4^* \times L \times B \times D$
   (P-A view, TSD $= 2$ m.; lateral view, 1.5 m.)

Relative Heart Volume (RHV) $= \dfrac{\text{PHV}}{\text{Body surface area}}$ (BSA in m.²)

	RHV (ml./m.²)
Significant difference between sequential exams	90 or more
Female adults (maximum normal)	450–490
Male adults (maximum normal)	500–540
Birth to 3 months (maximum normal)†	284–311
3 months to 2 years (maximum normal)†	334–371

Roentgenologic Heart Volume in Infants (Lind)

Actual volume preferred as determined by nomogram.
Heart Volume (HVRTG; *BD* = B above; LD = L above; DDH = D above.
                    For nomogram see Figure 22–7C.
   * Varies, as noted in text, by different investigators.
   † Antero-posterior recumbent, at least 3 hours after eating.

Figure 22–5   Summary of concepts of relative heart volume determination and roentgenologic heart volume in infants according to Amundsen and Lind respectively.

NOMOGRAM FOR THE DETERMINATION OF BODY SURFACE AREA OF ADULTS

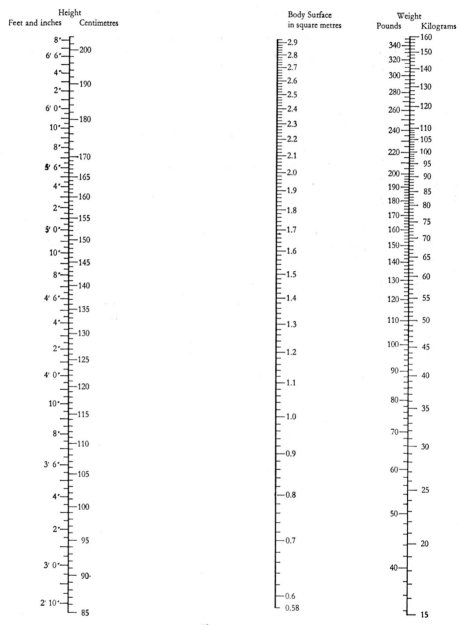

Figure 22–6

NOMOGRAM FOR THE DETERMINATION OF BODY SURFACE AREA OF CHILDREN

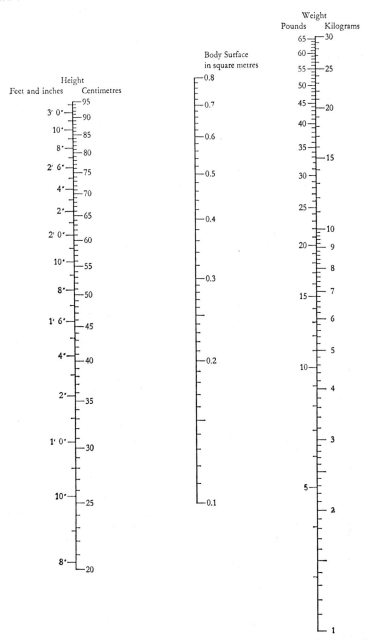

Figure 22–7   Key: The body surface area is given by the point of intersection with the middle scale of a straight line joining height and weight.

TABLE 22–1   NORMAL HEART VOLUMES IN CHILDREN*

Age	Volume per Square Meter of Body Surface (Relative Heart Volume)	Standard Error of the Mean
0– 30 days	196	22.6
30– 90 days	217.8	33.9
90–360 days	282	35.8
1– 2 years	295	30.4
2– 4 years	304	41.5
4– 7 years	310	36.2
7– 9 years	324	28.6
9– 12 years	348	33.6
12– 14 years	369	53.8
14– 16 years	398	61.9

*Adapted from Mannheimer, in Keats, T. E., and Enge, I. P.: Radiology, *85*:850, 1965.

Factors Affecting Cardiac Size and Contour (Figure 22–8)

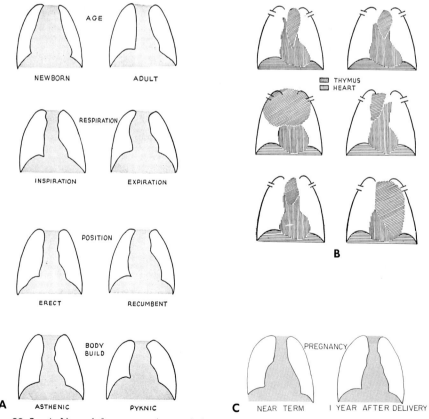

Figure 22–8   *A.* Normal factors causing variation in the supracardiac shadow and cardiac contour. *B.* Variations in size and position of supracardiac thymic shadow in the infant, which must be considered when measuring the infant's heart. *C.* Changes in cardiac size and contour which occur in hypervolemia of pregnancy.

Valsalva Maneuver.   If the glottis is closed after a deep inspiration and positive pressure is maintained against the closed glottis, there is a gradual diminution in cardiac size for several cardiac cycles. This is called a "positive pressure study," and has been proposed for differentiating compressible vascular structures from noncompressible mass lesions in the chest.

Thoracic Deformities.   Thoracic deformities will alter the position of the heart, as well as its size and contour. For example, a dorsal lordosis, a funnel chest, or pectus excavatum may produce a rotation of the heart toward the left or a flattened appearance with displacement posteriorly; a kyphoscoliosis will produce a rotation of the heart toward the side opposite the scoliosis.

Intrathoracic Pulmonary or Pleural Pathological Processes.   These very often affect cardiac size and contour.

Phase of Cardiac Cycle.   In sustained deep inspiration, cardiac systole is accompanied by a smaller frontal area of the heart than in full expiration. Changes in systole and diastole will produce detectable differences in cardiac size; indeed, heart rate will likewise produce slight differences in cardiac contour and size, so that the slow hearts of athletes tend to appear somewhat larger in frontal area than hearts of an unselected normal population.

RADIOGRAPHIC CARDIAC CONTOUR CHANGES IN RELATION TO SPECIFIC CHAMBER ENLARGEMENT

Indicators of Specific Chamber Enlargement

Left Ventricle

Rounded; extends farther laterally and posteriorly.
In relation to the inferior vena cava in the lateral view: 2 cm. cephalad to the diaphragm, the horizontal measurement of the left ventricle is greater than 18 mm.

Right Ventricle

In Infants: "Coeur en sabot" with squared elevated apex.
In Adults: Encroaches on the anterior and superior mediastinal clear space and the ventricle appears to be climbing the sternum.

Left Atrium

Double-contoured right cardiac margin in P-A view.
Prominence in the left auricular appendage.
Slight elevation of the left bronchus.
Esophagus selectively displaced posteriorly and usually to the right.
Encroachment upon the aortic window.

Right Atrium

Right cardiac margin farther to the right than normal.
In the lateral view it may appear to fill the retrocardiac space, producing a double-contoured appearance with the left ventricle.

Left Ventricular Enlargement

POSTERO-ANTERIOR

LEFT ANTERIOR OBLIQUE

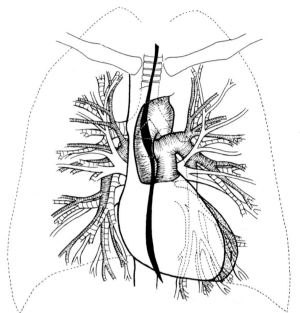

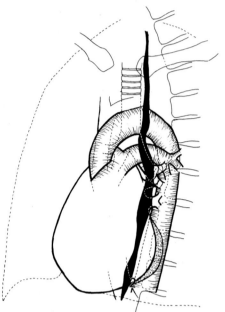

A

1. Left ventricular contour is rounded, extends farther laterally, and left diaphragm is depressed; rounding due to hypertrophy, distension to left due to dilatation.

B

2. Left ventricle extends beyond retrocardiac space and cannot "clear the spine" readily; is rounded.

LATERAL

Anterior pleura

Posterior pleura

$\dfrac{AB}{AC} > 0.42$

C

DISTANCE FROM INF. V. CAVA > 1.5 CM. (EYLER ET. AL.)

Figure 22–9   *See legend on opposite page.*

RIGHT ANTERIOR OBLIQUE

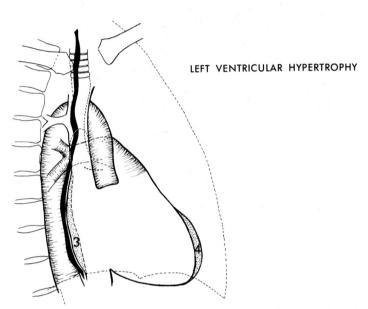

LEFT VENTRICULAR HYPERTROPHY

3. Heart as a whole is displaced posteriorly and comes close to spine.

4. Anterior apical portion of heart extends farther anteriorly.

Heart intersects left leaf of diaphragm.

Figure 22–9 Diagrams showing changes in appearance of cardiac contour with left ventricular hypertrophy and dilatation.

Right Ventricular Enlargement

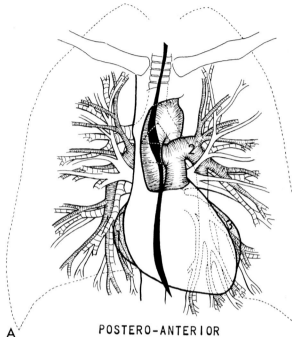

POSTERO-ANTERIOR

A

1. Enlarged right atrium.
2. Enlargement and dilatation of pulmonary arteries.
3. Increased convexity in left pulmonary sector.
4. Right ventricle bulges convexly on anterior aspect.

Note: "Wooden shoe" shape associated with right ventricular hypertrophy in tetralogy of Fallot not included here.

Figure 22–10 Changes in appearance of cardiac contour with right ventricular enlargement.

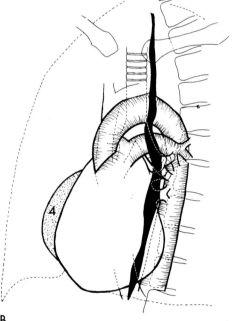

B   LEFT ANTERIOR OBLIQUE

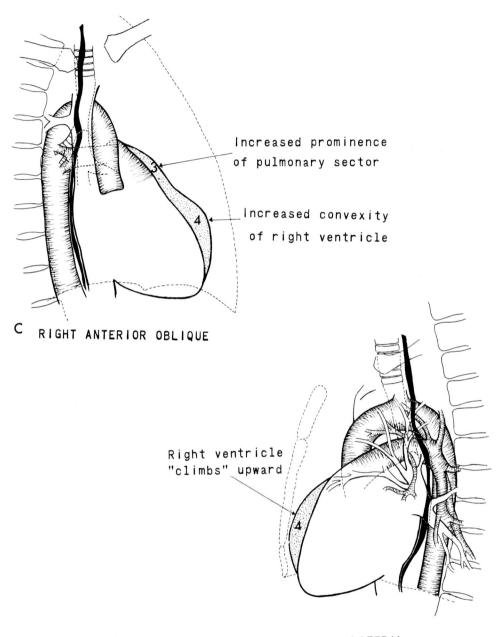

Increased prominence
of pulmonary sector

Increased convexity
of right ventricle

C   RIGHT ANTERIOR OBLIQUE

Right ventricle
"climbs" upward

LATERAL

Right ventricle enlargement
and encroachment on
mediastinal clear space

D

Figure 22–10 (*Continued*)   *See legend on opposite page.*

Left Atrial Enlargement

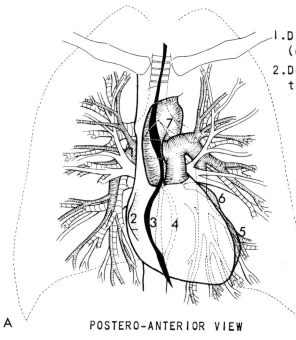

1. Dilated pulmonary arteries (especially right).
2. Double contour of right border due to left atrium.
   3. Esophagus usually displaced to right, but occasionally to left, as (4).
   5. Usually associated variable enlargement of left ventricle.
   6. Prominence of left auricular appendage and increased convexity of pulmonary sector.
   7. Left bronchus displaced upward.

A   POSTERO-ANTERIOR VIEW

(Dilatation element great; hypertrophy minimal; seldom unassociated with other pathology.)

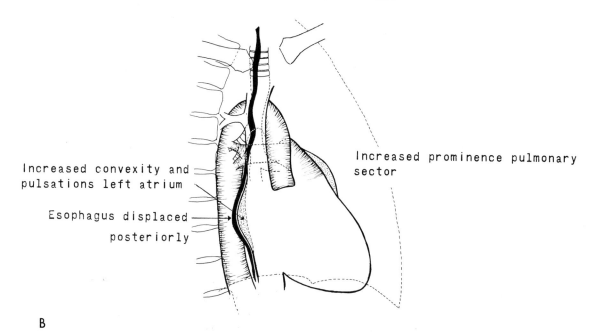

Increased convexity and pulsations left atrium

Esophagus displaced posteriorly

Increased prominence pulmonary sector

B

RIGHT ANTERIOR OBLIQUE

Figure 22-11   *See legend on opposite page.*

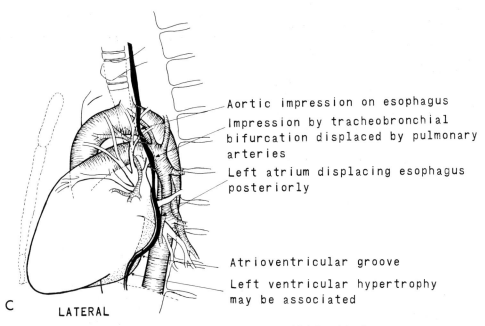

Aortic impression on esophagus

Impression by tracheobronchial bifurcation displaced by pulmonary arteries

Left atrium displacing esophagus posteriorly

Atrioventricular groove

Left ventricular hypertrophy may be associated

C   LATERAL

Figure 22–11   Changes in cardiac contour with left atrial enlargement.

Right Atrial Enlargement

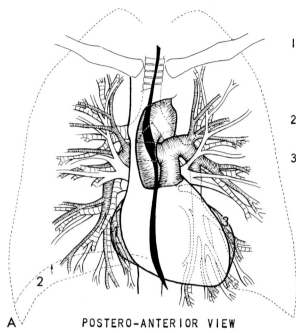

1. Extension to right of right atrial border, with increased convexity. Occasionally enlarged right ventricle does this.
2. Elevated diaphragm from enlarged liver.
3. Usually left-sided heart enlargement, since mitral and aortic valvular disease are associated with tricuspid.

A   POSTERO-ANTERIOR VIEW

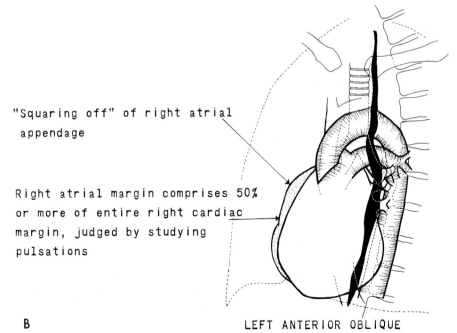

"Squaring off" of right atrial appendage

Right atrial margin comprises 50% or more of entire right cardiac margin, judged by studying pulsations

B   LEFT ANTERIOR OBLIQUE

Figure 22-12 *See legend on opposite page.*

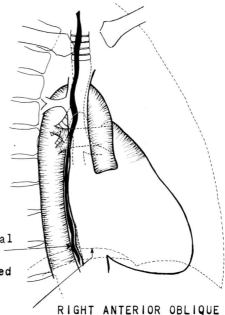

May see slight posterior
convexity in right atrial
sector and slight esophageal
displacement, but this is
usually obscured by elevated
right hemidiaphragm from
enlarged liver.

C

RIGHT ANTERIOR OBLIQUE

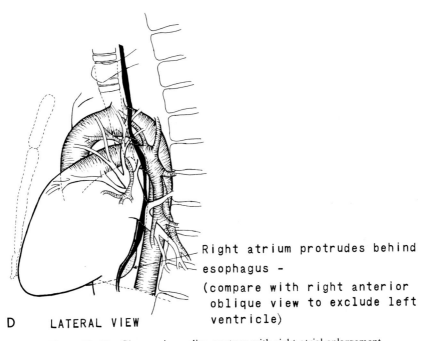

Right atrium protrudes behind

esophagus -

(compare with right anterior
oblique view to exclude left
ventricle)

D   LATERAL VIEW

Figure 22–12   Changes in cardiac contour with right atrial enlargement.

CARDIAC CHAMBER ENLARGEMENTS AND THEIR ASSOCIATED DISEASE STATES

LEFT SIDE OF HEART

Left Atrium

Congenital Diseases
> Ventricular septal defects
> Patent ductus arteriosus
> Coarctation of the aorta (adult type)

Acquired Diseases
> Rheumatic heart disease, with mitral or aortic valvular disease (aortic stenosis—30 per cent of cases)
> Bacterial endocarditis (mitral disease involved)
> Tumors of the left atrium (myxoma)

Left Ventricle

Congenital Diseases
> Aortopulmonary window
> Patent ductus arteriosus
> Endocardial fibroelastosis
> Coarctation of the aorta (adult type)
> Supra-aortic valvular stenosis
> Tricuspid atresia

Acquired Diseases
> Hypertensive heart disease
> Aortic or supra-aortic valvular stenosis
> Aortic insufficiency from any cause
> > Syphilitic heart disease
> > Rheumatic heart disease (especially aortic valve involved)
> > Bacterial endocarditis
> > Repeated episodes of cardiac failure in arteriosclerotic heart disease

RIGHT SIDE OF HEART

Right Atrium
   Congenital Diseases
      Ebstein's disease (low implantation of tricuspid valve)
      Tricuspid insufficiency
   Acquired Diseases
      Virtually any disease which can produce right ventricle dilatation
      and hypertrophy
Right Ventricle
   Congenital Diseases
      Ventricular septal defects
      Atrial septal defects
      Transposition of the great vessels
      Tetralogy of Fallot
      Eisenmenger complex
      Anomalous pulmonary venous return
   Acquired Diseases
      Cor pulmonale—acute
      Cor pulmonale—chronic
         Diffuse pulmonary disease
            Emphysema
            Chronic bronchitis
            Chronic fibrous tuberculosis
            Diffuse sarcoid
            Diffuse fibrosing pulmonary diseases
         Pulmonary vascular diseases
            Multiple thrombi and emboli
            Vasculitides (collagen disease)
         Chronic alveolar hypoventilation
            Massive pleural thickening
            Neuromuscular diseases
            Myasthenia gravis
            Muscular dystrophies
            Kyphoscolioses
         Any causes of pulmonary hypertension
            Congenital disease
            Acquired diseases: valvular, endocardial, myocardial, pericardial

Pitfalls in the Evaluation of Chamber Enlargement on Conventional Chest Radiographs

Changes Occurring in the Presence of a Greatly Enlarged Left Atrium. As a cardiac chamber continues to enlarge, secondary changes in the shape of the heart caused by displacement of other cardiac chambers may lead to misinterpretation in some cases.

A greatly enlarged left atrium may be responsible for a counter-clockwise rotation of the heart due to limitation in its movement to the left by the markedly enlarged left ventricle with which it is often associated. The left atrium is also restricted posteriorly by the spine. Thus, the left atrium enlarges to the right and anteriorly. The right atrium is thereby displaced anteriorly and to the right, accentuating the appearance of this chamber. Eventually, the left atrium forms the right heart border and approaches the right chest wall.

Changes Occurring in the Presence of a Massively Enlarged Right Ventricle. The right ventricle also is limited in its outward expansion by the sternum, and as it enlarges, it displaces the left ventricle in a counter-clockwise direction. It thereby produces exactly those changes which are produced by the left ventricle when it enlarges. This may lead to special confusion when the left ventricle is itself enlarged (Dinsmore et al.).

Similarly, a massively enlarged right ventricle may form the right heart border if there is an associated left ventricular enlargement. Usually, the enlarged right ventricle displaces the right atrium to the right and upward. This in itself does not usually lead to confusion, since the right atrial enlargement often accompanies right ventricular enlargement.

A massively enlarged right ventricle may also displace the left ventricle posteriorly and lead to a wrong evaluation.

Evaluation of Right Atrial Size. Evaluation of right atrial size also poses a special problem (Klatte et al., 1963).

Actually, no specific configuration of the right cardiac border in the posteroanterior view is reliable in the determination of right atrial size.

Enlargement of the right atrium can be best determined on the basis of the following criteria:

1. Differentiation of the right atrium fluoroscopically in the left anterior oblique view. There is a point of differential pulsation of the right atrium and the right ventricle in this projection along the right cardiac margin with an obliquity of 45 degrees or greater. If under these circumstances the right atrial margin comprises 50 per cent or more of the entire right cardiac margin, it is enlarged.

2. In the left anterior oblique view, the right atrial appendage may be identified on the upper right cardiac border. "Squaring" of the border at this site is a fairly good index (although not absolute) of right atrial enlargement.

3. Of lesser value is the right anterior oblique view. The posterior cardiac border is often behind the esophagus when the right atrium is enlarged. The obliquity for this view must be at least 45 degrees.

4. The lateral view may be similarly employed. When the right atrium enlarges, it forms a cardiac margin which protrudes behind the esophagus. However, if this is not corroborated on the right anterior oblique view, it is likely that the posteriorly protruding chamber is the left ventricle and *not* the right atrium.

Lastly, in Pectus Excavatum Deformities of the sternum and chest, the entire heart may be rotated counter-clockwise and toward the left, and the entire heart may be displaced posteriorly. The heart may also be "flattened" by such chest deformities. Ordinarily, volumetric studies of the heart continue to be reliable under these circumstances, but accurate individual chamber analysis is not feasible.

RADIOGRAPHIC CARDIAC CONTOUR CHANGES IN RELATION TO VALVULAR ABNORMALITIES

Aortic Valve Abnormalities

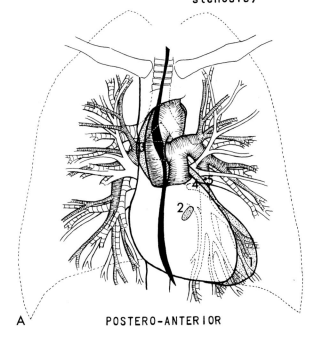

CARDIAC PATHOLOGY: VALVULAR DISORDERS
(Rheumatic, syphilitic, arterio-
   sclerotic) (aortic valve insuffiency and
   stenosis)

1. Enlargement left ventricle
      Apex directed to left,
      Apex rounded,
      Pulsations markedly increased.
2. Aortic valve and/or ring may be
      calcified.
3. Aorta is diffusely enlarged with
      increased amplitude of pulsations,
      especially in syphilis; slight
      enlargement with rheumatic aortic
      heart disease.
4. Cardiac waist deeper.
5. "Mitralization" occurs secondarily
      with damming back of blood and
      approaching failure.

A   POSTERO-ANTERIOR

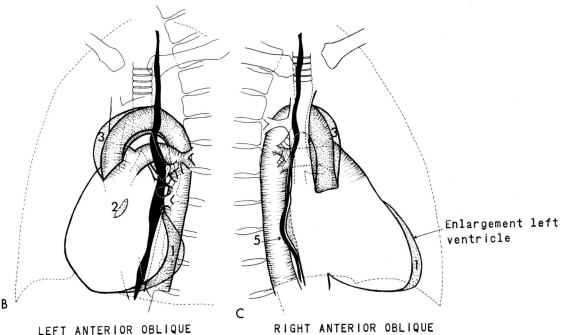

Enlargement left
ventricle

B

C

LEFT ANTERIOR OBLIQUE   RIGHT ANTERIOR OBLIQUE

Figure 22-13 Diagrams illustrating alterations in cardiac contour with aortic valve abnormality.

MITRAL VALVE ABNORMALITIES

Stenosis

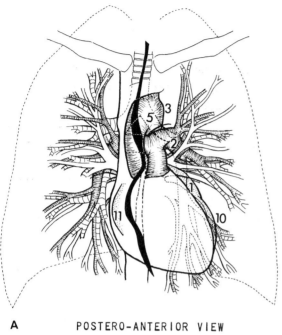

A   POSTERO-ANTERIOR VIEW

1. Prominence of left atrium with increased pulsatory activity.
2. Distension of pulmonary arteries (diminishes when right heart failure supervenes)
3. Loss of aortic incisura; heart rotates to left.
4. Left atrium border moves upward and posteriorly.
5. Left bronchus moves upward.
6. Left atrium bulges posteriorly.
7. Esophagus displaced posteriorly to right.
8. Increased distension of pulmonary veins.
9. Right ventricular hypertrophy (late)
10. In practically pure stenosis, left ventricle remains small.
11. Double contoured appearance due to large left atrium extending to right.
12. Left atrial enlargement becomes more prominent with Valsalva test, unlike normal.

Figure 22–14   Cardiac configuration changes with mitral stenosis.

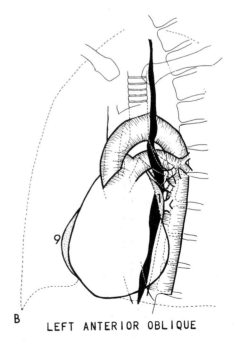

B   LEFT ANTERIOR OBLIQUE

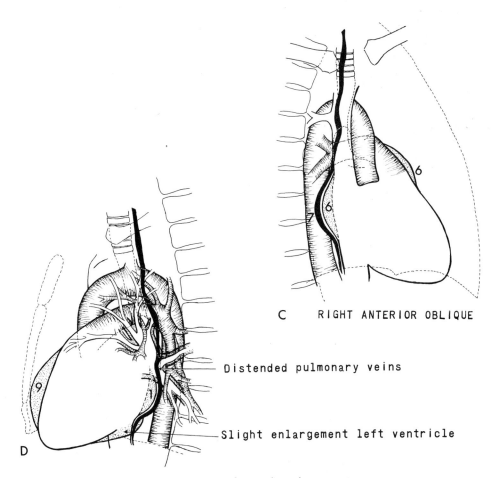

C   RIGHT ANTERIOR OBLIQUE

Distended pulmonary veins

Slight enlargement left ventricle

Figure 22–14 (*Continued*)   *See legend on opposite page.*

Mitral Insufficiency

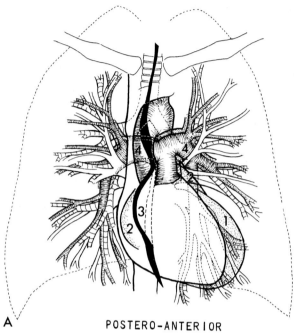

MITRAL INSUFFICIENCY
(Rheumatic)

Usually combined with stenosis*

1. Left ventricle enlarged to left and becomes rounded.
2. Left atrium enlarged to right, slightly upward and posteriorly.
3. Esophagus displaced to right and posteriorly.
4. Enlarged pulmonary arteries, until right heart failure supervenes.

Mitral regurgitation may occur in conjunction with aortic valve defects or hypertensive hearts, but changes are much less marked.

*See section on stenosis of mitral valve for other changes which also occur here.

A   POSTERO-ANTERIOR

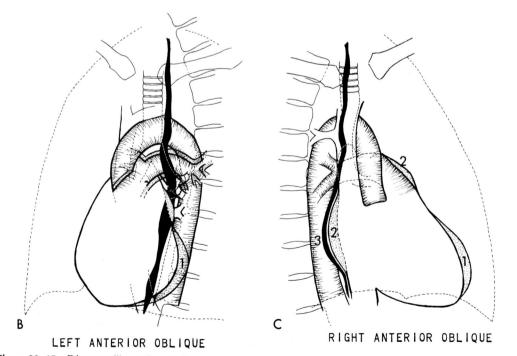

B   LEFT ANTERIOR OBLIQUE   C   RIGHT ANTERIOR OBLIQUE

Figure 22–15   Diagrams illustrating cardiac contour changes in the conventional views with mitral insufficiency.

Tricuspid Valve Abnormalities

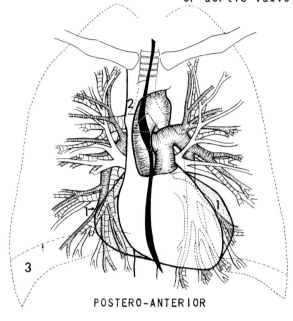

TRICUSPID REGURGITATION AND STENOSIS
Almost always combined with mitral
or aortic valve disease (rheumatic).

POSTERO-ANTERIOR

A. No characteristic roentgen signs.

   So-called "tricuspid configuration"
   is not pathognomic.

B. Regurgitation is pre-eminent in
   three fourths of cases.

1. Large bulge to right of right atrium
   and right ventricle enlarges.
2. Distending and pulsating vena cava

   (retrograde pulsations)

3. Elevated right hemidiaphragm due to
   engorged liver pulsating.
4. Little or no pulmonary stasis.

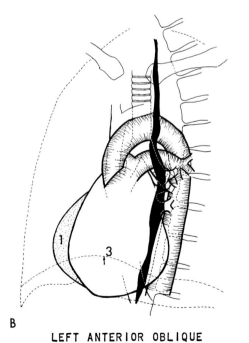

B

LEFT ANTERIOR OBLIQUE

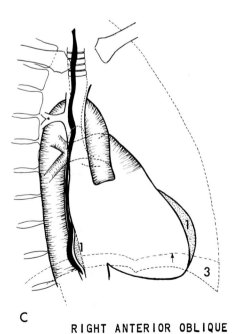

C

RIGHT ANTERIOR OBLIQUE

Figure 22–16 Diagrams illustrating cardiac contour changes with tricuspid regurgitation and stenosis (almost always combined with mitral or aortic valvular disease).

Combined Valvular Lesions

COMBINED VALVULAR LESIONS

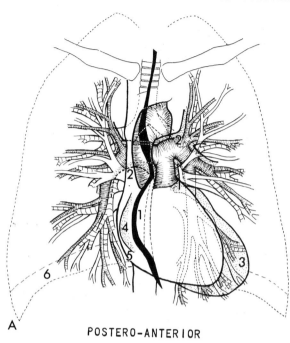

1. Esophagus displaced to right and posteriorly.
2. Distended pulsating pulmonary arteries.
3. Enlarged, rounded left ventricular arc.
4. Enlarged left atrium.
5. Enlarged right atrium and right ventricle.
6. Elevated right hemidiaphragm.

*When heart is in failure differentiation is virtually impossible, since enlargement of left atrium may occur in failure from any cause (hypertension, emphysema, etc.)

** When hydropericardium present, distinction may be impossible by these contour studies.

A   POSTERO-ANTERIOR

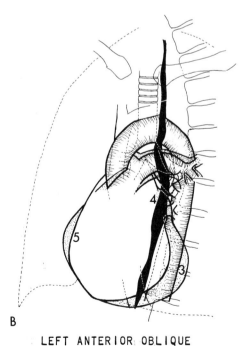

B   LEFT ANTERIOR OBLIQUE

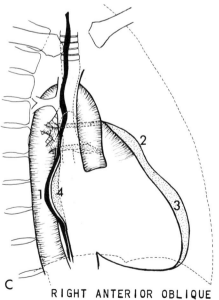

C   RIGHT ANTERIOR OBLIQUE

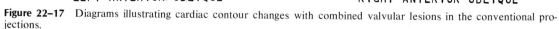

Figure 22–17 Diagrams illustrating cardiac contour changes with combined valvular lesions in the conventional projections.

INDICATORS OF VALVULAR ABNORMALITIES

Aortic Valve

Supravalvular Stenosis

Enlargement of left ventricle in 90 per cent of patients
Enlargement of left atrium in 30 per cent of patients

Subvalvular Stenosis

Heart is usually not enlarged
Poststenotic dilatation of the aorta in 70 to 84 per cent of patients

Aortic Stenosis—Valvular

Calcification present in 85 per cent of patients with acquired disease, but rarely detected in patients under 20 years of age
Heart is usually not enlarged

Aortic Insufficiency

Elongation and descent of the left ventricular apex
Relative narrowness of cardiac waist
Dilatation of the entire ascending aorta

With Chronic Failure

Pulmonary hypertension (see Chapter 19)

Mitral Valve

Prominence of left auricular appendage
Displacement of esophagus to right and posteriorly
Distention of upper lobe veins and diminution in lower lobe veins
Later, right ventricular hypertrophy and pulmonary hypertension occur

Stenosis

Left ventricle remains small
Kerley's "B" lines
Bone formation in lungs—3 to 5 per cent (Kerley)

Insufficiency

Usually combined with some stenosis
Left ventricle markedly enlarged
Valvular calcification in 30 to 40 per cent, more often when stenosis and insufficiency are combined

Triscuspid Valvular Disease

Almost always combined with aortic and mitral disease
Right atrium and right ventricle may enlarge
Superior vena cava distended
Elevation of right hemidiaphragm
Little or no pulmonary stasis

Pulmonary Valve

Stenosis

Primarily as a congenital lesion (Chapter 23)

Insufficiency

Usually with endocarditis and rare
Dilatation and hypertrophy of right ventricle and right atrium
Hilar vessels "dance"
Cardiac waist enlarged
Both cardiac borders appear to pulsate in collapsing fashion
Repeated pulmonary emboli are frequently present

Combined Valvular Lesions

Diffuse cardiac enlargement
Distended and pulsating pulmonary arteries
Esophagus displaced posteriorly and to the right
Right hemidiaphragm elevated
Contour simulates cardiac failure and hydropericardium

Figure 22–18 *A*. Diagrammatic radiograph showing evidence of pulmonary capillary hypertension. For enumeration of roentgen signs, see text. *B*. Tabulation of roentgen signs of pulmonary venous hypertension, capillary hypertension, and arterial hypertension.

Cephalization of Flow Concept

Kerley has summarized the findings in mitral valvular disease as follows: "Distended upper lobe veins, contracted lower lobe veins, and marked interstitial lines mean that mitral stenosis is dominant over mitral incompetence; distended upper lobe veins plus interstitial lines and small peripheral arteries indicate predominant mitral stenosis with pulmonary hypertension; distended upper and lower lobe veins indicate a low pulmonary pressure so that **whenever the lower lobe veins are visible it is safe to assume a low pressure**" (Figure 22–18).

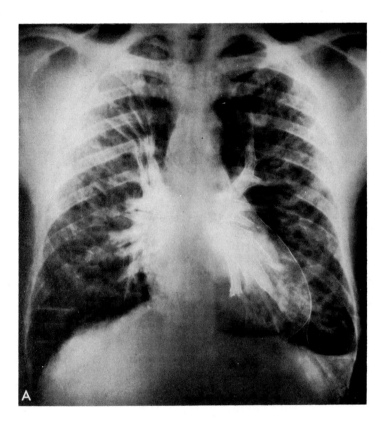

Pulmonary Venous Hypertension:
1. Normal or narrowed pulmonary veins in lower lung fields.
2. Prominent pulmonary veins in upper lung fields.
3. Dilated veins in hili.
4. Pulmonary root shadows indistinct.
5. Obliteration of right pericardiac space.

Pulmonary Capillary Hypertension:
1. Kerley's "A and B" lines.
2. Perivascular haziness.
3. Reticulation of pattern in lower lobes.
4. Loss of translucency in lung bases.

Pulmonary Arterial Hypertension:
1. Straightening or bulging of pulmonary artery segment.
2. Pulmonary arteries near hili enlarged, particularly more so in upper lobes.
3. Narrowing of pulmonary arteries in lower lobes.
4. Tortuosity of smaller pulmonary arteries.
5. Rapid tapering of midzone arteries.

B

Figure 22–18 *See legend on opposite page.*

ROENTGEN SIGNS OF ABNORMALITY OF THE AORTA

AORTA ELONGATION AND TORTUOSITY WITH SLIGHT DIFFUSE DILATATION

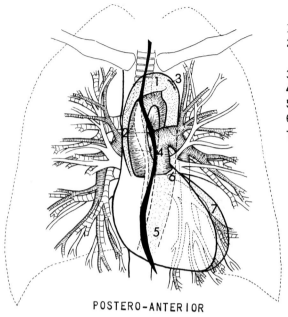

1. Transverse part of arch cephalad.
2. Ascending aorta rotates anteriorly and to right.
3. Calcium plaques*.
4. Esophagus drawn to left.
5. Descending aorta moves to left.
6. Cardiac waist becomes narrower.
7. Usually left ventricle also enlarged.

*Due to aortic sclerosis which is often associated

ABOVE CHANGES MAY BE EITHER ARTERIO-SCLEROTIC OR LUETIC IN ORIGIN.

PULSATIONS ARE USUALLY INCREASED IN AMPLITUDE, PARTICULARLY IN LUETIC AORTITIS.

POSTERO-ANTERIOR

Figure 22–19 Diagram illustrating changes in cardiac and aortic contour, with aortic elongation and tortuosity and slight diffuse dilatation.

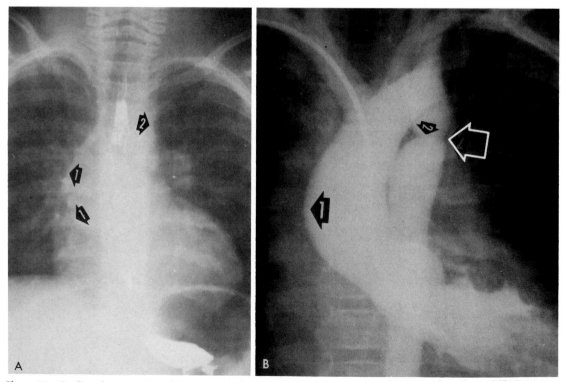

Figure 22–20 Pseudocoarctation of the aorta. *A.* Postero-anterior view of the chest. Arrow 1 points to the somewhat dilated ascending aorta and arrow 2 points to the infolding of the pseudocoarctation as seen in frontal perspective. Ordinarily a slight scalloped appearance of the knob of the aorta in this location can be seen. *B.* Antero-posterior view of the chest following the injection of contrast agent into the left heart showing an excellent delineation of the left ventricle and ascending and descending thoracic aorta. Arrow 1 points to the dilated ascending aorta and arrow 2 points to the pseudocoarctation site.

ROENTGEN SIGNS OF ABNORMALITIES OF THE PULMONARY ARTERIES

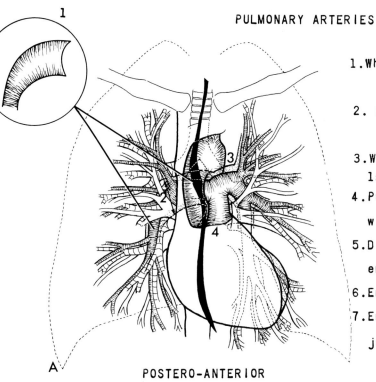

PULMONARY ARTERIES

1. When right pulmonary enlarges ⇨ "reverse comma."
2. Measurement normally less than 15 mm. (Assman).
3. When left pulmonary enlarges large "knob" below aortic knob.
4. Pulmonary conus is concealed within the heart.
5. Dilated left pulmonary artery encroaches on aortic window.
6. Enlarged right ventricle.
7. Enlarged pulmonary artery just below bifurcation.

A   POSTERO-ANTERIOR

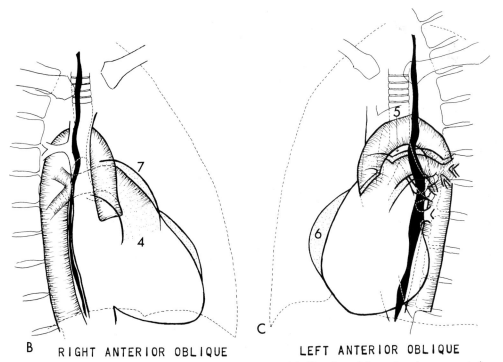

B   RIGHT ANTERIOR OBLIQUE

C   LEFT ANTERIOR OBLIQUE

Figure 22–21   Diagrams illustrating roentgen appearances with dilatation of the main pulmonary arteries.

Roentgen Signs of Abnormality of the Main Pulmonary Artery and its Immediate Branches

1. Enlargement with associated dilatation of the peripheral branches
   a. Congenital
      - (1) With intracardiac or extracardiac shunts (see Chapter 23)
      - (2) Without shunts
         - (a) Pulmonary stenosis (poststenotic dilatation)
         - (b) Coarctation of pulmonary artery or its branches
         - (c) Pulmonary vein stenosis
         - (d) Idiopathic dilatation of pulmonary artery
   b. Acquired
      - (1) Cardiac diseases
         - (a) Mitral valve disease
         - (b) Left atrial tumors
         - (c) Chronic left ventricular failure
      - (2) Pulmonary diseases
         - (a) Parenchymal
         - (b) Vascular
            - 1, Primary pulmonary hypertension
            - 2, Secondary pulmonary hypertension due to repeated pulmonary emboli, collagen diseases, schistosomiasis
            - 3, Syphilis
      - (3) Hyperkinetic circulatory states
         - (a) Anemia
         - (b) Hyperthyroidism
         - (c) Paget's disease
         - (d) Beriberi
         - (e) Systemic A-V fistulas
2. Enlargement with rapid tapering and no associated enlargement of the peripheral branches
   a. Pulmonary hypertension
3. Diminution in size or absence
   a. Congenital heart lesions (Chapter 23)
   b. Bronchopulmonary hypoplasia
   c. Unilateral hyperlucent lung (Swyer-James or MacLeod's syndrome)
   d. Peripheral pulmonary artery stenoses
4. Irregular and somewhat bizarre appearances
   a. Arteriovenous malformations
5. Large "inverse comma" right pulmonary artery
   a. Patent interatrial septum
   b. With "pruned branch" appearance—pulmonary artery thrombosis

ROENTGEN SIGNS OF ABNORMALITY OF THE PERICARDIUM

1. Diffuse "bulging" enlargement of cardiopericardial silhouette
   a. Pericardial effusion
   b. Cardiac failure
   c. Nephrosis
2. Localized "bulging"
   a. This is usually due to a myocardial aneurysm rather than a pericardial abnormality
3. "Shagginess" of the cardiopericardial silhouette
   a. Mediastinitis
   b. Pertussis
4. Calcification ("armored heart")
5. "Notching"
   a. Partial or complete absence of the pericardium
6. Diverticulum
   a. Cyst of the pericardium or coelomic cyst

Pericardial Effusion

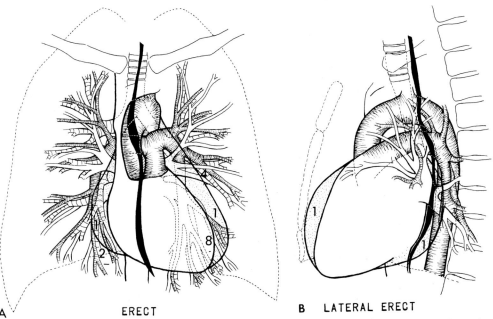

A   ERECT   **B**   LATERAL ERECT

Figure 22-22 Diagram illustrating roentgen changes with pericardial effusion. (1) Outpouchings bilaterally, (2) increased acuity of cardiophrenic angle, (3) cardiac pulsations reduced or absent, (4) cardiac indentation effaced (requires 400 cc. minimum), (5) no inspiratory movement,* (6) shape more globular in recumbent, (7) base of heart widens in recumbent, (8) *with image amplifier, epicardial fat may be seen inside the pericardial space, if more than 2 mm. thick.*

Pathology: (a) inflammatory, serous, or fibrinous; (b) hemorrhagic; (c) purulent; (d) transudate (uremia, collagen disease, protein deficiency).

Differential diagnosis is very difficult. Failing enlarged heart with myocardial edema or myxedema may be impossible to differentiate. Will require aspiration of fluid and production of pneumopericardium for proof.

Angiocardiography is helpful also.

*In sustained inspiration, shadow tends to move inward normally.

Chronic Adhesive Pericarditis

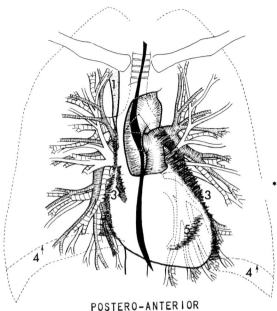

1. Superior vena cava distended.
2. Pulsations diminished or absent.
3. Thickened shaggy pericardium fills out indentations in contour
4. Diaphragm elevated due to ascites and enlarged liver.
5. Calcium plaques in pericardium.

*Triad: a) Quiet small heart (occasional enlargement).

        b) Venous pulse markedly increased.

        c) Pulse pressure small.

POSTERO-ANTERIOR

Figure 22–23   Diagrams illustrating roentgen changes with chronic adhesive pericarditis.

Pericardial Fat Pads

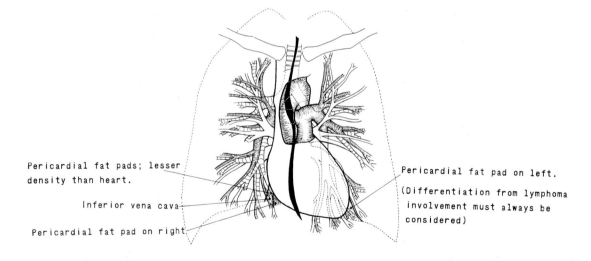

Pericardial fat pads; lesser density than heart.

Inferior vena cava

Pericardial fat pad on right

Pericardial fat pad on left.

(Differentiation from lymphoma involvement must always be considered)

POSTERO-ANTERIOR VIEW

Figure 22–24   The pericardial fat pad, diagrammatic illustration in frontal projection.

ROENTGENOLOGIC ALTERATIONS IN CERTAIN CARDIAC DISEASES (EXCLUDING CONGENITAL HEART DISEASE—CHAPTER 23)

Introduction

Inferences in regard to etiology are based upon alterations of size, contour, position, pulsations, density (calcification), and changes in sequential film studies in respect to time and therapy.

It is hazardous to attempt an etiological consideration when the heart is in failure, and all discussions of etiology under our consideration refer only to the compensated heart.

Coronary Heart Disease

Roentgenologic Alterations

1. Fibrocalcific changes in the valves occasionally in the more chronic forms.

2. Ventricular aneurysm, where a myocardial infarction has occurred and left the myocardium fibrotic, thin, and distensible. These occur predominantly in the anterior apical and posterior basilar portions of the heart. Paradoxical pulsations may be seen fluoroscopically at the site of such aneurysms.

3. Coronary angiography is utilized to analyze problems related to angina pectoris and coronary arteriosclerosis from the standpoint of potential surgical intervention and treatment, but these special procedures are outside the scope of this text.

4. The heart is usually small, unless the disease is accompanied by the hypertensive disease (as it is in about 25 per cent of cases), and the myocardium is ischemic, fibrotic, and atrophic.

Hypertensive Heart Disease (Figure 22–25)

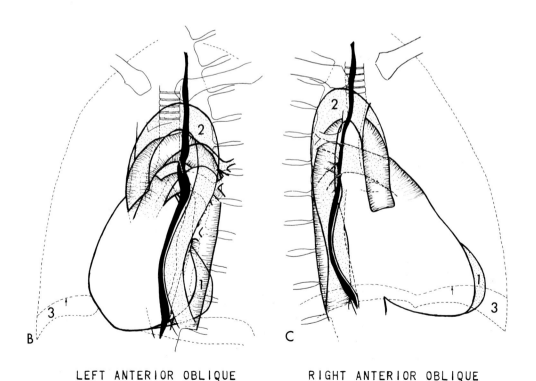

CARDIAC PATHOLOGY:HYPERTENSIVE
HEART DISEASE

(Nephritic; Essential; Arterial;
Arteriolar)

1. Left ventricle enlarges to left
   and becomes rounded.
2. Aortic knob becomes more prominent
   and cardiac waist narrowed; aorta
   elongated.
3. Diaphragm is usually elevated.
4. Pulsations regular; vary in
   amplitude.

Note: Pleural effusion, pulmonary
   edema, cardiac failure, etc,
   may be associated.

A

POSTERO-ANTERIOR

B

LEFT ANTERIOR OBLIQUE

C

RIGHT ANTERIOR OBLIQUE

Figure 22–25 Diagrams illustrating cardiac contour changes with hypertensive heart disease in the conventional projections.

Rheumatic Heart Disease

Principal Morphologic Changes

Rheumatic nodules in myocardium, epicardium, or pericardium.

During the acute phase acute pericarditis may develop, but otherwise the manifestations and disturbances are difficult to detect roentgenologically, since the changes are largely microscopic.

The endocardial involvement may produce mural plaques in the atria or damage to the heart valves. The distribution of involvement of the valves is as follows:

    a. Mitral valve alone, 40 per cent.
    b. Mitral and aortic valves together, 40 per cent.
    c. Aortic valves alone, 10 to 15 per cent.
    d. Aortic, mitral, and tricuspid involvement is next in frequency.
    e. Pulmonic valve is very seldom involved.

Roentgenologic Features

Pericardial effusion as such is not common but may occur.

Mitral, aortic, and tricuspid valvular alterations occur as previously described.

Mural thrombus within the fibrillating left atrium will produce a markedly increased prominence of the left auricular appendage.

Changes in the vasculature of the lungs as described in the text are distention of upper lobe veins, contraction of lower lobe veins (followed by contraction of all veins), accentuation of Kerley's "A" and "B" lines, tortuosity of veins, pulmonary edema, pleural effusion, and pulmonary hypertension.

Terminally the result is cardiac failure usually. However, embolization (especially to the lungs from the radiologic standpoint), bronchopneumonia, and bacterial endocarditis may also occur terminally and have their radiologic manifestations.

Cor Pulmonale

Roentgenologic Changes

Alterations in the lung—vessels, interstitium, alveoli.

Enlargement of main and central pulmonary arteries. Rapid tapering of pulmonary arteries near the third and fourth subdivision.

Right ventricular hypertrophy.

Radiologic evidence of right ventricular failure is ascites with elevation of the diaphragm, hepatosplenomegaly, pleural effusion, and peripheral edema (Harvey and Ferrer; Mack et al.).

Syphilitic Heart Disease

Roentgenologic Features

Marked left ventricular enlargement with collapsing pulsations and large pulse pressure manifestations.

Dilatation of the ascending aorta to aneurysmal proportions.

Collapsing pulsations in the ascending aorta, unless obscured by aneurysmal clot formation.

Laminated layers of calcification in the ascending aorta.

MISCELLANEOUS INTRACARDIAC CALCIFICATION

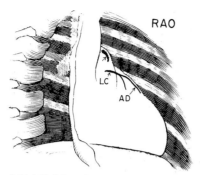

CALCIFIED LEFT CORONARY A.

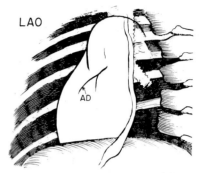

CALCIFIED LEFT CORONARY A.

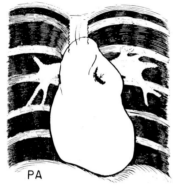

CALCIFIED PATENT DUCTUS

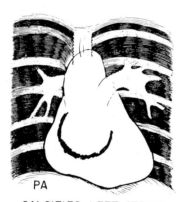

CALCIFIED LEFT ATRIUM

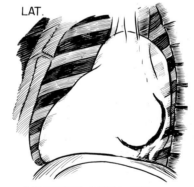

CALCIFIED LEFT ATRIUM

Figure 22–26 Cardiopericardial structures which may contain calcium as depicted radiographically.

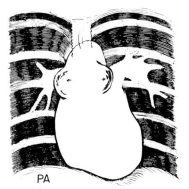

CALCIFIED SINUS OF VALSALVA
ANEURYSM

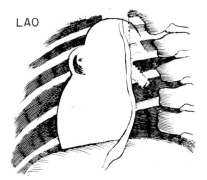

CALCIFIED SINUS OF VALSALVA

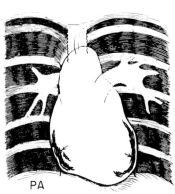

CALCIFIED PERICARDIUM

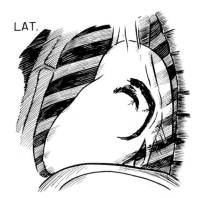

CALCIFIED LEFT ATRIUM
WITH CALCIFIED THROMBUS

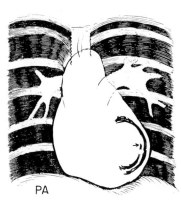

CALCIFIED
MYOCARDIAL INFARCT

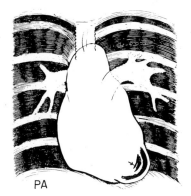

CALCIFIED
LEFT VENTRICULAR ANEURYSM

Figure 22–26 (*Continued*)

Questions – Chapter 22

See questions following Chapter 23.

23

Congenital Heart Disease: Plain Film Interpretation

Our emphasis in this abbreviated text will be devoted to plain film interpretation and no effort will be made to include interpretation of special catheterization studies or angiographic procedures. Many congenital diseases lend themselves to plain film analysis and interpretation, but many do not.

For greatest simplicity, this subject has been presented in outline form for emphasis.

SUMMARY OUTLINE*

A. Increased Pulmonary Vascularity without Cyanosis
1. Intracardiac shunts
   a. Interatrial shunts
   b. Interventricular shunts
   c. Ventriculoatrial shunts
   d. A-V communis defect (endocardial cushion defect)
2. Extracardiac shunts
   a. Aortopulmonary window
   b. Patent ductus arteriosus
   c. Peripheral arteriovenous malformation

B. Increased Pulmonary Vascularity with Cyanosis
1. Total anomalous pulmonary venous return
2. Persistent truncus arteriosus
3. Complete transposition of the great vessels
4. Incomplete transposition of the great vessels as with Taussig-Bing syndrome

---

*Only the more frequent of the entities listed will be considered in greater detail.

     5. Double outlet right ventricle
     6. Single ventricle with no pulmonary stenosis (cor triloculare biatriatum)
     7. Tricuspid atresia with transposition and no pulmonary stenosis (really similar to a two-chambered heart)

C. Decreased Pulmonary Vascularity
     1. Obstruction at the tricuspid valve level
        a. Tricuspid atresia or stenosis
        b. Ebstein's anomaly with low implantation of the tricuspid valve
     2. Obstruction at the level of the pulmonary valve
        a. Pulmonary valve atresia
        b. Pulmonary valve stenosis with intact atrial and interventricular septum
        c. Pulmonary valve or infundibular stenosis with a ventricular septal defect (tetralogy of Fallot)
        d. Pulmonary valve stenosis with interatrial septal defect, but no interventricular septal defect
        e. Pulmonary artery coarctation (or hypoplasia more peripherally)
     3. Absence of a pulmonary artery (persistent truncus communis, Type 4)
     4. Transposition with a single ventricle and pulmonary stenosis

D. Normal Pulmonary Vasculature When No Failure Is Present
     1. Corrected transposition of major vessels
     2. Aortic stenosis
     3. Aortic insufficiency
     4. Coarctation of the aorta (may show failure in the newborn)
     5. Hypoplastic left heart syndrome (usually shows left heart failure)
     6. Congenital mitral stenosis (usually shows left heart failure)
     7. Cor triatriatum (usually shows left heart failure)

E. Normal Pulmonary Vasculature with Diffuse Cardiac Enlargement Due to Endomyocardial Abnormalities
     1. Endocardial fibroelastosis (usually shows failure)
     2. Aberrant left coronary artery (usually shows failure)
     3. Glycogen storage disease (usually shows failure)

F. Cardiac Malpositions
     1. Situs inversus, mirror image dextrocardia
     2. Dextroversion of the heart
     3. Levoversion of the heart

G. Vascular Anomalies in Major Branches at the Arch of the Aorta (Swischuk)
     1. Producing no symptoms
        a. Anomalous right subclavian artery
        b. Right aortic arch, right descending aorta
        c. Right aortic arch, right descending aorta, anomalous left subclavian
        d. Right aortic arch, left descending aorta
        e. Left aortic arch, right descending aorta
     2. Producing symptoms
        a. Right or left double aortic arch
        b. Right aortic arch, right descending aorta, left ductus arteriosus
        c. Left aortic arch, left descending aorta, right ductus arteriosus
        d. Anomalous innominate artery
        e. Anomalous left common carotid artery
        f. Vascular sling—aberrant left pulmonary artery

H. Hypoplastic Pulmonary Artery and Ipsilateral Lung

ROUTINE OF ANALYSIS OF FILMS (POSTERO-ANTERIOR, LATERAL, AND BOTH OBLIQUES WITH ESOPHAGRAMS)

1. Study pulmonary vasculature, centrally and peripherally (it may be normal, increased, decreased, or bizarre)
2. Identify the chambers comprising the cardiac contour, if possible (Chapter 22)
3. Aortic knob and descending thoracic aorta: identify, study position and contour in relation to esophagus and trachea
4. Note postion of stomach gas bubble
5. Note bones of the thoracic cage (ribs, especially)

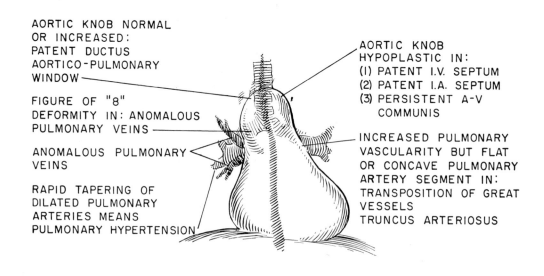

AORTIC KNOB NORMAL OR INCREASED:
PATENT DUCTUS
AORTICO-PULMONARY WINDOW

FIGURE OF "8" DEFORMITY IN: ANOMALOUS PULMONARY VEINS

ANOMALOUS PULMONARY VEINS

RAPID TAPERING OF DILATED PULMONARY ARTERIES MEANS PULMONARY HYPERTENSION

AORTIC KNOB HYPOPLASTIC IN:
(I) PATENT I.V. SEPTUM
(2) PATENT I.A. SEPTUM
(3) PERSISTENT A-V COMMUNIS

INCREASED PULMONARY VASCULARITY BUT FLAT OR CONCAVE PULMONARY ARTERY SEGMENT IN:
TRANSPOSITION OF GREAT VESSELS
TRUNCUS ARTERIOSUS

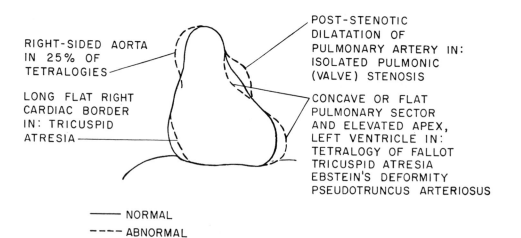

RIGHT-SIDED AORTA IN 25% OF TETRALOGIES

LONG FLAT RIGHT CARDIAC BORDER IN: TRICUSPID ATRESIA

POST-STENOTIC DILATATION OF PULMONARY ARTERY IN:
ISOLATED PULMONIC (VALVE) STENOSIS

CONCAVE OR FLAT PULMONARY SECTOR AND ELEVATED APEX, LEFT VENTRICLE IN:
TETRALOGY OF FALLOT
TRICUSPID ATRESIA
EBSTEIN'S DEFORMITY
PSEUDOTRUNCUS ARTERIOSUS

———— NORMAL
– – – – ABNORMAL

Figure 23–1 *A.* Differential features of main entities with increased pulmonary artery vascularity. *B.* Changes in cardiac contour in relation to various congenital heart lesions.

AREAS OF PREDOMINANT CHANGE IN VARIOUS CONGENITAL CARDIAC LESIONS

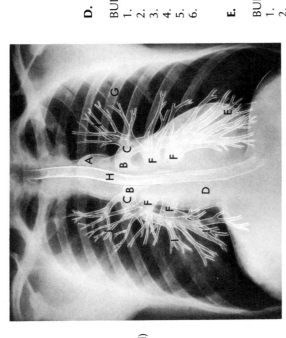

Figure 23–2

A. AORTIC KNOB

ALTERED IN:
1. Complete Transposition Major Blood Vessels (small)
2. Double Aortic Arch
3. Right-Sided Aortic Arch
4. Absence of Aortic Arch
5. Coarctation of Aorta

INCREASED IN:
6. Patent Ductus Arteriosus (with left to right flow)
7. Tetralogy of Fallot (on rt. – 1/4)
8. Tricuspid Atresia (except with transposition where it is decreased)
9. Aortic and Subaortic Valve Stenosis

DECREASED IN:
10. Ventricular Septal Defect (inversely proportional to left atrium size)
11. Atrial Septal Defect (secundum type)
12. Anomalous Pulmonary V. Return
13. Truncus Arteriosus
14. Pulmonary Stenosis
15. Fibroelastosis

OBSCURED IN:
16. Anomalous Pulmonary Venous Return (by overlying sup. v. cava or persistent left v. cava)

B. PULMONARY ARTERY

DECREASED IN:
1. Truncus Arteriosus Communis
2. Fallot Tetralogy

C. PULMONARY ARTERY and OUTFLOW TRACK

INCREASED IN:
1. Patent I.A. Septum
2. Patent I.V. Septum
3. Completely Absent I.V. Septum
4. Tricuspid Atresia with Transposed Vessels
5. Pure Pulmonary Stenosis
6. Taussig-Bing Syndrome
7. Eisenmenger Complex
8. Patent Ductus Arteriosus

D. RIGHT ATRIAL BORDER

BULGE TO RIGHT IN:
1. Combined I.A. and I.V. Septum Defects
2. Complete Transposition Major Blood Vessels
3. Taussig-Bing Syndrome
4. Eisenmenger Complex
5. Situm Viscerum Inversus
6. Absence of Aortic Arch

E. LEFT CARDIAC CONTOUR

BULGE TO LEFT IN:
1. Patent I.A. Septum
2. Tricuspid Atresia
3. Pulm. Stenosis with I.A. Septal Defect
4. Aortic Stenosis
5. Truncus Art. Communis
6. Complete Transposition Major
7. Fallot Tetralogy
8. Eisenmenger Complex
9. Coarctation of Aorta

F. PULMONARY VEINS

G. RIB NOTCHING

H. INDENTATIONS ON ESOPHAGUS

I. PULMONARY FLOW, PRESSURE RESISTANCE INCREASED

TABLE 23–1 MOST FREQUENT CONGENITAL HEART CONDITIONS

Most Frequent Congenital Heart Disease in Newborn Infants	Most Frequent Congenital Heart Disease in 7 to 10 Day Old Infants, Leading to Congestive Heart Failure	Most Frequent Congenital Heart Disease in Adults		
		PULMONARY VASCULAR ENGORGEMENT	PULMONARY VASCULATURE MARKEDLY DECREASED	NORMAL PULMONARY VASCULATURE
Hypoplastic left heart syndrome	Coarctation of the aorta	Atrial septal defect	Tetralogy of Fallot	Coarctation of aorta
Hypoplastic right heart syndrome with tricuspid atresia or pulmonary atresia		Patent ductus	Ebstein's anomaly	Aortic stenosis
Total anomalous pulmonary venous return				Isolated pulmonary stenosis
Most common cause of cyanosis in the first days of life: complete transposition of great vessels.		Ventricular septal defect		Small ventricular septal defect
Most marked cardiomegaly with or without associated cardiac failure— no cardiac murmurs: endocardial fibroelastosis.				

WHICH CARDIAC CHAMBERS WILL BE ENLARGED?

A. Right Ventricle

Roentgen Appearance: Elevated left apex on postero-anterior view; best evaluated on left anterior oblique and lateral views in which the right ventricle appears to "climb the sternum"

"Coeur-en-sabot" or wooden shoe appearance

    1. With intracardiac shunts:
        a. Patent interatrial septum
        b. Patent interventricular septum
    2. With pulmonic valvular or infundibular stenosis:
        a. Tetralogy of Fallot
    3. When the pulmonary veins in whole or in part empty into the right heart (anomalous pulmonary venous return)
    4. When the left ventricle ejects its blood into the pulmonary circulation:
        a. Transposition of great vessels
        b. Persistent truncus arteriosus
        c. Single ventricle

B. Left Ventricle

Roentgen Appearance: "Boot-shaped heart" but toe is not squared-off in P-A view. Best evaluated in the left anterior oblique view and the lateral view, in which it protrudes posteriorly toward the spine, far beyond the reflection of the inferior vena cava

    1. With extracardiac shunts:
        a. Patent ductus arteriosus
        b. Aortopulmonary window
    2. With mitral valvular insufficiency
    3. With aortic valvular disease
    4. With endocardial fibroelastosis

C. Right Atrium

Roentgen Appearance: In the P-A view, the right cardiac margin extends to the right; in left anterior oblique and lateral views, the chamber protrudes posteriorly somewhat like the left ventricle.

    1. Tricuspid valvular low implantation (Ebstein's disease)

D. Left Atrium

Roentgen Appearance: In the P-A view, the esophagus is displaced to the right and the left auricular appendage is prominent.

Esophagus is displaced posteriorly and a "notch" is evident at the junction of the right and left atria.

The left bronchus appears somewhat elevated:

    1. Mitral stenosis
    2. Endocardial fibroelastosis
    3. Patent interventricular septum
    4. Patent ductus arteriosus
    5. Aortopulmonary window
    6. In aortic valvular disease, when the left ventricle becomes markedly dilated and the mitral valve is also insufficient

E. Diffuse Cardiac Enlargement

Roentgen Appearance: The heart is diffusely enlarged in all its chambers and appears globular.

    1. Diffuse infiltrative disorders such as glycogen storage disease
    2. Aberrant left coronary artery
    3. Endocardial fibroelastosis

Positional Abnormalities of the Heart (Figure 23–3)

1. **The Position of the Heart and Viscera** ("gas bubble" of the stomach) are related as follows:
    a. Left-sided heart and normal position of viscera: *Levocardia*
    b. Left-sided heart and right-sided gas bubble: *Levoversion*
    c. Right-sided heart and situs inversus viscera: *Mirror-image dextrocardia*
    d. Right-sided heart and normal position of viscera: *Dextroversion*
2. **Statistical Associations**
    a. Overall incidence of associated heart disease is 5 per cent
    b. There is a much higher incidence of associated heart disease in infants and children
    c. Associated respiratory tract disease is common, especially in adults
        (1) 16.5 per cent incidence of bronchiectasis (Olsen)
        (2) Kartagener's triad, consisting of mirror-image dextrocardia with situs inversus, sinusitis, and bronchiectasis
3. **Dextroversion With Viscera in Normal Position: Situs Solitus**
    a. The right heart border resembles the normal left heart border, but is not usually the same. The aortic arch is usually on the left
    b. Increased incidence of associated congenital anomalies, especially in infants and children—perhaps as much as 85 to 90 per cent (Elliott et al.; Gasul et al.)
    c. The most common associated abnormality of the heart is the corrected transposition of the great vessels
4. **Levoversion:** Left-sided heart and right-sided gas bubble
    a. 74 per cent incidence of asplenia and 10 per cent incidence of polysplenia (Keith et al.)
    b. The aortic arch is usually on the right
    c. Atrial inversion also occurs in one-third to one-half of the cases (Gasul et al.)
    d. This is a serious abnormality with many other associated cardiac and extracardial abnormalities
5. **The Complete Radiologic Approach to Positional Abnormalities of the Heart and Abdominal Viscera is as Follows:***
    a. Rule out secondary dextrocardia. . . .
    b. Determine the visceral status. . . .
    c. Determine the cardia and apical position. . . .
    d. Localize the (cardiac) atria. . . .
    e. Localize the (cardiac) ventricles. . . .
    f. Determine the relationship of the atria to the ventricles. . . .
    g. Determine the presence and type of transposition of the great vessels. . . .
    h. Determine the "aortic arch—gastric air bubble" relationship. . . .

---

*From Meszaros, W. T.: *Cardiac Roentgenology. Plain Films and Angiocardiographic Findings.* Springfield, Ill., Charles C Thomas, 1969.

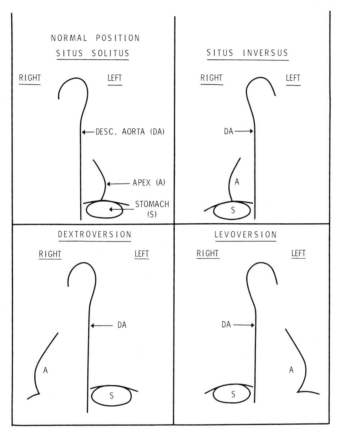

Figure 23–3 Schematic illustration of the alignment of descending aorta, apex and stomach in the four basic cardiac positions. The line drawings are shown as they would be projected in the frontal view of a chest x-ray.

In situs solitus (normal position) the descending aorta, apex and stomach are all on the *left*.

In situs inversus (mirror image dextrocardia) the descending aorta, apex and stomach are all on the *right*.

In dextroversion the descending aorta and stomach are on the *left* (as in the normal), but the apex is on the right.

In levoversion the descending aorta and stomach are on the right (as in situs inversus), but the apex is on the *left*. (From Perloff, J. K.: *The Clinical Recognition of Congenital Heart Disease*. Philadelphia, W. B. Saunders Co., 1970.)

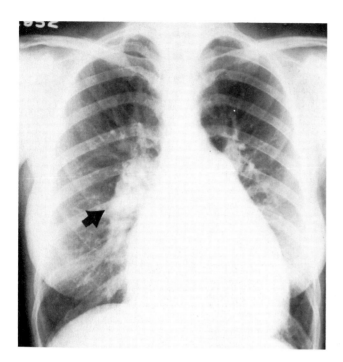

Figure 23–4 Atrial septal defect. Postero-anterior view of the chest in a patient with a patent interatrial septum. The large, comma-shaped right pulmonary artery is quite characteristic of many cases.

Figure 23–5 Pulmonic stenosis. Postero-anterior view of the chest in a patient with pure pulmonic valvular stenosis. The white arrow points to the poststenotic dilatation of the left pulmonary artery. Note the relative avascularity of the more peripheral portions of the lung.

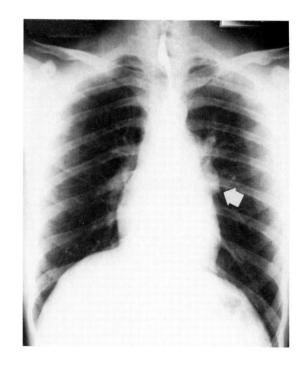

34. What disease states produce an enlarged right atrium in congenital and acquired heart diseases?

35. Indicate the most frequent lesions responsible for increased pulmonary vascularity without cyanosis in the congenital heart disease group.

36. Indicate the most frequent lesions responsible for increased pulmonary vascularity with cyanosis in the congenital heart disease group.

37. Indicate the most frequent lesions encountered in the decreased pulmonary vascularity group in congenital heart disease.

38. Indicate the most frequent diseases encountered in the congenital heart disease group in which the pulmonary vasculature is normal and there is no evidence of cardiac failure.

39. Indicate those diseases in the congenital heart disease group most frequently manifested by normal pulmonary vasculature but with diffuse cardiac enlargement due to endomyocardial abnormalities.

40. Indicate those diseases of congenital origin related to cardiac malpositions.

41. Categorize and describe the vascular anomalies in the major branches at the arch of the aorta. Which of these are apt to produce symptoms? Which ordinarily produce no symptoms?

42. What is a good routine for analysis of films in respect to congenital heart disease?

43. Suggest a convenient classification of the pulmonary vasculature in congenital heart disease.

44. What is the roentgen appearance of an enlarged right ventricle?

45. What is the roentgen appearance of an enlarged left ventricle?

46. What is the roentgen appearance of an enlarged right atrium?

47. What is the roentgen appearance of an enlarged left atrium?

48. What is the typical roentgen appearance of diffuse cardiac enlargement?

49. What is the importance of the esophagram and "tracheogram" in a study of the aortic knob?

50. Why is the position of the stomach gas bubble important in congenital heart disease?

51. Why is a careful study of the bones of the thoracic cage important for an understanding of congenital heart lesions?

52. Indicate the various types of anomalous pulmonary venous return.

53. What is meant by the "snowman appearance" and what anatomical aberrations are responsible for this appearance?

54. What is the most characteristic radiologic appearance of a patent ductus arteriosus? At what age is the characteristic appearance of a patent ductus arteriosus most apt to occur?

55. What are the various types of tricuspid stenosis or atresia, and what roentgenographic appearances are associated?

56. What are the various types of pulmonic stenosis and what are the various roentgenographic appearances associated?

57. Indicate the various elements in the diagnosis of tetralogy of Fallot. What are the most characteristic roentgenographic appearances?

58. Describe the basic pathologic alteration in transposition of great vessels and indicate the most frequently encountered roentgenographic appearances.

59. Indicate the types of persistent truncus arteriosus. Which are the most frequent? What are the most frequent roentgenographic appearances encountered in this disorder?

60. Indicate the various types of aortic stenosis. What are the most frequent roentgenographic appearances encountered?

61. Indicate the various types of endocardial fibroelastosis and describe the roentgenographic findings most frequently encountered.

62. What is meant by "Ebstein's anomaly"? What is the most characteristic roentgenographic appearance?

63. What are the various types of coarctation of the aorta? Indicate the roentgenographic appearances of each type.

24

Radiologic Study of the Abdomen Without Added Contrast Media

ROUTINE FILMS

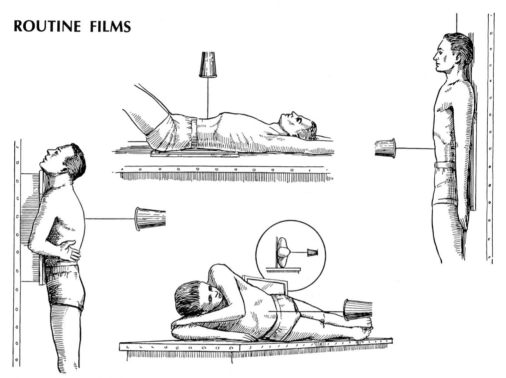

Figure 24–1 Routine film studies obtained for plain film survey of abdominal disease. Note that a P-A chest film is part of this routine. (Decubitus left lateral may be preferable.)

Purpose of These Films

In the plain film survey for abdominal disease, three different views of the abdomen are usually obtained:

1. **Anteroposterior supine film (KUB).** Shows maximal detail of roentgenologic anatomy and pathology.
2. **Upright film** demonstrates
   a. Fluid levels.
   b. Better detail of intestinal wall.
   c. Separation of loops and thickness of bowel wall.
   d. Mobility of bowel loops or air in the change from supine to erect.
   e. Free air beneath the diaphragm.
3. **Decubitus films** help corroborate erect studies and demonstrate free air in another projection.

In addition, a **chest film** is obtained in cases of

1. Possible chest abnormality with symptoms referred to the abdomen.
2. Free air beneath the diaphragm.

Method of Study of Routine Films

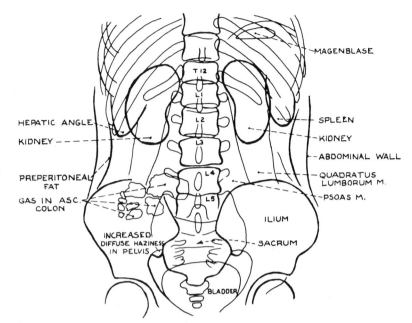

Figure 24-2 Routine for examination of the recumbent film of the abdomen.

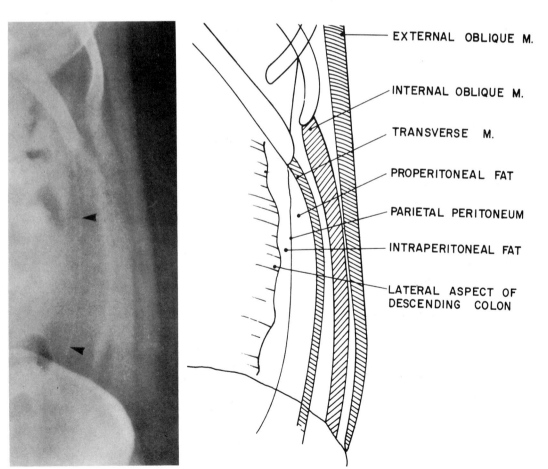

Figure 24-3 Radiograph and diagram showing normal roentgenographic anatomy in the flank. There is unusually extensive visualization of parietal peritoneum (arrows). (From Budin, E., and Jacobson, G.: Amer. J. Roentgen., 99:62, 1967.)

Normal Gas Patterns as Seen in the Abdominal Survey

In the *newborn*, no gas shadows are seen in the abdomen. Air appears in the stomach when the infant cries and swallows air in the process. Progression of intestinal gas results in complete filling of the small intestine, usually in two hours from birth, and of the large intestine in three to six hours. In the neonate, gas should be visible in the entire gastrointestinal tract by the end of 24 hours.

In the *adult,* gas shadows normally are recognized only in the stomach and colon.

Stomach. In the erect position the gas is retained largely in the fundus of the stomach but it may be distributed throughout the stomach in the supine or prone positions. In the erect position, gas in the fundus is normally closely applied to the left hemidiaphragm and this space measures approximately five millimeters. Increases in measurement of the distance between the top of the left hemidiaphragm and the gas bubble of the stomach in the erect position may indicate certain conditions which will be described subsequently (hepatomegaly, splenomegaly, subdiaphragmatic abscesses, mass in the fundus of the stomach).

Small Intestine. Normally, the small bowel does not contain gas. However, in aged patients or patients with pain, a small amount of gaseous distention of the small intestine is not unusual and may in itself not have great significance.

Ordinarily, reflex distention of the small intestine is only moderate.

Colon. An admixture of gas with fecal material usually produces a speckled appearance which is present unless special effort has been made to cleanse the colon. The gas pattern of the colon shows an indentation of the serosal coat of the colon as well as its mucosal coat, and thus, ordinarily, can be differentiated from the small intestine. However, when the ileum is markedly distended, the valvulae are not clearly demonstrated. In such instances clear differentiation between large and small intestine is not possible except by barium enema.

Rectal Gas is important for identification. Although highly variable in size, when it is impressed upon, diminished in distensibility, or tubular in appearance, it becomes a "pathology indicator." In the lateral view, the distance between the posterior margin of the rectum and the anterior surface of the sacrum is called the "retrorectal soft tissue space." This measurement approximates 5 to 15 mm. In presacral mass lesions from any cause, this measurement may be increased.

The colon when moderately distended may rise to the level of the fundus of the stomach and overlap the gaseous shadow of the fundus under the left hemidiaphragm. The hepatic flexure of the colon, however, even when distended with gas, is usually contained beneath the right lobe of the liver. In some circumstances the hepatic flexure and adjoining transverse colon may be interposed between the right lobe of the liver and the right hemidiaphragm. This *interposition* may be recognized by noting the haustrations of the colon. Interposition of the colon beneath the right hemidiaphragm (also called *hepatoptosis*) is without pathologic significance.

In the presence of eventration of the left hemidiaphragm, paralysis of the left hemidiaphragm, or atelectasis in the left hemithorax when the left hemidiaphragm is markedly elevated, the splenic flexure may rise immediately beneath the left hemidiaphragm and simulate gas in the peritoneal space. Careful identification of the haustral pattern of the colon will differentiate normal colon from free air in this position.

ROENTGEN SIGNS OF ABNORMALITY

The Psoas Shadows (Figure 24–2)

1. **Abnormality in size and contour** suggests a fluid or mass lesion such as hemorrhage, inflammation, or tumor of either a fatty or solid nature (Figure 24–5).
2. **Abnormality in density or architecture:** Although retroperitoneal, the abdominal aorta is ordinarily not reflected in the psoas or iliacus regions. However, when the abdominal aorta becomes enlarged or tortuous and partially calcified, an ellipsoid shadow may be projected over the iliacus muscle to the left of the midline, indicating either tortuosity or aneurysm formation in the abdominal aorta. Circumlinear calcification in the wall of the abdominal aortic aneurysm is virtually pathognomonic of this condition.
3. **Obscuring of the psoas shadow:** When the fatty envelope of the psoas muscle becomes infiltrated by inflammatory or neoplastic tissue, the normal psoas stripe may be obliterated ("unit density" material replacing "fat density"). This sign must be interpreted with caution since overlying gas or intestinal content may give a false impression of such obliteration (Figure 24–5). Occasionally, only one psoas shadow may be identified clearly.

Flank Area and Abdominal Wall

The flank anatomy is illustrated in Figure 24–3. Except in obese individuals, the flank shadow is concave inward on either side and a black stripelike shadow representing extraperitoneal fat (pre- or properitoneal fat) may be demonstrated on either side. This is continuous with another fatty shadow which usually delineates the hepatic angle on the right side, and usually delineates the inferior tip of the spleen on the left. This extraperitoneal fat is continuous with the tela subserosa throughout the entire body and is also continuous with the fascia surrounding the kidneys and the retroperitoneal musculature.

Alterations which may affect the fat shadow may be outlined as follows:
1. **Increase in size** such as occurs in rectus sheath hematoma.
2. **Alteration in shape** as in:
   a. Bulging of the flank asymmetrically from a contiguous retroperitoneal, intraperitoneal, or subhepatic inflammatory or mass lesion. Under these circumstances the flank shadows are usually asymmetrical.
   b. Bulging of the flanks symmetrically and bilaterally by a large intraperitoneal tumor such as might arise out of the pelvis (an ovarian cyst) (Figure 24–7) or by ascites.
3. **Alterations in density.** These may be of two types:
   a. A complete obliteration of the fat stripe as produced by an inflammatory process of the peritoneum (peritonitis) or by an edema of the abdominal wall.
   b. An accentuation of the appearance of the flank stripe that may be related to obesity, a pneumoperitoneum, or an adjoining lipomatous tumor mass such as a liposarcoma of the retroperitoneal space, or occasionally, a hematoma (Figure 24–6).
4. **Alterations in architecture.** Instead of the stripelike appearance noted above, there may be a "bubbly" appearance of the flank area. These bubbles of air gain access (1) by an external break or incision in the abdominal wall; (2) from an abscess or gas-producing organism; or (3) by communication with a gastrointestinal fistula. The abscess may be pericecal, subhepatic, or perisigmoidal in origin.

Some Examples of Abnormalities of Psoas Shadows, Flank Area, and Abdominal Wall

INTRAPERITONEAL AND RETROPERITONEAL ABSCESSES

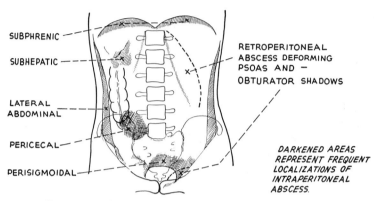

Figure 24–4   Usual localization of intra-abdominal abscesses.

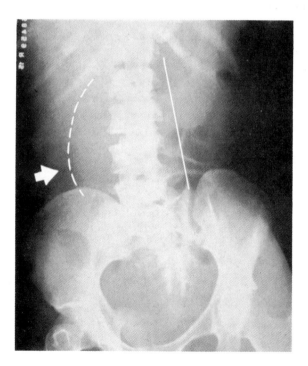

Figure 24–5   Radiograph demonstrating the appearance of the widened psoas shadow resulting from a large retroperitoneal abscess. Note the loss of detail in the flank shadow region. (Lines added to show psoas margins.)

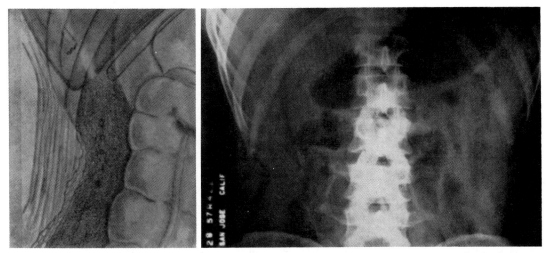

Figure 24–6 *A* and *B*. Irregularity of the properitoneal fat line and fracture of the right lower ribs indicating impact over the liver. Blood is present in the flank between the fat line and the ascending colon. A mild adynamic ileus is present. At operation there were three lacerations of the liver and a large amount of free blood in the peritoneal cavity. (From McCort, J. J.: Radiology, *78*:49, 1962.)

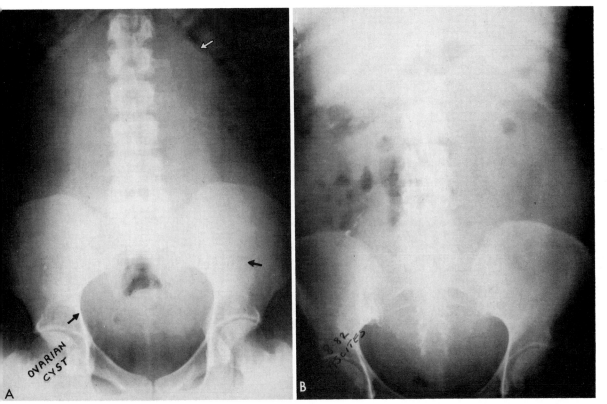

Figure 24–7 *A*. Displacement of all gastrointestinal loops, including rectum and sigmoid to some extent, by a huge ovarian cyst. *B*. The gas-containing loops of bowel "float" centrally with ascites. Note the following in ascites:

1. Separation and floating of bowel loops.
2. Fuzziness or obliteration of the psoas muscle shadows.
3. Overall abdominal haziness.
4. Poor definition of major abdominal organs.
5. Medial displacement and increased width of the flank stripe (normal range 1 to 2 mm.).

In ovarian cyst, note upward displacement of loops of bowel, and sharp circumscription superiorly, as well as bulging of the flanks.

Roentgen Signs of Abnormality of Gas Patterns in the Abdominal Survey

Absence or Diminution in Abdominal Gas. Feeble and premature infants as well as infants with severe respiratory distress may have delayed appearance of normal intestinal gas. Likewise, newborn infants under the influence of respiratory depressant drugs may lack normal intestinal gas patterns on a nonobstructive basis (Burko).

In the Infant the following causes of deficient intestinal gas pattern can be identified:

1. Mechanical obstruction.
2. Mechanical obstruction with dehydration.
3. Dehydration from causes unrelated to obstruction.
4. Interference with normal gas transit associated with respiratory distress.

The site of the mechanical obstruction may be identified at the point of cessation of progress of intestinal gas. Thus, if the entire stomach is outlined with no gas beyond, obstruction at the level of the pylorus may be postulated; if there are two distended foci of gas ("double bubble" appearance) the site of obstruction is either duodenal or jejunal in origin. Under these circumstances, the obstruction may be caused by an atresia, a web across the duodenum, abnormal mesenteric attachment of fibrous band, or small bowel volvulus (Figure 24–8).

At times the gas progress is "cut off" in the region of the pelvis, and this may be an indication of an atresia of the rectum or an imperforate anus. The "cut-off" appearance of the gas in the pelvis minor may be accentuated by turning the infant upside down and placing a thermometer or other opaque object in the anal dimple or by introducing an opaque medium into the vagina or urinary bladder where a communication with the obstructed colon may usually be identified.

In the Adult there may be an almost complete absence of gas in the intestines as the result of a thorough cleansing or purgative process. On such occasions only a small amount of gas in the stomach may be identified. Usually an enema will introduce gas into the colon along with its cleansing process.

A site of mechanical obstruction can usually be identified by the farthermost extent of gaseous distention in the gastrointestinal tract.

Excessive Gas, Either Diffuse or Regional, in the Gastrointestinal Tract

Gaseous Distention of the Stomach (Figure 24–9). Gaseous distention of the stomach can be readily recognized by virtue of its position and shape. It is seen with

1. Advanced pyloric stenosis (coupled with "tit" sign with barium)
2. Pyloric obstruction from any cause (most commonly from longstanding pyloroduodenal bulbar ulcerative disease)
3. Acute reflex gastric dilatation
4. Diabetic gastric atony or post-vagotomy syndrome (stomach shows no peristalsis and contains retained food and fluid)
5. Gaseous distention with uremia

Gaseous Distention of the Duodenum. When this is present, it is usually accompanied by gaseous distention of the stomach (Figure 24–8).

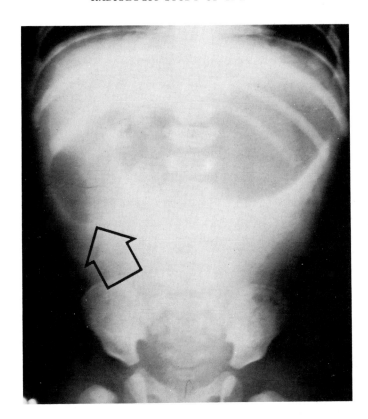

Figure 24–8 Radiograph of the abdomen of a newborn infant showing the appearance of gas in the stomach, duodenum, and proximal jejunum in association with a jejunal atresia. Note complete absence of gas distal to this point of obstruction.

Figure 24–9 Acute gastric dilatation. The arrow points to the junction of the markedly dilated stomach with the duodenal bulb in the region of the pyloric canal.

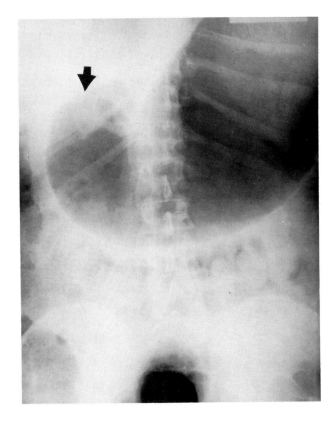

In infants it is related to duodenal atresia, stenosis, weblike obstructions of the duodenum or jejunum, or small bowel volvulus. There may be a characteristic "double bubble" appearance — one of the bubbles being the distended stomach and the other the markedly distended duodenum (Figure 24–8).

In adults marked duodenal distention may be due to:

1. An atony which may accompany obstruction of the duodenum by a long-standing band, mesenteric attachment, or superior mesenteric artery syndrome.
2. A tumor of the third part of the duodenum or proximal jejunum.
3. Internal herniation in the region of the ligament of Treitz.
4. Nontropical sprue, in which a coarsening of the folds, not only of the duodenum but often in the jejunum, may also be identified when barium is administered.

Distention of the Small Intestine. This is readily recognized by the demonstration of the *coiled-spring appearance* of the small intestine and its valvulae conniventes (Figure 24–10 B). If such distention is present without distention of the large intestine a mechanical obstruction of the small intestine must be suspected. By contrast, a *reflex ileus* will usually involve both small and large intestines. Occasionally, however, when a mechanical obstruction has persisted for a considerable period of time, a reflex ileus becomes superimposed. Under these circumstances, the identification of the mechanical obstruction is completely obscured. In these patients both the reflex and mechanical obstruction will be present, and the true nature of the process cannot be clearly identified.

With a reflex ileus the *diameter of the small intestine* does not become as great as with the mechanical obstruction.

Also, *fluid levels* are usually not present in the erect position or with a horizontal beam study.

Diffuse, Marked Overdistention of the Large Intestine may be recognized by:

1. The identification of the distended loops of bowel in the distribution of the colon even though redundancy is present. The lower the site of a mechanical obstruction, the greater the length of distended large intestine (Figure 24–10).

2. The lack of valvulae conniventes, and the presence of the valvulae semicirculares characteristic of the large intestine.

Combined Distention of the Small Intestine and Proximal Part of Colon (Figure 24–10). This appearance has often been ascribed to:

1. Mesenteric vascular occlusion.
2. Paralytic ileus.
3. Obstructing neoplasms of the splenic flexure of the colon.
4. Toxic ulcerative colitis.
5. Pancreatitis.

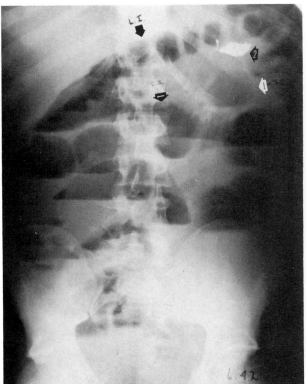 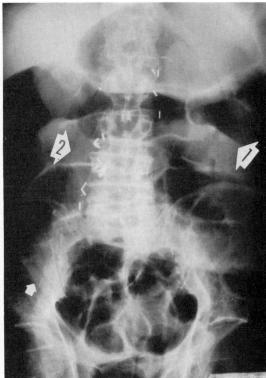

Figure 24–10 *A*. Radiograph demonstrating the stepladder (circular staircase) pattern often produced by air-fluid levels with markedly distended small intestine in mechanical obstruction (arrow 1, small intestine; LI, large intestine; arrow 2, mercury bag of Cantor tube). *B*. Mesenteric thrombosis demonstrating edematous valvulae conniventes in the right lower quadrant (unnumbered arrow), the "cut-off" sign of gas in the distal transverse colon (arrow 1), and the layered arrangement of the markedly dilated small bowel loops (arrow 2). If the patient were erect (as in *A*) these would produce a "stepladder" appearance.

IN MESENTERIC VASCULAR OCCLUSION, the distention corresponds closely to the distribution of the superior mesenteric artery, with a rather *abrupt demarcation of the distended intestines near the splenic flexure of the colon* (Figure 24–11).

Other *roentgen signs of mesenteric vascular occlusion are*

1. Gas in the portal vein (Wolfe and Evans).
2. Gas in the intramural portion of the bowel (Wiot and Felson).
3. Crescentic shadows of air in the wall of the intestine that are different from pneumotosis intestinalis (Schorr).
4. The presence of minimal roentgen signs despite a serious abdominal crisis (Rigler and Pogue).
5. A solitary loop of greatly distended bowel with an excessive quantity of fluid within it (Mellins and Rigler).
6. Presence of several loops of bowel in which the lumen is greatly reduced but the wall is markedly thickened (Nelson and Eggleston).
7. Ringlike shadows surrounding the bowel in a semicircular fashion (Schorr).
8. Long linear areas of lesser density appearing in the wall of the colon in patients with toxic megacolon secondary to ulcerative colitis (Wolfe and Marshak).
9. Additional adjunctive signs (Dunbar and Nelson).
   a. Thickening of the bowel wall of the infarcted segment.
   b. Fluid-filled small bowel loops creating a soft tissue mass (the "pseudo-tumor" of Frimann-Dahl).
   c. The rigid thick loops of bowel containing minimal gas unchanged in distribution from upright to recumbent positions. This finding suggests mesenteric venous obstruction.
   d. Localized or generalized bowel distention with an abrupt demarcation at the hepatic or splenic flexure in the distribution of the superior mesenteric vessels.

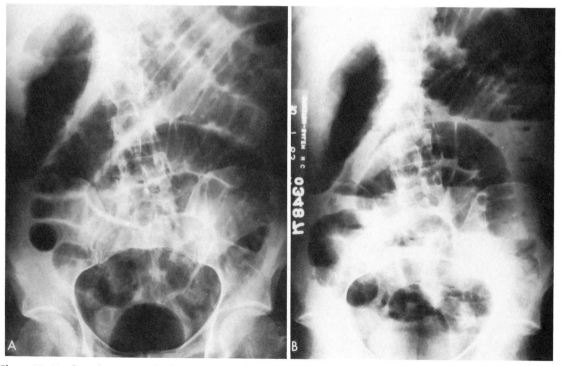

Figure 24–11 Superior mesenteric thrombosis. *A.* Recumbent KUB film showing massive distention of small intestine with only moderate distention of proximal one-half of colon in the distribution of the superior mesenteric artery. *B.* Erect film of the abdomen showing fluid levels in massively dilated small intestinal loops with only moderate distention in large intestine (proximal one-half).

ISOLATED DISTENTION OF LOOPS OF SMALL INTESTINE.   Isolated distention of loops of small intestine may occur with

1. Internal herniation of the small intestine through the foramen of Winslow (into the lesser omental bursa).
2. Volvulus of a segment of the small intestine.
3. Incarceration of a loop of small intestine either from internal herniation or by a fibrous band (Figure 24–12).
4. Overlying local peritoneal inflammatory process.

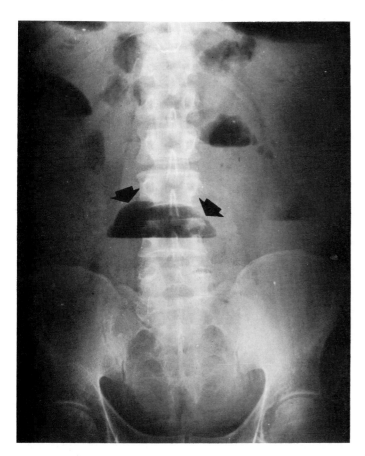

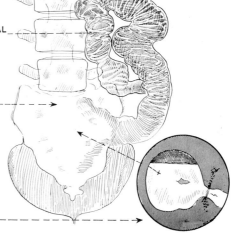

Figure 24–12 Strangulation of a loop of small intestine producing mechanical obstruction. The strangulation was due to internal herniation. Erect study.

STRANGULATION
(SUPINE APPEARANCE)

SMALL INTESTINAL
ILEUS

Figure 24–13 Line tracing. Note the complete absence of gas in the pelvis minor (pseudotumor appearance). The gas in the strangulated bowel is best seen in the erect position.

COMPLETE ABSENCE
OF GAS, GIVING
TUMOR-LIKE
APPEARANCE
DUE TO FLUID;
FLUID LEVEL
OBTAINED IN
ERECT POSITION

ISOLATED DISTENTION OF SMALL PORTIONS OF THE LARGE INTESTINE. Marked distention of the transverse colon occurs with:

1. Acute pancreatitis.
2. Toxic dilatation of the transverse colon in association with ulcerative colitis (Figure 24–15).
3. The colon "cut-off" sign at or just beyond the splenic flexure in relation to pancreatic disease has already been described (Aronson and Davis; Schwartz and Nadlehaft; Glenn and Baylin; Price; Stuart). Various inflammatory processes such as diverticulitis, tuberculosis, and amebiasis may produce somewhat similar appearances.
4. The large balloon-shaped distention of the sigmoid colon or cecum occurs with volvulus of the sigmoid or cecum, respectively (Figure 24–14), and with Hirschsprung's disease (Figure 24–16).
   (a) When the sigmoid undergoes volvulus (Figure 24–14) it usually extends upward in the midline or into the right upper quadrant.
   (b) The open end of an inverted U points downward toward the pelvis in volvulus of the sigmoid.
   (c) When the cecum undergoes volvulus (Figure 24–14), it usually extends toward the midline and the left upper quadrant.

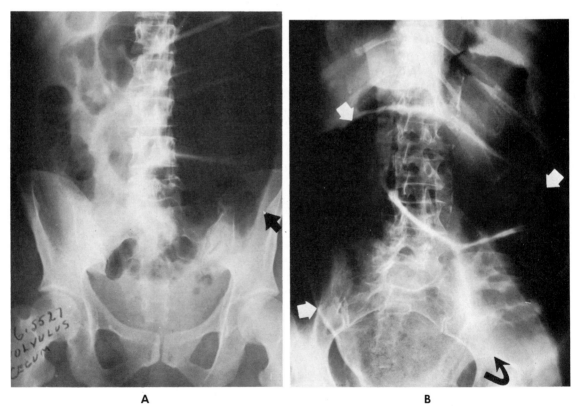

A   **B**

Figure 24–14   *A*. Radiograph demonstrating a rather typical appearance of volvulus of the cecum. Note the tremendously dilated, rather isolated loop of bowel in the left upper quadrant and left midabdomen. *B*. Volvulus of the sigmoid. The open end of the inverted U of distended bowel points toward the pelvis.

Figure 24–15 Distention of the large intestine, particularly its proximal one-half, with toxic ulcerative colitis. →

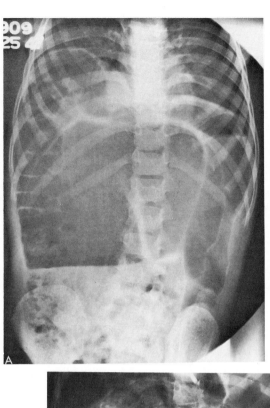

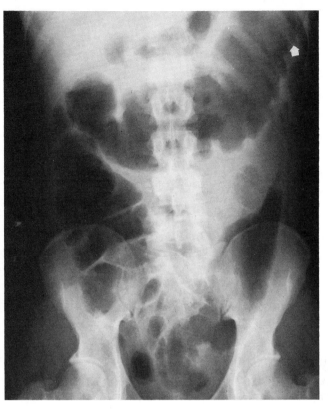

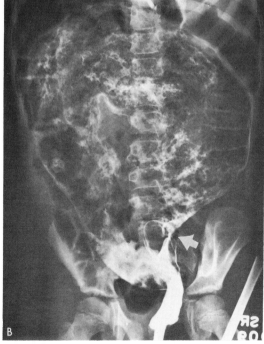

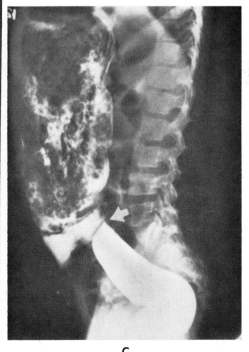

C

Figure 24–16 Hirschsprung's disease—congenital megacolon. *A*. Plain film of the abdomen showing tremendous dilatation of the sigmoid colon with inspissated fecal content. The dilated loops of bowel displace the right hemidiaphragm upward. *B*. A barium enema examination with filling of the rectum and dilated sigmoid. The arrow points to the aganglionic site. The barium enema examination is discontinued when this site is demonstrated. A small amount of barium escapes past the point of constriction into the dilated sigmoid, intermixing itself with the fecal contents therein. *C*. Lateral view, once again demonstrating the aganglionic site. The rectum below this level is of normal caliber. The tremendously dilated sigmoid containing a small amount of barium now is once again visualized.

415

Abnormalities of Contour of Gas-Containing Loops of Bowel

Stomach

The stomach gas bubble may be absent or impressed as a result of constriction by an infiltrating carcinoma.

The stomach gas bubble may also be displaced or impressed as a result of extragastric causes. The impression may arise from the region of the left hemidiaphragm beyond a usual normal of approximately 5 mm. It may be related to enlargement of the left lobe of the liver or spleen, splenic rupture, tumor masses of this region, accumulation of peritoneal fluid, or a subphrenic abscess.

At times the entire stomach may be constricted as with a linitis plastica.

Small and Large Intestines

The contour of the small and large intestines may be altered by:

1. Neoplastic or inflammatory lesions inside or adjoining the intestines.

2. Intraperitoneal or retroperitoneal abscesses.

3. Fibrinous or exudative responses of the peritoneal or serosal surfaces of the bowel.

4. Fibrous adhesions such as might occur with a pelvic peritonitis, causing marked constriction and narrowness of the rectum or the adjoining sigmoid colon.

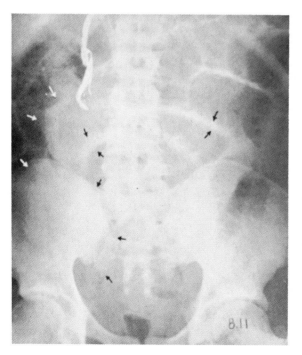

Figure 24–17   Radiograph of the abdomen in association with a fibrinous peritonitis which produces a considerable thickening of the wall of the small bowel and causes an inordinate separation of the various loops of small intestine. This separation is indicated by the arrows. Normally the distance between such distended loops should not exceed 3 or 4 mm.

Thickening may be produced by granuloma, peritonitis, or neoplasia.

The valvulae conniventes of the small intestine in the markedly dilated loops may be identified also.

Abnormalities of Position of Abdominal Gas Shadows

Alterations of position of abdominal organ gas shadows can be categorized as follows:

1. Gastrointestinal malrotations.
2. Herniations.
3. Hepatodiaphragmatic interpositions.
4. Displacements.

The Stomach

Gastrointestinal Malrotations

The stomach is situated on the right side of the abdomen in *situs inversus*.

As noted in Chapter 23, the position of the stomach is of considerable importance in relation to congenital diseases of the heart.

In *organoaxial rotation of the stomach* (Chapter 27) the stomach swings forward and upward on its two points of fixation (apex of duodenal bulb and esophagocardiac junction), so that the lesser curvature faces caudad. The greater curvature of the stomach is, under these circumstances, in contact with the anterior margin of the diaphragm in the region of the foramen of Morgagni, and there may be an associated herniation of greater omentum through these foramina. The greater omentum is drawn upward under these circumstances, resulting in an inverted V appearance of the transverse colon. Organoaxial rotation of the stomach may occur intermittently. There are no characteristic symptoms of this condition, but abdominal pain, nausea, and vomiting may result.

Frequent Sites of Intra-abdominal Herniations

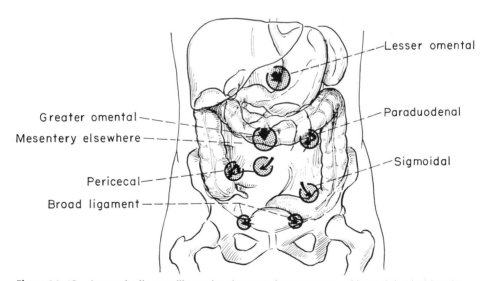

Figure 24–18   Anatomic diagram illustrating the more frequent types of intra-abdominal hernia.

Herniation of the stomach through the diaphragm may occur through any of the orifices of the diaphragm or through a traumatic orifice. They are most accurately identified with barium (Chapter 28). The herniated stomach may often be identified without additional contrast materials in the stomach as a confined gas-containing structure, usually behind the heart, and usually with a fluid level in the erect position.

Extragastric Displacement. Stomach abnormalities of position and shape due to extragastric displacements are illustrated in Figure 24–19.

STOMACH ABNORMALITIES OF POSITION AND SHAPE DUE TO EXTRAGASTRIC DISPLACEMENT

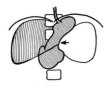

THIS TYPE OF DISPLACEMENT TO THE RIGHT MAY BE DUE TO:

1. RETROPERITONEAL TUMOR
2. SPLENIC ENLARGEMENT
3. SUPRARENAL TUMORS
4. RENAL TUMORS (LEFT)

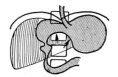

DISPLACEMENT OF STOMACH BY CYST OF GREATER OMENTUM

Figure 24–19 Abnormalities of position and shape of the stomach due to displacement by extragastric forces.

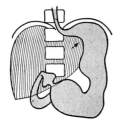

DISPLACEMENT OF STOMACH TO LEFT AND POSTERIORLY BY ENLARGED LIVER OR MASS IN LIVER.

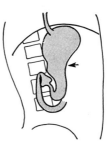

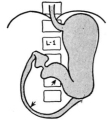

INDENTATION ON ANTRUM BY TUMOR IN BODY OF PANCREAS; ENLARGED HEAD OF PANCREAS INDICATED BY SPREADING OF DUODENAL LOOP(C LOOP FORMATION.)

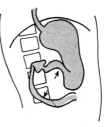

P-A VIEW

LEFT LAT. ERECT VIEW

THIS TYPE OF LAT. AND ANTERIOR DISPLACEMENT OF BODY OF STOMACH IS DUE TO:

1. *ABDOMINAL AORTIC ANEURYSMS (OFTEN WITH LAMINATED CALCIUM AND EROSION OF VERTEBRAE)*
2. *RETROGASTRIC TUMOR (BODY OF PANCREAS, RETROPERITONEAL SARCOMA, TUMORS OF ADRENAL AND KIDNEY)*

WHERE EROSION FROM ANEURYSM OCCURS

INDENTATION OF GREATER CURVATURE AND POSTERIOR WALL OF STOMACH BY TUMORS OR PSEUDOCYSTS OR CYSTS IN VICINITY OF TAIL OF PANCREAS.

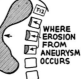

Small and Large Intestine

Generally, barium studies are essential for detection of many of the abnormalities of position of the gastrointestinal tract.

Displacements of Gas-Containing Small or Large Intestine Within the Abdomen

Displacement may be produced by an enlarged adjoining solid organ; an inflammatory mass; a cyst or neoplasm; a hematoma (within the wall of the intestine, intraperitoneal or retroperitoneal).

Fluid-containing masses arising out of the anatomic pelvis such as ovarian cysts, may be so extensive at times as to produce an appearance which closely resembles that of ascites (Figure 24–7). Ordinarily, however, the sharp circumscription of the tumor mass immediately beneath the displaced loops of bowel permits important differential indications (Figure 24–7).

When extensive *ascites* is present there is a tendency for the loops of bowel to float in the abdomen when the patient is supine; these tend to have air-containing loops of bowel centrally placed; and the flanks bulge with the intermediate density fluid (Figure 24–7).

Hematomas may occur in the lesser omental bursa, in the peritoneal space retroperitoneally, or within the intestine proper. The roentgen appearance depends upon the position of the hematoma in relation to the displaced gastrointestinal loops (intramural hematomas ordinarily deform the wall of the bowel, producing a "picket fence" or a "stacked coin" appearance. This is best recognized following the administration of barium (see Chapter 29).

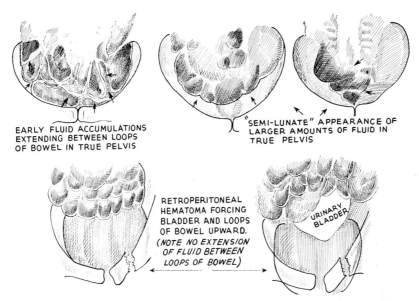

EARLY FLUID ACCUMULATIONS
EXTENDING BETWEEN LOOPS
OF BOWEL IN TRUE PELVIS

"SEMI-LUNATE" APPEARANCE OF
LARGER AMOUNTS OF FLUID IN
TRUE PELVIS

RETROPERITONEAL
HEMATOMA FORCING
BLADDER AND LOOPS
OF BOWEL UPWARD.
(NOTE NO EXTENSION
OF FLUID BETWEEN
LOOPS OF BOWEL)

URINARY
BLADDER

Figure 24–20 Diagrammatic sketches from radiographs demonstrating the appearance of intraperitoneal and retroperitoneal fluid accumulations in the true pelvis. (Modified from Frimann-Dahl: *Roentgen Examinations in Acute Abdominal Diseases.* Springfield, Charles C Thomas, 1951.)

Alterations in Density of Gas Within the Loops of Bowel

Free fluid intermixed with air within the bowel produces negative shadows of intermediate density, readily identified in the erect position as *fluid levels,* with the fluid settling to the bottom of each hollow viscus by gravity, and the air interfaced at the top.

Feces or meconium intermixed with gas produces a *speckled gas appearance* (Figure 24–16). A similar speckled gas appearance may be produced by intra-abdominal abscesses. These can be differentiated as follows:

1. An abscess usually remains constant in its relationships in the abdomen irrespective of the position of the patient.

2. When bowel is delineated by either air or barium, the speckled appearance of an abscess is identified outside the bowel.

Fatty or Sebaceous Material contained within dermoid or teratomatous cysts in the pelvis and elsewhere in the peritoneal space may at times simulate a gas-containing loop of bowel. This can be recognized by the absence of a fluid level with a horizontal beam study, and by the fact that the density is slightly greater than that of gas in the bowel. Occasionally such cysts may contain calcific masses representing either teeth or portions of an incompletely developed embryo.

Architectural Appearance of Gas Outside the Bowel

1. In the wall of any organ (Figure 24–26)
    a. Linear or crescentic (with intestinal infarction at times)
    b. Pseudocystic with pneumatosis of the stomach or intestine, gall bladder, urinary bladder (cystitis emphysematosa), vaginitis emphysematosa
2. In the circulatory system — tubular
    a. Portal venous system or inferior vena cava
3. In the biliary tree — tubular (Figure 24–23)
    a. Gas is centrally disposed near the porta hepatis and in the liver
4. In the liver —
    a. Tubular in the biliary tree or portal venous system — more peripheral in the latter
    b. Speckled in an abscess (Figure 24–22)
    c. Circumlinear with a cyst
5. Subdiaphragmatic — large pocket, semilunate (Figures 24–21, 24–24)
6. In the fascial planes of the abdominal wall — appears streaky or bubbly
7. Bulging against the flanks — "football" sign (Figure 24–25)
8. In the urinary tract — pneumaturia in a diabetic
9. Just outside the ureter or renal pelvis — rupture of ureter during catheterization
10. Perirenal air — perirenal abscess
11. Coiled or tubular air in the gastrointestinal tract of worms (ascariasis)

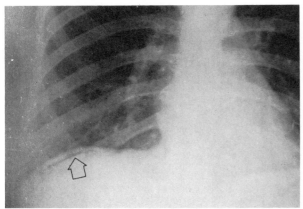

Figure 24–21 Free air beneath the right hemidiaphragm producing a crescentic shadow.

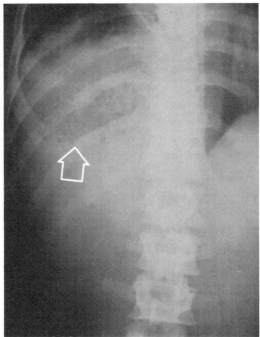

Figure 24–22 Speckled gas appearance projected over liver in patient with subhepatic abscess.

SUBDIAPHRAGMATIC ABSCESS

Roentgenologic Findings (In Decreasing Order of Frequency)

Diaphragm elevated
Blunted costophrenic angle
Pleural effusion
Pulmonary infiltrations
Pulmonary atelectasis
Subphrenic gas (air fluid level)
Ileus
Diminished diaphragmatic movement
A fixed diaphragm
Pneumothorax

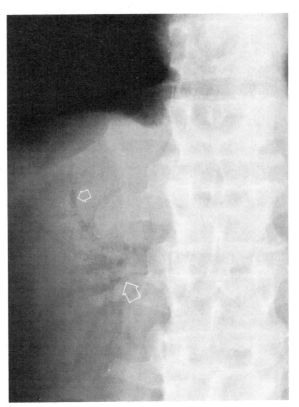

Figure 24–23 Free air in the biliary tract resulting from a surgical communication produced between the gallbladder and the duodenum.

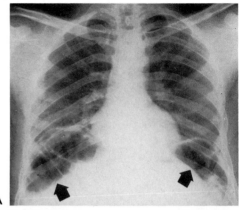

Figure 24-24 *A*. P-A film of the chest demonstrating the appearance of interposition of colon under the right hemidiaphragm. This appearance must not be confused with free air under the diaphragm and can usually be distinguished by the appearance of haustrations within the gas pattern. *B*. Free air on the lateral decubitus film study. The free air is above the liver and beneath the right hemidiaphragm.

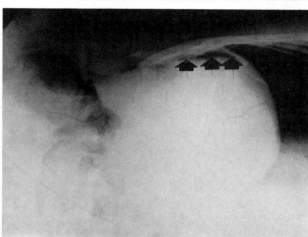

A

B

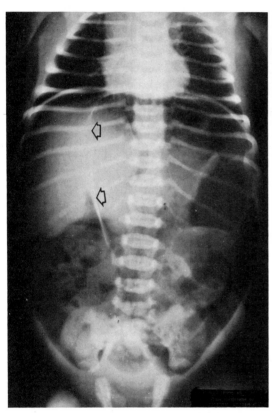

Figure 24-25 "Air dome" or "football sign" indicating a large amount of free air in the abdomen. Arrows point to falciform ligament—the "lacing" on the "football."

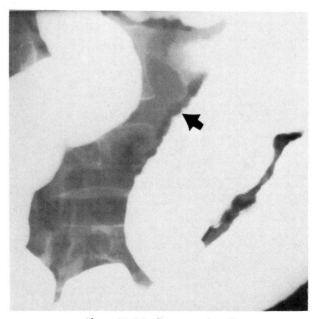

Figure 24-26 Pneumatosis coli.

Identification of Calcific Shadows in the Abdomen

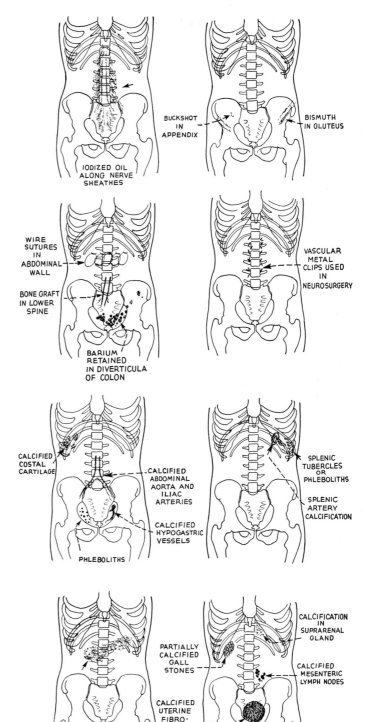

Figure 24–27 Diagrammatic sketches illustrating various calcific abdominal extra-urinary shadows and other opacities in the abdominal and periabdominal regions.

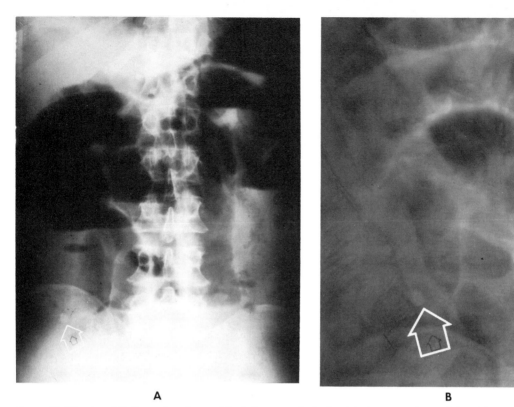

A   **B**

Figure 24–28 *A* and *B*. Examples of coprolith of the appendix in the right lower quadrant of the abdomen. Absence of free air in the biliary tree and the clinical findings of appendicitis will usually differentiate these from gallstones in the ileocecal junction producing a gallstone ileus.

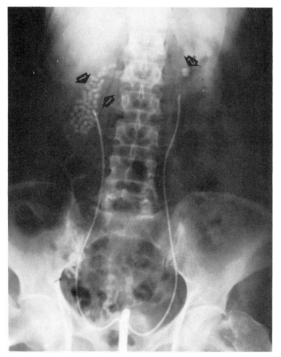

Figure 24–29 Radiograph demonstrating various types of calcific shadows in the abdomen. In the left renal region there is a left renal calculus in the kidney pelvis. There are innumerable small calcific stones in the gall-bladder. Projected over the inferior margin of the right sacroiliac joint are calcified lymph nodes. In the extreme left upper quadrant there is a small phlebolith or tubercle in the spleen.

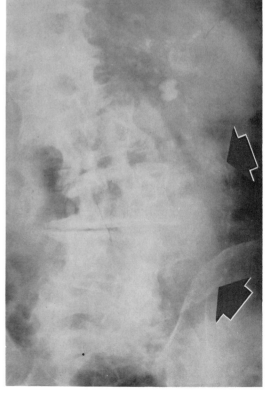

Figure 24–30 Calcified abdominal aortic aneurysm. Note the tendency to lamination of the calcium in the aneurysm (arrows).

424

SPECIAL PROBLEMS IN RELATION TO CHILDREN

Abdominal Calcification

1. Gallbladder *gallstones* usually indicate the presence of hemolytic anemia and are associated often with sickle cell anemia.
2. *Intrahepatic calcifications* may represent primary tumors such as hepatomas, hepatoblastomas, and hemangioblastomas. Hepatic hamartomas, usually seen in females under the age of two years, are frequently cystic and calcified, while neuroblastomas may at times be calcified and primary in the liver.
3. Calcifications in the left upper quadrant in children include *granulomas of the spleen, teratomas,* and *dermoids* of the stomach.
4. Apart from *renal and suprarenal calcifications,* non-neoplastic retroperitoneal calcification in children usually involves the *pancreas.*
5. *Retroperitoneal neoplasms in children.*
    a. The most important retroperitoneal tumors are *Wilms' tumor* (renal embryoma) and *neuroblastoma.*
    b. A Wilms' tumor is most common in the right upper pole of the kidney but may be located anywhere in the kidney; it displaces the kidney downward, medially, or upward. A Wilms' tumor is rare after the age of six but may occur even in adults.
    c. Neuroblastomas arise frequently from the lumbar sympathetic chain or from the adrenal glands and usually displace the kidney downward and outward. *About 50 per cent of all neuroblastomas show calcification, in contrast to Wilms' tumors which calcify in some 8 to 12 per cent of cases.* The calcification of the neuroblastoma tends to be flocculent or punctate, whereas the calcification of a Wilms' tumor tends to be peripheral and cystic in appearance.
    d. The benign ganglioneuroma shows calcification very similar to that found in neuroblastoma.
    e. Retroperitoneal teratomas are ordinarily located in the midline of the upper abdomen or across the midline only slightly. Renal function is intact and unimpaired but the kidneys may be displaced laterally and downward. Most teratomas have calcified spicules of cartilage or bone and sometimes teeth.
    f. Adrenal cortical carcinomas also calcify frequently in children.
    g. A cavernous hemangioma is recognized by its many phleboliths scattered throughout the tumor mass. These are small concentric rings of calcification usually 5 to 8 mm. in diameter.
    h. In the right lower quadrant, calcified appendiceal fecaliths (coproliths) account for at least half the calcifications recorded in children. They have been observed as early as 23 months.
    i. In the pelvis, the most important calcification of childhood is the vesical calculus.
    j. Ovarian dermoids with radiolucency and calcification occur in children and adults and have been described previously.
    k. The calcification of meconium peritonitis has already been described.
    l. Widespread colonic calculi may be seen in Hirschsprung's disease also.

ABDOMINAL MASSES—THE MOST COMMON ENTITIES

1. Every mass in a child must be considered malignant until proved otherwise.
2. Approximately 50 per cent of the masses are genitourinary in origin, including polycystic kidneys, Wilms' tumor, and neuroblastoma adjoining the kidney.
3. Unilateral multicystic kidneys do occur in about 0.1 per cent, and they are usually noted in the first year of life.
4. Calcification is present in at least one-half of the neuroblastomas and may assume any form. It is relatively rare in Wilms' tumor (Emmett and Witten).
5. The neuroblastoma tends to be extrarenal and the Wilms' tumor intrarenal.
6. Bony metastases are apt to occur in neuroblastoma.
7. Destructive and reactive lesions of the skull with spreading of the sutures are almost pathognomonic of neuroblastoma.
8. Positive biochemical tests of the urine or aspiration biopsy of the bone marrow or both may provide conclusive evidence of neuroblastoma.
9. Neuroblastoma is the most common abdominal tumor in infants and children. The most common site for metastasis is bone.
10. More than 90 per cent of cases of Wilms' tumor are encountered before the eighth year of life. However, the incidence of metastasis increases from approximately 25 per cent of children under two years of age to nearly 50 per cent of older children.
11. The most common renal lesion in infants is hydronephrosis.
12. "In the newborn infant with an enlarged nonfunctioning kidney and a patent vena cava, the possibility of multicystic kidney must be kept in mind" (Emmett and Witten).
13. Urographic changes with Wilms' tumor:
    a. Renal mass, which may have indistinct borders.
    b. Bizarre distortion of renal pelvis or calyces.
    c. Anterior displacement of the kidney in lateral view. (A lateral view is essential for all these cases.)
    d. Displacement and compression of the ureter may occur with either Wilms' tumor or neuroblastoma.

Abdominal Masses — Some Differential Features

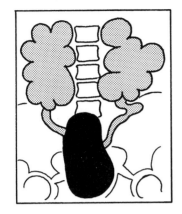
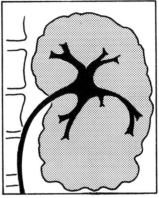
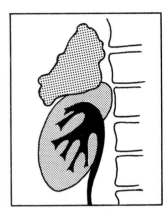

	Multi-or Polycystic Disease	Wilm's Tumor	Neuroblastoma
	MOST COMMON ABDOMINAL TUMOR IN YOUNG INFANTS		
CALCIFICATION	UNCOMMON	5 - 10%	APPROXIMATELY 50%
SITE	RENAL (ENLARGED)	RENAL	30 TO 50% SUPRARENAL
BONE METASTASES	NONE	NONE	FREQUENT
DIASTASIS OF SKULL SUTURES	NONE	NONE	FREQUENT
AGE	NEWBORN	1/3 IN FIRST YEAR OF LIFE	90% LESS THAN 8 YEARS OF AGE
DISPLACEMENT OF KIDNEY	KIDNEY ENLARGED AND LOBULATED	ANTERIORLY (LATERAL VIEW ESSENTIAL)	CAUDAD USUALLY "DROOPING LILY" ON IVP

APPROXIMATELY 50% OF ALL ABDOMINAL MASSES IN CHILDREN ARE GENITOURINARY IN ORIGIN

Figure 24–31   Abdominal masses in children: some differential features.

THE LIVER

Roentgen Signs of Abnormality of the Liver

Enlargement of the Liver (See Figures 24–32, 24–33, and 24–34)

Diminution in Size of the Liver. This is very difficult to evaluate on plain films and ordinarily would require special contrast studies.

Abnormalities of Position

Occasionally the liver may *herniate* into the chest because of markedly enlarged pleuroperitoneal hiati or foramina of Bochdalek, or because of traumatic laceration of the diaphragm.

The liver may be *ptotic,* and in such circumstances the colon or other gastrointestinal loops may be interposed between the liver and the diaphragm.

Abnormalities in Shape

These may be associated with benign or malignant tumors involving the liver or adjoining the liver. Of the benign tumors, cavernous hemangioma is a frequent concomitant of carcinoma of the liver.

Alcoholic cirrhosis may produce a markedly irregular liver.

At times the liver appears to be V-shaped, in which case there appear to be two symmetrical lobes on the right and left side of the abdomen. This is particularly true with *Ivemark's syndrome* in which dextrocardia and asplenia are usually associated.

Abnormalities in Density

Accumulations of gas in the bile ducts.

Accumulations of gas in the portal venous system.

Accumulations of gas in abscesses, within or adjoining the liver. *Gas gangrene* of the liver may be recognized by the presence of numerous bubbles of gas throughout the entire right lobe of the liver. This differs from gas in the portal system or gas in the biliary tree since in this instance the gas distribution is diffuse, widespread, and does not follow any definite channel as it does in the other two circumstances (Wiot and Felson; Sisk; Susman and Senturia, Elson).

Increased density within the liver. The liver may be diffusely increased in density as a result of (1) *hemachromatosis;* (2) *calcification in the parenchyma of the liver.*

These two conditions may be observed with:

1. Cavernous hemangiomas
2. Phleboliths
3. Cysts such as Echinococcus cysts
4. Tuberculous granulomas
5. Primary and secondary carcinomas. Calcification of a very fine, diffuse, granular type may occur with diffuse metastases from carcinoma of the colon. Also, calcification from metastatic melanoma may occur in the liver which may show nodular and shell-like calcifications scattered throughout (Karras et al.).
6. Occasionally, intrahepatic calcified gallstones can be seen in the biliary duct

7. Shell-like calcifications overlying the liver may occur in association with long-standing subphrenic abscesses
8. Rarely, calcification may develop as a sequel to eclampsia or other diseases which give rise to hepatic necrosis

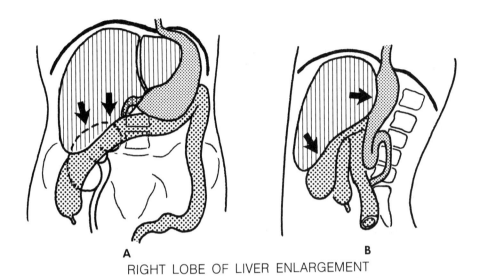

A   B

RIGHT LOBE OF LIVER ENLARGEMENT

DISPLACEMENT OF STOMACH TO LEFT AND POSTERIORLY
DOWNWARD DISPLACEMENT OF RIGHT KIDNEY
NO DISPLACEMENT OF SECOND PART OF DUODENUM
DOWNWARD DISPLACEMENT OF TRANSVERSE COLON
DOWNWARD AND POSTERIOR DISPLACEMENT OF HEPATIC FLEXURE
NO DISPLACEMENT OF DUODENOJEJUNAL FLEXURE

Figure 24–32

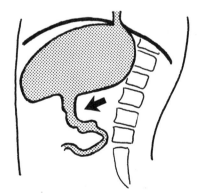

Figure 24–33 Displacement of stomach and duodenum with caudate lobe of liver enlargement.

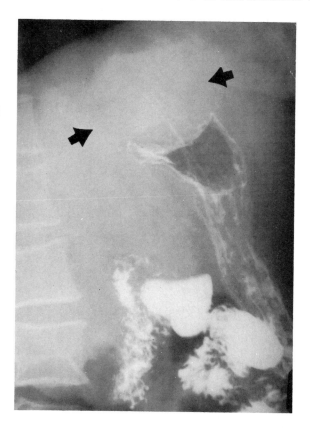

Figure 24-34 Carcinoma of the liver displacing the fundus of the stomach downward from the left hemidiaphragm. This carcinomatous involvement of the liver was thought to be secondary to a carcinoma of the pancreas.

Left Lobe (Figure 24–34) (Enlargement or Involvement by Tumor)

1. A central upper abdominal mass extending toward the left lateral abdominal wall and inseparable from the liver outline.
2. Downward displacement of the splenic flexure.
3. Anterior displacement of the transverse colon, which may be pushed upward or downward around the mass.
4. Marked displacement of the entire stomach toward the left.
5. No displacement ordinarily of the second part of the duodenum.
6. Downward displacement of the duodenojejunal flexure.
7. Normal position of the right kidney.
8. Downward and posterior displacement of the left kidney.

In any case, there may be calcification within the liver related to tumor calcification. Approximately 30 per cent of carcinomas of the liver in infants contain calcification (Sorsdahl and Gay; Margulis, Nice, and Rigler).

37. What is the significance of streaky gas along fascial planes in the abdomen?

38. What is meant by the "air dome" or "football" sign?

39. Describe the roentgen findings in pneumatosis intestinalis. What is its special significance in infants and in adults?

40. How may worm infestation manifest itself on plain films of the abdomen?

41. What are some of the main primary and metastatic malignancies that may undergo calcification within the abdomen?

42. In infants, what may cause calcification of the peritoneal space?

43. What are the various causes of abdominal calcification in infancy and early childhood?

44. What differences are there in the calcification pattern and incidence of Wilms' tumor and neuroblastoma in infants?

45. What is the characteristic calcific pattern of a cavernous hemangioma?

46. What is the characteristic appearance of vascular calcifications within the abdomen? In what vessels are these most apt to occur and what is their relative significance?

47. What may cause mass shadows within the abdomen?

48. What in particular may cause abdominal masses in children?

49. Describe the various roentgen techniques for examination of the liver.

50. Describe the roentgen signs of abnormality of the liver.

51. What are some of the abnormalities of radiodensity as projected over the liver? Indicate the causes of radiolucent density. Also indicate the most frequent causes of radiopaque densities over the liver.

52. What are some of the associated findings in the lung, pleural space, or properitoneal fat in respect to the liver?

53. Describe the technique for examination of the spleen.

54. What is the normal roentgen appearance of the spleen on an antero-posterior view of the abdomen?

55. How can normal size of the spleen be judged? What is the significance of an enlarged splenic shadow?

56. What are some adjunctive evidences of the acutely ruptured spleen?

25

Radiology of the Urinary Tract and Suprarenal Glands

RADIOLOGIC METHODS OF STUDY OF THE URINARY TRACT

1. Preparation of patient
2. Plain film, patient supine (KUB)
   a. Prone film in infants
3. Single injection intravenous excretory urogram—high dose
4. Infusion excretory urogram
5. Hypertension study pyelogram—rapid sequence dehydrated urogram, combined with a hydrated pyelogram
6. Nephrotomography
7. Retrograde pyelography
8. Cystography and cystourethrography
   a. With voiding urethrogram
   b. Retrograde urethrogram
   c. Cystogram (with excretory or retrograde pyelogram)
   d. With double contrast (air)
   e. Triple contrast—angiography plus pneumocystogram plus interstitial air in wall of urinary bladder—especially useful for staging carcinoma of the urinary bladder
   f. "Chain" cystourethrogram—investigation of stress incontinence
9. Renal arteriography and aortography
10. Phlebography and inferior vena cavography
11. Roentgen evaluation of the surgically exposed kidney
12. Cineradiography of the upper urinary tract and cystourethrography
13. Perirenal air insufflation
14. Seminal vesiculography
15. Cyst puncture
16. Ultrasound

Uses and Limitations of Each Method of Study

Plain Film of Abdomen (KUB). Baseline study for contrast examinations. Opacities which might become obscured by the contrast are visualized.

Intravenous Excretory Urogram. Single Injection. A single high dose of contrast agent may delineate the collecting systems, ureters, and urinary bladder with such clarity that additional, more invasive studies are unnecessary. This method is often combined with tomography during any phase of the study, particularly the nephrographic, so that parenchymal and pelvicalyceal lesions are clearly delineated. Patients with compromised renal function may also at times be satisfactorily studied, especially if delayed films are included in the examination.

Infusion Excretory Urogram. The major advantage of this technique is the increased clarity with which the collecting system and ureters may be identified. Nephrotomography as an adjunct to this technique is especially useful. If excretion and concentration are decreased, delayed films (up to 24 hours) can be helpful.

Hypertensive Pyelogram. In patients with renovascular hypertension, there is a decrease in urinary flow and a tendency to hyperconcentration in the affected kidney. When films are obtained in rapid sequence during the first few minutes following intravenous injection of contrast agent, differences in excretion between the two kidneys can be documented. In addition, a delay of more than three minutes in both kidneys suggests this physiologic disorder. In the washout phase, hyperconcentration may persist in an abnormal kidney.

Nephrotomography is particularly useful when overlying shadows obscure renal detail. In addition, cysts can frequently be differentiated from solid neoplasms.

Retrograde Pyelography is useful for detailed examination of the pelvicalyceal collecting system, ureters, and urinary bladder. Its disadvantages are (1) potential infection; (2) distortion of the calyces by overdistention; (3) back flow phenomena which obscure detail; (4) stenosis and stricture formation; (5) potential rupture of the collecting systems and ureters; (6) the need for anesthesia.

Cystography and Cystourethrography permit accurate visualization of the urinary bladder and its mucosal pattern when the bladder is distended. The voiding urethrogram may be combined with this study, allowing anatomic visualization of the urethra. In addition, reflux into the ureters (either prior to or during voiding) may be detected.

Renal Arteriography and Aortography are particularly useful for delineation of the renal arterial and venous systems, especially in relation to renovascular hypertension and renal neoplasia. It has become an extremely accurate tool for distinguishing benign from malignant tumors, except for hamartomas.

Phlebography and Inferior Vena Cavography. Phlebography is useful for obtaining samples for renal vein renin assays. The technique is also useful for determining the extent of malignant neoplasms. A malignant neoplasm which has invaded the inferior vena cava is inoperable.

Roentgen Evaluation of the Surgically Exposed Kidney is utilized to determine the extent of removal of previously demonstrated calculi.

Cineradiography. Contraction of the kidney and peristalsis of the ureter, as well as urinary bladder emptying may be documented.

Perirenal Air Insufflation is used to delineate the adrenal glands.

Seminal Vesiculography is used to determine invasion of the seminal vesicles by carcinoma of the prostate.

Cyst Puncture is used to obtain fluid for pathologic analysis and, following the instillation of contrast media, to delineate the inner margins of the cyst. A thick wall indicates malignancy.

Ultrasound is a noninvasive technique useful in differentiation of cystic masses from solid masses involving the renal bed.

NORMAL ANATOMY

Gross Anatomy

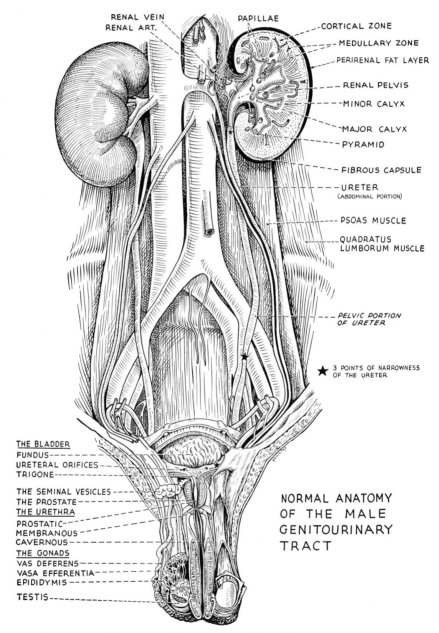

Figure 25–1   Gross anatomy of the urinary tract.

Radiographic Anatomy

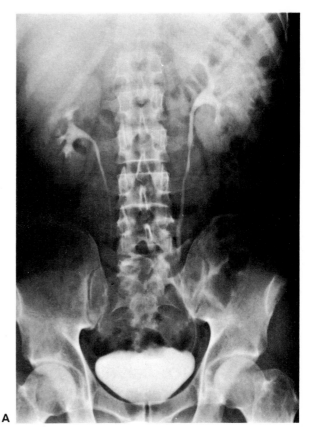

Figure 25–2 *A* and *B*   Representative excretory urogram (also called intravenous pyelogram) obtained 15 minutes after the intravenous injection of a suitable contrast agent.

A

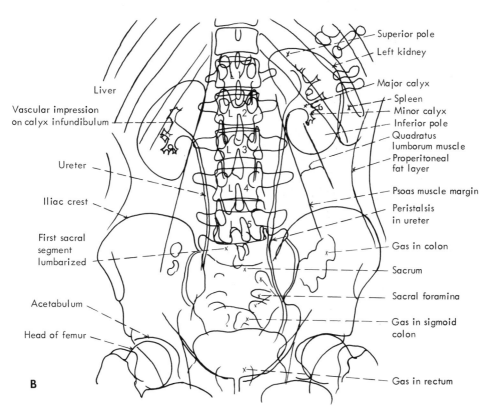

B

A

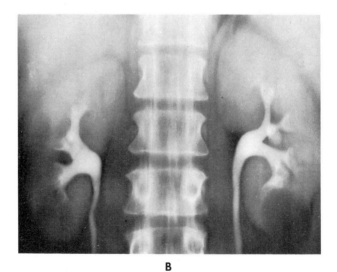

B

Figure 25–3 *A* and *B*. Value of drip-infusion urogram with tomogram. *A*. Excretory urogram. Poor visualization of renal pelvis and calyces. *B*. Drip-infusion urogram with tomogram. Excellent visualization of renal parenchyma and collecting system. Previously unsuspected mass (simple cyst) is present in lower pole of left kidney. (From Emmett, J. L., and Witten, D. M., *Clinical Urography*, Vol. 1. 3rd Ed. Philadelphia, W. B. Saunders Co., 1971.)

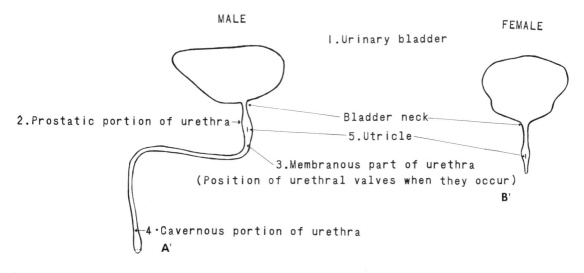

MALE

FEMALE

1.Urinary bladder

2.Prostatic portion of urethra→

Bladder neck

5.Utricle

3.Membranous part of urethra
(Position of urethral valves when they occur)

B'

4·Cavernous portion of urethra

A'

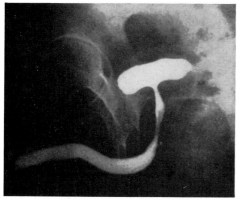

A

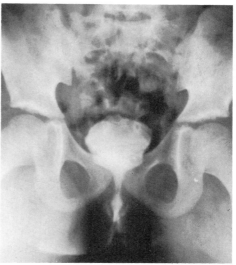

B

Figure 25–4 *A* and *A'*. Normal male urethrogram. *B* and *B'*. Female urethrogram.

Reactions to Contrast Media

General Comments. Reactions to the intravenous injection of contrast media are common. Mild reactions include warmth and flushing, nausea, vomiting, tingling, numbness, cough, and local pain in the arm, especially if the injection is carried out slowly. Serious reactions may include conjunctivitis, rhinitis, urticaria, facial edema, glottic edema, and even shocklike reactions with dyspnea, convulsions, cyanosis, shock, and even occasional death. It has been estimated that there has been an incidence of 6.6 deaths per million examinations (Pendergrass et al., 1958). Approximately 90 per cent of fatal reactions occurred during or immediately after injection, and hence it is vital that medications to counteract reactions be immediately available to the physician who performs the injection.

Some Basic Concepts of Anatomy Requiring Special Attention

Normal Kidney Size

The right kidney is normally slightly smaller than the left and accurate measurements within two standard deviations are indicated in Table 25–1. Differences between the two kidneys of 1.5 cm. or more are significant.

Simon has reported the ratio of renal adult cephalocaudad lengths to the height of the second lumbar vertebral body (plus disk) to be 3.7 ± 0.37 with a statistical range of normal values between 3.0 and 4.4 (Meschan; Martin).

TABLE 25–1 NORMAL ADULT RENAL SIZE (THE MEAN PLUS OR MINUS TWO STANDARD DEVIATIONS)* (Modified after Moell)

Male:	Right kidney	Vertical: 11.3–14.5 cm.
		Width: 5.4– 7.2 cm.
	Left	Vertical: 11.6–14.8 cm.
		Width: 5.3– 7.1 cm.
Female:	Right kidney	Vertical: 10.7–13.9 cm.
		Width: 4.8– 6.6 cm.
	Left	Vertical: 11.1–14.3 cm.
		Width: 5.1– 6.9 cm.

*Standard deviation = 0.8 cm. for vertical dimension

Kidney Position

The kidneys are retroperitoneal, lying on either side of the vertebral column. The upper poles lie approximately 1 cm. closer to the midline than do the lower, and ordinarily the right kidney is lower in position than the left. In about 15 per cent of cases, however, the left kidney is the lower one.

The kidneys correspond in position with the last thoracic and upper three lumbar vertebrae in the recumbent position. A maximum excursion of 5 cm. or 1½ vertebral bodies occurs in the change from the recumbent to the erect position.

Renal Shape

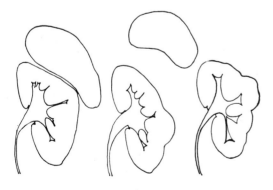
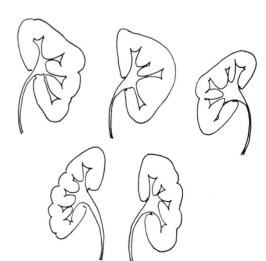

Figure 25–5 Various types of lobulated renal contours. (From Cooperman, L. R., and Lowman, R. M.: Amer. J. Roentgenol., 92:273, 1964.)

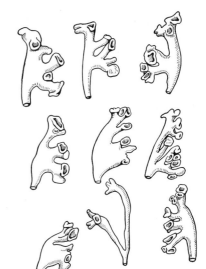

Figure 25–6 Variations in configuration in normal renal pelvis and calyces.

ROUTINE METHOD OF STUDY OF THE UROGRAM

EXAMINATION OF THE KIDNEY

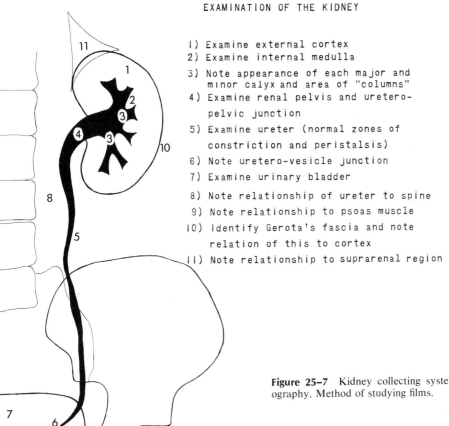

1) Examine external cortex
2) Examine internal medulla
3) Note appearance of each major and minor calyx and area of "columns"
4) Examine renal pelvis and uretero-pelvic junction
5) Examine ureter (normal zones of constriction and peristalsis)
6) Note uretero-vesicle junction
7) Examine urinary bladder
8) Note relationship of ureter to spine
9) Note relationship to psoas muscle
10) Identify Gerota's fascia and note relation of this to cortex
11) Note relationship to suprarenal region

Figure 25–7 Kidney collecting system with excretory urography. Method of studying films.

ROENTGEN SIGNS OF ABNORMALITY OF THE KIDNEY

Variations in Renal Size or Number

VARIATIONS IN RENAL SIZE OR NUMBER

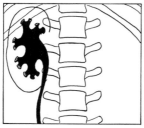

ABSENCE OF KIDNEY
(Look for ectopia)

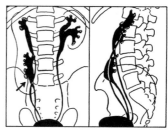

SUPERNUMERARY KIDNEY

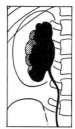

DILATATION
(See causes
of dilatation
separately)

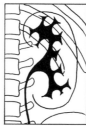

POLYCYSTIC
KIDNEY

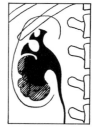

RENAL TUMOR
(Cyst more sharply
demarcated)

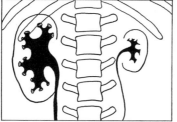

COMPENSATORY HYPERPLASIA
OF ONE KIDNEY WITH APLASIA
OF THE OTHER

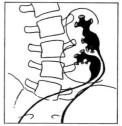

UNILATERAL FUSED
KIDNEY

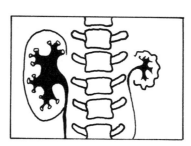

SMALL SCARRED KIDNEY
(End-stage kidney)

Figure 25–8

Changes in Position of the Kidney

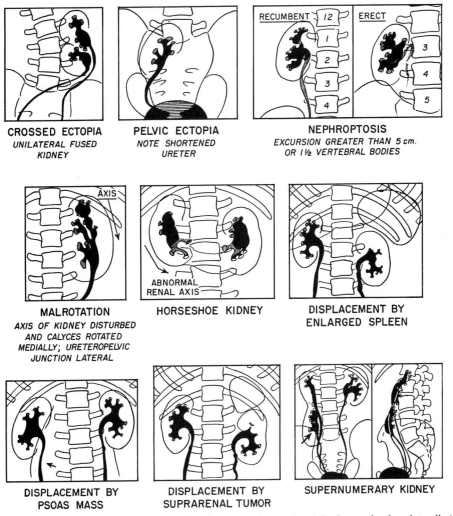

Figure 25–9 (Ureters in "horseshoe kidney" are not shown; they join the renal pelves laterally.)

Abnormalities in Renal Contour

1. Prior to the age of four years, lobulation of a kidney is normal but this may persist into adult life without pathologic significance (Figure 25–5).

2. Occasionally a "dromedary" or humped left kidney may be noted as a normal variant which must be differentiated from tumor or "pseudotumor," cyst, or abscess (Figure 25–10).

3. Irregularity in kidney contour may be due to (a) pyelonephritis; (b) renal infarction; (c) kidney rupture (Figure 25–10); and more rarely (d) hemangioma, or (e) hamartoma. The latter occurs especially in patients with tuberous sclerosis. Renal angiography is particularly helpful in diagnosis of these latter conditions.

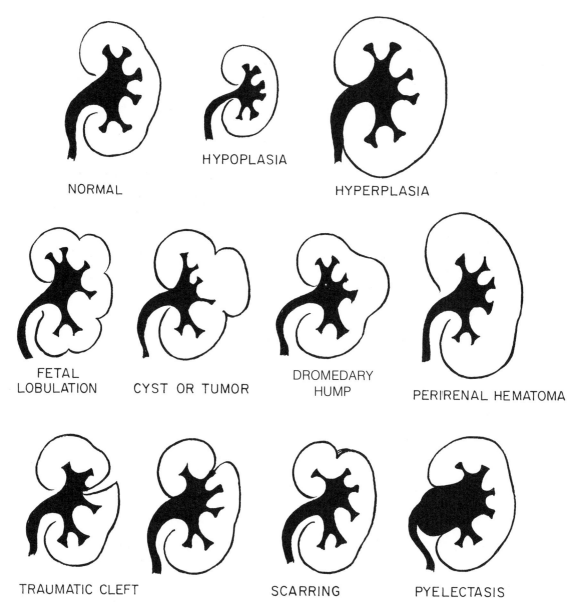

NORMAL

HYPOPLASIA

HYPERPLASIA

FETAL LOBULATION

CYST OR TUMOR

DROMEDARY HUMP

PERIRENAL HEMATOMA

TRAUMATIC CLEFT

SCARRING

PYELECTASIS

Figure 25–10 Alterations in renal contour with various diseases.

4. Distention of the renal pelvis predominantly is associated with ureteropelvic obstruction from any cause. This produces a "ball type" rounded, masslike appearance on the medial aspect of the renal shadow, which, with the aid of contrast material, can be identified as the distended renal pelvis. The ureteropelvic junction may be higher than usual and sharply angulated; a partial obstruction may be postulated due to either an aberrant vessel, fibrous band, or congenital constriction (Figure 25–10).

Variations in Renal Density

Renal Calcification

Figure 25–11 Line diagram showing how determination of the location of a calculus may help to elucidate the basic disease process.

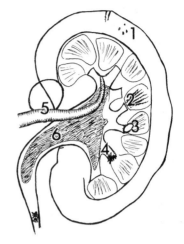

1. Calcification in renal cortex
   a. Granuloma infection
   b. Infarction
   c. Xanthogranuloma
   d. Neoplasm
      Calcification may be punctate, powdery, amorphous, mulberry, or circumlinear
2. Calcification in renal pyramids
   a. Medullary sponge kidney
   b. Nephrocalcinosis
   c. Renal tubular acidosis
3. Renal papillary necrosis
4. Calcification in calyces, pelvis, or ureter common in hypercalcemic states
   a. Hyperparathyroidism
   b. Sarcoidosis
   c. Cushing's disease
5. Renal artery calcification (aneurysm)
6. Staghorn calculus—not common with hypercalcemic states
7. Calcification in tuberculosis often occurs throughout kidney or ureter

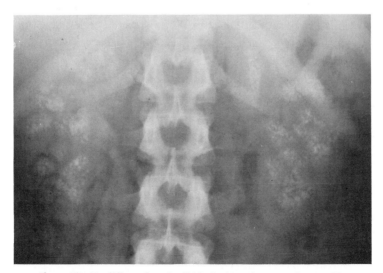

Figure 25–12 Bilateral nephrolithiasis throughout renal pyramids.

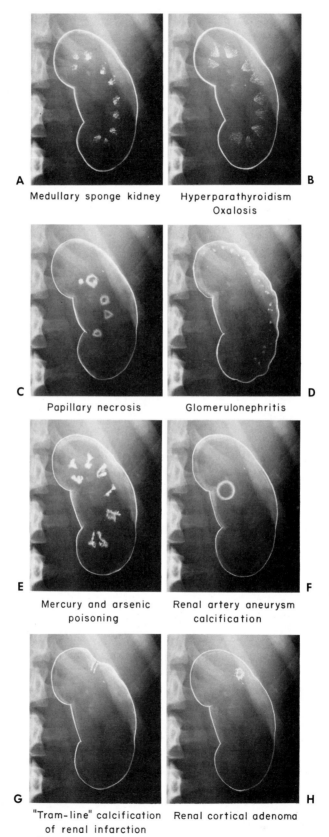

A Medullary sponge kidney

B Hyperparathyroidism
Oxalosis

C Papillary necrosis

D Glomerulonephritis

E Mercury and arsenic
poisoning

F Renal artery aneurysm
calcification

G "Tram-line" calcification
of renal infarction

H Renal cortical adenoma

Figure 25–13 *A* to *H*. Diagrams superimposed upon radiographs illustrating different types of renal calcification.

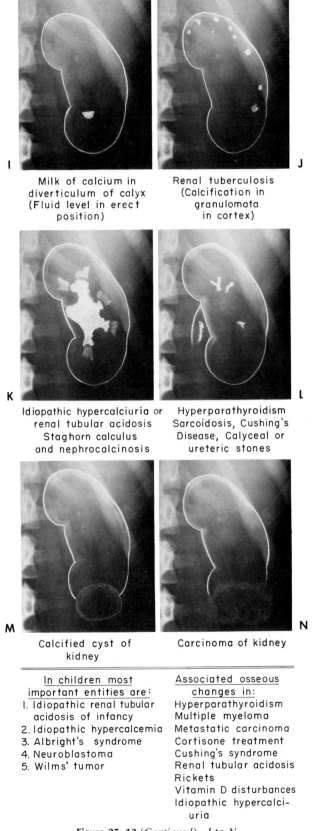

I — Milk of calcium in diverticulum of calyx (Fluid level in erect position)

J — Renal tuberculosis (Calcification in granulomata in cortex)

K — Idiopathic hypercalciuria or renal tubular acidosis Staghorn calculus and nephrocalcinosis

L — Hyperparathyroidism Sarcoidosis, Cushing's Disease, Calyceal or ureteric stones

M — Calcified cyst of kidney

N — Carcinoma of kidney

In children most important entities are:	Associated osseous changes in:
1. Idiopathic renal tubular acidosis of infancy	Hyperparathyroidism
2. Idiopathic hypercalcemia	Multiple myeloma
3. Albright's syndrome	Metastatic carcinoma
4. Neuroblastoma	Cortisone treatment
5. Wilms' tumor	Cushing's syndrome
	Renal tubular acidosis
	Rickets
	Vitamin D disturbances
	Idiopathic hypercalciuria

Figure 25–13 (*Continued*) *I* to *N*.

Summary of Types of Urinary Calculi

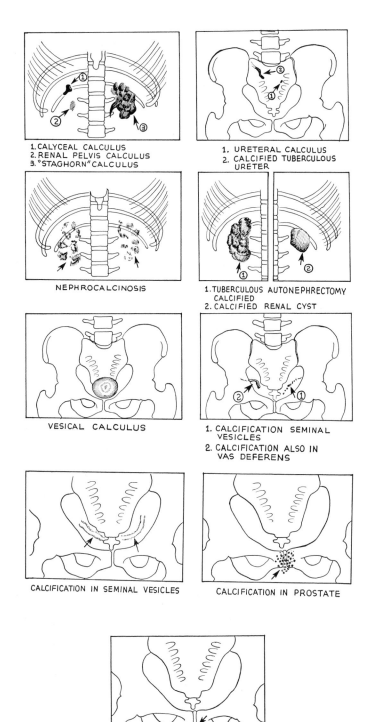

1. CALYCEAL CALCULUS
2. RENAL PELVIS CALCULUS
3. "STAGHORN" CALCULUS

1. URETERAL CALCULUS
2. CALCIFIED TUBERCULOUS URETER

NEPHROCALCINOSIS

1. TUBERCULOUS AUTONEPHRECTOMY CALCIFIED
2. CALCIFIED RENAL CYST

VESICAL CALCULUS

1. CALCIFICATION SEMINAL VESICLES
2. CALCIFICATION ALSO IN VAS DEFERENS

CALCIFICATION IN SEMINAL VESICLES

CALCIFICATION IN PROSTATE

URETHRAL CALCULUS

Figure 25–14 Miscellaneous groups of urinary calculi.

SPECIAL COMMENTS ON RENAL CALCIFICATION

Ringlike or rimlike calcification occurs with relatively high frequency in renal cell carcinoma and is suggestive of a malignancy in a renal mass (Kikkawa and Lasser).

Diffuse calcification may be present rarely in multilocular renal cysts, thus simulating renal cell carcinoma (Brown, Cornell, and Culp).

Renal calcification following renal necrosis tends to increase gradually until a dense band of heavy calcification is seen throughout the cortical area of the kidney, completely sparing the medullary portions which appear as relatively lucent pyramids. As the cortical density increases, there is a progressive decrease in the cortical thickness with an eventual significant decrease in renal measurement. No change in the medullary area is noted (Riesz and Wagner).

Renal calcification occurs rarely with chronic glomerulonephritis. The kidneys are then small (10 cm. or less) and retain a normal shape. The calcifications are granular and diffusely scattered throughout the cortex, sparing the medullary portions of the kidney. The calcium is in the lumina of the tubules of the cortex and not in the glomeruli.

Differential Diagnosis: (a) In nephrocalcinosis of hyperparathyroidism or hyperchloremia calcification is pyramidal. (b) In medullary sponge kidney, calcification is near the apices of the pyramids and is small and round or oval (Lalli). (c) In chronic pyelonephritis, calcification is seen in large deposits and is more unequal in distribution (Esposito).

Abnormalities in the Architecture of the Collecting System

The architecture of these structures is described in relation to (1) the edge pattern; (2) the internal pattern.

The Edge Pattern alterations may be described as (a) dilatation; (b) fraying; (c) elongation and thinning; (d) cicatricial change; (e) outpouching; (f) linear streaking.

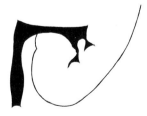

The "pinched infundibulum" from cicatricial change (pyelonephritis)

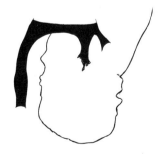

Loss of part of cup (malignant tumor;tuberculosis)

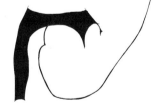

Loss of cup and infundibulum (tuberculosis; pyelonephritis)

A

Figure 25–15   *See legend on following page.*

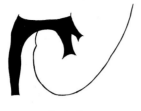

Normal

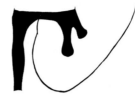

Rounding of edge and
flattening of cup

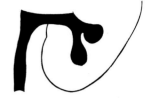

Clubbing

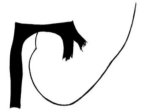

Fraying

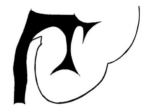

Thinning of infundibulum and
flattening of cup
(polycystic disease)

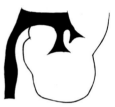

Flattening of cup
(simple cyst)

B

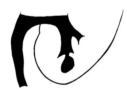

Calyceal diverticulum -
smooth outpouching

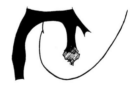

Frayed outpouching
(papillary necrosis; abscess)

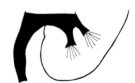

Streaking from cup of calyx
(medullary sponge kidney;
pyelotubular backflow)

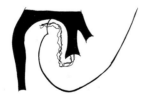

Backflow-pyelolymphatic
Calyx intact

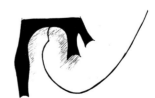

Pyelointerstitial backflow

C   Calyx intact

Figure 25–15 (*Continued*)   Diagrams illustrating the various alterations in the edge pattern of a calyx.

ALTERATIONS OF "INTERNAL STRUCTURE" OF THE CALYX AND PELVIS

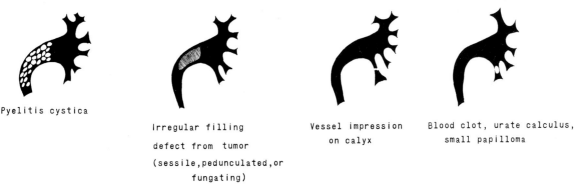

Pyelitis cystica

Irregular filling
defect from tumor
(sessile,pedunculated,or
fungating)

Vessel impression
on calyx

Blood clot, urate calculus,
small papilloma

Figure 25–16   Line diagrams illustrating alterations of the internal architecture of a calyx or renal pelvis.

The Internal Pattern alterations within a calyx or the pelvis may be related to (Figure 25–16):

1. Blood clots.
2. Calculi (such as uric acid or urate calculi which are nonopaque and comprise about 4 per cent of all urinary tract concretions.
3. Neoplasms.
4. Leukoplakia (sometimes termed renal cholesteatoma).
5. Granulomatous lesions (infectious granulomas or xanthogranulomatous pyelonephritis).
6. Papillary excrescences, sessile or fungating.
7. Extrinsic impressions (blood vessels, fibrous bands). Vascular impressions on a calyx will ordinarily produce a tubular, sharply circumscribed "cut-off" appearance of the calyx, usually in its infundibular portion.
8. Pyelitis cystica (usually associated with ureteritis cystica). Accompanies long-standing infections.
9. Air bubbles (from retrograde pyelography). These may change from one film to the next.

The Utilization of the Excretory Urogram as a Study of Renal Function

Those media which are derived from benzene derivatives such as the diatrizoates (Hypaque and Renografin) or the iothalamates (such as Conray) are excreted predominantly by glomerular filtration. The clearance ratio, for example, of inulin to Renografin is approximately 0.9 (Meschan et al.).

However, the rapid sequence or "minute" pyelogram combined with a washout type pyelogram does render significant physiologic information.

In the rapid sequence study, the appearance of the calyceal collecting system is normal when the nephrogram phase tends to fade (three minutes or less). Any disparity between the two kidneys may be of pathologic significance (Elkin et al.).

CONFUSING PYELOGRAPHIC APPEARANCES

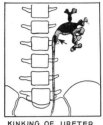

KINKING OF URETER
WITHOUT OBSTRUCTION

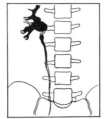
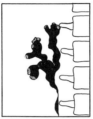

ATYPICAL URETEROPELVIC JUNCTIONS
NORMAL VARIANTS

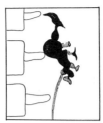

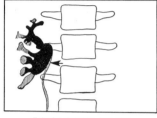

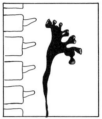

Figure 25–17

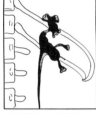

EXTRARENAL PELVIS

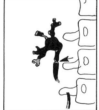
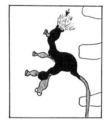

NORMAL VARIANTS OF RENAL CALYCES

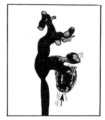

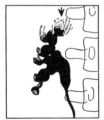

CALYCEAL NORMAL
VARIANTS

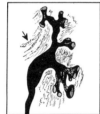

PERISTALSIS IN URETER

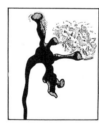

PYELOTUBULAR BACKFLOW

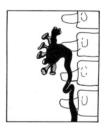

PYELOSINOUS TRANSFLOW

PYELOVENOUS BACKFLOW   PYELOLYMPHATIC BACKFLOW   PYELO-INTERSTITAL
BACKFLOW   URETERAL KINKING
WITHOUT OBSTRUCTION

ROENTGEN SIGNS OF ABNORMALITY OF THE URETER

Abnormalities of Number

The ureter may be either partially or completely duplicated when duplication of the renal pelvis occurs. In complete ureteral duplication, the ureter which descends from the uppermost renal pelvis empties caudad to its mate. Sometimes such emptying is anomalous and occurs in the urethra, in which case enuresis results—this may escape detection sometimes until adulthood.

The upper or lower half of such a duplicated renal system is particularly subject to renal infection, with resulting pyelonephritis and loss of function. The need for alertness to this possibility is emphasized, particularly since ordinary excretory urograms will not reveal such an anomaly.

Abnormalities of Size of the Ureter

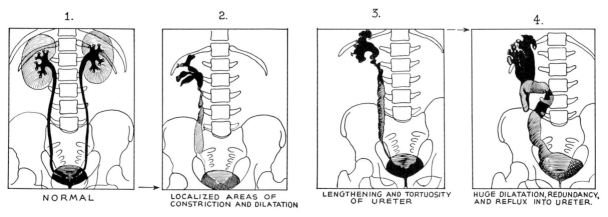

Figure 25–18 Urographic changes in ureterectasis.

Abnormalities of Position of the Ureter

TABLE 25–2 CHARACTERISTIC URETERAL DEVIATIONS*

Upper Third of the Ureter (Renal Area)
    A. Commonly associated with renal displacement
    B. Lateral displacement
        1. Commonest cause: Retroperitoneal lymph node enlargement
        2. Malrotation of the kidney
        3. Peripelvic cyst
        4. Pyelectasis
    C. Medial deviation: uncommon and nonspecific
        1. Most commonly on the left side with splenomegaly
        2. With cysts or tumors of the lower pole of the kidney
        3. Retroperitoneal tumors located lateral to the ureter. (There is usually no distortion of the kidney collecting system associated with this)

Middle Third of the Ureter
    A. Lateral deviation is more common than medial
    B. Lateral deviation
        1. Most common cause: Enlarged retroperitoneal lymph nodes from any cause
        2. Malignant lymphomas
    C. Medial deviation: tends to be nonspecific
        1. Retrocaval ureter: Deviates maximally at L-3 and returns to a relatively normal position after producing a plateau-like appearance near the transverse process of L-5
        2. Retroperitoneal fibrosis—usually bilateral, and usually associated with obstruction
        3. Retroperitoneal tumors

Lower Third of the Ureter—the Pelvic Ureter
    A. Lateral deviation
        1. Central pelvic lesion, such as an ovarian cyst or uterine fibroid
    B. Medial deviation
        1. Diverticulum of the bladder—sharply near the bladder
        2. Pelvic carcinoma (from colon)
        3. Tortuous redundancy from low obstruction
        4. Mass lesion in the lateral retroperitoneal area, of aneurysm of the iliac artery, or inflammatory abscesses

*Modified from Ney, C., and Friedenberg, R. M.: *Radiographic Atlas of the Genitourinary System.* Philadelphia, J. B. Lippincott Co., 1966.

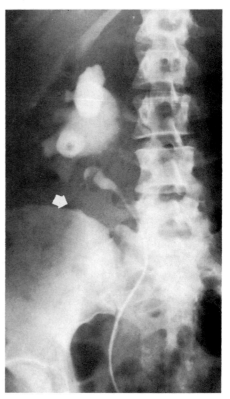

Figure 25-19 Retrograde pyelogram demonstrating marked displacement of the ureter by a large psoas abscess. Note the marked broadening of the psoas shadow. There is a partial obstruction of the upper ureter with an associated hydronephrosis on the right side. Note also that in this instance there happens to be a papilloma in a minor calyx.

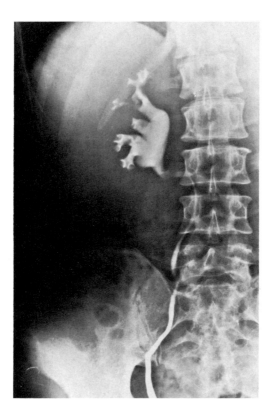

Figure 25-20 Retrocaval ureter.

Abnormalities in Architecture of the Ureter

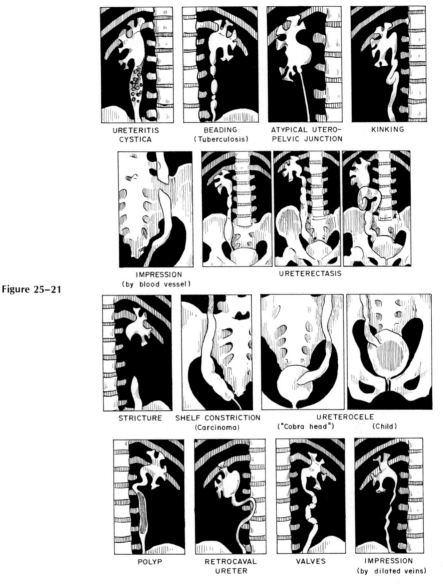

Figure 25–21

Abnormalities in Density of the Ureter

These, for the most part, have already been described.

Opacities have been previously discussed

Gas in the Ureter

Gas in the Fascial Planes Surrounding the Ureter ("ureter in uretero" appearance)

Air in the ureter will be discussed with pneumaturia and air in the urinary bladder. In diabetics it may be derived spontaneously without instrumentation if fermentation of glucose in the urine occurs.

Air in the fascial planes surrounding a ureter is derived in two ways—from perforation (usually during catheterization), or by erosion of a calculus through the wall of the ureter by superimposed gas-reproducing infection or by introduction of air at the time of ureteral catheterization.

Abnormalities of Ureteral Function

Abnormalities of ureteral function can be categorized as (a) spasm, and (b) atony and abnormal reflux from the urinary bladder. These are best studied by cineradiography coupled with fluoroscopy with image amplification.

ROENTGEN SIGNS OF ABNORMALITY OF THE URINARY BLADDER AND URETHRA

Abnormalities in Size
  a. Increased size
  b. Diminished size with trabeculation

Abnormalities in Shape
  a. Bladder ears
  b. Indentations after micturition from Hunner's ulcer
  c. Tumors
  d. The neurogenic bladder and its various types of deformity
  e. Posterior urethral valves
  f. Urethral fistulas
  g. From prostatitis
  h. Inflammation of urethral and Cowper's glands
  i. Nodular masses of urethra
  j. Developmental anomalies

Abnormalities in Position
  a. Exstrophy
  b. Displacement
  c. Cystocele
  d. Impression by extravasation
  e. Tumor masses or adjoining organs, or both

Abnormalities in Architecture
  a. Edge pattern altered by trabeculation, indentations, or diverticula
  b. Internal pattern altered by filling defects, or edema of the interureteric ridge

Abnormalities in Density
  a. Cystitis emphysematosa
  b. Pneumaturia
  c. Calcification of urinary bladder wall
  d. Urinary bladder calculi
  e. Urethral calculi

Abnormalities in Function
  a. Urinary bladder retention
  b. Vesicoureteric reflux
  c. Stress incontinence

Abnormalities of Size

Increase in Size.   The urinary bladder may be markedly distended with atony from any cause such as bladder neck or urethral obstruction.

The Urinary Bladder Distended from Neurogenic Causes is often associated with chronic infection. Even though there may be distention, the edge pattern of the urinary bladder is somewhat thickened and trabeculated and the urinary bladder contour is altered so that it has a "pine cone" appearance.

Diminution of Urinary Bladder Size usually results from chronic infection, such as tuberculosis. Here, the edge pattern of the urinary bladder is altered with irregular thickened rugae called trabeculation.

Alterations in Shape of the Urinary Bladder or Urethra

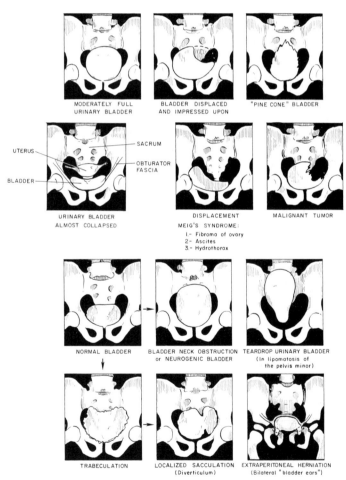

Figure 25–22

Bilateral "Bladder Ears" have been described as characteristic of extraperitoneal herniation of the urinary bladder into the internal inguinal ring and canal (Figure 25–22).

Abnormalities in Position

1. Exstrophy

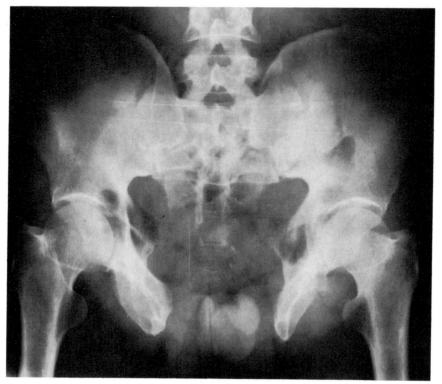

Figure 25–23

2. Cystocele—protrusion into the vagina
3. Displacement by extrinsic tumor or adjacent organ
4. Elevation by extravasation—ruptured urethra

Abnormalities in Architecture

1. Edge pattern altered by entities included under shape
2. Internal pattern: (1) Filling defects; (2) interureteric ridge (normal)

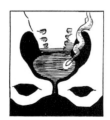

URETEROCELE
ADULT
(Cobra-head sign)

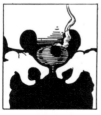

URETEROCELE
INFANT

Figure 25–24

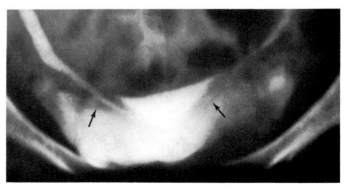

Figure 25–25

Alterations in Density

Cystitis Emphysematosa has been described in Chapter 24. A discontinuous layer of gas is observed within the bladder wall.

Pneumaturia may result from the fermentation of sugar contained in the urine if gas-producing organisms are found in the urine or if there is stasis with secondary infection by appropriate gas-producing organisms. Thus, pneumaturia may occur especially in patients with diabetes and marked glycosuria. The pneumaturia may produce negative shadows within the entire collecting system inclusive of the urinary bladder (Figure 25–26).

Urinary Bladder Wall Calcification. Calcification of the urinary bladder may occur with (1) bilharziasis, or (2) precipitation of calcification on a tumor surface within the urinary bladder. Vesical calculi may also be associated (Ney and Duff).

Urinary Bladder Calculi comprise major alterations in density of the urinary bladder. The calculi may originate in the urinary bladder or be passed down from the urinary structures above. They are usually composed of uric acid coupled with calcium salt. A bladder stone may lie in a diverticulum, and this must be differentiated by cystography.

Urinary Calculi May at Times Lodge in the Urethra Proper, and when seeking a urinary calculus which has not been recovered in strained urine, it is well to be certain that the calculus has not been detained in the urethra.

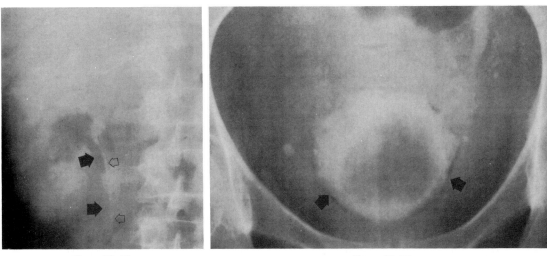

Figure 25–26   **Figure 25–27**

Figure 25–26   Gas in the fascial planes around and in the ureter, giving a *ureter in uretero* appearance.

Figure 25–27   Cystitis emphysematosa of the urinary bladder.

Alterations in Function

Vesicoureteric Reflux is a result of deficient closure of the ureter and its orifice due to inflammatory changes in the bladder wall, with partial stricture and rigidity of the orifice or anomalous development.

CYSTOURETHROGRAPHY

Normal and Normal Variants

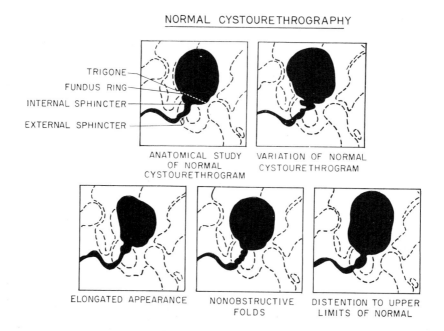

Representative Abnormalities

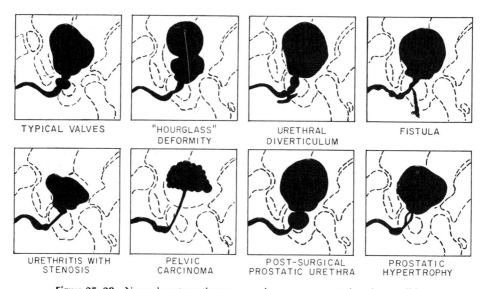

Figure 25–28 Normal cystourethrograms and some representative abnormalities.

ROENTGEN ABNORMALITIES IN SPECIFIC DISEASES OF THE URINARY TRACT

Enlarged Kidney (cf. Figure 25–8)

Renal Cysts

Classification. Classification may be highly complex; for example, Wahlqvist enumerated 29 varieties. A classification we have found most useful follows.

1. Simple cysts, which may be solitary or multiple, unilateral or bilateral, serous or hemorrhagic.
2. Peripelvic cysts.
3. Calyceal diverticulum.
4. Cysts associated with neoplastic diseases.
5. Cysts secondary to non-neoplastic renal pathology.
6. Congenital renal cystic disease, including the following:
   a. Unilateral multicystic disease.
   b. Multilocular cysts.
   c. Polycystic disease (1) in infants or children; (2) in adults.
   d. Medullary sponge kidney.
7. The perinephric cyst (Spence et al.).

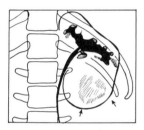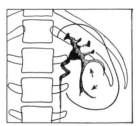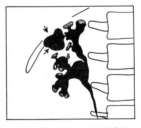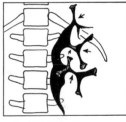

PYELOGENIC CYST OR CALYCEAL DIVERTICULUM

BILATERAL POLYCYSTIC DISEASE

Figure 25–29 Sketches illustrating the radiographic changes in association with renal cysts as they affect the calyceal pattern particularly.

The Duplex Kidney: The Problem of Nonvisualization of the Upper Pole

A duplex kidney is usually 1 to 3 cm. longer than normal. Vesicoureteral reflux and obstruction are increased in incidence. Obstruction more commonly affects the upper pole ureter because often its orifice is ectopic, since it is located in the vesical neck, urethra, or even in an extra-urinary position (Emmett and Witten). Since nonvisualization of the upper pole pelvis may also result, diagnosis of this condition becomes difficult.

It is essential that on plain films of the abdomen correlated with excretory urograms the entire kidney be carefully delineated.

Ureteropelvic Obstruction

Pyelectasis and Hydronephrosis.   In advanced cases of pyelocaliectasis, the calyces become markedly club-shaped and the pelvis becomes dilated, at times to huge proportions. The contrast agent may settle in the dilated calyces, forming crescentic collections of contrast material overlying the nonopacified dilated calyces and producing a so-called *crescent sign of hydronephrosis.* This sign may also be attributed to the accumulation of contrast material in collecting tubules that have been flattened and displaced by the hydronephrotic calyces so that they lie parallel to the renal convexity and close to its surface (LeVine et al.).

In very advanced hydronephrosis where function is markedly impaired, excretory urography even on prolonged or delayed films may be unsuccessful. At times, however, 4 hour or even 24 hour delayed films are helpful in delineating the extent of the hydronephrosis.

GENERAL COMMENT.   A hydronephrotic kidney from obstruction at the ureteropelvic junction is the most common cause of an upper abdominal mass in a child (Emmett and Witten).

ETIOLOGY.   The following possible causes have been suggested: (1) anomalous vessels crossing the ureteropelvic junction; (2) obstructive lesions such as stenoses, strictures, bands, or adhesions; (3) nonobstructive dilatation due to infection and significant reflux from the urinary bladder into the ureter, and from the ureter into the renal pelvis exceeding the ability of the upper urinary tract to empty itself into the urinary bladder (Shopfner 1965; 1966a; 1966b).

ROENTGENOLOGIC FEATURES

The calyces are club-shaped.

The renal pelvis is distended and ball-shaped with a high ureteral pelvic junction usually.

The ureter may or may not be dilated (if dilated it is likely that infection and reflux are contributing to the cause of this condition).

The ureter may be markedly dilated and tortuous.

Vesicoureteral reflux may be demonstrated on voiding cystourethrography.

UROGRAPHIC CHANGES IN PYELOCALIECTASIS

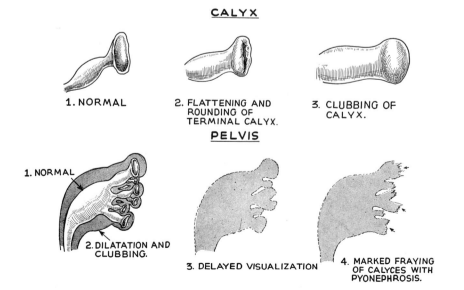

Figure 25–30

Tumors of the Kidney and Renal Pelvis

Classification. These tumors may be classified as (1) those arising from the renal cortex or parenchyma; and (2) those arising from the renal pelvis.

The tumors may be of either epithelial or mesenchymal origin.

Embryonal tumors are derived from the embryonic renal tissues and comprise the Wilms' tumor group.

In general, the benign tumors are small and rare, and with two possible exceptions, rarely come into consideration in relation to roentgen diagnosis. These two benign tumors are hemangiomas and hamartomas.

Tumors of the renal pelvis and ureter are benign or malignant. The benign tumors are usually nonepithelial, whereas the epithelial tumors are most frequently transitional cell carcinomas or epitheliomas, carcinomas of squamous cell or epidermoid origin, adenocarcinomas, secondary tumors, or mesenchymal tumors (sarcomas).

Benign Tumors of the Renal Cortex. Very few benign lesions become large enough to produce clinical signs and symptoms and permit recognition during life although they are found with a high order of frequency (15 to 20 per cent) during routine autopsy.

The benign adenoma may reveal no changes by urography and angiography shows no evidence of neovascularization, puddling, or tumor staining. The nephrotomogram may reveal a relatively radiolucent mass with a smooth regular outline suggesting a simple cyst. The distinguishing factor is the thick capsule. Under these circumstances a malignant tumor with cystic degeneration would be difficult to exclude.

Two types of hamartomas are recognized —

1. The small, multifocal medullary fibromas usually involving both kidneys and associated with tuberous sclerosis; and

2. The single larger tumor of mixed mesenchymal origin not associated with tuberous sclerosis (angiomyolipoma) (Seabury et al.).

Adenocarcinoma of the Kidney (hypernephroma; clear cell carcinoma; Grawitz tumor of the kidney) (Figure 25–2).

GENERAL COMMENT. Adenocarcinoma of the renal parenchyma comprises approximately 85 per cent of all renal tumors (Emmett). Almost all clear cell carcinomas are highly vascular neoplasms showing considerable necrosis and hemorrhage and some will show well-defined hemorrhagic cysts within the tumor mass.

ROENTGEN SIGNS OF ABNORMALITY OF ADENOCARCINOMA OF THE KIDNEY

Polar enlargement of a kidney is one of the four most frequent pyelographic changes (Evans). Unilateral enlargement of a kidney may likewise be the only manifestation of abnormality.

The mass involving the kidney may become so large that it causes a rotation of the renal shadow and an impression upon the adjoining ureter sufficient to displace the ureter.

The renal outline may be altered and markedly irregular.

Calcification of renal carcinoma is not common but may occur and may simulate renal lithiasis or calcification of a renal cyst.

The architecture of the collecting system is markedly altered. This varies from simple deformity of a calyx and splaying or spreading of the calyces simulating a cyst to outright destruction of one or more calyces with bizarre amputation. Usually, retrograde pyelography allows a more detailed study than does excretory urography.

The invasion of the renal pelvis may make it difficult to distinguish this lesion from a primary tumor of the renal pelvis or from blood clots contained within this structure.

One of the most difficult differentiations is that between a malignant neoplasm and a benign cyst. The nephrotomogram may help differentiate a solid neoplastic structure from the annular radiolucent cyst, and the renal arteriogram may differentiate the abnormal vascularity of a renal tumor with more staining from the displaced blood vessels secondary to a benign cyst. Whereas conventional radiography may be accurate in predicting the diagnosis in perhaps 50 per cent of cases, nephrotomography has improved this accuracy to at least 94 per cent (Evans et al.). As previously indicated, renal cystography by aspiration of cyst contents and injection of contrast media into the cyst may help further in the differentiation in that the contents of a malignant cyst are often bloody. Likewise, the demonstration of a filling defect or thick wall within the cyst (greater than 5 mm.) is a further important roentgen sign. Horizontal x-ray beam studies of the opacified cyst are required with the patient lying supine, prone, and on his right and left side as well as erect, so that the profile of the cyst will be demonstrated in all projections.

Rarely, there may be no urographic abnormalities despite extensive tumor of the renal parenchyma.

Arteriography has been shown to detect renal carcinoma in 97 per cent of cases (Watson, Fleming, and Evans).

RADIOGRAPHIC CHANGES WITH TUMORS OF THE KIDNEY

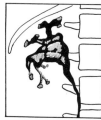

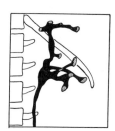

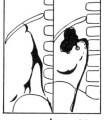

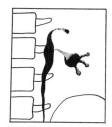

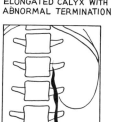

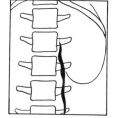

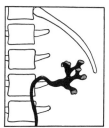

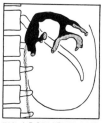

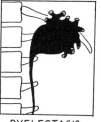

ENLARGEMENT AND IRREGULARITY OF RENAL OUTLINE

ELONGATED CALYX WITH ABNORMAL TERMINATION

NARROWING OR COMPLETE OBLITERATION OF A CALYX

ENCROACHMENT ON RENAL PELVIS

DEFORMITY OR OBSTRUCTION AT URETEROPELVIC JUNCTION

PYELECTASIS
(*TUMOR OBSCURED BY CONTRAST MATERIAL*)

CALCIFICATION

WILMS' TUMOR

ABNORMAL POSITION

Figure 25–31

A

B

C

D

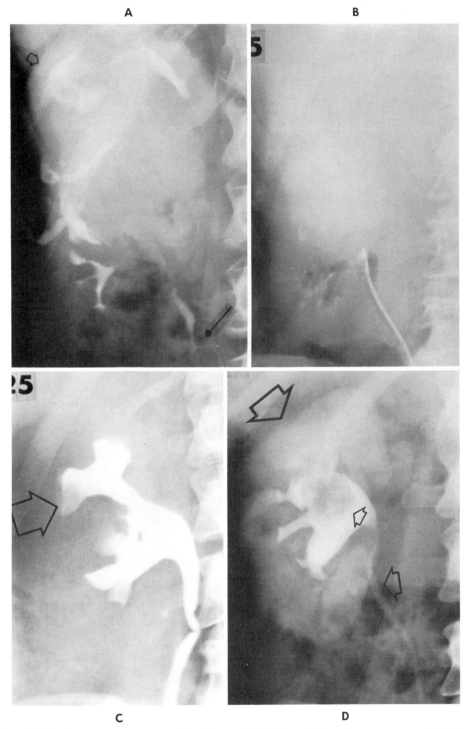

Figure 25–32 Roentgen appearances of carcinoma of the kidney. *A.* Excretory urogram, and *B.* Retrograde pyelogram. Upper pole carcinoma invading the perihilar region and displacing the upper ureter laterally. *C.* Carcinoma invading a calyx. *D.* Transitional cell carcinoma, primary in the renal pelvis, growing outward to involve the renal cortex.

Embryonal Tumors (Wilms' tumor of the kidney) (see Chapter 24 also).   These tumors are of embryonal origin—usually cortical—and distort the kidney in many different ways.

They are usually unilateral but may be bilateral in 1 to 10 per cent of cases (Bishop and Hope; Scott).

GENERAL COMMENT.   The three most common abdominal mass lesions in an infant are hydronephrosis, Wilms' tumor, and neuroblastoma. Approximately 50 per cent of abdominal masses in infants are renal in origin (Lattimer et al.).

Wilms' tumor is rare in adults. The average age at diagnosis is three years, although it may occur in older children and the prognosis is then more favorable.

ROENTGEN SIGNS OF WILMS' TUMOR

Plain films: usually a large tumor mass in a renal site can be demonstrated.

The pelvis and calyces may or may not be deformed or partially destroyed.

A special attempt must be made to differentiate neuroblastoma and hydronephrosis from this entity.

A lateral view is essential when anterior displacement of the kidney has been emphasized (Lalli et al.).

Although calcification is common in neuroblastoma, it is rare in Wilms' tumor.

Bony metastases are common with neuroblastoma and rare with Wilms' tumor.

An inferior vena cavagram has been recommended to exclude, especially in the newborn infant, the possibility of spontaneous renal thrombosis, which may yield a somewhat similar clinical and roentgen picture otherwise (Rubin et al., 1968).

Renal Trauma

Roentgenographic Features

On a KUB film the renal outline may be indistinct.

The psoas shadow may be broad, depending on retroperitoneal hemorrhage.

There may be a bulging of the flank, depending upon seepage of either blood or urine into the flank.

The plain film may reveal fractures of rib, spine, or pelvis.

The excretory urogram may reveal changes ranging from none whatsoever to complete lack of renal function. Extravasation of contrast agent may be demonstrated (Figure 25–33).

Renal arteriography is important for disclosure of the full extent of the damage (Figure 25–33). The nephrographic phase following renal arteriography is particularly helpful in showing the extent of the fracture contained in the kidney.

A traumatized kidney may heal ultimately to show little or no evidence of injury if the parenchymal fracture has not been a major one requiring surgical intervention.

If there is a persistent leak which gradually distends the capsule, a so-called **renal hydrocele** may result. This may be recognized by excretory urography by the increasing density in the renal cortical area.

Following healing of a renal rupture or injury, "tramline" calcification (better called "train track" calcification), which is characteristic of small healed areas in the kidney, may occur in this instance also.

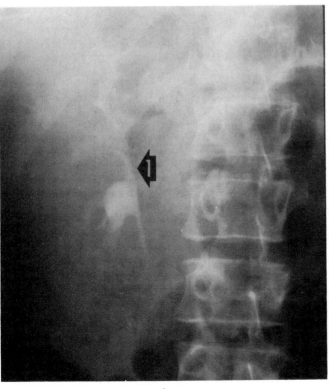

A

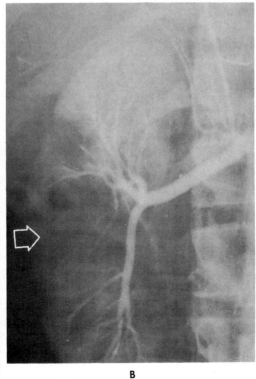

B

Figure 25–33 *A.* Excretory urogram following fracture of the kidney. Note the elongation of the superior pole calyx at the fracture site. *B.* Renal arteriogram, arterial phase. The arrow points to the fracture in the kidney.

(*Illustration continued on the following page*)

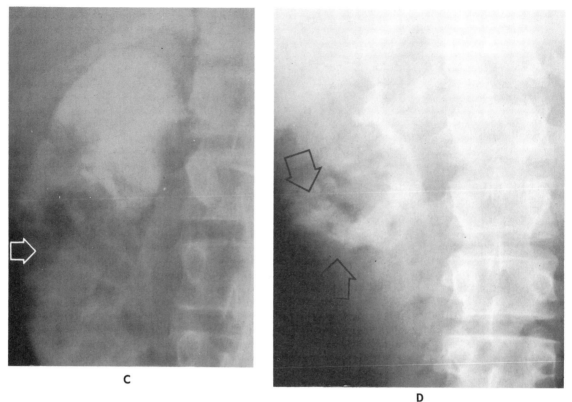

Figure 25–23 (*Continued*) *C*. Nephrogram phase. *D*. Excretory phase showing the escape of contrast agent better than in *A*.

Nontuberculous Infections of the Genitourinary Tract

Chronic Pyelonephritis

General Comment. The routes of infection may be hematogenous, ascending via the ureter or lymphatic. The changes which are observed radiologically are directly related to bacterial, nontuberculous infections.

Roentgenologic Findings

There may be linear striations of the mucosa of the pelvis and upper ureters (Gwinn and Barnes).

There may be a coarse localized renal scarring with clubbing and irregularity of the underlying calyx.

The infundibular portions of the calyx may become scarred and constricted.

The cortical scarring may give rise to irregularities and thickness of the cortex.

There may be localized areas of normal parenchyma remaining in grossly scarred calyces that are undergoing compensatory hypertrophy resulting in a pseudotumor (Figure 25–34 A and B).

In infants with chronic pyelonephritis there is a high incidence of vesicoureteral reflux—thus the voiding cystogram is an essential part of this investigation in children.

RADIOGRAPHIC CHANGES WITH ASCENDING PYELONEPHRITIS AND PYONEPHROSIS
(NONTUBERCULOUS)

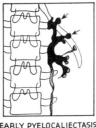

EARLY PYELOCALIECTASIS
(MINIMAL CLUBBING)

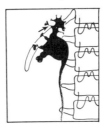

CICATRICIAL CHANGES
IN CALYCES

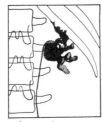

"FUZZY" PYELO-
CALIECTASIS

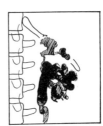

COMBINED PYELO-
CALIECTASIS AND
CICATRICIAL CHANGES
AND URETERAL IRREG-
ULARITY AND DILATA-
TION

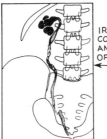

IRREGULAR
CONSTRICTION
AND DILATATION
OF URETER

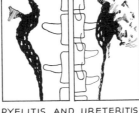

PYELITIS AND URETERITIS
CYSTICA

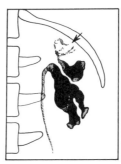
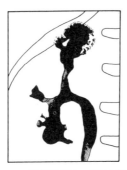
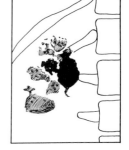

ATROPHIC
PYELONEPHRITIS
(SMALL CONTRACTED
KIDNEY)

A

Figure 25–34 *A.* Sketches illustrating the radiographic changes in association with nontuberculous pyelonephritis and pyonephrosis, particularly in the calyces. *B.* Urograms demonstrating some of the more typical findings in association with pyelonephritis. *Left,* there is evidence of cicatricial change in the infundibular portions of several of the calyces, with slight dilatation of the calyces and pelvis. *Right,* the changes are predominantly localized to the superior pole region of the right kidney.

IRREGULAR FILLING
OF CALYX

CORTICAL DESTRUCTION, ABSCESS
CALCIFICATION, CICATRIX FORMATION.

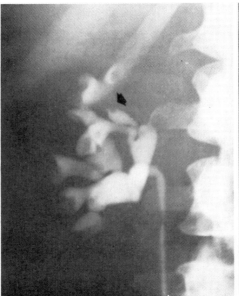
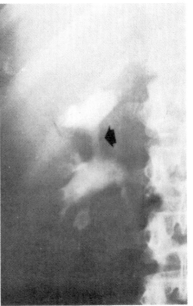

B

Renal Parenchymal Abscess Formation or Infection Surrounding the Renal Cortex

General Comment. Cortical abscesses may be single or multiple and may involve the cortex either primarily or secondarily from a perirenal origin.

RADIOGRAPHIC CHANGES WITH HEMATOGENOUS RENAL AND PERIRENAL CORTEX INFECTIONS

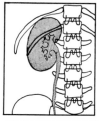

DISTURBED EXCRETORY FUNCTION

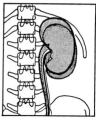

FIXATION OF KIDNEY MOBILITY LESS THAN 4-5 CM. WITH DEEP INSPIRATION.

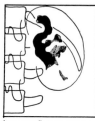

"FUZZY" CALYCEAL OUTLINE

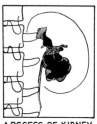

ABSCESS OF KIDNEY CORTEX

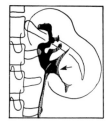

PRESSURE ON A CALYX

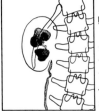

PERINEPHRIC ABSCESS MAY LEAD TO:

1. PSOAS ABSCESS.
2. SUBPHRENIC ABSCESS.
3. SKIN FISTULA.
4. BRONCHIAL FISTULA.
5. PERIRENAL GAS.

DISPLACED KIDNEY AND LUMBAR SCOLIOSIS BY CORTICAL ABSCESS WHICH HAS ERODED INTO PERINEPHRIC SPACE.

Figure 25–35

Urinary Tract Tuberculosis

Roentgen Findings

Urogram°

Early
May be normal
Dilatation of calyces
  or pelvis, localized or
  generalized
Destruction of the fornix of
  the calyx because of
  communicating abscess
Advanced
Localized stricture of
  infundibulae
Multiple abscesses
Parenchymal calcifications
Localized mass lesions
  (tuberculoma)
Nonfunctioning kidney
Massive ulcerating
  cavernous tuberculosis

Ureterogram°

Early
Dilated ureter
Ulcerative ureteritis
Advanced
Long segments of ulcer-
  ating ureteritis
Strictures (frequently
  multiple)
Beaded or corkscrew
  ureter
Pipestem ureter
Calcified ureter

Cystogram°

Early
Mucosal irregularity
Trabeculation
Late
Reflux
Distal ureteral constriction
Fibrosis with thickening
  of bladder wall
Decreased bladder
  capacity

---

*From Friedenberg, R. M. (slightly modified): Seminars in Roentgenology, 6:310–322, 1971.

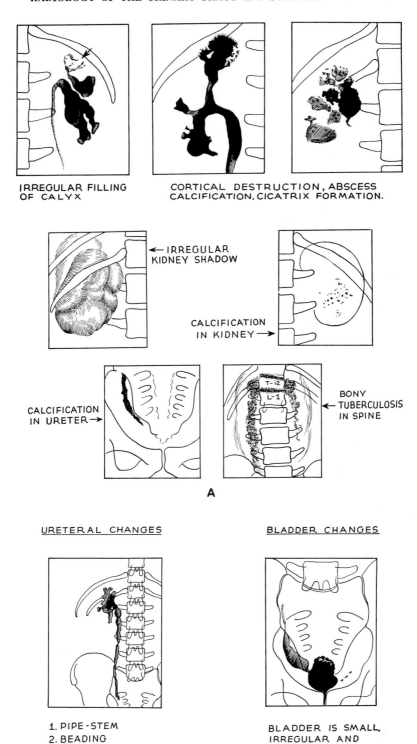

Figure 25–36 *A.* Sketches illustrating the radiographic changes in association with renal tuberculosis, particularly in the calyces. *B.* Diagram of radiographic findings with renal tuberculosis, particularly in the region of the ureter and urinary bladder.

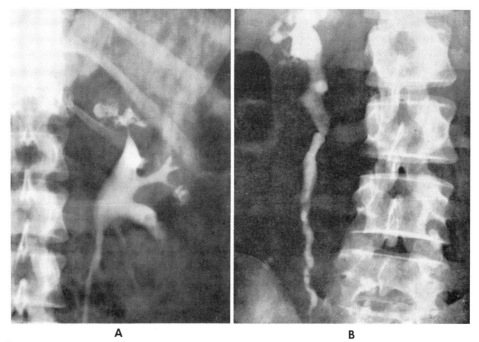

A   **B**

Figure 25–37 *A*. Pyelogram illustrating the irregularity of calyces and cortical destruction with caseation found in renal tuberculosis. *B.* Right retrograde pyelogram, demonstrating advanced right renal tuberculosis with irregularity and cortical necrosis of some calyces and with some obliteration of others. There is a marked involvement of the ureter, which is tortuous, thick-walled, and rigid, with irregular areas of dilatation and constriction (Part *C* from Emmet, J. L., and Witten, D. M.: *Clinical Urography*, Vol. 2, 3rd Ed. Philadelphia, W. B. Saunders Co., 1971.)

Renal Papillary Necrosis (Renal Medullary Necrosis; Necrotizing Papillitis) (Figure 25–38)

Importance of Associated Disease.   It is probable that diabetes is still the most frequent cause of papillary necrosis; next in order of frequency are analgesic abuse and sickle cell disease (Harrow; Harrow et al. 1963 a and b; Sanerkin).

Pathologic Considerations.   Two types of necrosis may be distinguished—the *medullary*, which is centrally situated in the pyramid, and the *papillary*, which involves the whole papilla and sometimes the greater part of the pyramid. After sloughing has occurred, the wound surface may be epithelialized, but there is no new regeneration of the elastic membrane or the muscular layer. The detached necrotic tissue may then remain in the cavity, shrink and be absorbed, or be passed in the urine as a whole or in fragments. It may also form the nucleus of a concretion. The kidneys may either enlarge or shrink.

Roentgenologic Features consist of two types—a **ring shadow** (sling shadow) and a **rounded cavity** (flask appearance) of small and large sizes (Figure 25–38). The papillary form of renal papillary necrosis is differentiated by involvement and destruction of the entire fornix of the calyx. The typical ring sign is due to the sloughing edge of the necrotic medulla separated from the viable portion of the kidney. Radiographs then show a triangular cavity pointing medially with absence of any calyceal fornix. At times the necrotic portions of the pyramid remain in the pelvis or calyces and become calcified. **The x-rays outline triangular or rounded rings of calcification with a radiolucent center.**

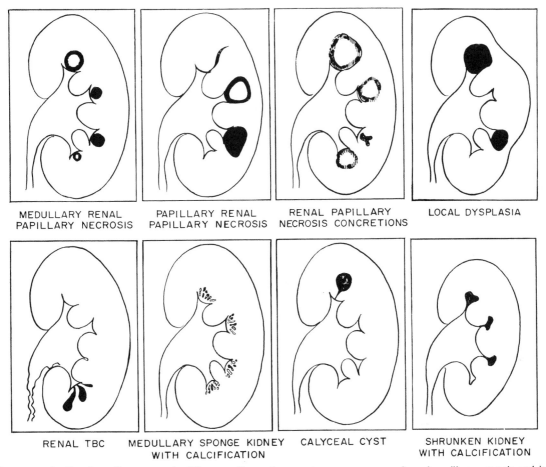

Figure 25–38 Renal papillary necrosis. Diagrams illustrating roentgen appearances of renal papillary necrosis and its differential diagnosis. (Modified from Harrow, Sloane, and Liebman: J.A.M.A., *184*:445, 1963.)

Row 1 labels:

MEDULLARY RENAL PAPILLARY NECROSIS

PAPILLARY RENAL PAPILLARY NECROSIS

RENAL PAPILLARY NECROSIS CONCRETIONS

LOCAL DYSPLASIA

Row 2 labels:

RENAL TBC

MEDULLARY SPONGE KIDNEY WITH CALCIFICATION

CALYCEAL CYST

SHRUNKEN KIDNEY WITH CALCIFICATION

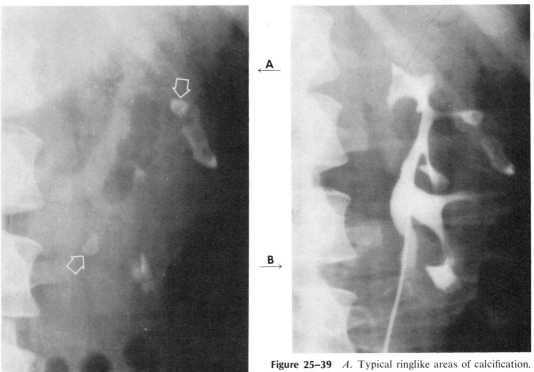

A

B

Figure 25–39 *A.* Typical ringlike areas of calcification. *B.* Retrograde pyelogram.

Renovascular Hypertension

General Comment.   Radiologic aids have come to the fore in recognition and diagnosis of renovascular hypertension. These have included the rapid sequence (minute) pyelogram, the pyelogram following hydration (washout), the radioisotopic renogram, the renal arteriogram, and the radioisotopic renal scan.

Major Roentgen Findings on Rapid Sequence Intravenous Pyelogram

A discrepancy in size of the kidneys on either side, or a kidney which is unusual in size either because of diminution or increase.

Lobulation in a kidney contour in the adult which appears excessive.

A delay in the appearance of the medium in an unobstructed upper urinary tract, beyond the three minute film on the rapid sequence study.

Nonvisualization of an entire unobstructed upper urinary tract.

Persistent segmental nonvisualization of one or more unobstructed calyces which on retrograde study may be demonstrated to fill normally (renal infarction).

Persistent or increasing differences in the apparent concentration of the medium in one upper urinary tract or a portion thereof. This has been called hyperconcentration, or hypoconcentration.

Persistent unilateral delicacy and thinness of a completely visualized upper urinary tract and ureter. This has been termed the spidering, spastic, or low-flow pattern.

Localized atrophy of a portion of the renal mass observed on serial examinations but not due to a healing abscess.

Vascular calcification in the region of the renal pedicle or a portion of the renal mass.

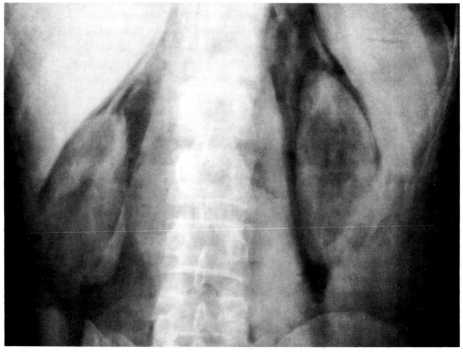

Figure 25–40   Normal retroperitoneal pneumogram. (From McLelland, R., Landes, R. R., and Ransom, C. L.: Radiol. Clin. N. Amer., *3*:115, 1965.)

THE SUPRARENAL GLANDS

The normal suprarenal gland may vary considerably in size, its shape is fairly well-preserved and its margins are practically always concave (Meyers). Occasionally the normal medial border of the left suprarenal gland may be minimally convex.

Abnormality in Contour and Density of the Suprarenal Glands

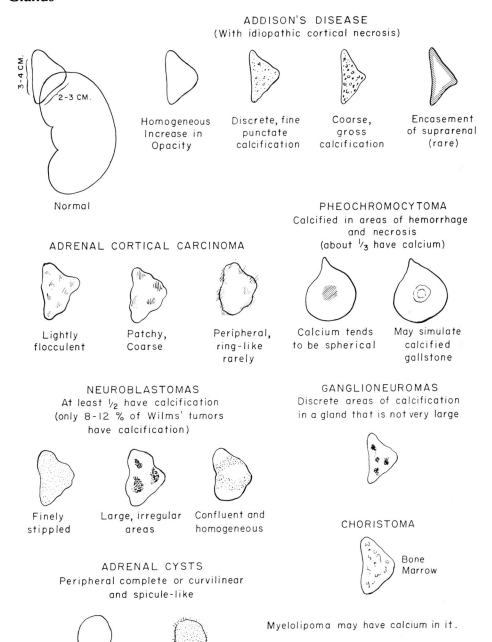

Figure 25–41   Abnormalities of density and contour of the suprarenal gland, diagrammatically illustrated.

Related Comments Regarding Suprarenal Tumor Masses

Metastases to the adrenal gland comprise the most frequent tumor involvement of the adrenals (Herbut). Melanoblastoma comprises about 60 per cent of this group; carcinoma of the breast, 58 per cent; carcinoma of the kidney, 45 per cent; and lung carcinoma, 36 per cent (Meyers).

Neuroblastomas are the most common neoplasm of infancy and childhood next to leukemia. About one-third of these arise and are detected in the first year of life. In the abdomen they are second in frequency only to Wilms' tumors, and in some series equal in frequency to Wilms' tumor. About 30 to 50 per cent of neuroblastomas arise in the adrenal medulla. Any portion of the sympathetic nervous system, however, may give rise to this neoplasm.

Only about 12 per cent of ganglioneuromas are found in the suprarenal gland, with the majority being abdominal in location and about 16 per cent lumbar. The ganglioneuroma may secrete norepinephrine and dopamine, giving rise to corresponding clinical symptomatology.

Adrenal cysts are more commonly hemorrhagic and lymphangiomatous. They vary considerably in size even up to 30 cm. in diameter.

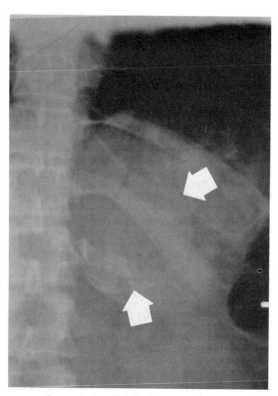

Figure 25–42   Calcified suprarenal cyst.

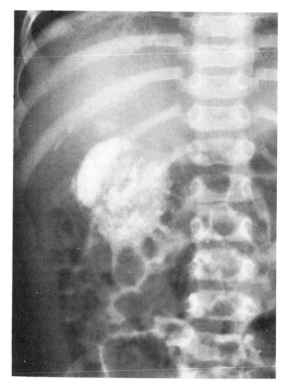

Figure 25–43   Extensive calcium deposits in a neuroblastoma overlying the right kidney.

Questions — Chapter 25

1. How would you prepare a patient for an intravenous pyelogram?

2. Describe the technique for single injection excretory urograms.

3. What would be the purpose of delayed films with excretory urograms? How long a delay would you recommend?

4. What is the difference between infusion excretory urography and single injection intravenous pyelography?

5. Describe the technique for rapid sequence dehydrated excretory urograms. What is the main purpose of this study?

6. Indicate the main purpose of nephrotomography and how it is done.

7. What are the advantages and disadvantages of retrograde pyelography in comparison with intravenous pyelography?

8. Indicate various types of cystography and cystourethrography. What is the main purpose of each?

9. What is the advantage of a retrograde urethrogram over the voiding type? What is the main disadvantage of cineradiography in connection with cystourethrography?

10. Indicate some of the main purposes of renal arteriography either selective or via the aorta.

11. Indicate some of the main purposes of renal vein phlebography. Under what circumstances would it also be helpful to demonstrate the inferior vena cava?

12. Indicate the main purposes of perirenal air insufflation. Why might this be an advantageous procedure over a suprarenal or renal arteriogram?

13. Describe some of the common unfavorable reactions to contrast media and how they should be managed. Indicate in sequence the treatment of a reaction to the injection of a contrast agent used in the urinary tract.

14. Indicate a technique for examination of films of the upper urinary tract.

15. How would you describe the normal kidney size?

16. What is the normal position of the kidney? How may this vary without significance to the patient? What is meant by the normal "renal axis" and what is the significance of this axis in diagnosis?

17. Describe the normal mobility of the kidney. How would you indicate abnormal mobility and what is the significance of it?

18. Indicate some of the abnormalities of renal shape and their pathologic significance.

19. Indicate the significance of the "edge pattern" of the kidney in respect to normal anatomy and pathology.

20. Describe the internal architecture of the kidney.

21. Describe the normal anatomic relationship of the ureter.

22. Describe the normal anatomy of the male and female urethra.

23. Describe the normal blood supply and venous drainage of the kidney.

24. Tabulate the various functions performed by the kidney, and indicate which of these are frequently investigated by roentgenologic methods.

25. Indicate some of the roentgen signs of abnormality in respect to kidney size or number.

26. Indicate some of the abnormalities in position of the kidney.

27. Describe the abnormalities in renal contour and how they may be significant in respect to certain disease entities.

28. Indicate some of the variations and abnormalities in renal density from the standpoint of decreased density as well as of increased density.

29. Describe various types of renal calcification and indicate the significance of accurate localization of these calculi in respect to final diagnosis.

30. What is meant by the term nephrocalcinosis and how would you categorize the causes of this disorder?

31. What are the important entities to be considered in nephrocalcinosis in children?

32. Indicate some of the abnormalities in the architecture of the renal calyces.

33. What are some of the causes of calyceal fraying, elongation and thinning, cicatricial change, outpouching, and linear streaking?

34. What is meant by the term papillary necrosis? What are some of the roentgen appearances of this disorder?

35. Indicate some of the alterations of the internal architecture of the renal calyces or pelvis.

36. Summarize the utilization of the excretory urogram as a study of renal function.

37. What are some of the roentgen abnormalities of number in respect to the ureter?

38. How would you catalogue the abnormalities of the ureter in respect to size, and what are some of the clinical causes of these abnormalities?

39. What is meant by the term achalasia of the ureter?

40. What is meant by the term idiopathic retroperitoneal fibrosis? How may it appear? Describe correlative findings in this entity.

41. Indicate some of the causes for abnormalities of position of a ureter.

42. What is meant by the term retrocaval ureter?

43. How would you describe some of the abnormalities in architecture of the ureter?

44. What are some of the causes of abnormalities in density of the ureter, both lucent and opaque?

45. How would you explain pneumaturia?

46. What are some of the abnormalities of size of the urinary bladder?

47. How would you catalogue changes which might be seen in the neurogenic bladder?

48. How may abnormalities of position of the urinary bladder be recognized? Indicate some of the causes of this roentgen abnormality.

49. Indicate some of the causes of alterations in shape of the urinary bladder or urethra.

50. Where are posterior urethral valves situated and what types of valvular obstruction are noted?

51. Indicate some of the causes of alteration in the "edge pattern" in respect to the architecture of the urinary bladder.

52. How may endometriosis at times affect the urinary bladder?

53. Indicate the roentgen appearance of cystitis emphysematosa of the urinary bladder.

54. Indicate the clinical significance of air within the urinary bladder lumen. How is this produced physiologically or clinically?

55. Indicate the structural alterations which occur in the urinary bladder as a result of neurogenic disturbance.

56. What is the importance of vesicoureteric reflux? How would you recognize this roentgenologically?

57. Describe some of the more confusing pyelographic appearances which must be borne in mind in order to avoid pitfalls in roentgen diagnosis of the urinary tract.

58. Describe the gross anatomy of the suprarenal gland—in particular how this is related to size and shape as seen roentgenologically.

59. What is the major blood supply of the suprarenal glands?

60. Indicate the main methods of examination of the suprarenal glands.

61. Indicate some of the abnormalities of the suprarenal gland in respect to its (1) size and (2) contour. Describe some of the disease entities which might alter the contour of the suprarenal gland. Are any of these fairly specific?

62. Indicate some of the abnormalities of density of the suprarenal gland. In what percentage of cases might one expect to see calcification in pheochromocytoma; in neuroblastoma; in a Wilms' tumor of the kidney?

63. In what percentage of suprarenal glands involved in Addison's disease is calcification noted?

64. How may the fundus of the stomach interfere with the diagnosis of suprarenal glandular abnormalities?

65. What are some of the other areas of the body which should be studied in patients with Cushing's syndrome, apart from the suprarenal region? What might be seen roentgenologically?

66. How often is the adrenal gland involved with metastases from tumors elsewhere and what are some of the most common tumors which do metastasize to adrenals?

67. When is neuroblastoma most frequently discovered in infancy? What are some of the

other abdominal tumors which must enter into differential diagnosis and how would you go about differentiating these?

68. Indicate a useful classification of renal cysts. What are the most common causes for an enlarged kidney?

69. What is meant by a "calyceal diverticulum"?

70. What is a useful classification of congenital renal cystic disease?

71. What relationship exists between renal cystic disease and hepatic cystic disease?

72. Why is it important to anticipate a duplex kidney? In the event of nonvisualization of either the upper or lower pole what further expedient must be employed?

73. What is meant by the term "renal pseudotumor"?

74. What are the roentgenologic features of adenocarcinoma of the kidney?

75. List criteria for differentiating a renal cyst from a neoplasm by any radiologic means. What special radiologic examinations are necessary?

76. What are the roentgen signs associated with a high incidence of unresectability of carcinoma of the kidney?

77. What are the roentgen signs of a Wilms' tumor?

78. Which are the most important renal masses in the pediatric age group, and what differential features can you elicit among them? What is their order of frequency?

79. What are the radiologic features of chronic pyelonephritis?

80. What are the radiologic features of pyelitis and ureteritis cystica?

81. What are the roentgen findings in perirenal abscess?

82. What are the roentgenologic features of renal tuberculosis?

83. What are the radiologic features of renal papillary necrosis?

84. How would you go about studying a patient in respect to renovascular hypertension? What are the major roentgen findings in the several studies?

85. Where are the congenital urethral valves situated and what types of these may be encountered? What are the roentgenographic features of cystourethrography in this condition?

26

Roentgenology of the Biliary System

ORAL CHOLECYSTOGRAMS

Physiological Basis

The Telepaque is absorbed in the gastrointestinal tract, and then is delivered to the liver. It is excreted in the bile, and if the extrahepatic biliary passages are open, it finds its way to the gallbladder. In the gallbladder the contrast agent and bile are concentrated above the level of the original bile. If, however, the gallbladder is inflamed, or its mucosa is otherwise pathological, the contrast medium is absorbed from the gallbladder, and concentration of the agent does not occur sufficiently for roentgenologic visualization. When Cholografin is used, it accumulates in the gallbladder in the same form in which it is administered in sufficient concentration usually for visualization, although it is not as opaque as Telepaque.

Selection of Patients and Dose Considerations

Selection of Patients

TABLE 26–1 SELECTION OF PATIENTS FOR ORAL CHOLANGIOGRAPHY AND CHOLECYSTOGRAPHY

Test	Values	Probability of Success
Serum bilirubin (Mandel)	< 5 mg.% >10 mg.%	Worth trying Failure
(Shehadi)	< 1 mg.% < 2 mg.% 3 mg.% or> > 4 mg.%	Excellent Satisfactory Poor or unlikely Not possible
Bromsulphalein (BSP) retention (Etess and Strauss)	5–20% >20–23%	Should not interfere Failure
(Blornstrom and Sandstrom)	>40%	Failure

Dose Considerations. Three grams of Telepaque are usually sufficient for all adults irrespective of weight. With some patients we have used doses as high as 6 grams (12 tablets) within a period of 24 hours. Different studies on the renal toxicity of contrast medium in patients with hepatorenal damage have called attention to the danger of larger doses of oral cholecystographic media. It has therefore been recommended that a dose of 6 grams not be exceeded within a period of 24 hours. and if such a dose has been employed, that it not be repeated for a period of at least one week.

Pediatric patients may be given proportionately smaller doses.

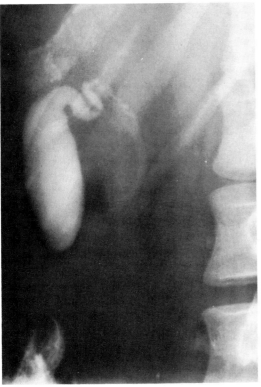

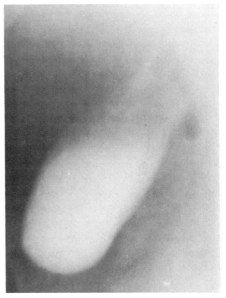

Figure 26–2 Layering of Telepaque which may occur normally in the gallbladder, patient erect.

Figure 26–1 Representative scout film of the gallbladder region extending from the iliac fossa to the diaphragm and from the left portion of the spine to the outer flank region.

Upright or lateral decubitus films are also obtained routinely to determine possible stratification or mobility of filling defects within the gallbladder (Figure 26–2). Fluoroscopy with compression spot film studies may be employed for this purpose.

Side Effects. Whitehouse and Martin* have reported the following side effects from 3 gram doses of Telepaque in 400 patients: diarrhea, 25.3 per cent (of which 2.5 per cent were severe); dysuria, 13.7 per cent; mild nausea, 5.8 per cent; and mild vomiting, 1.5 per cent. There were other side effects in 2.8 per cent of the cases and no side effects were noted in 62.5 per cent of the cases.

Patients with hepatorenal dysfunction constitute a potential hazard group for oral cholecystography.

---

*Whitehouse, W. M., and Martin, O.: Clinical and roentgenologic evaluation of 3 gram Telepaque dosage in cholecystography. Radiology, *65*:422, 1955.

RADIOGRAPHIC SIGNS OF ABNORMALITY

ROENTGEN SIGNS OF ABNORMALITY OF THE BILIARY SYSTEM BY ORAL CHOLECYSTOGRAPHY

1. Nonvisualization of the gallbladder as an indicator of abnormality is probably better than 90 per cent accurate.
2. Increased size: greater than 35 square cm. frontal area or 5 cm. in width.
3. Fixed papillary filling defects in the gallbladder.
4. Multiple filling defects in the gallbladder due to hyperplastic cholecystoses.
5. Emphysematous cholecystitis.
6. Supernumerary gallbladder.
7. Gallstone filling defect—abnormality in density
   a. 15 to 20 per cent of gallstones are partially or completely radiopaque.
   b. "Crowfoot" sign on plain film studies.
8. Calcification within the gallbladder as:
   a. Stones.
   b. Milk of calcium bile.
   c. Calcified plaques in wall or calcified wall of gallbladder.
9. The reappearing gallbladder or re-formed gallbladder following cholecystectomy.

The Significance of Nonvisualization of the Gallbladder in Patients with Intact Gallbladder. Abnormality of Function.   There are certain basic assumptions that must be verified as far as possible in order to interpret oral cholecystograms:

1. That the patient actually has taken the contrast agent.
2. That adequate absorption of the agent has occurred (no esophageal, gastric, or intestinal obstruction).
3. That the liver function is adequate for secretion of the test compound.
4. That the ductal system above the level of the gallbladder is not obstructed.
5. That the common bile duct is not obstructed (in which case there may be some associated gallbladder disease).

The oral cholecystogram is fundamentally a function test. It must not, however, be assumed that nonvisualization necessarily indicates abnormal function in certain rare instances. Complete absence of the gallbladder is a rare anomaly but can occur.

A surprisingly high proportion of men with cholelithiasis are asymptomatic (70 per cent of men with stones and 86 per cent of a control group have no symptoms) (Wilbur and Bolt).* Of 30 per cent of patients with gallstones, two-thirds had only the unreliable signs and symptoms of dyspepsia and epigastric pain, symptoms which are found in 10 per cent of normal controls. Also, typical biliary colic can be a misleading description, since it is found in about 3.6 per cent of those with no stones and in 0.9 per cent of normal men.

---

*Wilbur, R. S., and Bolt, R. J.: Gastroenterology, 36:251–255, 1959.

Variations in Shape. The gallbladder may be ovoid, spheroidal, or elongated and the shape in itself does not indicate a diagnosis of abnormality. The mucosal or serosal fold (phrygian cap) in the fundus of the gallbladder is a normal variant (Fig. 26–3).

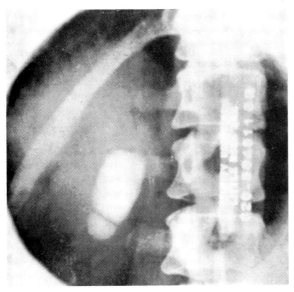

Figure 26–3 Mucosal or serosal fold of gallbladder, known as a phrygian cap.

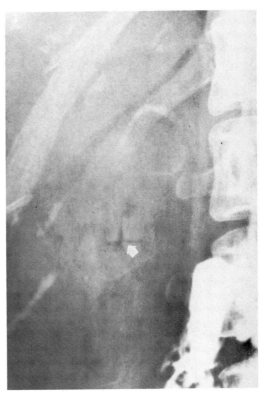

Figure 26–4 "Crowfoot" sign showing crevices which appear radiolucent in a gallstone and giving the appearance of a crow's foot.

Abnormalities of Density

Gallstone Filling Defect. Approximately 85 per cent of gallstones are radiolucent (Figure 26–6). Approximately 15 to 20 per cent of gallstones are partially or completely radiopaque (Figure 26–5).

Occasional Gallstones May be Fissured and appear radiolucent in the fissures. These fissures may be demonstrable even though the stone itself is not visible ("crowfoot" sign) (Figure 26–4).

Gallstones Prior to Puberty. When gallstones appear prior to puberty, they are almost invariably associated with a hemolytic anemia and are due to excessive excretion of blood pigment.

Papillary Filling Defects Due to Papilloma.   Papillomas of the gallbladder usually measure about 3 mm. in diameter, are circular or slightly ovoid in shape, and constant in all positions.

Multiple Filling Defects Due to Hyperplastic Cholecystoses (Figures 26–7, 26–8, 26–9, 26–10).

Multiple filling defects within the gallbladder may be produced by the *hyperplastic cholecystoses* (Jutras). Jutras has included nine separate disease entities among the hyperplastic cholecystoses. The most important among these are cholesterolosis, adenomyomatosis, and the neuromatoses. Jutras has also proposed a synergistic concept for this group of disorders, so that there is a corresponding hyperfunctional triad—hyperconcentration, hyperexcitability, and hyperexcretion.

Cholesterolosis is manifest radiographically as a radiolucent defect of varying size but ordinarily larger than a papilloma of the gallbladder. Whereas the true papilloma and granuloma of the gallbladder are more frequent in the middle third of the gallbladder, these cholesterol "polyps" may be found in all parts of the gallbladder, even in the fundus. Cholesterol polyps are multiple, in contrast to papillomas which are usually single. At times, the cholesterol polyp is set free into the gallbladder and becomes the nidus for a gallstone. It usually does not exceed 1 cm. in diameter.

Adenomyomatosis of the gallbladder is characterized by (1) proliferation of the epithelium; (2) increased thickness of the muscle layers; (3) the formation of out-pouchings of the mucosa into small sinuses called Rokitansky-Aschoff sinuses (Figure 26–9 C). The radiologic appearance is based upon the visualization of minute intramural diverticula, and hence these will be more properly described later under "Abnormalities in Architecture."

The term neuromatosis refers to a non-neoplastic proliferation of the autonomic nerve fibers in the gallbladder, either superficial or deep. Each form of the above described cholecystoses may exist singly or conjointly with or without stones and with or without mucosal congestion.

Emphysematous Cholecystitis (Blum and Stagg) (Figure 26–11).   Emphysematous cholecystitis is characterized by gas within the wall of the gallbladder, in the pericholecystic tissues, and usually within the lumen of the gallbladder as well. The offending organisms most frequently found are *Clostridium welchii, Clostridium oedematiens,* and *E. coli.* Diabetes mellitus may be associated in some cases. Radiologically, the diagnosis on plain films may be suspected by a mottled or homogeneous, round or pear-shaped gas shadow in the right upper quadrant of the abdomen, resembling the gallbladder and in the position of this organ. There may or may not be an associated fluid level in the erect position. At times, calculi may also be seen within the gallbladder. Although the gas surrounding the gallbladder is at first smooth, in later stages of the disease the appearance becomes more bubblelike and streaked. In this latter phase there is an actual separation of the muscularis layer of the gallbladder from the mucous membrane (Heifetz and Wyloge).

Care must be exercised to distinguish air within the gallbladder wall from air within the gallbladder itself as a result of a biliary gastrointestinal fistula or incompetent sphincter of Oddi. Likewise, one must exclude extrabiliary subhepatic abscesses and gas in the gastrointestinal tract without involvement of the gallbladder.

Calcification may be recognized within the gallbladder as: (1) stones; (2) milk of calcium bile; (3) a calcified plaque or wall in the gallbladder proper (Figure 26–12).

Biliary Calculi

In the presence of biliary stasis, infection, or increased concentration of one or more of the biliary constituents, a supersaturation may result, and gallstones may form. It is thought that hypercholesterolemia may predispose to the formation of calculi. In hemolytic disease, bilirubin may precipitate in various compounds and form the basis for stones.

The inflammation of the gallbladder may either be of physical origin or follow bacterial infection.

In any case, the density, number, and configuration of biliary calculi vary widely. Pure cholesterol calculi are ordinarily radiolucent. Some calculi have an admixture of opaque constituents.

In the erect or decubitus position, the gallstones may stratify, depending upon the specific gravity of the stones in relation to that of the surrounding liquid substance in the gallbladder. The detection of such stratification, however, is important.

On occasion, small gallstones may be obscured in the prone or supine position and become manifest by virtue of the stratification in the erect or decubitus position. Stratification of gallstones must not be confused with the normal sedimentation of the contrast agent within the gallbladder (Figure 26–2).

MILK CALCIUM BILE represents a polarization or emulsion of bile stones. These may layer out in the erect position. When the patient is recumbent, milk calcium bile may be indistinguishable from a gallbladder filled with dye—hence, scout films and erect films are necessary for detection of this abnormality.

Calcified Plaques in the Gallbladder or completely calcified walls of the gallbladder are related to chronic cholecystitis. They may be associated with gallstones and have been found to be associated with carcinoma of the gallbladder. The frequency of coexistent calcification and carcinoma in the wall of the gallbladder is such that operation should be undertaken in patients with roentgenographic evidence of calcification of the gallbladder who are acceptable operative risks (Ochsner and Carrera).

Calcification of the wall of the gallbladder occurs apparently in two different forms:

1. Calcification in the muscular coat of the gallbladder extending lengthwise in relation to the wall of the gallbladder. Grossly and radiographically, this calcification looks like large flakes or plaques of calcification in the wall of the gallbladder.

2. Multiple small calculi or microliths in the glandular spaces of the mucosa of the gallbladder. These are actually small calculi scattered in the mucosa and submucosa in small Rokitansky-Aschoff sinuses. Some of this calcification may be found in the muscularis. The gallbladder under these circumstances has a denuded mucosa which grossly resembles sandpaper, and radiographically a fine granular and plaquelike calcification of the wall of the gallbladder is observed.

Calcification of the wall of the gallbladder is also found with the so-called "petrified" gallbladder and distinction between the two usually is not clearly made.

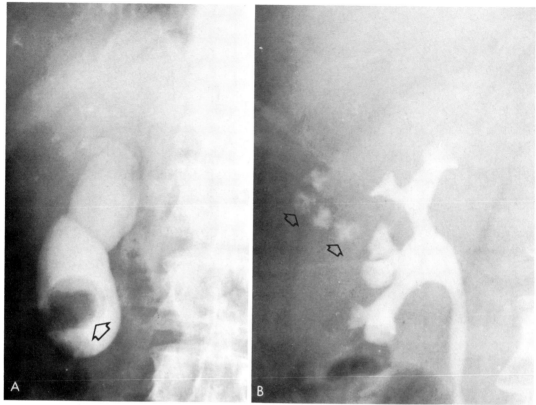

Figure 26–5 *A.* Large cholesterol stone in the gallbladder. *B.* Calcified gallstones in the gallbladder, assuming a "mulberry" appearance.

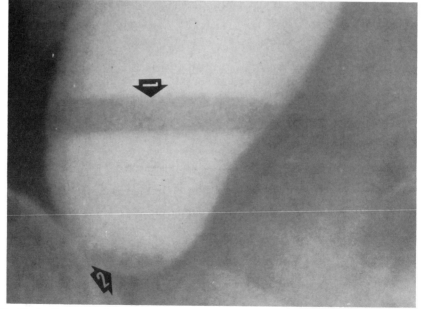

Figure 26–6 Stratified gallstones in the gallbladder in the erect position: (1) showing that the gallstones may float in the center of the gallbladder, and (2) demonstrating that some gallstones will settle to the bottom of the gallbladder since they are heavier than bile.

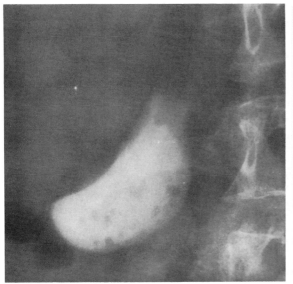

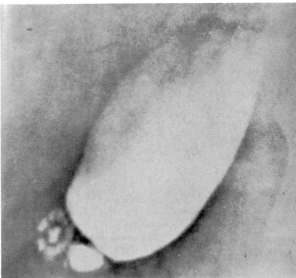

Figure 26–7 Cholesterolosis of the gallbladder (example of hyperplastic cholecystosis).

Figure 26–8 Extraluminal adenomyoma.

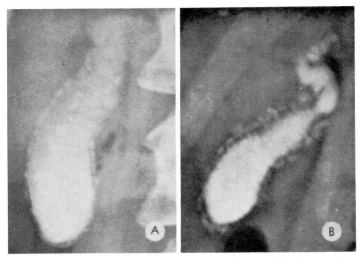

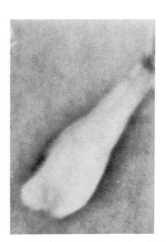

Figure 26–9 Adenomyomatosis, generalized type. *A.* A fully distended and normally shaped gallbladder presenting numerous diverticula over the surface and around the edge. *B.* Same gallbladder exhibiting a contraction ring that gives a piriform shape to the shadow. The annular narrowing obviously is not an organic abnormality. (From Jutras, J. A.: Amer. J. Roentgenol., *83*:807, 1960.)

Figure 26–10 Intraluminal adeno-myoma showing pseudocalculus ap-pearance. After partial evacuation the appearance changes into one of the trans-marginal types. (From Jutras, J. A.: Amer. J. Roentgenol., *83*:815, 1960.)

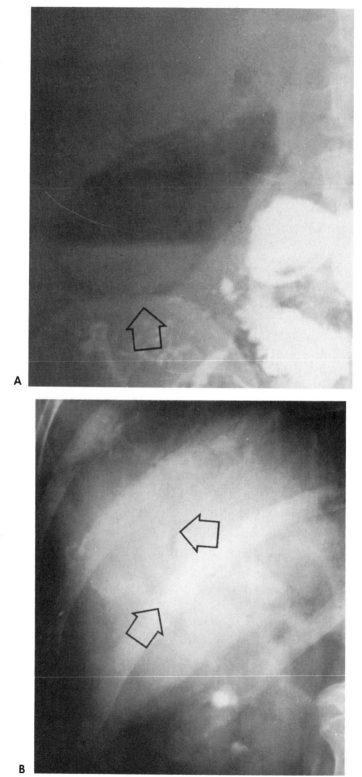

Figure 26–11 *A.* Emphysematous cholecystitis. *B.* Ruptured gallstone producing free air in the biliary tree.

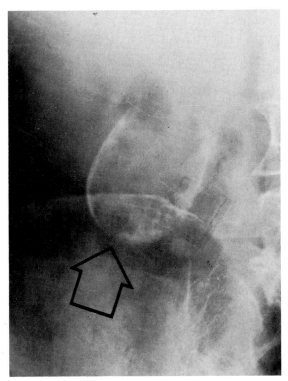

Figure 26–12 Calcification of the wall of the gallbladder.

Abnormalities of Architecture

The "Reappearing" Gallbladder (Lipton and Soule) presents an interesting problem. The dilated cystic duct remnant is one of the common causes of recurrent symptoms in the postcholecystectomy patient. This has been called the "reappearing" or "reformed" gallbladder. It is thought that the dilated stump is unable to contract, and stagnation of bile may occur with subsequent infection, inflammation, and possible calculus formation.

On roentgenograms, the reappearing gallbladder resembles a miniature gallbladder in the right upper quadrant. Its size varies from 0.5 cm. to 7 cm. in length and from 0.5 to 3 cm. in width, as compared with the normal cystic duct diameter of 0.2 to 0.3 cm.

The ratio of opaque to nonopaque calculi is higher in this entity than in primary gallbladder disease.

In certain instances, the reformed gallbladder may be related to saccule formation which occurs at the site of spillage of bile through the surgical opening in a common hepatic or common bile duct, following removal of T-tube drainage after cholecystectomy.

INTRAVENOUS CHOLANGIOGRAPHY

Criteria and Indications for Intravenous Cholangiography

With *serum bilirubin levels of 1 mg. per 100 ml. or less*, opacification of the ducts may be expected in 92.5 per cent of cases. If serum bilirubin values are above 4 mg. per 100 ml., opacification may be expected in only 9.3 per cent.

With BSP (bromsulphalein) retention level below 10 per cent after 45 minutes, opacification may be expected in 96 per cent of injections, but if retention level is above 40 per cent, opacification may be expected in 26.2 per cent.*

With these basic criteria in mind, *intravenous cholangiography is indicated in the following situations:*

1. Nonvisualization by the oral route. According to Wise, 12 per cent of these patients were found to have gallbladders without visualized calculi and appearing normal. Among 201 patients with intact gallbladders not visualized by the oral route, visualization was accomplished in 70 by the intravenous method and 24 of these were considered normal. All those with nonvisualization by the intravenous method turned out to have disease.
2. Differentiation of gallbladder disease and obstructive disease of the distal common duct.
   a. If the common duct is less than 7.0 mm. in diameter, nonvisualization of the gallbladder is due to cystic duct obstruction or primary gallbladder disease.
   b. If the common duct is dilated, the cause of non-opacification may be common duct obstruction alone or combined with cystic duct obstruction.
3. Postcholecystectomy syndrome.
4. Preoperative cholangiography to demonstrate calculi in the common bile duct before cholecystectomy.
5. In infants and children with appropriate biliary histories.
6. In emergencies when speed is a factor.
7. If a tumor is suspected near the porta hepatis.
8. In recent or subsiding jaundice when bilirubin and BSP levels are appropriate to help differentiate between infective hepatitis and common duct stones.
9. In functional biliary disorders in which a study of the duct system may help differentiate organic disease.

Radiographic Signs of Abnormality in Intravenous Cholangiography

In Patients With an Intact Gallbladder and Nonvisualization by Oral Cholecystography Wise visualized 35 per cent of 201 gallbladders. In 12 per cent the gallbladder was considered normal by this technique.

When the bile ducts were visualized but the gallbladder was not, approximately 70 per cent of the patients were shown to have primary gallbladder disease. Approximately 10 per cent were shown to have primary common duct or pancreatic disease and 20 per cent had combined gallbladder and common duct or pancreatic disease.

---

*Wise, Robert E.: *Intravenous Cholangiography.* Springfield, Illinois, Charles C Thomas, Publishers, 1962.

Abnormalities in Size of the Common Bile Duct

In unoperated biliary tracts, the upper limit of normal when magnified approximately 30 per cent is probably 10 mm.

In the postcholecystectomy state, the normal limit is variable, and may be as great as 19 mm.

Abnormalities of Architecture

Edge Pattern. A saclike communication, at the site of the cyst duct following cholecystectomy or at the site of a T-tube entry into the common duct, has given rise to the concept of a "reformed" gallbladder or "cystic duct remnant." These remnants may at times contain filling defects due to calculi.

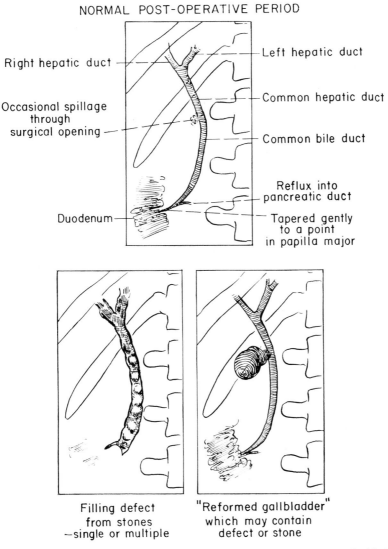

NORMAL POST-OPERATIVE PERIOD

Right hepatic duct

Occasional spillage through surgical opening

Duodenum

Left hepatic duct

Common hepatic duct

Common bile duct

Reflux into pancreatic duct

Tapered gently to a point in papilla major

Filling defect from stones —single or multiple

"Reformed gallbladder" which may contain defect or stone

Figure 26–13   Abnormalities in cholangiograms following cholecystectomy, compared with the normal.

PATTERNS OF INCREASED PATULENCE, SPINDLING, OR OBSTRUCTION

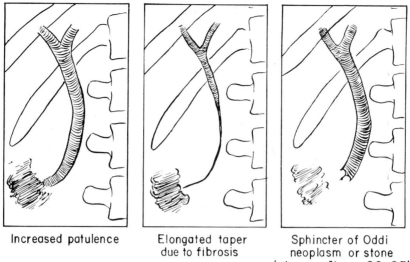

Increased patulence

Elongated taper
due to fibrosis

Sphincter of Oddi
neoplasm or stone
(also see Figure 26-25)

ALTERATION OF POSITION

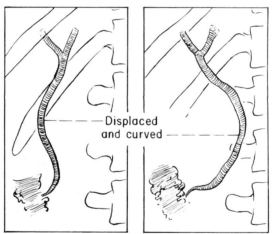

—Displaced
and curved —

Figure 26-13 *(Continued)*

CARCINOMA VS. STONE IN COMMON DUCT

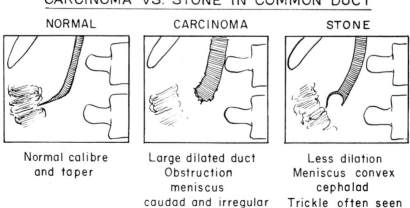

NORMAL

CARCINOMA

STONE

Normal calibre
and taper

Large dilated duct
Obstruction
meniscus
caudad and irregular
Nipple inferiorly

Less dilation
Meniscus convex
cephalad
Trickle often seen
around stone

Figure 26-14   Roentgen signs which may be helpful in differentiating carcinoma and stone in the common duct in cholangiography.

PERCUTANEOUS CHOLANGIOGRAPHY

Introduction

Under normal circumstances, puncture of the liver with an exploratory needle will fail to produce bile. Bile is obtained if extrahepatic obstruction is present. Percutaneous cholangiography may be employed in the differential diagnosis of jaundice in certain selected cases, provided normal clotting factors are present and broad spectrum antibiotics are given for a day in advance in case operation is necessary (Flemma et al., Mujahed and Evans). It is contraindicated in hemorrhagic diathesis and vitamin K resistant hypoprothrombinemia or in patients with febrile cholangitis.

The *main indications* for percutaneous cholangiography are (Mujahed and Evans):

1. To differentiate between obstructive and nonobstructive jaundice.
2. To demonstrate the presence and site of carcinoma of the biliary system.
3. To demonstrate the number of calculi in the biliary system and their location.
4. To study the biliary tree in congenital biliary atresia.
5. To decompress the biliary tree prior to surgery.

The procedure is restricted to patients scheduled for surgery and it is performed an hour or two beforehand.

Roentgen Signs of Abnormality in Percutaneous Cholangiography

1. Calculi producing filling defects.
2. Obstructed duct (convexity upward) is usually due to a calculus.
3. Smooth narrowness of a short segment indicates stricture.
4. Duct rigid and irregular indicates carcinoma.
5. Dilatation of the duct with an uneven and ragged obstruction pattern indicates carcinoma of ampulla or pancreas (dilatation usually greater with pancreas).
6. Smooth, flat shallow obstruction with dilatation of the duct indicates ampullary carcinoma.
7. Tortuous and marked dilatation of ducts indicates pancreatic carcinoma. Obstructed end may be rounded, bulbous, tapered, or notched.

DIRECT CHOLANGIOGRAPHY

Introduction

There are two types of direct cholangiography: (1) operative cholangiography (at the time of operation); or (2) postoperative or T-tube cholangiography (during the postoperative period).

Cholangiography at the Time of Surgery should be performed in all cholecystectomy patients except in those who are seriously debilitated.

The T-tube Cholangiogram allows a study of the common bile duct in the postoperative period prior to removal of the T-tube. In this way, a determination of patency of the common bile duct is determined.

Questions — Chapter 26

1. List the various roentgenologic methods of study of the biliary system.

2. What is the value of the plain film of the abdomen in respect to the study of the biliary tract?

3. Describe the technique of oral cholecystography in respect to (1) contrast agent employed; (2) physiology of the procedure; (3) basic anatomy of radiographic visualization; (4) the interpretation of nonvisualization; (5) the preparation of the patient for oral cholecystography.

4. Describe briefly the film and fluoroscopic technique for oral cholecystography.

5. Describe the side effects to be anticipated with oral cholecystography.

6. What is the size of the normal gallbladder?

7. What is the interpretation of nonvisualization of the gallbladder based upon?

8. What are filling defects in the gallbladder due to? Indicate the various disease entities.

9. What is meant by "hyperplastic cholecystoses"?

10. What interpretation can you render for calcification of the gallbladder?

11. What is meant by the term "reappearing" or reformed gallbladder?

12. What is the relationship of gallbladder carcinoma to gallstones?

13. Indicate the accuracy of cholecystography in respect to patients' symptomatology. What morbidity might be anticipated following oral cholecystography?

14. Indicate the criteria and indications for intravenous cholangiography.

15. Describe the technique of intravenous cholangiography.

16. In what percentage of patients with an intact gallbladder and nonvisualization by oral cholecystography would you expect to visualize the gallbladder by the intravenous study?

17. How would you diagnose abnormalities in the size of the common bile duct and what interpretation would you render?

18. What are some of the abnormalities of contour of the common bile duct and their significance?

19. Describe different filling defects which might be expected within the common bile duct. How would they be interpreted?

20. How would you evaluate the contribution of intravenous cholangiography to diagnosis in patients with intact gallbladders?

21. How would you evaluate the contribution of intravenous cholangiography to diagnosis in postcholecystectomy patients?

22. Indicate the hazards of intravenous cholangiography.

23. Describe the technique of percutaneous cholangiography and its clinical indication.

24. Describe the roentgen signs of abnormality that might be anticipated with percutaneous cholangiography.

25. Indicate the evaluation of percutaneous cholangiography as a diagnostic or therapeutic method.

26. What techniques are available to us for direct cholangiography? Describe each briefly.

27. What complications might be anticipated from direct cholangiography?

28. Indicate the value of direct cholangiography in respect to clinical diagnosis.

27

Upper Alimentary Tract: Oropharynx, Laryngopharynx, and Esophagus

ROENTGEN SIGNS OF ABNORMALITY IN LATERAL SOFT TISSUE FILMS OF THE NECK

1. **Abnormalities in Size of the Soft Tissues.** The relative widths of the posterior oropharynx, the soft tissues of the neck, and the vertebral bodies are indicated in Figure 27–2. This is important in detection of inflammatory and neoplastic processes affecting these areas.

   Other soft tissues which may be increased in size in this area are
   a. the posterior tongue.
   b. the lymphoid tissues in the posterior oropharynx as well as the nasopharynx.
   c. the uvula.
2. **Alterations in the Size of the Air Space.** Increase in the size of the soft tissues of the oropharynx will inevitably encroach on the air space, clearly delineated on the soft tissues. These encroachments may occur adjoining the soft palate, adjoining the tongue, or extending into the vallecula.
3. **Abnormalities of Contour of the Soft Tissues or Air Space.**
4. **Abnormalities in the Architecture or Edge Pattern.** Even minimal irregularities of the tongue, the vallecula, and the oropharynx can be detected in good air space studies.
5. **Abnormalities of Function**
   a. Mobility studies of the soft palate in phonation have proved to be of value in the analysis of speech defects especially. They may be supplemented by cineradiographic examination and an associated study of the swallowing function, depending upon advisable exposure to radiation.
   b. The act of swallowing is best studied by cineradiography. Since swallowing involves not only an oral component but a pharyngeal and esophageal stage as well, this will be described in relation to the esophagus. Movements of the tongue, soft palate, and oropharyngeal muscles form a very important part of the act of swallowing. Video tape recording may be used if desired (less radiation exposure than cineradiography), but a kinescopic permanent record is preferable.

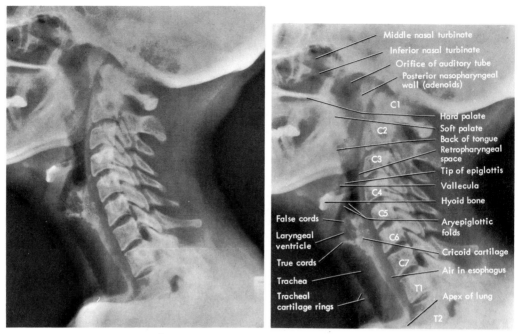

Figure 27–1 Lateral soft tissue film of neck.

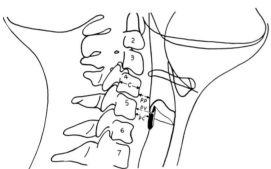

UPPER NORMAL LIMITS OF SOFT TISSUE SPACES OF NECK				
AGE	POSTPHARYNGEAL SOFT TISSUE		POSTLARYNGEAL SOFT TISSUE	
0–1	1.5 c		2. c	
1–2	.5 c		1.5 c	POSTVENTRICULAR
2–3	.5 c		1.2 c	
3–6	.4 c		1.2 c	
6–14	.3 c		1.2 c	
ADULT	MALE .3 c	FEMALE .3 c	MALE .7 c	FEMALE .6 c	POSTCRICOID

PV = POSTVENTRICULAR SOFT TISSUE
PP = POSTPHARYNGEAL SOFT TISSUE   PC = POSTCRICOID SOFT TISSUE
C = ANTERO-POSTERIOR DIMENSION OF C-4 VERTEBRAL BODY AT ITS MIDDLE

Figure 27–2 Relative widths of the posterior oropharynx and the soft tissues of the neck posterior to the larynx. (After Hay, P. D.: Ann. Roentgenol. *9*, 1930.)

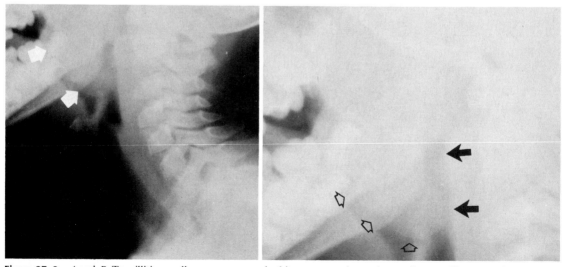

Figure 27–3 *A* and *B.* Tonsillitis: small open arrows and white arrows point to the swollen tonsillar mass. Closed black arrows show that this mass is distinct from the retropharyngeal space.

ROENTGEN SIGNS OF ABNORMALITY OF THE LARYNGOPHARYNX

Abnormalities of Size in respect to the air space or the adjoining soft tissues. This sign may be related to either inflammatory or neoplastic processes.

Abnormalities in Contour may be due to an increased rigidity of the laryngopharynx from invasion by an inflammatory or neoplastic process or by scarring. For example, scarring may be associated with certain skin disorders such as dermatomyositis and scleroderma.

Abnormalities in Architecture. Here as elsewhere these abnormalities may involve the edge pattern or the internal structure.

The Major Abnormalities of Edge Pattern include (1) diverticula of the pharynx, and (2) pharyngoceles.

PHARYNGEAL DIVERTICULA. True lateral pharyngeal diverticula are rare, although pseudodiverticula protruding between the thyroid cartilage and the hyoid bone at the level of the vallecula may frequently be noted (Fowler).

The muscle in this region is quite relaxed and bulging may occur under pressure, particularly in older people, in glass blowers, and in patients with choanal atresia.

The most frequent diverticula observed are the posterior hypopharyngeal pouches, also known as Zenker's or pulsion diverticula. They originate in the midline or the posterior wall in an area of weakness at the site of the cricopharyngeal muscles. When these diverticula become enlarged and retention of food results, symptoms of dysphagia and regurgitation of undigested food appear. A typical posterior hypopharyngeal diverticulum is shown in Figure 27–4.

Lateral pharyngeal diverticula are best shown during the pharyngeal phase of swallowing a thick barium suspension and by contrast oral laryngography while blowing through the closed lips. Ordinarily, they cause no symptoms and may measure up to 1.5 cm. in diameter. This diverticulum is best visualized in the frontal view.

Pharyngoceles at the level of the pyriform sinuses may be demonstrated by the Valsalva maneuver during laryngography. These are two diverticula-like extensions from the pyriform sinuses and must not be confused with marked distention of the pyriform sinuses that may occur normally under these circumstances.

As mentioned earlier, a distortion of the edge architecture of the pharynx may be associated with certain skin and ductal mucous membrane disorders. These include Behçet's disease, pemphigus, lichen planus, and occasionally collagen diseases such as dermatomyositis. Here, the marked irregularity and narrowness of the hypopharynx may be noted during the swallowing act.

Internal Architectural Abnormalities of the laryngopharynx may be either:
1. Intraluminal, or
2. Infiltrating.

NEOPLASMS are by far the most frequent etiologic agents. Laryngography plays a very important role in the demonstration of these lesions, since direct and laryngoscopic inspection of these lesions do not ordinarily demonstrate their full extent as well as laryngography.

WEBS may also distort the internal architecture of the upper esophagus or hypopharynx. Many seem to be situated at the pharyngoesophageal junction. They are best demonstrated by cineradiography at frame speeds of 15 to 30 frames per second (Seaman). The web appearance is of very short duration. The typical web arises on the anterior wall of the hypopharyngeal wall and thus may be differentiated from incompletely relaxed cricopharyngeal muscles that arise posteriorly. Even multiple webs may occur (Seaman).

The posterior cricoid impression is probably a normal variant and should not be confused with a web (Titman and Frazer). The clinical significance of webs is not clear, nor is the validity of the Plummer-Vinson syndrome sometimes said to be associated with this (Seaman). Indeed, every aspect of the Plummer-Vinson syndrome—dysphagia, esophageal web, and anemia—has been seriously questioned.

Functional Disorders of the Hypopharynx. Similar radiographic and spot film studies of this region are very helpful in respect to **phonatory abnormalities.** The **swallowing function** is best studied by single and multiple swallows of barium. The swallowing function and its derangements will be described in conjunction with the esophagus.

Cricomuscular esophageal spasm in patients with bulbar or pseudobulbar palsy from any cause (neuronitis or diphtheria among others) will frequently

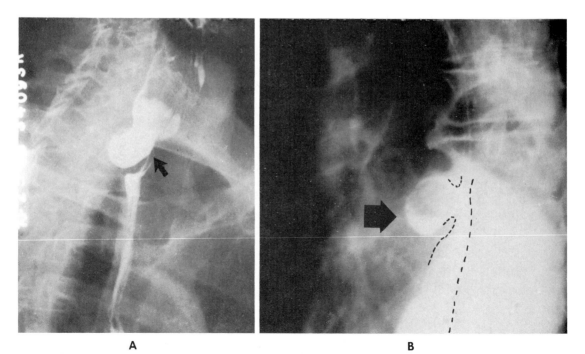

A   **B**

Figure 27–4   *A*. Radiograph demonstrating a pharyngeal pulsion diverticulum in the oblique projection. *B*. Pulsion-traction type diverticulum involving the lower one-third of the esophagus.

cause marked difficulty in swallowing. If the patient is encouraged to attempt swallowing, the barium streak is deflected at the level of the cricopharyngeal muscle and aspiration of the barium into the tracheoesophageal tree will result.

THE ESOPHAGUS

Normal Anatomy

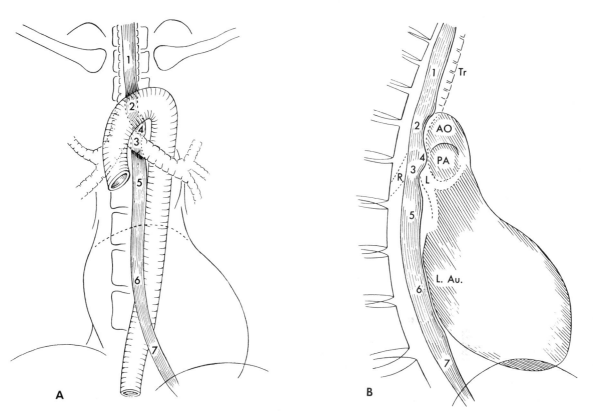

Figure 27–5   Segments of the esophagus. *A*. The segments of the thoracic esophagus (antero-posterior view): (1) paratracheal segment, (2) aortic segment, (3) bronchial segment, (4) interaorticobronchial triangle, (5) interbronchial segment, (6) retrocardiac segment, (7) epiphrenic segment.

   B. The segments of the esophagus (right anterior oblique view). Shown are: trachea (Tr), right (R) and left (L) main bronchi, pulmonary artery (PA), left auricle (L. Au), and the different segments of the paratracheal (1), aortic (2), bronchic (3), interaorticobronchial (4), interbronchial (5), retrocardiac (6), and epiphrenic (7) esophagus. (From Margulis, A. R., and Burhenne, H. J., (Eds.): *Alimentary Tract Roentgenology*. St. Louis, C. V. Mosby Co., 1967.)

   The *sites of normal constriction* in the esophagus are frequently areas of disease predilection. These are:

   At the pharyngoesophageal junction.

   At the bifurcation of the trachea and the indentation of the esophagus produced by the aortic knob (to the right and slightly posteriorly).

   At the minimal indentation and deflection produced by the left pulmonary artery and its close relationship to the left bronchus.

   At the slight area of narrowness of the esophagus as it passes through the esophageal hiatus of the diaphragm.

Basic Anatomic Concepts Regarding the Lower Esophagus.　There has been great interest and considerable confusion in relation to that segment of the esophagus just above the diaphragm and extending to the stomach (Lerche; Johnstone, 1959).

In an effort to clarify terminology in respect to this area, Wolf* has referred to the long narrow segment as the "submerged segment" and he further refers to A and B rings (Figure 27–6). In this terminology, the cardia (CO) is the orifice at the junction between the esophagus and the diaphragm and is normally situated beneath the diaphragm. The A ring was originally referred to by Lerche as the inferior esophageal sphincter and is an inconstant constriction at the superior margin of the esophageal ampulla. The B ring refers to the true mucosal junction between the esophagus and stomach when there is a hernia of the stomach above the diaphragm. The "submerged segment" is defined by the constrictor cardiae of the diaphragm.

The submerged segment functions most effectively when a portion of the esophagus lies beneath the diaphragm (esophageal vestibule), where the diaphragmatic contraction assists it in establishing a high pressure zone to prevent reflux from the stomach to the esophagus. It is when the fundus slides above the diaphragm through a patulous hiatus to create a hiatal hernia, that the function of this segment is most vulnerable and the barrier furnished by it to regurgitation may be inadequate to protect the lower esophagus from the refluxing digestive enzymes from the stomach.

---

*Wolf, B. S.: Amer. J. Digestive Dis., 5:751–769, 1960.

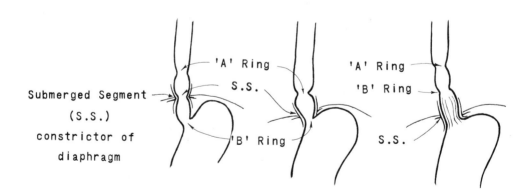

A　Ring – junction of esophagus
　　　　with esophageal
　　　　ampulla

'B' Ring –　gastroesophageal
　　　　junction

Appearance with sliding hiatal hernia

Figure 27–6　Anatomic concept of lower esophagus, modified from Wolf.*

Roentgen Signs of Abnormality in the Esophagus as Visualized in the Course of the Study

1. Prior to the introduction of barium:
   a. Increased density—indicates foreign body.
   b. Decreased density—indicates
      (1) Gaseous distention with scleroderma.
      (2) Gas in the upper part of an esophageal atresia.
      (3) Gas (and possibly fluid level) in diverticula, especially of the upper esophagus.
2. When barium is administered, the esophagus may be interrupted in its continuity by
   a. Esophageal atresia.
   b. Stenoses, strictures, carcinoma.
   c. Cricopharyngeal spasm (pseudobulbar palsy).
3. The esophagus may be shorter than normal due to
   a. Congenital shortening.
   b. Acquired shortening from inflammation, as in esophagitis, esophageal ulceration, scleroderma, hiatal herniation.
4. The esophagus may be larger than normal from
   a. Achalasia.
   b. Longer than normal with presbyesophagus, esophageal curling, hypertrophic esophageal musculature.
   c. Chalasia.
5. The esophagus may undergo segmental spasm in the upper or lower esophagus.
6. The esophagus may be displaced by local indentations that are abnormal:
   a. Enlarged thyroid.
   b. Vertebral body spurs.
   c. Pulmonary fibrosis.
   d. Mediastinal tumors.
   e. Aberrant vessels arising from the aortic arch or in the region of the pulmonary outflow tract.
   f. An enlarged left atrium.
   g. Aortic aneurysm.
   h. Elongated aorta, or pseudocoarctation of the aorta.
   i. Coarctation of the aorta.
   j. Intramural esophageal tumors.
7. The esophagus may not join the stomach in normal fashion due to:
   a. Hiatal herniation.
   b. Esophageal ulceration with local irregularity.
   c. Schatzki ring.
   d. Esophagogastric carcinoma.
   e. Fistulation, or esophageal rupture.
   f. Epiphrenic diverticulum.
8. A careful study of the intrinsic architecture of the rugae of the esophagus may show:
   a. Cobblestone effect from varices or esophageal moniliasis.
   b. Esophageal ulcer.
   c. Benign or malignant tumor.
9. A careful study for gastroesophageal reflux may show excessive reflux to or above the carina or a positive water test.

Abnormalities in Size

Esophageal Atresia

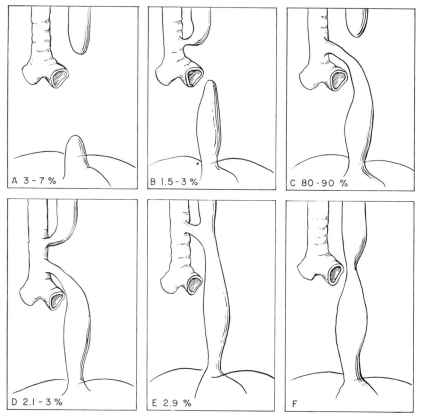

Figure 27–7 *A* to *F*. Classification of esophageal atresia by gross statistical incidence. (From Jones, J. D.: South. Med. J., *52*:1485, 1959.)

The Acquired Abnormally Short Esophagus.   A shortened esophagus may also result from chronic inflammatory disease of the lower esophagus such as may occur with peptic ulceration of the esophagus, caustic ulceration or scleroderma (Chunn and Geppert).

Abnormalities of Diameter

1. Marked dilatation of the esophagus in association with an over-active esophagogastric junction—*achalasia or megaesophagus* (Figure 27–8).

2. *Chalasia*—widely patent esophagogastric junction, with no barrier to regurgitation from the esophagus to the stomach (Figure 27–9).

3. *Cicatricial stenoses or strictures,* resulting from caustic ulceration of the esophagus and scar formation (Figure 27–10).

4. *Esophageal spasm* (Figure 27–11).

5. Diminutions of diameter of the esophagus by *tumor encroachment,* either benign or malignant, sometimes associated with dilatation of the esophagus above the level of partial obstruction. (This discussion is deferred to another section in this chapter.)

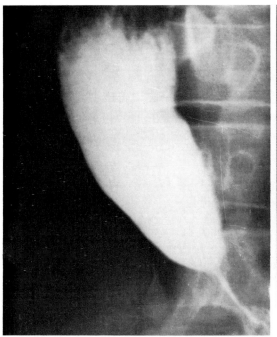

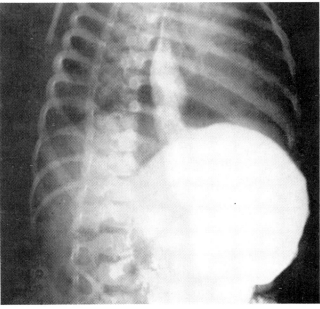

Figure 27–9 Radiograph demonstrating esophageal chalasia.

Figure 27–8 Radiograph demonstrating the esophagus in achalasia. Note the fusiform tapered distal end of the esophagus and the redundancy and dilatation of the esophagus above this level.

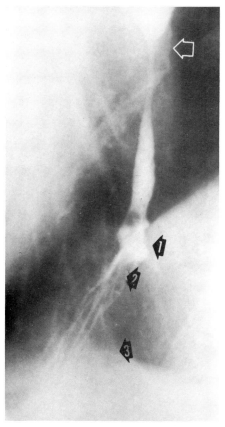

Figure 27–10 Esophageal narrowness following esophageal ulceration with hiatal hernia. Open arrow shows esophageal stricture and thickened wall of the esophagus; (1) site of esophageal ulceration; (2) hiatal hernia; (3) left hemidiaphragm.

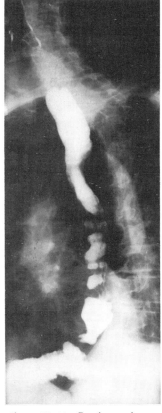

Figure 27–11 Presbyesophagus.

Abnormalities of Position

Displacement by Contiguous Structures

Indentations or displacements by vertebral body spurs. This is particularly apt to occur in the cervical portion of the esophagus.

Displacement by an enlargement of the thyroid. Enlargement of the thyroid gland (goiter) may at times displace the esophagus either to the right or to the left, or at times the goiterous thyroid may be situated between the trachea and esophagus, in which case the esophagus is displaced posteriorly. Substernal extension of the thyroid gland in particular may be associated with dysphagia (also see Chapter 21).

Displacement of the esophagus by pulmonary fibrosis. Long-standing fibrotic alterations in the lung such as may occur with chronic infectious granulomas or marked thickening of the pleura, may cause a deflection of the esophagus.

Displacement by mediastinal tumors (lymphomas and others). See Chapter 21.

Displacement by an aberrant right subclavian artery produces a compression of the trachea or esophagus which may result from impression by vascular bands or rings in association with malformation of the aortic arch.

Displacement by a right-sided aortic arch. (See also Chapter 23.) Here, the esophagus in the region of the aortic knob is displaced to the left instead of to the right. It may or may not descend completely on the left side of the aorta posteriorly.

Displacement by an enlarged left atrium. See Chapter 22.

Displacement by an aortic aneurysm. See Chapter 22.

Displacement by an elongated aorta. See Chapter 22.

Abnormalities of Density

Since for the most part examination of the esophagus involves the administration of barium, the abnormalities of this structure have not been related to density. However, simple density alterations may be manifest in three ways:

1. Alteration in the posterior mediastinal esophageal line or stripe.
2. Increased thickness of the esophageal wall.
3. Increased and persistent air content in the esophagus or a portion of it.
4. Foreign bodies in the esophagus (discussed subsequently).

Abnormality of Esophageal Position Resulting from Hiatal Hernia

Hiatal hernia may be of three types (Figure 27–12):

1. Related to a congenitally short esophagus (previously discussed).
2. Para-esophageal hernia—encased in a peritoneal envelope, the esophagogastric junction remains near the diaphragm.
3. Sliding hiatal hernia.

HERNIATIONS

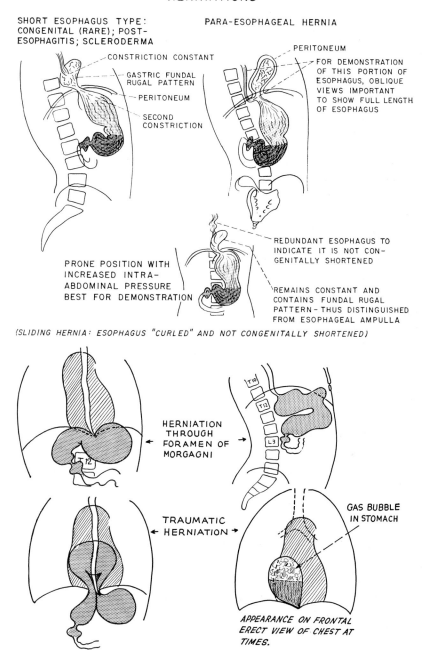

SHORT ESOPHAGUS TYPE:
CONGENITAL (RARE); POST-
ESOPHAGITIS; SCLERODERMA

CONSTRICTION CONSTANT

GASTRIC FUNDAL
RUGAL PATTERN

PERITONEUM

SECOND
CONSTRICTION

PARA-ESOPHAGEAL HERNIA

PERITONEUM

FOR DEMONSTRATION
OF THIS PORTION OF
ESOPHAGUS, OBLIQUE
VIEWS IMPORTANT
TO SHOW FULL LENGTH
OF ESOPHAGUS

PRONE POSITION WITH
INCREASED INTRA-
ABDOMINAL PRESSURE
BEST FOR DEMONSTRATION

REDUNDANT ESOPHAGUS TO
INDICATE IT IS NOT CON-
GENITALLY SHORTENED

REMAINS CONSTANT AND
CONTAINS FUNDAL RUGAL
PATTERN - THUS DISTINGUISHED
FROM ESOPHAGEAL AMPULLA

(SLIDING HERNIA: ESOPHAGUS "CURLED" AND NOT CONGENITALLY SHORTENED)

HERNIATION
THROUGH
FORAMEN OF
MORGAGNI

TRAUMATIC
HERNIATION

GAS BUBBLE
IN STOMACH

*APPEARANCE ON FRONTAL
ERECT VIEW OF CHEST AT
TIMES.*

Figure 27–12 Summary diagram illustrating herniations of the stomach through the diaphragm.

Whenever a hiatal hernia is demonstrated, it is important to determine whether or not free reflux from the stomach into the esophagus, at least to the level of the bifurcation of the trachea, occurs in the recumbent position under ordinary gravitational circumstances (Texter et al.).

Abnormalities in Contour and Architectural Pattern of the Esophagus

The Internal and Edge Architecture and Contour of the esophagus are not actually separable roentgen signs, since often the edge architecture may also alter contour; and intrinsic architecture may be altered along with the edge architecture of the esophagus.

STENOSES have previously been considered as an alteration in size (diameter) of the esophagus.

DIVERTICULA OF THE ESOPHAGUS (Figure 27–13). These are usually classified into three types (a fourth type is listed here as "intramural diverticulosis").

The Pharyngeal or Zenker Type Diverticulum has been previously described in the section dealing with the pharynx.

ESOPHAGEAL DIVERTICULA   (APART FROM PHARYNGEAL TYPE)

TRACTION TYPE

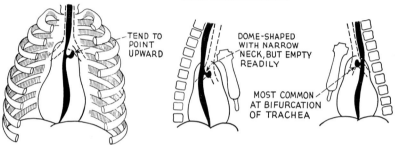

EPIPHRENIC TRACTION-PULSION TYPE

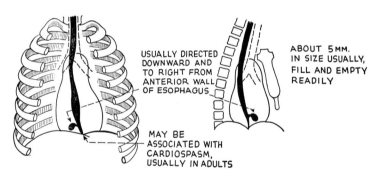

Figure 27–13

Esophagitis

ACUTE ESOPHAGITIS. Trauma from an indwelling tube, infection by a bacterial or mycotic invader, or perhaps even hypersensitivity processes may produce a marked irregularity of the esophagus with numerous indentations occurring along the wall and a "cobblestone" appearance throughout its length (Figure 27–14). The thickened, disorganized and cobblestone appearance of the entire esophagus resembles closely the changes in architecture which occur primarily in the lower third with esophageal varices (esophageal moniliasis).

PEPTIC OR REFLUX ESOPHAGITIS, with or without hiatus hernia. This may be associated with esophageal ulceration and ultimately fibrosing stenosis or shortening of the esophagus. The irregularity, ulceration, and alteration in architecture at times is difficult to distinguish from invasive carcinoma. Ordinarily, however, the esophagus is not quite as rigid, the tapering of the esophagus is gradual and smooth and there is an associated hiatal herniation, which does not frequently occur with carcinoma of the esophagus.

Esophageal Ulcer (Figure 27–10). An ulcer of the esophagus is demonstrated as a persistent niche with irregularities usually present in the adjoining esophageal architectural pattern. Esophageal ulcers are of three types:

1. Ulcerations occurring with duodenal or gastric ulcer.

2. Ulcers situated at the esophagogastric junction, usually in association with hiatus hernia.

3. Ulcers in heterotopic gastric mucosa in the lower esophagus (Barrett's ulcer) (Wolf, Som, and Marshak; Wright).

Esophageal Varices (Figure 27–16). Esophageal varices are related to an increased portal venous pressure, most often resulting from cirrhosis of the liver. Hematemesis is frequent. The fundus of the stomach may also be involved.

The venous drainage of the lower one-third of the esophagus passes to the coronary vein of the stomach, and the latter vein empties into the portal vein. Higher up, the veins of the esophagus empty into the azygos system and thyroid veins, which in turn empty into the superior vena cava. Thus, the lower esophagus and upper stomach form a communicating link between the portal circulation on the one hand, and the systemic veins on the other.

An increase in portal venous pressure will reflect itself in the formation of esophageal varices. Any procedure which accentuates intra-abdominal pressure will produce an accentuated appearance of the esophageal (and gastric) varices. The varices may disappear completely in the presence of a negative intrathoracic pressure. *The radiographic appearance and disappearance of these cobblestone filling defects in the lower one-third of the esophagus is pathognomonic of esophageal varices.*

Radiographically, varices appear as small, rounded translucent, irregular wormlike defects in the wall of the lower esophagus, causing a disruption of the parallel rugal pattern. Ordinarily, the dilated veins are less prominent when the patient is erect and most prominent when the patient is prone, particularly when Valsalva and Müller maneuvers are employed.

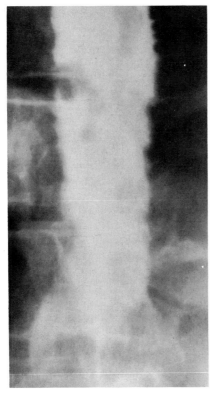

Figure 27–14 Monilial esophagitis producing the irregular "coiled worm" appearance.

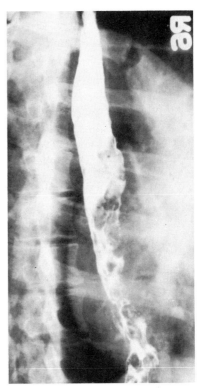

Figure 27–15 Esophagram demonstrating marked irregularities due to esophageal varices.

ESOPHAGEAL   VARICES

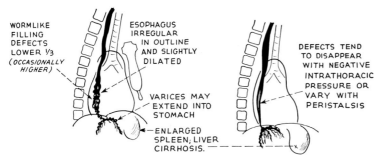

WORMLIKE
FILLING
DEFECTS
LOWER ⅓
(OCCASIONALLY
HIGHER)

ESOPHAGUS
IRREGULAR
IN OUTLINE
AND SLIGHTLY
DILATED

VARICES MAY
EXTEND INTO
STOMACH

ENLARGED
SPLEEN; LIVER
CIRRHOSIS.

DEFECTS TEND
TO DISAPPEAR
WITH NEGATIVE
INTRATHORACIC
PRESSURE OR
VARY WITH
PERISTALSIS

FORCED EXPIRATION
WITH INCREASED
INTRA ABDOMINAL PRESSURE

INSPIRATION WITH
NEGATIVE INTRATHORACIC
PRESSURE

Figure 27–16 Diagrams illustrating the radiographic appearances in association with esophageal varices. Note that with forced expiration there is increased intrathoracic pressure and an accentuation of the appearance of the esophageal varices, which may virtually disappear when the negative intrathoracic pressure is restored.

ETIOLOGY : 1. PORTAL VEIN OBSTRUCTION.
           2. THROMBOSIS SPLENIC VEIN.

SPECIAL TECHNIQUE : 1. MODERATELY THICK BARIUM (NOT TOO THICK).
               2. RADIOGRAPHS IN FORCED EXPIRATION and FULL
                  INSPIRATION.
               3. ALWAYS COMBINE FLUOROSCOPY WITH SPECIAL FILMS.
               4. PATIENT PRONE.

Foreign Bodies. Eighty to ninety per cent of foreign bodies become lodged in the upper third of the esophagus (Terracol and Sweet). If the foreign body persists without removal, cough may supervene due to aspiration of esophageal fluids or saliva into the tracheobronchial tree.

If the foreign body is discoid in type it will usually occupy a position in the coronal plane of the esophagus and can be readily differentiated from a similar discoid object lodged in the trachea, where usually it occupies a position in the sagittal plane. There are exceptions to this rule, and further careful study is necessary.

With small foreign bodies, an air bubble may be observed in the esophageal lumen above or surrounding the object.

Perforation of the esophagus by the foreign body with resultant para-esophageal abscess and mediastinitis may result.

Benign Tumors of the Esophagus (Figure 27–17)

These may be intramural, extramural, or both, and they include polyps, lipomas, myomas, hemangiomas, and neurofibromas. They may have a long pedicle and protrude directly into the stomach.

When the lesions are extramural, an increased soft tissue density adjoining the esophagus can usually be seen with some evidence of impression upon, or filling defect within, the lumen of the esophagus. The margins are usually smooth. Sometimes the stream of barium flowing through the esophagus at the level of the lesion produces a "forked-stream" appearance, the barium stream being diverted on either side of the defect (Gibbon et al.).

Malignant Tumors of the Esophagus may be of three general types (Figure 27–17):
1. Papillary or fungating.
2. Ulcerating.
3. Infiltrating.

PRIMARY SARCOMAS OF THE ESOPHAGUS are rare and are usually of smooth muscle origin (leiomyosarcoma). In rare instances, tumors in the upper third of the esophagus may arise from striated muscle tissue (rhabdomyosarcoma).

RADIOLOGIC FINDINGS OF CARCINOMA OF THE ESOPHAGUS (Fig. 27–18):
1. Soft tissue mass lesions surrounding the carcinoma site.
2. Deficient peristalsis.
3. Irregularities of the esophageal wall or rugal pattern.
4. Partial or complete obstruction of the flow of barium at the level of the carcinoma.
5. Dilatation may occur above the level of the carcinoma although this is not universal and occurs much less than with stricture or achalasia.
6. The invasive carcinoma will, in addition, usually produce a napkin-ring-like, irregular tumefaction encroaching on the wall of the esophagus with a shelf above and below the involved region.

FILLING DEFECTS OF THE ESOPHAGUS

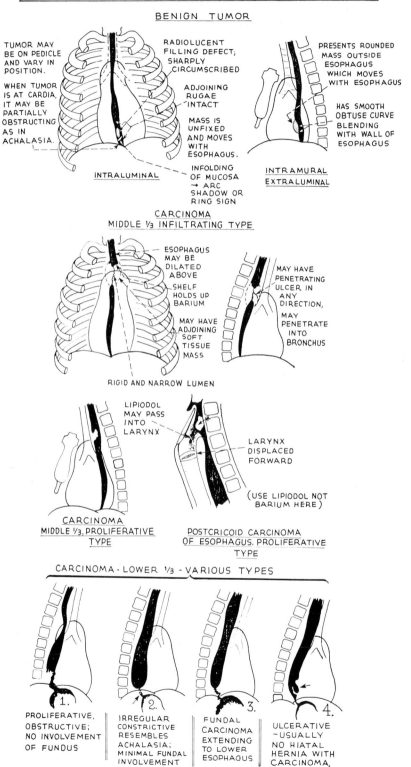

BENIGN TUMOR

TUMOR MAY BE ON PEDICLE AND VARY IN POSITION.

WHEN TUMOR IS AT CARDIA, IT MAY BE PARTIALLY OBSTRUCTING AS IN ACHALASIA.

RADIOLUCENT FILLING DEFECT; SHARPLY CIRCUMSCRIBED

ADJOINING RUGAE INTACT

MASS IS UNFIXED AND MOVES WITH ESOPHAGUS.

INTRALUMINAL

INFOLDING OF MUCOSA → ARC SHADOW OR RING SIGN

PRESENTS ROUNDED MASS OUTSIDE ESOPHAGUS WHICH MOVES WITH ESOPHAGUS

HAS SMOOTH OBTUSE CURVE BLENDING WITH WALL OF ESOPHAGUS

INTRAMURAL EXTRALUMINAL

CARCINOMA
MIDDLE ⅓ INFILTRATING TYPE

ESOPHAGUS MAY BE DILATED ABOVE

SHELF HOLDS UP BARIUM

MAY HAVE ADJOINING SOFT TISSUE MASS

MAY HAVE PENETRATING ULCER IN ANY DIRECTION, MAY PENETRATE INTO BRONCHUS

RIGID AND NARROW LUMEN

LIPIODOL MAY PASS INTO LARYNX

LARYNX DISPLACED FORWARD

(USE LIPIODOL NOT BARIUM HERE)

CARCINOMA
MIDDLE ⅓, PROLIFERATIVE TYPE

POSTCRICOID CARCINOMA OF ESOPHAGUS, PROLIFERATIVE TYPE

CARCINOMA - LOWER ⅓ - VARIOUS TYPES

1. PROLIFERATIVE, OBSTRUCTIVE; NO INVOLVEMENT OF FUNDUS

2. IRREGULAR CONSTRICTIVE RESEMBLES ACHALASIA; MINIMAL FUNDAL INVOLVEMENT

3. FUNDAL CARCINOMA EXTENDING TO LOWER ESOPHAGUS

4. ULCERATIVE -USUALLY NO HIATAL HERNIA WITH CARCINOMA,

Figure 27–17

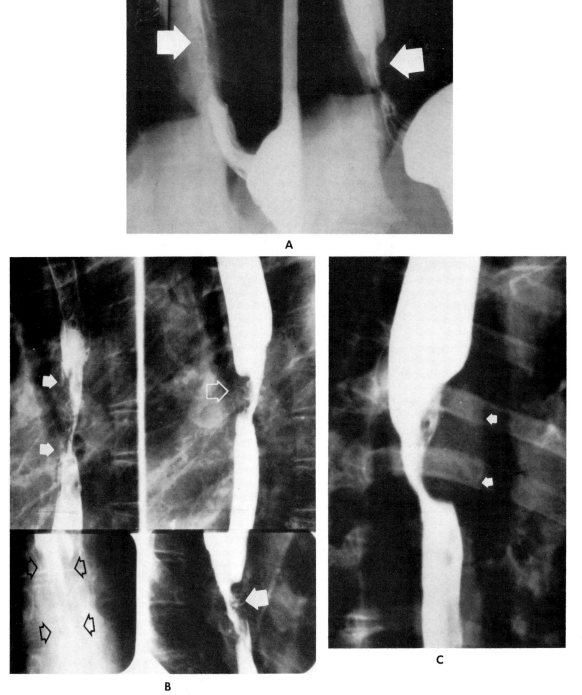

Figure 27–18 *A* and *B*. Representative radiographs of carcinoma of the esophagus. *C*. Carcinoma of esophagus simulating somewhat an intramural esophageal tumor of the upper third.

Abnormalities of Function of the Esophagus

Pharyngo-esophageal Spasm (has been described earlier in relation to the pharynx).

Gastroesophageal Reflux. This is usually associated with hiatal hernia.

Scleroderma. In scleroderma, there is diminished or absent peristalsis of the esophagus and esophageal emptying occurs virtually by gravity (Tatelman and Keech; Treacy). The pathologic sequence is as follows: swelling of the esophagus, induration, atrophy, stricture, and ultimately shortening of the esophagus, sometimes associated with hiatal herniation. In these latter circumstances, a stricture may form above the level of the diaphragm (Figure 27–19).

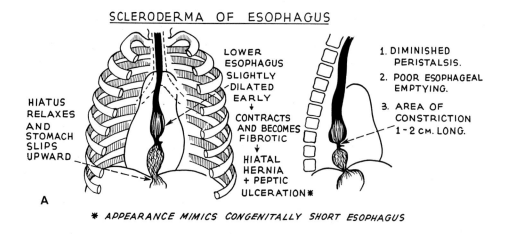

SCLERODERMA OF ESOPHAGUS

LOWER ESOPHAGUS SLIGHTLY DILATED EARLY
↓
CONTRACTS AND BECOMES FIBROTIC
↓
HIATAL HERNIA + PEPTIC ULCERATION *

HIATUS RELAXES AND STOMACH SLIPS UPWARD

1. DIMINISHED PERISTALSIS.
2. POOR ESOPHAGEAL EMPTYING.
3. AREA OF CONSTRICTION 1-2 CM. LONG.

A

* APPEARANCE MIMICS CONGENITALLY SHORT ESOPHAGUS

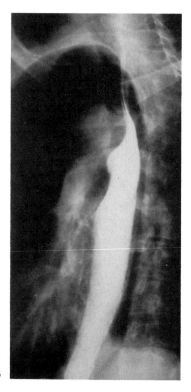

Figure 27–19 *A.* Line diagrams demonstrating the radiographic appearances in association with scleroderma of the esophagus. *B.* Scleroderma of the esophagus. The tubular appearance of the esophagus without peristalsis with mild or moderate dilatation is characteristic.

B

Prior to this period, the esophagus presents a tubular immobile appearance radiographically.

Somewhat similar changes have been recorded in a lesser number of patients with systemic lupus erythematosus but not in long-standing rheumatoid arthritis.

These diseases are closely related collagen disorders and may even be combined in one patient (Stevens; Alarcon-Segovia and Osmundson).

Questions — Chapter 27

1. What is the importance of the width of the soft tissue space in the retropharynx?

2. Where are the normal indentations upon the esophagus found? What is the significance of barium in the esophagus in respect to the delineation of mediastinal structures?

3. What is meant by the following terms: esophageal vestibule; A ring; B ring; esophageal ampulla; Schatzki's ring; esophageal lip; submerged segment of the esophagus; gastro-esophageal reflux?

4. Describe the roentgen findings in esophageal atresia.

5. What are some of the causes of an acquired abnormally short esophagus? What sequelae may be anticipated as the result of such findings?

6. What is the roentgen appearance of achalasia of the esophagus? of chalasia?

7. What is the roentgen appearance of esophageal spasm? Where are segmental spasms usually located?

8. What is meant by the following terms: esophageal curling; presbyesophagus; elevator esophagus?

9. What are some of the reasons which produce displacement of the esophagus? What is their clinical importance?

10. What type of displacement might be anticipated from the following: an aberrant right subclavian artery; a right sided aortic arch; an enlarged left atrium; an aortic aneurysm; an elongated aorta; pseudocoarctation of the aorta?

11. What are the three types of hiatal hernia and what is their pathologic significance? Which of these are most apt to be associated with symptoms?

12. What are the four types of diverticula of the esophagus? What is their pathologic significance?

13. Describe the various types of esophagitis which can be identified. What is the roentgen appearance of esophageal moniliasis?

14. Describe the roentgen appearances which may be associated with esophageal ulcer.

15. Describe the roentgen appearances which may be associated with esophageal varices.

16. Describe the roentgen appearances associated with intramural tumors of the esophagus.

17. Describe the roentgen findings in malignant tumors of the esophagus. What varieties are there? What are the general roentgen signs of carcinoma in particular?

18. Classify the various abnormalities of function of the esophagus.

19. Describe the roentgen appearance of scleroderma involving the esophagus.

28

Stomach, Duodenum, and Pancreas

STOMACH — NORMAL ANATOMY

Gross Anatomy

Subdivisions of the Stomach and Duodenum. Generally accepted subdivisions of the stomach into fundus, body, antrum, prepyloric and pyloric regions, duodenal bulb, and duodenum are indicated in Figure 28–1.

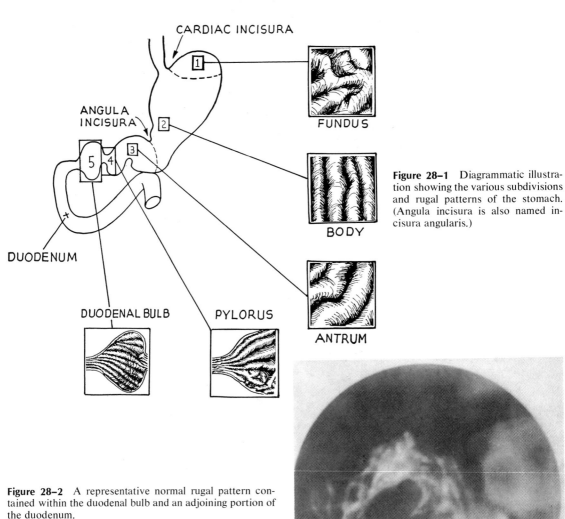

Figure 28–1 Diagrammatic illustration showing the various subdivisions and rugal patterns of the stomach. (Angula incisura is also named incisura angularis.)

Figure 28–2 A representative normal rugal pattern contained within the duodenal bulb and an adjoining portion of the duodenum.

Radiographic Anatomy

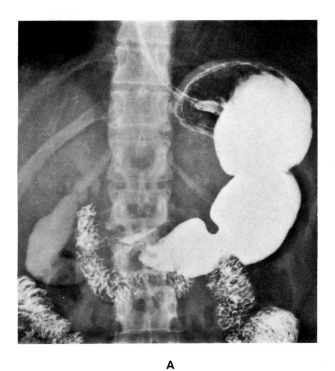

A

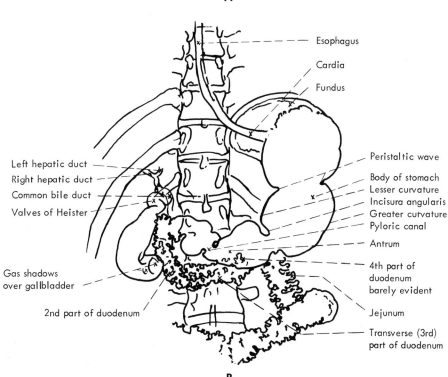

B

Figure 28–3 *A*. Recumbent postero-anterior projection of stomach and duodenum. (An oral cholecystogram was also obtained at this time in the film illustrated.) *B*. Tracing of *A*.

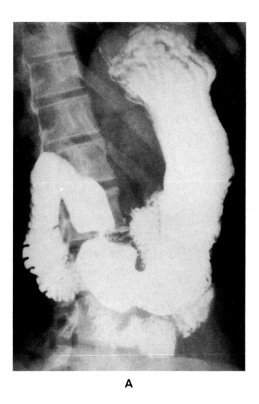

A

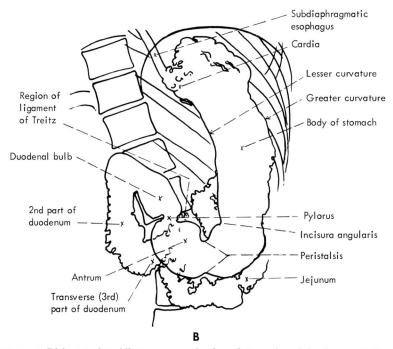

B

Figure 28–4 *A*. Right anterior oblique prone projection of stomach and duodenum. *B*. Tracing of *A*.

DUODENUM

Normal Gross Anatomy

Figure 28–5 Normal relationships of the bile ducts to the duodenum, and the normal mucosal patterns of the duodenum proper.

Radiographic Anatomy

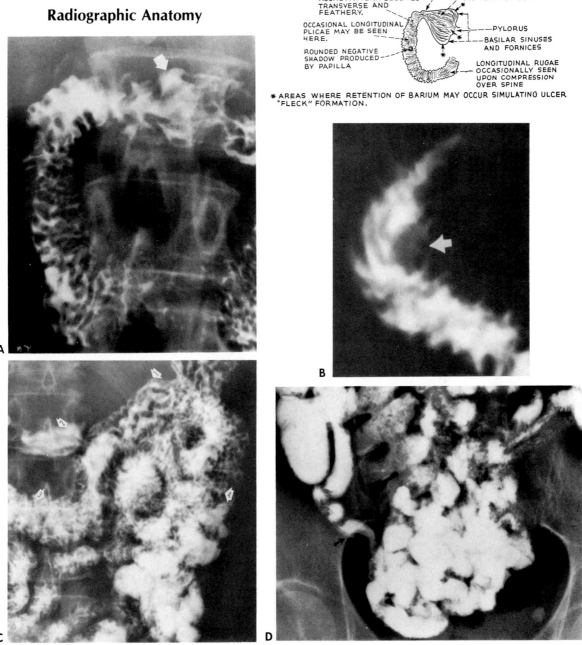

Figure 28–6 *A.* The mucosal pattern of the second and third parts of the duodenum are magnified to show good detail. There is, however, an ulceration in the superior aspect of the duodenal bulb (arrow).

B. Magnified coned-down view of the major papilla in the midportion of the second part of the duodenum and the adjoining rugae of the second part of the duodenum. Occasionally the only manifestation of pancreatic abnormality may be an enlargement of the shadow of the major papilla.

C. Mucosal pattern of the jejunum in the left upper quadrant. Arrow 1 points to the mucosal pattern of the stomach; arrow 2, to the duodenal bulb; arrow 3, to the transverse part of the duodenum; and arrow 4, to the jejunal pattern per se.

D. The clumped normal pattern of the ileum. The terminal ileum as it arises out of the pelvis minor is indicated by the arrow.

Roentgen Signs of Abnormality of Gastroduodenal Disease

Abnormalities in Size

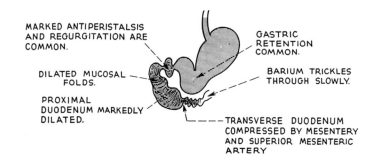

MARKED ANTIPERISTALSIS AND REGURGITATION ARE COMMON.

GASTRIC RETENTION COMMON.

DILATED MUCOSAL FOLDS.

BARIUM TRICKLES THROUGH SLOWLY.

PROXIMAL DUODENUM MARKEDLY DILATED.

TRANSVERSE DUODENUM COMPRESSED BY MESENTERY AND SUPERIOR MESENTERIC ARTERY

1. MAY PREDISPOSE TO DUODENAL ULCER.
2. CLINICAL HISTORY: RECURRING DIGESTIVE DISTURBANCES AND EVIDENCE OF UPPER GASTROINTESTINAL OBSTRUCTION.

A

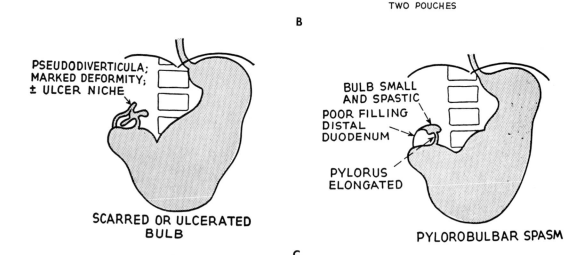

MID-DUODENAL DIAPHRAGM

DILATED

NARROWED AND MAY BE COLLAPSED

MID-DUODENAL CORDLIKE ATRESIA

NO GAS

MID-DUODENAL AGENESIS

NO GAS

NO VESTIGE OF BOWEL BETWEEN TWO POUCHES

B

PSEUDODIVERTICULA; MARKED DEFORMITY; ± ULCER NICHE

SCARRED OR ULCERATED BULB

BULB SMALL AND SPASTIC

POOR FILLING DISTAL DUODENUM

PYLORUS ELONGATED

PYLOROBULBAR SPASM

C

Figure 28–7 *A.* Radiographic appearance associated with duodenal stasis from compression by mesenteric vessels. *B.* Various types of duodenal atresia. *C.* Note that the first sign of obstruction is a downward "bulge" of the greater curvature of the antrum.

THE ENLARGED STOMACH

1. Atony or ileus
2. Vagotomy
3. Benign pyloric obstruction (as with peptic disease or hypertrophic pyloric stenosis)
    a. Gastric rugae persist despite hypersecretion
    b. Retained fluid is homogeneous and barium layers out
4. Pyloroantral malignancy with secondary obstruction
    a. Hyposecretion
    b. Rugae tend to become obliterated
    c. Retained fluid is nonhomogeneous, with less tendency to layering of barium
5. Achlorhydria and gastric atrophy
6. Foreign bodies within the stomach
    a. Bezoars
7. Secondary to duodenal abnormalities beyond the bulb
    a. Hereditary megaduodenum
    b. Superior mesenteric ileus (secondary to Ladd's bands or anomalous superior mesenteric artery)
    c. Duodenal web
    d. Duodenal and jejunal atresias and stenosis

THE SMALL, CONTRACTED STOMACH

1. Microgastria
2. Postoperative subtotal gastric resection
3. Linitis plastica from any cause (malignancy or chronic inflammatory diseases)

Abnormalities of Position — Intrinsic

Transposition of the Viscera, Situs Inversus (See Chapter 23)

Cascade Stomach

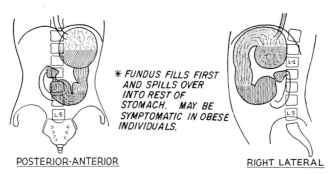

* *FUNDUS FILLS FIRST AND SPILLS OVER INTO REST OF STOMACH. MAY BE SYMPTOMATIC IN OBESE INDIVIDUALS.*

POSTERIOR-ANTERIOR   RIGHT LATERAL

Figure 28–8

Organoaxial Rotation

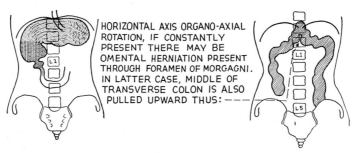

HORIZONTAL AXIS ORGANO-AXIAL ROTATION, IF CONSTANTLY PRESENT THERE MAY BE OMENTAL HERNIATION PRESENT THROUGH FORAMEN OF MORGAGNI. IN LATTER CASE, MIDDLE OF TRANSVERSE COLON IS ALSO PULLED UPWARD THUS: ———

Figure 28–9

Herniation of the Stomach.   Herniation of the stomach through the diaphragm may occur through any of the orifices of the diaphragm or through a traumatic orifice. Hiatal hernia has been previously described in Chapter 27.

Duodenal Anomalies

DEFECTIVE ATTACHMENT OF DUODENAL MESENTERY

MOBILE DUODENUM

DUODENUM APPEARS INVERTED AND BEGINS IN SECOND PART RECUMBENT

DUODENUM HAS NORMAL APPEARANCE

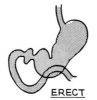

ERECT

REDUNDANCY – FIRST PART

INVERTED DUODENUM

MAY PREDISPOSE TO PANCREATITIS DUE TO TWIST OF BILE DUCT AND REFLUX INTO PANCREAS.

NONROTATION OF DUODENUM

LOWER DUODENUM CURVES TO RIGHT INSTEAD OF LEFT AND JOINS JEJUNUM IN RIGHT UPPER QUADRANT *(USUALLY NONROTATION OF JEJUNUM ALSO.)*

NOT INVOLVED *(ARISES FROM FOREGUT)*

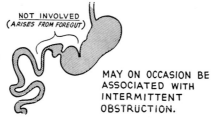

MAY ON OCCASION BE ASSOCIATED WITH INTERMITTENT OBSTRUCTION.

REDUNDANCY- 3rd PART

Figure 28–10

Abnormalities of Position — Extrinsic

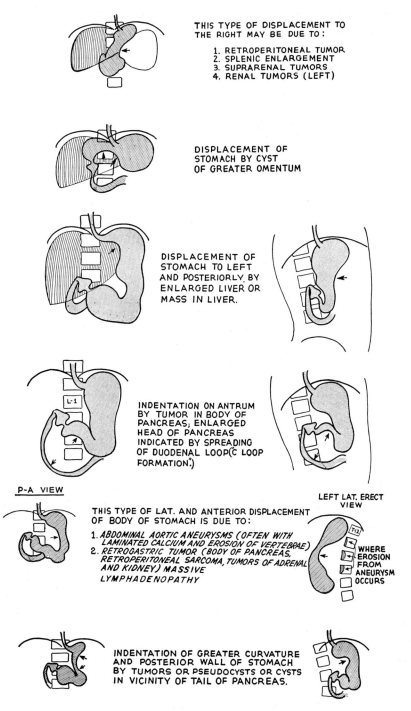

THIS TYPE OF DISPLACEMENT TO THE RIGHT MAY BE DUE TO:

1. RETROPERITONEAL TUMOR
2. SPLENIC ENLARGEMENT
3. SUPRARENAL TUMORS
4. RENAL TUMORS (LEFT)

DISPLACEMENT OF STOMACH BY CYST OF GREATER OMENTUM

DISPLACEMENT OF STOMACH TO LEFT AND POSTERIORLY BY ENLARGED LIVER OR MASS IN LIVER.

INDENTATION ON ANTRUM BY TUMOR IN BODY OF PANCREAS; ENLARGED HEAD OF PANCREAS INDICATED BY SPREADING OF DUODENAL LOOP (C LOOP FORMATION.)

P-A VIEW

LEFT LAT. ERECT VIEW

THIS TYPE OF LAT. AND ANTERIOR DISPLACEMENT OF BODY OF STOMACH IS DUE TO:

1. *ABDOMINAL AORTIC ANEURYSMS (OFTEN WITH LAMINATED CALCIUM AND EROSION OF VERTEBRAE)*
2. *RETROGASTRIC TUMOR (BODY OF PANCREAS, RETROPERITONEAL SARCOMA, TUMORS OF ADRENAL AND KIDNEY) MASSIVE LYMPHADENOPATHY*

WHERE EROSION FROM ANEURYSM OCCURS

INDENTATION OF GREATER CURVATURE AND POSTERIOR WALL OF STOMACH BY TUMORS OR PSEUDOCYSTS OR CYSTS IN VICINITY OF TAIL OF PANCREAS.

Figure 28–11 Abnormalities of position and shape of the stomach due to displacement by extragastric forces.

Abnormalities of Position—Predominantly Extrinsic Impressions on Duodenum

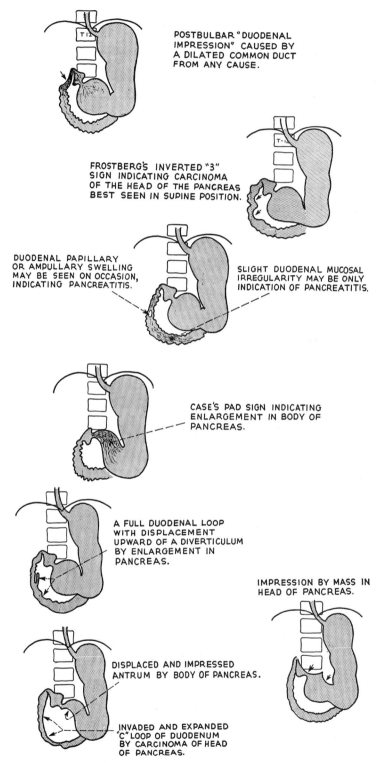

POSTBULBAR "DUODENAL IMPRESSION" CAUSED BY A DILATED COMMON DUCT FROM ANY CAUSE.

FROSTBERG'S INVERTED "3" SIGN INDICATING CARCINOMA OF THE HEAD OF THE PANCREAS BEST SEEN IN SUPINE POSITION.

DUODENAL PAPILLARY OR AMPULLARY SWELLING MAY BE SEEN ON OCCASION, INDICATING PANCREATITIS.

SLIGHT DUODENAL MUCOSAL IRREGULARITY MAY BE ONLY INDICATION OF PANCREATITIS.

CASE'S PAD SIGN INDICATING ENLARGEMENT IN BODY OF PANCREAS.

A FULL DUODENAL LOOP WITH DISPLACEMENT UPWARD OF A DIVERTICULUM BY ENLARGEMENT IN PANCREAS.

IMPRESSION BY MASS IN HEAD OF PANCREAS.

DISPLACED AND IMPRESSED ANTRUM BY BODY OF PANCREAS.

INVADED AND EXPANDED "C" LOOP OF DUODENUM BY CARCINOMA OF HEAD OF PANCREAS.

Figure 28–12 Extragastric duodenal displacements.

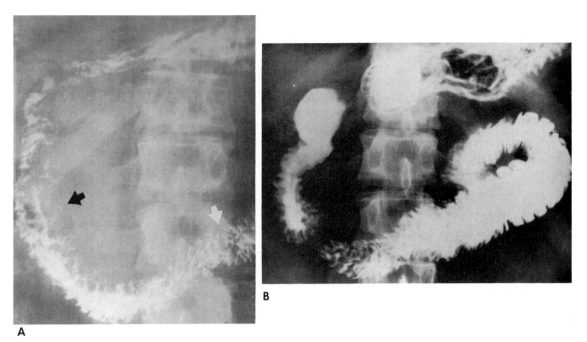

Figure 28–13 *A*. Radiograph demonstrating the duodenal loop in a patient with hemorrhage into the lesser omental bursa and pancreas. This patient had hemophilia. Note that there is a double-contoured appearance in the second part of the duodenum (dark arrow) with a broadened, coarsened mucosal pattern in this area. There is a tendency to a "brush" or "spike" pattern at the junction of the second and third parts of the duodenum, and the fourth part of the duodenum in the region of the duodenojejunal juncture is depressed.

B. Patient with pancreatitis. Note the depression of the fourth part of the duodenum in the region of the duodenojejunal juncture and upward displacement of the stomach. The gallbladder contains gallstones which can be visualized just to the left of the duodenal bulb.

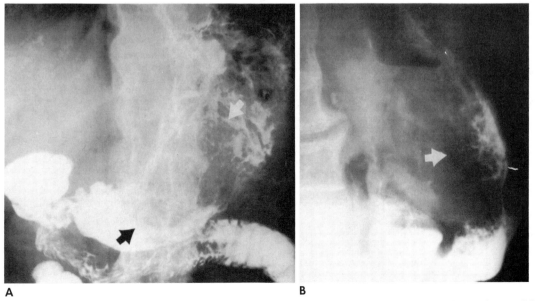

Figure 28–14 *A* and *B*. P-A and left lateral erect views of the stomach and duodenum in a patient with carcinoma of the tail of the pancreas. Note the irregular impression upon the stomach and its displacement anteriorly. There is also a downward displacement of the fourth part of the duodenum and alteration of the mucosal patterns at the duodenojejunal juncture.

Abnormalities in Contour of the Gastroduodenum

Stiffening and Narrowness of the Pyloric Antrum from Gastric Sarcoidosis, Syphilis, Tuberculosis, and Fungal Diseases (Granulomas; Eosinophilic Gastritis)

Linitis Plastica

Eccentricity of the Pylorus

Scarring of the Duodenal Bulb. Scar formation will deform the duodenal bulb in various ways, frequently presenting the appearance of a cloverleaf. Deformity of the duodenal bulb usually indicates that it has been the site of chronic or remote disease of an infiltrative type.

Elongation of the Pyloric Canal. Elongation and narrowness of the pyloric canal (frequently to the extent of 2 to 4 cm.) with hypertrophy of the musculature of the pylorus occurs in *pyloric hypertrophy* in the infant and the adult (Figure 28–15). The appearance resembles a napkin ring around the distal stomach, or, in conjunction with the base of the duodenal bulb, an open umbrella with a curved handle pointing toward the duodenum. The pyloric antrum proximal to the pyloric canal as well as the entire stomach may be markedly distended. This has been called the "pyloric string sign" and antispasmodics do not alter this appearance (Kleitsch).

Mucosal Prolapse into the Base of the Duodenal Bulb. Prolapse of prepyloric antral mucosa into the base of the duodenal bulb is thought to be caused by an increased mobility of the mucosa in respect to the underlying muscularis layer. Typically, the radiographic appearance resembles a mushroom impinging itself upon the base of the duodenal bulb, with the stem of the mushroom representing the pyloric canal. The pyloric canal, under these circumstances, is of normal width (Figure 28–16).

Annular Pancreas (Kjellman). The head of the pancreas may, at times, encircle the postbulbar portion of the duodenum. Symptomatology will vary depending upon the degree of constriction.

This encirclement of the postbulbar duodenum is indicated radiologically by a significant indentation and narrowness of this portion of the duodenum from its *lateral aspect* (Figure 28–19 A) (Dodd and Nafis; Truelsen; Moore; Hope and Gibbons).

Deformity of the Pyloric Antrum Due to Perigastric Adhesions or Bands

Incisura Formation. Localized areas of spasm on the greater curvature of the stomach opposite an ulcer on its lesser curvature produce an incisura of the greater curvature. This may impart an hourglass appearance to the stomach and suggests that the ulcer opposite is likely to be benign.

Diverticula of the Stomach and Duodenum (Figures 28–20 and 28–21)

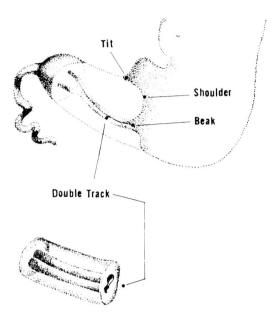

Tit

Shoulder

Beak

Double Track

Figure 28–15 Composite diagram illustrating the different radiographic signs of hypertrophic pyloric stenosis. (From Havan, P. J., Jr., Darling, D. B., and Sciammas, F.: Radiology *86*:723, 1966.)

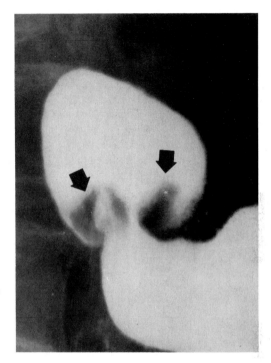

Figure 28–16 Umbilication at the base of the duodenal bulb with protrusion of pyloric mucosa.

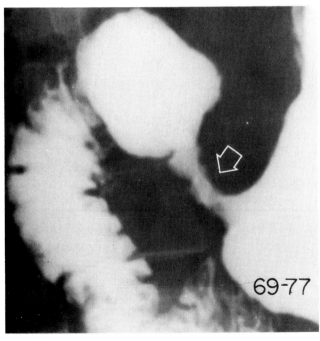

69-77

Figure 28–17 Hypertrophic gastritis producing stenosis of the distal antrum and elongation of the pyloric canal.

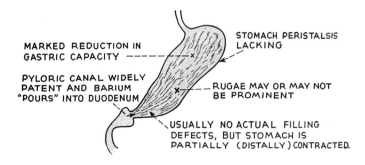

MARKED REDUCTION IN
GASTRIC CAPACITY ————

STOMACH PERISTALSIS
LACKING

PYLORIC CANAL WIDELY
PATENT AND BARIUM
"POURS" INTO DUODENUM

RUGAE MAY OR MAY NOT
BE PROMINENT

USUALLY NO ACTUAL FILLING
DEFECTS, BUT STOMACH IS
PARTIALLY (DISTALLY) CONTRACTED.

Figure 28–18   *A* and *B*. Linitis plastica due to carcinoma of the stomach.

PATHOLOGY: DIFFUSE SPREADING FIBROSIS OF THE
             SUBMUCOSA STARTING USUALLY AT PYLORUS

ETIOLOGY: 1. CARCINOMA (60%)
             2. CHRONIC INFLAMMATION (40%)
                (*AMONG THESE IS SYPHILIS*)

A

B

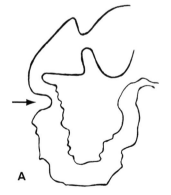

Annular pancreas

A

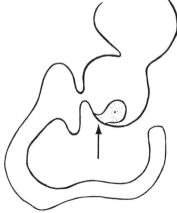

Ectopic pancreas in stomach.
(Note duct "dimple.")

B

Figure 28–19   *A*. Line drawings of radiographic appearance of annular pancreas (upper drawing) surrounding the postbulbar duodenum. Diagram at right *(B)* depicts ectopic pancreas in the stomach.

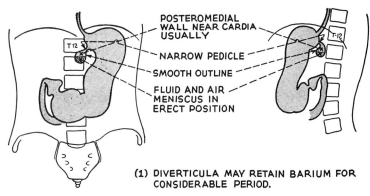

POSTEROMEDIAL WALL NEAR CARDIA USUALLY

NARROW PEDICLE

SMOOTH OUTLINE

FLUID AND AIR MENISCUS IN ERECT POSITION

(1) DIVERTICULA MAY RETAIN BARIUM FOR CONSIDERABLE PERIOD.

(2) OCCASIONALLY OCCUR ALSO AT PYLORUS, BUT VERY RARELY.

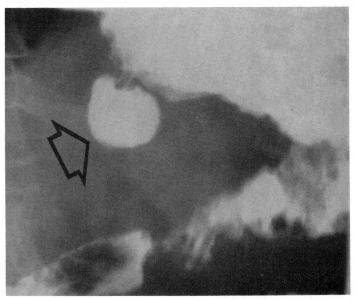

Figure 28–20 Diagram and radiograph showing a gastric diverticulum arising from the fundus of the stomach in typical fashion.

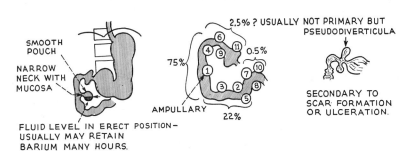

SMOOTH POUCH

NARROW NECK WITH MUCOSA

FLUID LEVEL IN ERECT POSITION— USUALLY MAY RETAIN BARIUM MANY HOURS.

AMPULLARY

75%

2.5%? USUALLY NOT PRIMARY BUT PSEUDODIVERTICULA

0.5%

22%

SECONDARY TO SCAR FORMATION OR ULCERATION.

1. INCIDENCE: ⅓ OF ALL G-I DIVERTICULA; AT AUTOPSY, 3.5%; BY X-RAY, 2%.
2. CLINICAL ASPECTS:
    a. USUALLY ASYMPTOMATIC.
    b. OCCASIONALLY MAY NOT EMPTY WELL, MAY CAUSE PRESSURE, BECOME INFLAMED OR NEOPLASTIC.
3. SIZE: FEW M M. TO 8.0 CM. DIAMETER.
4. SINGLE OR MULTIPLE.

5. COMPLICATIONS:
    1. INFLAMMATION;
    2. ULCERATION;
    3. PERFORATION;
    4. SITE OF NEOPLASM OR
    5. ABERRANT PANCREATIC OR GASTRIC TISSUE;
    6. LODGEMENT OF GALL-STONES.

Figure 28–21 Diagrammatic illustration of pertinent features regarding duodenal diverticula and duodenal bulbar pseudodiverticula.

527

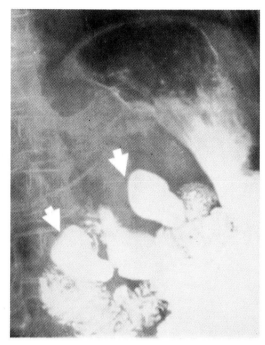

Figure 28–22   Radiograph demonstrating not only two large diverticula of the duodenum but a diverticulum arising from the proximal jejunum as well.

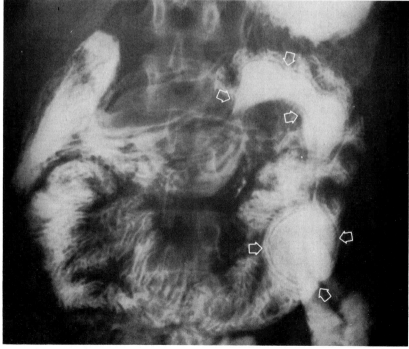

Figure 28–23   Intraluminal diverticulum of the duodenum.

Abnormalities of Internal Architecture in the Stomach and Duodenum

Foreign Bodies

Gastric Varices

Gastritis

GENERAL COMMENT.   Various classifications may be rendered: gastritis may be acute, subacute, or chronic, it may be atrophic or hypertrophic, or it may be classified on the basis of the causative agent or etiology.

1. Superficial gastritis.
2. Atrophic gastritis.
3. Gastric atrophy.
4. Giant hypertrophy of gastric mucosa (Menetrier's disease).
5. Hypertrophic glandular gastritis (Stempien et al.).

Superficial gastritis involves only the mucosa. *The radiological picture will vary considerably from no detectable alteration in the gastric appearance to severe irregularity of the gastric folds.* Occasionally ulceration may also be noted.

Atrophic Gastritis

RADIOLOGIC FINDINGS

The fundus of the stomach appears like a small dome with an absence of rugae and a very thin gastric wall (bald fundus sign) (Figure 28–26).

The greater curvature of the stomach is remarkably smooth when filled with barium and no rugae are manifest.

The stomach is usually rather long and tubular.

The gastric folds in the fundus or body of the stomach are very thin ("tissue paper folds").

When the thin-walled fundus becomes distended with air in the erect position or with barium in the supine position, this distention results in the mushroom appearance called the "H bomb" sign. When a small quantity of barium is given, the mucosal pattern may appear but completely disappears when the stomach is distended.

The barium mixes poorly with the gastric juices and produces a characteristic speckled appearance (Figure 28–26) (Laws and Pitman; Joske and Vaughan; Martin et al.).

Giant Hypertrophy of Gastric Mucosa (Menetrier's Disease) (Reese et al.)

RADIOLOGIC FINDINGS

Tremendous enlargement of the mucosal folds.

Irregularity of the greater curvature especially, and marked thickening of the gastric wall.

Peculiar reticular pattern of the barium which mixes poorly with large amounts of mucus.

The giant rugae appear especially localized to the greater curvature and very seldom if ever near the antrum and lesser curvature.

The mucous membrane measures up to 5 mm. in thickness and gastric glands are increased in number and length.

Differential diagnosis:

a. Diffuse infiltrating lymphoma.
b. Polypoid carcinoma of the cardia.
c. Chronic gastritis of other origin.

STOMACH: ABNORMALITIES OF SIZE

BEZOARS

1. MASS OFTEN FREELY MOVABLE EXCEPT WHEN ADHERENT TO ULCER.

2. LIGHTER AREA WITHIN THE STOMACH BARIUM

3. FILLING DEFECT MAY APPEAR WITHIN GAS BUBBLE IN ERECT POSITION

4. CONTOUR OF STOMACH NORMAL, BUT LARGE; PERISTALSIS PRESENT.

5. CAST OF BEZOAR COATED WITH BARIUM REMAINS AFTER STOMACH IS EMPTY (3 TO 8 hrs.)

TYPES:
    1. HAIR - TRICHOBEZOARS
    2. SEEDS OR PARTS OF PLANTS - PHYTOBEZOAR ESPECIALLY PERSIMMON. (14% GUM; 7% PECTIN)
    3. SHELLAC

ASSOCIATED GASTRIC ULCER:
    1. 24.4 to 77.8 %
    2. ALMOST INVARIABLY BENIGN

A

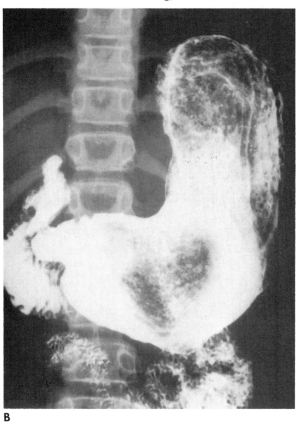

B

Figure 28–24 *A.* The stomach is not always enlarged when it contains a bezoar, but it is very often so. *B.* Hair ball in the stomach producing a trichobezoar.

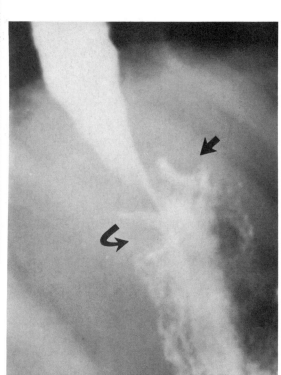

Figure 28–25 Gastric varices, producing large fundal and lower esophageal filling defects. These defects tend to change with intraluminal pressure changes. (From Kerr, et al.: Amer. J. Roentgenol., *113*:129–138, 1971.)

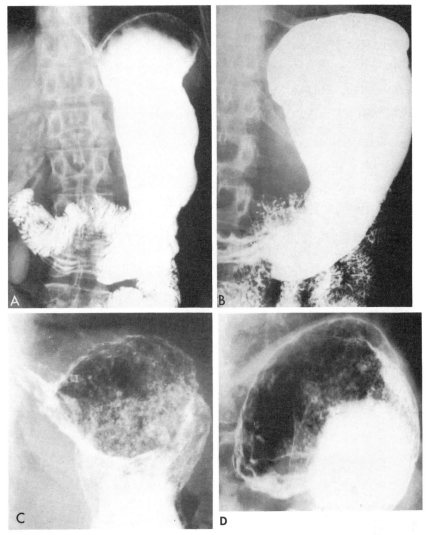

Figure 28–26 Atrophic gastritis. *A.* Relatively hypotonic stomach with thin-walled fundus and absent rugal pattern in fundus. *B.* Smooth greater curvature and sluggish peristalsis. *C.* "Speckled" appearance of the barium, suggesting flocculation in gastric mucosa. *D.* Bald, thin, speckled fundus with "crumpled paper" pattern also. (From Martin, J. F., et al.: Amer. J. Roentgenol., *94*:343–352, 1965.)

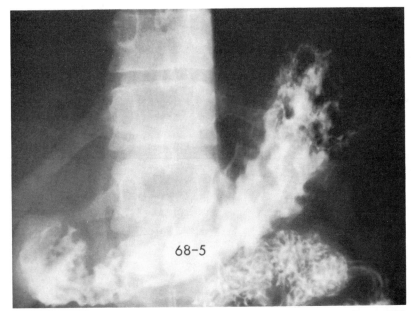

Figure 28–27 Hypertrophic rugation of the stomach. (From Kerr et al.: Amer. J. Roentgenol., *113*:129–138, 1971.)

Ulceration of the Stomach or Duodenum (Figure 28–41)

ROENTGEN SIGNS OF A BENIGN ULCER

Ulcer niche, or "fleck" (German for "spot").

Edematous ridge leads to the ulcer and surrounds it at its base. (Hampton's thin lucent line; "ulcer collar" and "mound" when thick.) The ulcer is central with respect to the mound; the mound is smooth, symmetrical, and gently shouldered.

Folds radiate from the ulcer like the spokes on a wheel — "cartwheel configuration." (This is probably the best single roentgen sign.)

There is often an incisura on the greater curvature opposite a gastric ulcer, usually indicating that the ulcer is benign.

The ulcer may be penetrating, and protrudes beyond the alignment of the lumen on either side.

When ulcers of the duodenum are associated with ulcers of the stomach, both are usually benign.

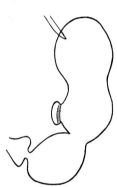

Wide band of edema
with parallel
margins. Collar
at ulcer base smooth.
Ulcer penetrating.

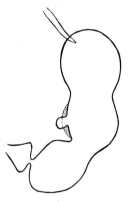

Peripheral edema
slopes smoothly
and gently.
Ulcer penetrates
beyond expected
lesser curvature.

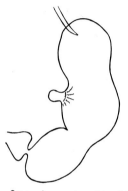

Greater depth than
diameter at base.
Smooth floor.

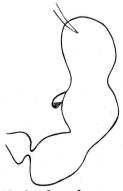

Fluid level

when upright.

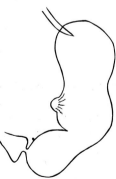

Regular radiating
folds to edge
of ulcer.

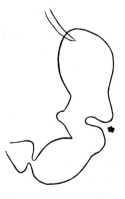

Incisura opposite
crater and
pointing to it.

Figure 28–28 Diagram illustrating various appearances of a probable benign gastric ulcer.

ROENTGEN SIGNS OF A MALIGNANT ULCER OF THE STOMACH (Figure 28–29)

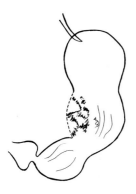

Ulcer edges irregular.
Crater does not extend
beyond expected
line of lesser
curvature.

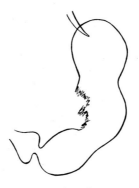

Ulcer within a
polypoid mass
in stomach.

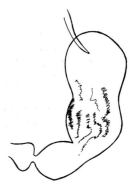

Shallow ulcer
surrounded by thick
rigid folds.
No peristalsis.

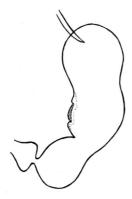

Carmen's meniscus sign.

Crater is crescentic
and when in body
curves away from lumen
of stomach.

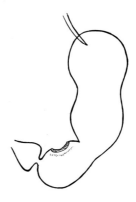

Carmen's meniscus sign in antrum.
Crater is crescentic
toward lumen
of stomach

Figure 28–29 Diagrams of gastric ulcers illustrating roentgen signs of malignancy.

The Size of the Ulcer is in itself no indication of malignancy.

Response of the Ulcer Under Good Treatment. Approximately 80 per cent heal within four weeks, leaving no trace pathologically (Keller et al.).

In the remainder, radiating folds may persist toward a small pit or scar. The ulcer mound and collar do disappear, and the folds which may still radiate are smooth and tapered. In the prepyloric region, there may be a transverse or "vertical" fold (Keller et al.) often associated with more proximal gastric dilatation. Deformity resembling hypertrophic pyloric stenosis may develop. The dimple or "fossette" may persist without change for years.

Location of the Ulcer Site in the Stomach. The site of the ulcer does not help in distinguishing a benign from a malignant ulcer. The association of a gastric ulcer with a duodenal ulcer suggests benignity. Multiplicity of gastric ulcers also suggests benignity.

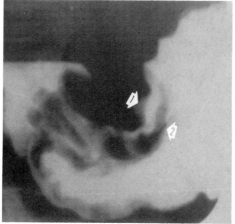

Figure 28–30 Antral ulcer with hypertrophic gastritis.

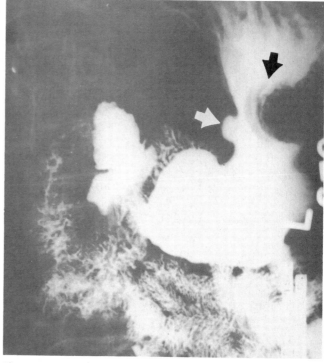

Duodenal Ulcer

Figure 28–31 Radiograph illustrating incisura opposite a benign gastric ulcer.

1.
ACUTE PENETRATING OR EROSIVE STAGE

EDEMATOUS MUCOSAL HALO

ULCER NICHE

THICK PYLORIC RUGA

MAY BE IRRITABLE SPASTIC

2.
BEGINNING SCAR FORMATION

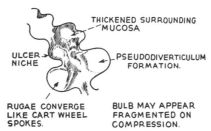

THICKENED SURROUNDING MUCOSA

ULCER NICHE

PSEUDODIVERTICULUM FORMATION.

RUGAE CONVERGE LIKE CART WHEEL SPOKES.

BULB MAY APPEAR FRAGMENTED ON COMPRESSION.

3.
LATE SCARRING STAGE

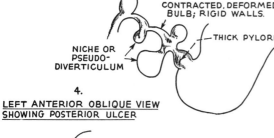

CONTRACTED, DEFORMED FIBROTIC BULB; RIGID WALLS.

THICK PYLORIC RUGA

NICHE OR PSEUDO-DIVERTICULUM

Figure 28–32 Summary diagrams showing the roentgen appearances of duodenal ulcer.

4.
LEFT ANTERIOR OBLIQUE VIEW SHOWING POSTERIOR ULCER

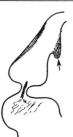

5.
POST-BULBAR ULCER (4%)

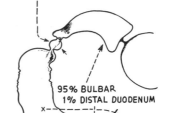

95% BULBAR
1% DISTAL DUODENUM

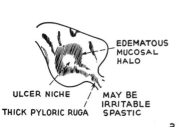

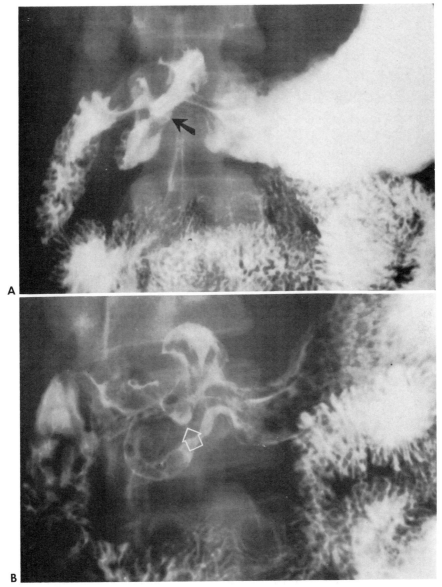

Figure 28–33   Duodenal ulcer showing the advantages of double contrast with barium and air, (*A*) erect, and (*B*) supine. Both views show the ulcer.

SYSTEMIC DISEASES ASSOCIATED WITH DUODENAL ULCER

These include adrenal cortical hyperplasia; pancreatic adenomas, islet cell hyperplasia and islet cell carcinoma; diseases of the central nervous system (hypothalamus, especially); and the Zollinger-Ellison syndrome or complex previously mentioned.

Stress may be a factor in the etiology of several of these entities, especially in relation to adrenal cortical hyperplasia and hypothalamic involvement (Long et al.; Fisher and Hicks).

Adenomatosis of endocrine glands such as the pituitary, thyroid, parathyroid, adrenals, and pancreas has given rise to the so-called "endocrine ulcer syndrome" (Wermer; Jackson; Cope et al.; Hellstrom). Lipomas extrinsic to the endocrine system are also associated very frequently in this syndrome. Villous adenomas and Menetrier's disease involving giant fold formation in the stomach with large ulcers have also been implicated.

The ulcers are frequently located at unusual sites such as the second or third parts of the duodenum (Schlaeger et al.).

The Ulcerogenic Tumor of the Pancreas. The Zollinger-Ellison Syndrome (Nelson and Christoforidis). In this syndrome, severe recurrent peptic ulcers, gastric hypersecretion, and hyperchlorhydria are associated with nonbeta islet cell tumors of the pancreas.

Primary Roentgen Findings

Evidence of gastric hypersecretion.
Large mucosal folds in the stomach, duodenum, or jejunum.
The peptic ulcers are in "unusual" locations.
The ulcers are multiple, often in bulb, or stomach and jejunum.
The mucosal fold pattern in the jejunum is abnormal, simulating regional enteritis.
Megaduodenum.

Postoperative Roentgen Findings

Recurrent large ulcers in site of anastomosis.
Large saucer-shaped multiple ulcers in jejunum.
Hypersecretion continues.

COMPLICATIONS OF GASTRODUODENAL ULCERATION

Gastric or Duodenal Hemorrhage is the cause of death in about 25 per cent of cases in which peptic ulcer is the precipitating cause.

Perforation or Penetration occurs in about 5 per cent of cases. The perforating ulcer may rupture into the peritoneal cavity. Penetration may occur into the pancreas or perigastric tissues or region of the lesser omental bursa. The signs here include the development of a fistulous tract with which an inflammatory mass may be associated. Free air may be localized in the lesser peritoneal sac in association with such penetration. A duodenal ulcer may penetrate into the biliary tract giving rise to free air in the biliary tree. Peritonitis causes 65 per cent of the deaths from peptic ulcer disease.

Development of Gastrocolic Fistula. Usually a barium enema is more satisfactory for demonstration of such fistulae than an upper gastrointestinal examination, despite the fact that diarrhea ensues.

Do Benign Ulcers of the Stomach Become Malignant? To quote from Robbins: "This has been hotly debated for years, but most would now agree that the incidence of malignant transformation in a gastric ulcer is in the order of one per cent or less (Paustian et al.)." Much of the controversy stems from the difficulty of ascertaining whether a cancer has actually developed in a previously benign lesion or whether a small mucosal carcinoma has ulcerated to produce an apparent peptic crater (Mallory).

Obstruction at the Pylorus. Obstruction is rarely a problem with gastric peptic ulcers except those that occur within the pyloric orifice.

Benign Tumors of the Stomach

The following benign tumors of the stomach are listed in their relative order of frequency: adenomas and leiomyomas—64 per cent; others are lipomas, aberrant pancreas, neurogenic inflammatory polyps, and even rarer entities such as angiomas, carcinoids, and fibromas.

Adenomas may be either single or multiple. They may be pedunculated or sessile (Marshak and Feldman). Leiomyomas are intramural tumors but project into the lumen of the stomach and may be readily detected radiologically when large. They may ulcerate centrally, hemorrhage, and undergo calcification in time (Crummy and Juhl).

Although benign tumors may arise in any part of the stomach, the site of preference is the pyloric portion, which is involved in 75 per cent of cases.

ROENTGENOLOGIC FEATURES

The gastrointestinal polyp generally is defined as a sharply circumscribed filling defect projecting within the lumen with a uniform translucent appearance (Figure 28–34).

The large leiomyoma very frequently has an ulcer niche sharply circumscribed within the filling defect (Figure 28–35).

Figure 28–34   Benign polyp.

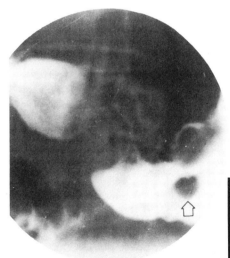

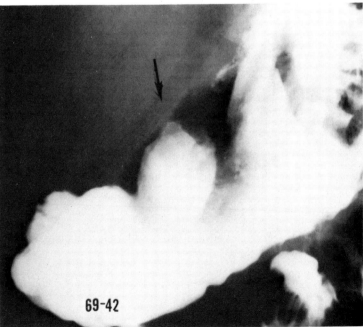

Figure 28–35   Ulcerating leiomyoma of the stomach.

Carcinoma of the Stomach (Figures 28–36 and 28–38)

Gastric carcinoma represents about 70 per cent of all stomach neoplasms (Robbins).

ASSOCIATED CONDITIONS of great importance are:

1. Chronic gastritis
2. Achlorhydria
3. Pernicious anemia
4. Adenomas

SITES OF PREDILECTION: more than half are in the pyloric and prepyloric regions.

GROSS MORPHOLOGIC TYPES:

1. Ulcerative, 28 per cent
2. Fungating or polypoid, 22 per cent
3. Spreading or infiltrating, 13 per cent
4. Remainder unclassifiable

USUAL HISTOLOGIC PATTERN: well-differentiated adenocarcinoma.

RADIOLOGIC APPEARANCES (Figures 28–36 and 28–38):

1. A mass projecting into the gas bubble in the erect position.
2. An ulceration of the stomach with irregular rolled edges which are not undermined.
3. A marked irregularity or nodular margination of the stomach.
4. An ulcer crater within a mass not extending outside the confines of the stomach.
5. A shallow crater which does not hold fluid in the upright position.
6. Rigidity of the area of the stomach involved.
7. An ulcer within a rigid area of the stomach.
8. An ulcer crater with a complete interruption of the rugae of the stomach toward the crater.
9. Evidence of a perigastric mass indenting the stomach.
10. A "leather bottle" type stomach suggesting scirrhous carcinoma.

CHRONIC GASTRITIS AND CANCER. Carcinoma develops more often in patients with achlorhydria or pernicious anemia than in the normal population (Schell et al.).

Lymphoma of the Stomach (Jenkinson et al., 1954)

In the stomach, this is usually of the diffuse or infiltrating variety, but occasionally it is nodular, polypoid, or pedunculated. Occasionally also there are large ulcerations or an annular defect in association with the lymphosarcoma.

ROENTGENOLOGIC ASPECTS

"Fingerprint impression" pattern due to diffuse intramural invasion (Figure 28–37).

Broad ulceration.

Moderate rigidity with loss of peristaltic activity. There may be a persistence of sluggish peristalsis despite extensive involvement of the wall of the stomach.

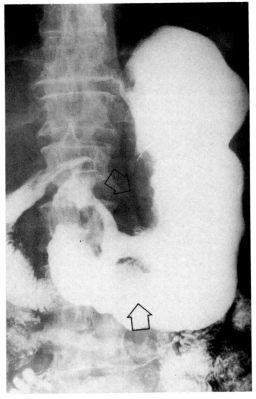

Figure 28–36 Radiograph demonstrating large irregular carcinomatous filling defects of the stomach.

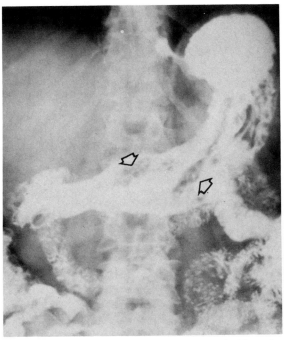

Figure 28–37 Lymphosarcoma of the stomach. Note the marked thickening of the gastric wall. "Hypertrophic rugation" is also present.

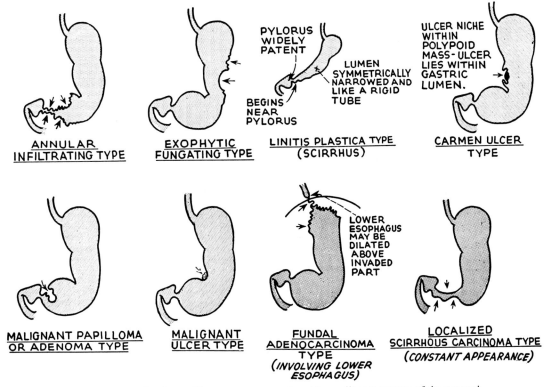

Figure 28–38 Radiographic appearances produced by malignant tumors of the stomach.

Benign Tumors of the Duodenum

Benign tumors of the duodenum are very rare and may occur as single smooth filling defects within the duodenum. They may at times be multiple. These are polypoid lesions which histologically prove to be adenomas, papillomas, lipomas, angiomas, fibromas, myomas, neurinomas, cysts, carcinoid tumors, ectopic pancreas, and villous tumor. Hypertrophic glands of Brunner must also enter into the differential diagnosis.

Occasionally, polyps on a long stalk will prolapse from the pyloric antrum through the pylorus into the duodenal bulb (Figure 28–39).

ROENTGENOLOGIC ASPECTS

Hypertrophic glands of Brunner produce a cobblestone appearance.

Ectopic pancreas produces the "sign of the duct" (Kjellman). This is a broad-based tumor defect in stomach or duodenum and central to the filling defect is a craterlike dimple, from the bottom of which fine lines may extend peripherally (Figure 28–19 B).

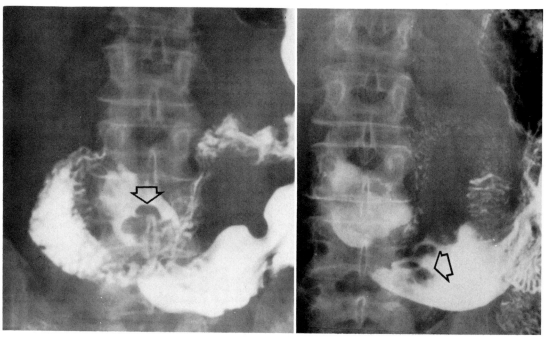

Figure 28–39 Spot film radiographs demonstrating a benign polyp of the pyloric antrum herniating from antrum (*right*) into duodenal bulb (*left*).

Malignant Tumors of the Duodenum. These are rare.

Duodenal malignancies occur above the papilla in about 15 per cent of the cases, at the same level in about 65 per cent, and below this level in about 20 per cent. Most often they are ulcerative, polypoid, or infiltrative and may encircle the duodenum, producing an obstruction or partial obstruction at this level. Primary malignancies of the duodenum are difficult to distinguish from those which involve the duodenum by extension from adjoining structures.

In general, malignant tumors of the upper levels of small bowel are more likely to be carcinomas or carcinoid tumors, and those of the lower level of the small intestine, lymphomas (Robbins).

Intramural Duodenal Hematoma and Retroperitoneal Rupture of the Duodenum (Figure 28–40)

Blunt abdominal trauma may produce retroperitoneal rupture of the duodenum. This occurs most frequently at the junction of the second and third portions of the duodenum but multiple perforations are possible.

Occasionally, intramural duodenal hematomas will occur with:

1. Treatment with anticoagulants.
2. Carcinoma of the pancreas.
3. Pancreatitis.
4. Obscure bleeding diathesis in infants.

ROENTGENOLOGIC FINDINGS

Plain film studies may reveal (1) retroperitoneal air; (2) extension of the air to the mediastinal and cervical regions; (3) a mass adjoining the spine.

When barium contrast is administered: (1) A coiled spring appearance of the mucosa overlying the mass occurs (Felson and Levin), owing to crowding of the valvulae conniventes by intramural hemorrhage. The appearance suggests intussusception except that there is no associated shortening of the bowel (Bruck and Caplan). There may also be an extrinsic pressure defect on the greater curvature of the stomach. (2) Less commonly, there may be complete obstruction of the duodenum or jejunum produced by the intramural mass (Butz and Tarnay), coming to a conical point at the site of obstruction.

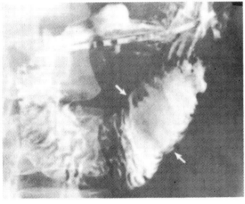
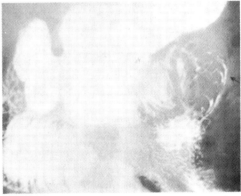

A   B

Figure 28–40 *A.* Preoperative roentgenogram showing defect indicative of intramural mass in distal duodenum which proved to be an intramural hematoma. *B.* Preoperative roentgenogram showing crowding of valvulae conniventes and coiled spring appearance due to an intramural hematoma in this region. (From Bruck, R. N., and Caplan, B.: J.A.M.A., *189*:326, 1964.)

THE POSTOPERATIVE STOMACH

Introduction. It is important to examine the stomach during the early post-operative period (that is, during the third or fourth week as opposed to several years later), in order to obtain a postoperative base line. Edema at an anastomosis usually subsides in about two weeks (Kim and Evans).

Common Terminology in Respect to Gastric Surgery (Figure 28–41)
Billroth I: partial gastrectomy with end-to-end gastroduodenostomy.

Billroth II: partial gastrectomy with end-to-side gastrojejunostomy.

Polya: a gastric resection in which the entire cut end of the stomach is used for anastomosis without restriction of the size of the stoma.

Hofmeister: a gastric resection with gastrojejunostomy (like Billroth II) with partial closure of the cut end of the stomach.

Roux-en-Y: partial gastrectomy; jejunojejunostomy with or without anastomosis with the esophagus, stomach, duodenum, gallbladder, bile duct, or pancreas.

Whipple: partial gastrectomy, gastrojejunostomy, and end-to-side choledochojejunostomy.

In each of these it is important to note the extent of gastric resection; whether the anastomosis is anterior, posterior, superior, or inferior; whether the anastomosis is right-to-left, or left-to-right; and if there is a gastrojejunostomy, whether it is anterior to the colon or posterior to the colon (antecolic or retrocolic) (Figure 28–41) (Burhenne, 1964).

The fundoplication procedure for repair of a sliding hiatal hernia produces a mass defect in the fundus of the stomach. This must be differentiated from neoplasms such as carcinoma or leiomyosarcoma.

Complications to be Excluded or Looked for in the Study of the Postoperative Stomach

1. *Persistent pneumoperitoneum* (Bevan). Ordinarily, only a very small amount of pneumoperitoneum may still be noted at the end of one week, depending upon the amount of air initially present. However, if 1000 ml. or more of air had been present originally, this may persist for two weeks.
2. *Paralytic ileus and gastric atony.* There is a very marked decrease in peristaltic activity following vagotomy and this may persist in one-third of the patients for an interval of six months (Isaac et al.).
3. *Acute gastric dilatation.*
4. *Pulmonary* complications (thromboembolism).
5. *Leakage* at the anastomotic stomal site or in the vicinity of a duodenal stump. This may occur as late as the 19th day postoperatively (Rudko and Price).
6. *Postgastrectomy hemorrhage.* Apart from hemorrhage into the gastrointestinal tract, hemorrhage into the peritoneal space or hemorrhage involving adjoining organs such as the spleen must be carefully eliminated.
7. *Obstruction*
   a. Stomal.
   b. Prolapse of gastric mucosa into the anastomotic opening.

     c. Intussusception, when the jejunum invaginates into the gastric pouch in retrograde fashion or direct antegrade gastrojejunal intussusception.

     d. Obstruction in the anastomotic jejunal loop may result from internal herniation. Internal herniation may occur particularly anterior or posterior to a mesocolon or through the defect in the mesocolon.

     e. Obstruction in the small intestine may occur anywhere from adhesions, intussusception, compression, or food bezoars.

In a review of the most common causes of postoperative deaths following gastrectomy, Carillo noted that duodenal leakage and proximal obstruction occurred most frequently.

    8. *Difficulties at the site of plication.* Ischemic necrosis, foreign body granulomas, pseudodiverticular deformities. Plication abnormalities may sometimes be difficult to differentiate from recurrent ulcers near the stomal margin.

    9. Gastroileostomy instead of gastrojejunostomy.

   10. *The afferent loop syndrome,* in which the afferent loop retains secretions, food, and barium for an inordinate period of time. This syndrome may also be related to preferential emptying of the stomach into the proximal (afferent) loop rather than the distal (efferent). In turn, this may lead to the "blind loop syndrome" in which lodgement of bacteria may impose a vitamin B-12 deficiency and resulting anemia (Figure 28–45).

   11. *The antral remnant syndrome.* If a portion of the gastric antrum is no longer in continuity with the remainder of the stomach and remains as part of the proximal loop, gastrin is elaborated, in turn stimulating any remaining parietal cells in the proximal stomach to secrete acid. There is a high incidence of marginal ulcer reformation under these circumstances (Figure 28–43).

   12. *Recurrent gastric ulcer.*

   13. *Marginal ulcer formation.* This ordinarily occurs in the jejunum just distal to the site of the anastomosis. The majority occur in the first 2 cm. of the anastomosed jejunum (Figure 28–44).

   14. *Persistent esophagitis, gastritis, or jejunitis.*

   15. *Gastrocolic fistula.* A barium enema is more diagnostic than the upper gastrointestinal study for this (Thoeny, Hodgson, and Scudamore).

   16. *Persistence of ulcerogenic tumors* (Zollinger-Ellison syndrome) (see previously).

   17. *Recurrence of gastric carcinoma after gastric resection.*

   18. *The dumping syndrome* (Figure 28–42). A theory for the proposed mechanism in the dumping syndrome is illustrated (Burhenne, 1964). Unfortunately, the roentgenologic findings in the dumping syndrome are not diagnostic.

   19. *Malabsorption syndrome.* This may result from a deficient production of intrinsic factor, decreased vitamin B-12 absorption, increased fat content in the stool, and iron deficiency anemia. Also, the calcium metabolism may be altered.

   20. *Postvagotomy alterations in function.* These will include marked gastric distention, diarrhea, and possibly impairment of gallbladder function. Gastroesophageal reflux and gastric atony have been previously described.

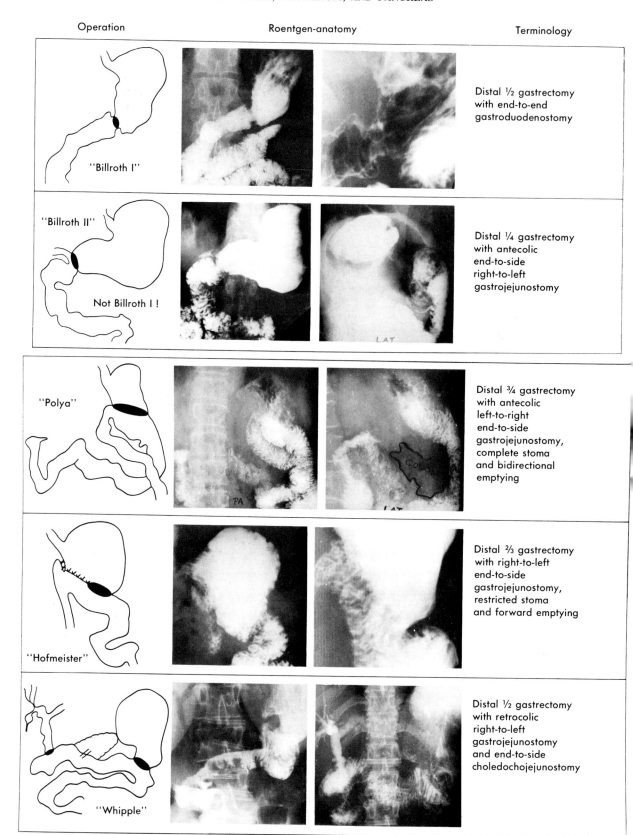

Figure 28–41 Roentgenographic appearances of the postoperative stomach. (From Burhenne, H. J.: Amer. J. Roentgen., 91:731, 1964.)

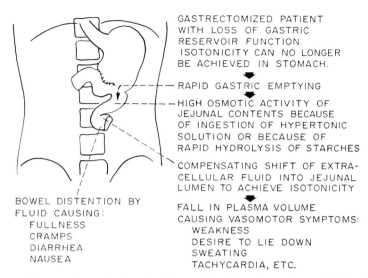

GASTRECTOMIZED PATIENT
WITH LOSS OF GASTRIC
RESERVOIR FUNCTION.
ISOTONICITY CAN NO LONGER
BE ACHIEVED IN STOMACH.

RAPID GASTRIC EMPTYING

HIGH OSMOTIC ACTIVITY OF
JEJUNAL CONTENTS BECAUSE
OF INGESTION OF HYPERTONIC
SOLUTION OR BECAUSE OF
RAPID HYDROLYSIS OF STARCHES

COMPENSATING SHIFT OF EXTRA-
CELLULAR FLUID INTO JEJUNAL
LUMEN TO ACHIEVE ISOTONICITY

FALL IN PLASMA VOLUME
CAUSING VASOMOTOR SYMPTOMS:
  WEAKNESS
  DESIRE TO LIE DOWN
  SWEATING
  TACHYCARDIA, ETC.

BOWEL DISTENTION BY
FLUID CAUSING:
  FULLNESS
  CRAMPS
  DIARRHEA
  NAUSEA

Figure 28–42 Diagram illustrating the physiology of the "dumping syndrome." (After Burhenne.)

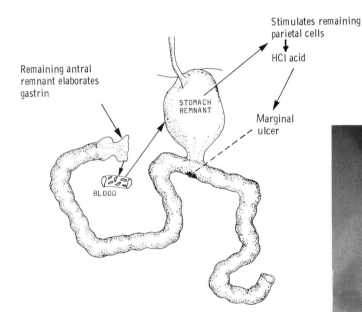

Stimulates remaining
parietal cells

HCl acid

Remaining antral
remnant elaborates
gastrin

STOMACH
REMNANT

Marginal
ulcer

BLOOD

Figure 28–43 Antral remnant syndrome.

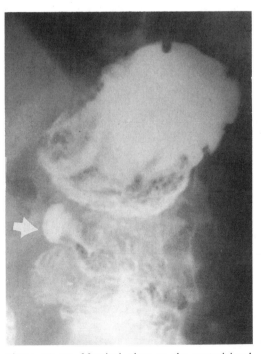

Figure 28–44 Marginal ulcer at the gastrojejunal anastomotic junction following gastric resection.

Symptoms

   (a) Loss of weight
   (b) Diarrhea
   (c) Macrocytic anemia
   (d) Multiple vitamin
       deficiencies
   (e) Occasionally
       steatorrhea

Diagnosis by
 Intestinal biopsy
 assisted by:
Roentgen Signs.
  (a) Isolated diverticulum
            or
  (b) anastomosal loop
       of bowel which becomes
  (c) progressively distended,
       and retentive of
       contents

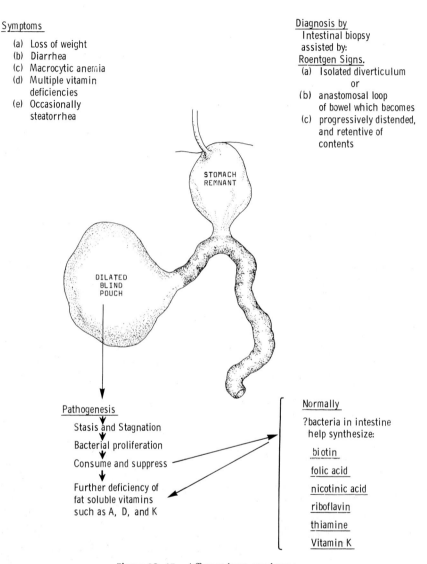

STOMACH REMNANT

DILATED BLIND POUCH

Pathogenesis

  Stasis and Stagnation

  Bacterial proliferation

  Consume and suppress

  Further deficiency of
  fat soluble vitamins
  such as A, D, and K

Normally

?bacteria in intestine
 help synthesize:

  biotin

  folic acid

  nicotinic acid

  riboflavin

  thiamine

  Vitamin K

Figure 28–45   Afferent loop syndrome.

THE PANCREAS

Introduction

Examination of the pancreas is largely by indirect means and radiologic diagnosis of pancreatic disease leaves much to be desired. The advent of newer techniques such as ductography may contribute to greater refinement in diagnosis.

Plain Films of the Abdomen. Antero-posterior and lateral views centered over the pancreas, with oblique views taken as necessary, may reveal the following:

Pancreatic Calcification (Figure 28–46). The calcification may consist either of (1) multiple small punctate areas in the distribution of the pancreas; or (2) larger, mulberry type areas of calcification in one or more foci.

Abnormal Gas Distribution. (1) The gas distribution may be segmental, diffusely reflex, or colon cut-off sign. (2) There may be free gas in the immediate vicinity of the pancreas or lesser omental bursa. The latter would, of course, indicate abscess formation or fat necrosis.

ROENTGEN SIGNS OF CARCINOMA OF THE PANCREAS BY UPPER GASTROINTESTINAL STUDIES

1. In 46 cases of body and tail of pancreas (Mani et al.):*
   a. Displacement of stomach, 67 per cent
   b. Invasion of stomach, 41 per cent
   c. Extrinsic mass impressing on stomach or splaying mucosal folds, 67 per cent
2. Duodenum
   a. Displacement, 43 per cent
   b. Invasion, 61 per cent
   c. Extrinsic mass, 50 per cent
3. Enlargement of the duodenal "sweep"
4. Bulbar and postbulbar defects including narrowness.
5. Mucosal changes of the duodenum: changes in shape, width, height, direction, brushlike configuration, flattening, irritability, fixation, rigidity, induration, divergence of folds, corrugation, elongation of folds with pseudodiverticulum formation
6. Inverted "3" sign of Forstberg
7. Impression on duodenal diverticulum if present
8. Fixation and wrap-around effects (rigidity, partial compression of stomach or duodenum)
9. Biliary tract signs (impression on duodenum by enlarged gallbladder, common duct sign)
10. Functional disturbances (marked spasticity, irritability, periodic retroperistalsis)
11. Swollen ampulla

---

*Mani et al.: Amer. J. Roentgenol., 96:429–446, 1966.

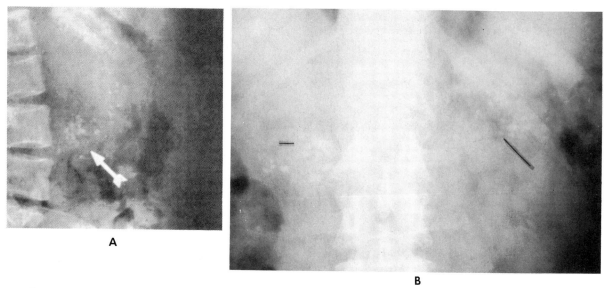

Figure 28–46 Pancreatic calculi. *A.* Lateral projection. The calcific shadows lie anteriorly to the second and third lumbar vertebrae. *B.* After the administration of an opaque meal. The calcific shadows are visualized within the loop of the duodenum (black arrow). (From Ritvo, M., and Shauffer, I. A.: *Gastrointestinal X-ray Diagnosis.* Philadelphia, Lea & Febiger, 1952, p. 685.)

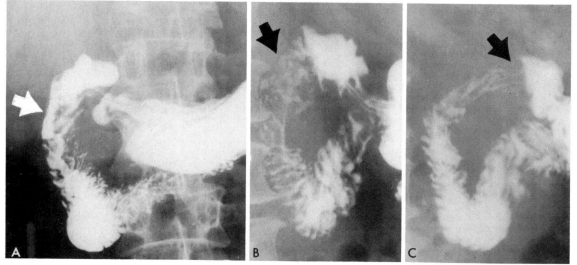

Figure 28–47 *A.* Carcinoma of the pancreas with the following roentgen changes to be noted: (1) Irregular, double-contoured appearance of the descending portion of the duodenum on its medial aspect. (2) Widened and irregular mucosal pattern in the upper half of the second part of the duodenum. (3) A faint "spike" or "brush" pattern on the medial aspect of the descending portion of the duodenum. (4) Impression upon the adjoining portion of the distal pyloric antrum.

B. Effacement of the normal mucosal pattern of the descending portion of the duodenum by carcinoma of the pancreas.

C. Radiograph demonstrating the effacement of the mucosal pattern in the postbulbar portion of the duodenum and the sharp line of demarcation between the postbulbar duodenum and the margin of the duodenal bulb produced by impression from a dilated common duct. This was due to a carcinoma of the pancreas. There is also a slight irregular indentation on the descending portion of the duodenum.

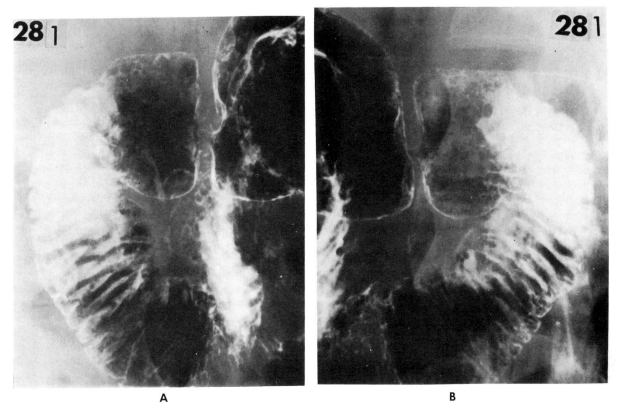

A

B

Figure 28–48 Hypotonic duodenography. *A* and *B*. Duodenum following hypotonic duodenography demonstrating the marked double contrast obtained in the duodenal bulb and duodenum.

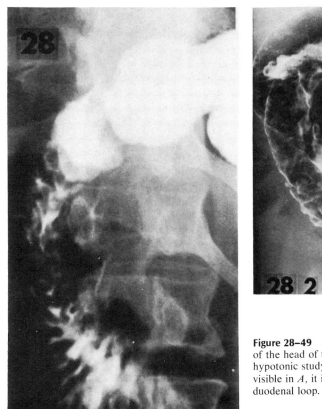

A

B

Figure 28–49 Hypotonic duodenography in a patient with carcinoma of the head of the pancreas. *A*. Prior to the hypotonic study. *B*. The hypotonic study. Although the rigid impression upon the duodenum is visible in *A*, it is better shown following the gaseous distention of the duodenal loop.

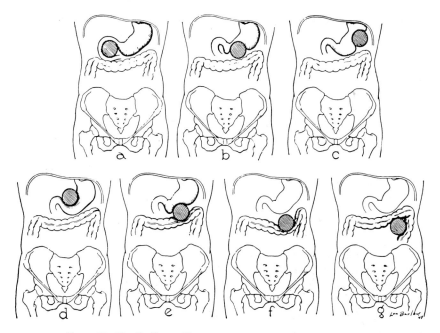

Figure 28–50 Radiographic appearance of cysts in various locations adjoining the pancreas. (From Poppel, M. H.: *Roentgen Manifestations of Pancreatic Disease.* Springfield, Illinois, Charles C Thomas, Publisher, 1951.)

Questions—Chapter 28

1. Indicate the important organs in the immediate vicinity of the stomach that may be studied for detectable pathology by upper gastrointestinal barium studies.

2. Describe the rugal pattern of the stomach and duodenum and indicate its general importance.

3. What is meant by the term cascade stomach? How is it important radiologically?

4. Describe the physiologic considerations in respect to the gastric glandular secretions. How are they important in respect to the following: gastroduodenal evacuation; postoperative complications following partial gastric resection; the Zollinger-Ellison syndrome?

5. What is the main normal function of the pyloric sphincter apparently?

6. What is the main disadvantage of water soluble contrast media for gastrointestinal study?

7. What is the primary disadvantage of oral barium in gastrointestinal studies?

8. What are the disadvantages of the so-called "emergency study of the upper gastrointestinal tract" and what are its limitations?

9. Indicate some of the abnormalities in size in respect to the gastroduodenal region.

10. How might you differentiate pyloric obstruction related to an old gastric ulcer from malignancy causing obstruction?

11. Indicate some of the abnormalities of position of the gastroduodenal region.

12. What are some of the abnormalities of position of the duodenum and how may they manifest themselves clinically?

13. What is the significance of eccentricity of the pylorus pathologically?

14. What is the influence of the biliary tract on the appearance of the duodenal bulb?

15. What is the significance of elongation of the pyloric canal? In what pathologic entities or variations of normal is this seen?

16. What is the significance of mucosal prolapse in the base of the duodenal bulb and how may this appear radiologically?

17. What is the meaning of the term "linitis plastica" and what are its causes? How may it manifest itself radiologically?

18. What is meant by the terms "annular pancreas" and "ectopic pancreas"? How may these abnormalities manifest themselves?

19. What is the significance of incisura formation on the stomach?

20. What are some of the causes of bezoars of the stomach and how may these be distinguished radiologically?

21. Indicate the most frequent sites of diverticula of the stomach. What is their pathologic significance?

22. Indicate the significance of pseudodiverticula of the duodenal bulb.

23. How do we classify gastritis? What are the various roentgen appearances of the different types of gastritis? Which are the most frequent types?

24. What are the roentgen signs of a benign ulcer of the stomach or duodenum?

25. What are the roentgen signs of a malignant ulcer of the stomach?

26. How would you judge radiologically the response of a gastric ulcer under good treatment?

27. What special problems of ulceration of the gastroduodenal area present themselves in infancy and childhood?

28. What are the most frequent complications of gastroduodenal ulceration? Which are most important in respect to the cause of death?

29. Indicate the most frequent benign tumors of the stomach and describe their radiographic appearances.

30. What are the important associated conditions in carcinoma of the stomach and why must we pay special attention to these?

31. What are the sites of predilection of carcinoma of the stomach and what are the usual gross morphologic types of histologic pattern?

32. Describe the radiologic appearances associated with carcinoma of the stomach.

33. Describe the radiologic appearances associated most frequently with lymphoma of the stomach.

34. What is the differential diagnosis of benign tumors of the duodenum?

35. Under what circumstances is intramural duodenal hematoma or retroperitoneal rupture of the duodenum most important? How would you recognize these entities radiologically?

36. How is the postoperative stomach examination different from the routine examination? When is the postoperative stomach best examined?

37. Define the following terms in respect to gastric surgery and indicate their importance radiologically: Billroth I, Billroth II, Polya, Hofmeister, Roux-en-Y, and Whipple.

38. What is the explanation for the "afferent loop syndrome"?

39. What is the explanation for the "antral remnant syndrome"?

40. Where are marginal ulcers most apt to occur following gastrojejunostomy?

41. What are the most likely radiologic findings with gastric cancer recurrence after gastric resection?

42. What explanation can you offer for the "dumping syndrome"?

43. What are the post-vagotomy alterations in function of the stomach and duodenum?

44. List the various methods for radiologic study of the pancreas.

45. What contribution does the plain film study make to a study of the pancreas radiologically?

46. Indicate the contributions that fluoroscopy and the opaque meal in the stomach and duodenum have to make in the study of the pancreas. What are the most significant roentgen findings?

47. How may the barium enema contribute to a study of the pancreas radiologically?

48. How may the cholecystogram or cholangiogram contribute to a study of the pancreas?

49. What is meant by the term "hypotonic duodenography"? How does this contribute to a study of pancreatic lesions?

50. What is the main purpose of direct pancreatography? What has been its application in roentgen diagnosis and treatment?

29

Radiology of the Small Intestine Beyond the Duodenum

INTRODUCTION

Related Gross Anatomy

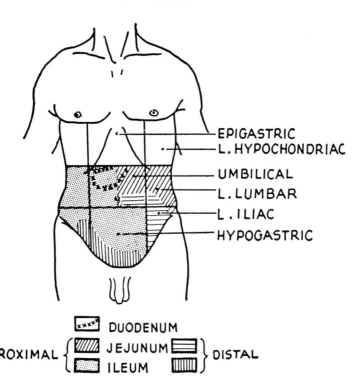

SCHEME OF NORMAL POSITION OF SMALL INTESTINE

- EPIGASTRIC
- L. HYPOCHONDRIAC
- UMBILICAL
- L. LUMBAR
- L. ILIAC
- HYPOGASTRIC

PROXIMAL { DUODENUM, JEJUNUM, ILEUM } DISTAL

Figure 29–1 Approximate distribution of the small intestine within the abdomen.

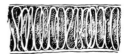

JEJUNUM
(NO INDENTED SEROSA; COILED SPRING APPEARRANCE)

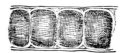

ILEUM
(NO INDENTED SEROSA)

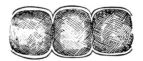

COLON
(NOTE INDENTED SEROSA BY HAUSTRA)

Figure 29–2 Schematic illustration of distended bowel, showing differences between jejunum, ileum, and colon.

Radiographic Anatomy

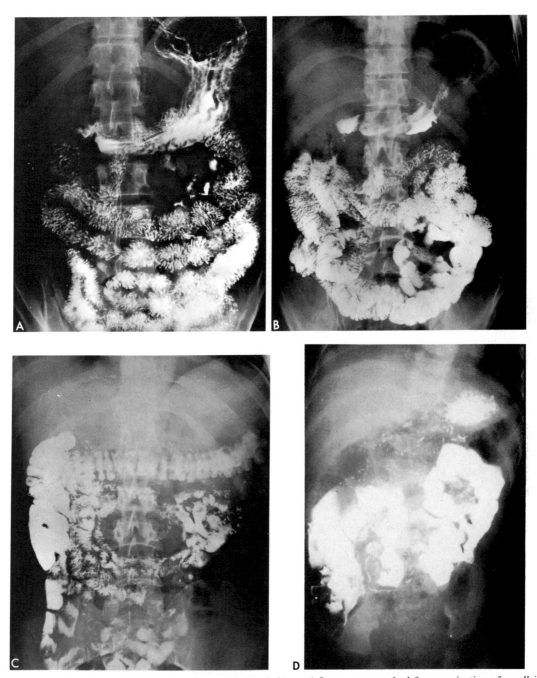

Figure 29–3 Illustrations to demonstrate frequent-interval film and fluoroscopy method for examination of small intestine: *A*, at one hour following administration of the barium; *B*, at two hours; *C*, at three hours. *D*. Representative small intestinal pattern of a normal infant on a predominantly milk diet. Note that the clumping and scattering are relatively normal for infants at this stage of development.

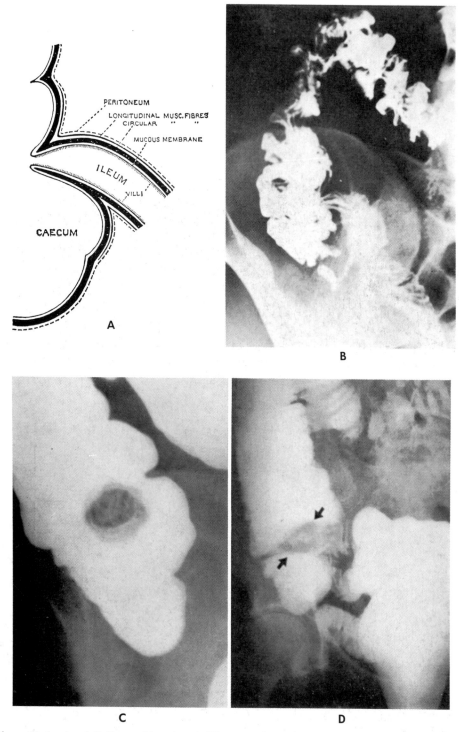

Figure 29–4   *A* and *B*. Ileocecal junction. *A*. Diagrammatic section. (From *Cunningham's Textbook of Anatomy,* London, Oxford University Press.) *B*. Spot film study. *C* and *D*. Difference between prolapse (*C*) and prominent ileocecal valves (*D*). In the former the central slitlike valve orifice is not filled with barium, whereas in the latter it stands out clearly. This is a posteriorly situated valve. (From Hinkel, C. L.: Amer. J. Roentgenol., *68*:171, 1952.)

ROENTGENOLOGIC VARIATIONS OF NORMAL

Variations With Age

During the first three or four months of life, while the infant is still on a milk diet, there is a tendency toward segmentation and lack of continuity of the barium column and delay of transit time. The stomach to colon time may be as long as nine hours in the newborn (Figure 29–3D).

Gas in the small bowel is abnormal except in the very young and the very old (when not excessive). In the young it is due to air swallowing and in the old to a relative hypotonicity of the small intestine. Such changes begin to be particularly manifest beyond the age of 60 years.

A persistent deficiency of gas in the small intestine of the newborn infant beyond the first day may be a cardinal sign of intestinal obstruction. However, there are other entities which may be responsible for this appearance, such as adrenal insufficiency, dehydration, diarrhea, and other interference with the normal transport mechanisms.

ROENTGEN SIGNS OF ABNORMALITY

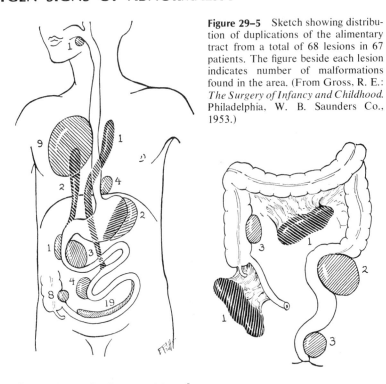

Figure 29–5 Sketch showing distribution of duplications of the alimentary tract from a total of 68 lesions in 67 patients. The figure beside each lesion indicates number of malformations found in the area. (From Gross, R. E.: *The Surgery of Infancy and Childhood.* Philadelphia, W. B. Saunders Co., 1953.)

Abnormalities in Relation to Number

Congenital Duplication or Triplication of the small intestine or the formation of elongated diverticula of the intestine may occur (Figure 29–5).

Enterogenous Cysts. When intestinal duplications do not communicate with the bowel, enterogenous cysts result. Under these circumstances, a cystic mass is found within the abdomen adjoining the small bowel and situated within the mesentery or in the omentum. Ordinarily, such cysts contain a clear fluid of mucoid consistency. Complications like volvulus and intussusception may occur with enterogenous cyst formation. Such a mass may produce intrinsic or extrinsic pressure upon the adjoining small bowel.

Abnormalities of Position

Abnormalities of Intestinal Rotation (Figure 29–6).   The foregut consists of the stomach and superior portion of the duodenum down to approximately the major papilla. The midgut consists of the remaining portion of the duodenum, the whole of the small intestine, and the proximal one-half of the colon. The hindgut consists of the distal one-half of the colon beyond the midtransverse colon to the rectum.

Anomalies of intestinal rotation are principally limited to the midgut. The most common problem is incomplete rotation. The cecum fails to migrate completely from the subhepatic area to the normal position in the right lower quadrant. The midgut hangs on the superior mesenteric artery. The cecum and terminal ileum are either free or attached in the subhepatic region by peritoneal bands. If the entire midgut is unattached volvulus may occur, usually in a clockwise direction. This not only occludes the blood supply to the midgut, but also increases the pressure on the duodenum. In most instances of malrotation, symptoms begin shortly after birth and are persistent, but sometimes they are intermittent and date from an early age only in retrospect.

In the adult, abnormalities of rotation may produce no symptoms and be recognized radiographically only when it is found that the entire small intestine beyond the midportion of the duodenum is situated in the right half of the abdomen and the entire colon is situated in the left half of the abdomen (common mesentery deformity) (Figure 29–6). The cecum, in these circumstances, is situated under the liver or in the left upper quadrant. Also, there is an absence of the usual duodenojejunal flexure, and the duodenum is in normal position only down to the region of the major papilla of Vater (Aldrich et al.).

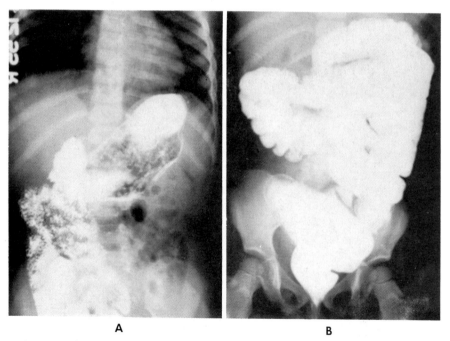

A   **B**

Figure 29–6   *A* and *B*. Common mesentery deformity showing the nonrotation of the small intestine. As a result, the colon is largely in the left half of the abdomen and the small bowel is in the right half of the abdomen.

Alteration in Position by Displacement.   The small intestine is subject readily to displacement because of the long small intestinal mesentery. Even an overdistended urinary bladder will displace the ileum upward.

Under these circumstances, an absence of gas in an area where normally some gas should be identified is easily recognized. When the small bowel is filled with barium, there are pressure defects on the small intestine produced by the adjoining mass.

Other lesions which may produce displacement of bowel are enlarged mesenteric lymph nodes either from inflammation or neoplasm, matted loops of bowel, pelvic cysts and tumors, enterogenous cysts, and omental or peritoneal cysts. Occasionally, retroperitoneal mass lesions are so large that they displace the small and large intestine anteriorly and to either side. Such retroperitoneal lesions may be neoplastic in origin or may be related to enlargement of existing organs.

Alterations in Position by Internal Herniation

Paraduodenal Hernias

Included here are hernias into the pockets and fossae in the region of the duodenum or duodenojejunal flexure, those under peritoneal folds or bands, and those, congenital or acquired, of the posterior wall. Hernias through the foramen of Winslow into the lesser peritoneal sac are also included (Figure 29–7 A and B).

RADIOGRAPHIC MANIFESTATIONS:

1. Localized air and fluid, intraluminal collections in the left upper quadrant in or adjoining the lesser peritoneal sac (Walker and Weens).
2. The aggregation of barium in the anatomic position of the lesser omental sac should lead to a suspicion of the diagnosis.
3. Associated partial or even complete obstruction with strangulation may occur (Parsons).
4. On plain films, a small bowel tumor may be simulated (Gardiner and Miller).

Differential diagnosis must include pneumoperitoneum, lesser omental bursal abscess, and pseudocysts of the pancreas.

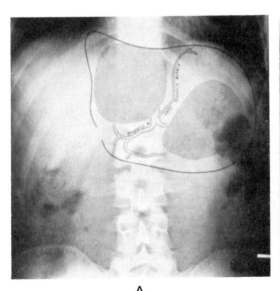
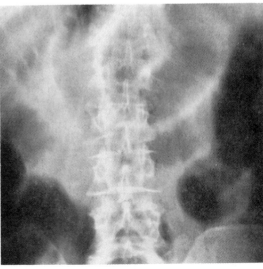

A   **B**

Figure 29–7   *A.* Diagrammatic presentation of location of abscess in the two compartments of the lesser sac. (From Walker, L. A., and Weens, H. S.: Radiology, *80:*727, 1963.) *B,* Lesser sac hernia. Coiled loops of dilated small bowel in region of lesser sac. The findings are striking in the lateral view. (Courtesy Dr. Taft Edenfield, Georgia Baptist Hospital, Atlanta, Ga.)

Abnormalities of Size: Dilated Loops of Small Intestine with Splayed-out Valvulae

Paralytic Ileus. This usually involves the entire gastrointestinal tract, although reflex changes may be localized to one area of bowel. The latter is particularly true of a response to sudden pain, when the small intestine may be moderately dilated in small or regional foci. (1) Usually there are no fluid levels. (2) When the ileus is regional, the distention is apt to be only moderate. (3) The bowel wall is thin, not thickened. (4) The valvulae, although distended, remain delicate in appearance.

Dynamic Ileus (Mechanical Obstruction). Usually the cause of a mechanical obstruction will have a more specific roentgen sign at the site of the obstruction. These signs will be described separately. The loops proximal to the site of the obstruction are diffusely and markedly dilated, and in addition (1) fluid levels are present; (2) the coiled-spring pattern of the distended bowel is most apparent; (3) there is a tendency to certain types of layering of the distended loops, so that in the erect position they assume either a *circular staircase pattern* (Figure 29–8 B) or a *herringbone pattern* (Figure 29–8 A).

MOST FREQUENT CAUSES OF SMALL INTESTINAL OBSTRUCTION IN ADULTS
(McIver—335 Cases)*

	Per Cent
Hernia (often strangulated)	44
Adhesions and bands (often postoperative)	30
Neoplasms (primary or secondary)	10
Intussusception	5
Volvulus	4
Mesenteric thrombosis	3
Miscellaneous (including gallstone ileus)	4

*McIver, M. A.: Amer. J. Surg., *19*: 163–206, 1933.

MOST COMMON CAUSES OF NEONATAL INTESTINAL MECHANICAL OBSTRUCTION
(Moore)*

Atresia of the duodenum, jejunum, or ileum

Atresia of the colon, rectum, or anus

Meconium ileus

Aganglionosis (Hirschsprung's disease)

Annular pancreas

Midgut volvulus

Internal herniation

Additional congenital defects are often present, as is ischemic necrosis.

*Moore, T. C.: J. Indiana Med. Assoc., *55*:607–613, 1962.

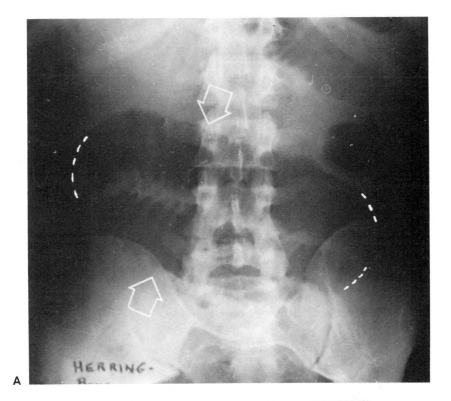

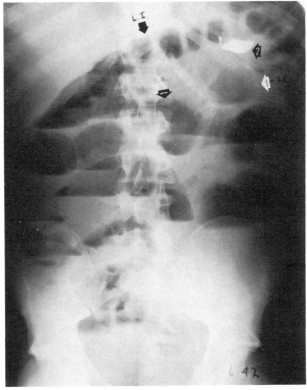

Figure 29–8   *A.* The "herringbone" pattern sometimes produced by distended small intestine. *B.* An erect film of the abdomen in association with small bowel obstruction, demonstrating a rather typical "step-ladder" small intestinal pattern. This is produced by fluid levels within the markedly distended small intestine. Note also the coiled spring appearance of this dilated small intestine.

Combined Abnormalities of Architecture, Size, Contour, and Function

1. Mucosal changes which may involve:
   a. Loss of villi with flattening of the mucosa
   b. Denudation by loss of the mucosal layer (ulceration) and often associated increased secretions in bowel
   c. Infiltration of the villi and valvulae conniventes by:
      (1) edema fluid
      (2) fat
      (3) exudate
      (4) tumor
      (5) lymphocytic infiltration predominantly
      (6) hemorrhage
      (7) granuloma
      (8) scar tissue (after prior insult)
      (9) amyloid
2. Submucosal and intramural infiltrative processes
   a. These may be hemorrhagic, acute inflammatory, granulomatous, or neoplastic in origin.
3. Predominantly serosal changes, such as occur with peritonitis or mesenteritis
4. Manifestations from extrinsic involvement adjoining the small intestine. These largely alter the position of the bowel and do not invade the bowel.
5. Complete obstruction

In so far as possible, an effort is made to relate these changes to roentgen signs (although this relationship is limited in scope) by the barium coating of the lumen of the bowel.

Function is impaired by abnormal secretions or muscular involvement in the wall of the bowel. It may also be impaired by an obstructing lesion, in which case extreme stretching and dilatation proximal to the obstruction may occur.

Mucosal Changes and Their Roentgen Appearances

Loss of Villi (as in Non-Tropical Sprue): Leads to a loss of the normal feathery pattern and a *smooth appearance* of the internal layer of bowel (so-called "intestinalization") (Figure 29–9).

There is a tendency also to *segmentation* and *clumping* of the barium (Figure 29–10). The barium is not propelled in normal fashion and tends to accumulate in scattered foci (so-called "scattering") and "sausagelike" or "moulage" accumulations (Figure 29–11). The bowel under these circumstances is either increased or decreased in its irritability—and hence motility may be increased or decreased in respect to transit time from the pylorus to the ileocecal region.

Denudation or Ulceration of the Mucosa leads to the *longitudinal* or *transverse streaking* (Figure 29–12) associated with the ulceration. If this is associated with deep penetration of the ulcer, *fistulation* may result and this gives rise to the appearance of an irregular channel of the barium into the peritoneal space or from one loop of bowel to another.

Ulcerations when seen in profile, particularly of the transverse type, lead to an appearance of "sawtoothing"; "punctate spiculation" is the descriptive term when seen *en face* (Figure 29–17).

Increased Secretions in the bowel lumen intermix with the barium, imparting a *hazy appearance* and *poor delineation* of the normal feathery pattern (Figure 29–13).

Infiltration of the Mucosa, irrespective of the cause, produces an increased prominence of the valvulae conniventes. They are spread apart and stand out more coarsely. Depending upon the view obtained and the extent of involvement, the mucosal pattern takes on the following appearances, described as (1) *"picket fence,"* (2) *"stacked coins,"* or (3) coarsening of the folds, with increased spacing between valvulae conniventes (Figures 29–14 and 29–24).

Outpouchings or Pseudodiverticula (Figure 29–15).   Disruption of the elastic tissue within the bowel wall with deposition of increased collagen (as in scleroderma) produces a relaxation of the musculature of the bowel wall and pseudodiverticulum formation.

"Cobblestone" Appearance (Figure 29–16).   Patchy infiltration of the bowel wall by a number of processes may produce this roentgen appearance. Thus, it may be produced by lymphocytic or granulomatous infiltration as in regional enteritis, lymphoid hyperplasia, neoplastic infiltration, amyloid, hemorrhage, or Whipple's disease. The hemorrhage may be associated with hemoglobinopathies, anticoagulant therapy, hemophilia, arteritis, infarction, or venous occlusion (venous infarction).

Depending upon the view obtained, this may give rise to the appearance called *"thumbprinting."*

Complete Disruption of the Normal Architecture (Figures 29–16 and 29–21).   Destruction of the mucosa by invasion of the bowel wall or by neoplasia produces a local rigidity of the wall, with ulceration or destruction of the mucosal pattern. An adjoining tumefaction may be identified. Adenocarcinoma, leiomyosarcoma, or occasionally lymphosarcoma may produce this change.

"Skip Areas" of Involvement.   Skip areas occur when a process involves scattered areas of the small intestine with normal bowel intervening, as found in regional enteritis.

Narrow, Rigid and Smooth Sites — Symmetrical or Asymmetrical.   Alterations which are predominantly intramural, or extrinsic to the bowel and effacing the mucosa of the bowel, make it appear locally rigid and immobile in the peritoneal space. This may occur with mesenteritis, panniculitis, lymphosarcoma, or tumor metastases (Figure 29–17).

Immobile Kink of Bowel with Dilated Proximal Loops (Figure 29–18). Scar formation for any reason may obstruct the bowel. If the scar is bound down to the peritoneal surface, this will produce the "immobile kink." If the scar encircles the bowel without binding it to the peritoneal surface, the dilatation proximal to the obstruction and the powerful contraction of the adjoining intestine will produce a modification called the "snake head appearance" (Nelson, Christoforidis, and Roenigk, 1965 A). (Figure 29–18).

Coiled Spring and Stalk Within (Figute 29–19).   With intussusception led by a diverticulum or polyp, the intestine which is distended around the intussus-cipiens has a coiled spring appearance. The intussuscipiens has the appearance of a stem within this. At times, when peroral barium is given, only the central canal will be visible (Carlson). In this case, the diagnosis is more subtle. Vascular insuf-ficiency may be impending.

"Bull's Eye" Appearance.   This is due to central necrosis in a polypoid mass protruding into the lumen of the bowel. Metastatic melanoma, leiomyomas, leio-myosarcomas, polypoid carcinomas, and carcinoid have a tendency toward this change. (See Chapter 30 for illustration.)

"Coiled Linear Streaking" (Figure 29–20).   Fine cylindrical or tubular shad-ows with a central fine line within the tube are suggestive of round worm infesta-tion. The worms ingest the barium, giving rise to this appearance.

The "String Sign."   This is thought to represent spasm due to irritability of the bowel. It has been used especially to describe the spasm with granuloma in regional enteritis.

Cobweb or Lacelike Reticulation and smudging of the intestinal feathery pat-tern (Figure 29–22) has been particularly described with the Zollinger-Ellison syndrome (Weber et al.; Marshak and Lindner). This pattern may in part be due to an increased motor irritability of the small intestine with rapid gastric emptying. The rapid passage of the barium leaves behind it a thin film of contrast to outline the valvulae conniventes (Morrison et al.; Haubrich et al., 1962).

Multiple Round Filling Defects.   This pattern is due to intramural or muco-sal nodular excrescences (Figure 29–23) such as may occur with carcinoid or polyposis.

ABNORMALITIES IN ARCHITECTURE IN DISEASE GROUPS

1. **Focal areas of dilated bowel with splayed-out valvulae.**
    a. Abrupt kinking of bowel leading to obstruction, with dilatation of the segment of bowel proximal to it.
    b. The "blind loop" syndrome, either in association with prior surgery or diverticula.
    c. Paraduodenal or other internal hernias.
    d. Volvulus.
    e. Intussusception, especially associated with tumors as in the Peutz-Jeghers syndrome or a Meckel's diverticulum.
    f. Mesenteric thrombosis.
    g. Aganglionosis.
   Some of these entities are summarized in the adjoining boxes.

2. **Scattered foci of dilated bowel without significant alteration of valvulae.**
    a. Diverticulosis of the small intestine.
    b. Minimal reflex ileus.

3. **Scattered filling defects in the bowel with no dilatation.**
    a. Amyloidosis.
    b. Polyposis (occasionally) without complicating intussusception.
    c. Carcinoid tumors of the small intestine.
    d. Metastatic carcinoma.
    e. Kaposi's sarcoma.

4. **Minimal foci of dilatation with thickening of the valvulae.**
    a. Giardiasis. This especially involves the duodenum and jejunum, and is associated with spasm, irritability, increased secretions, blurring, and thickened valvulae.
    b. Angioneurotic edema.
    c. Partial mechanical obstruction.
    d. Occasionally, in regional enteritis.

5. **Narrowness of the bowel lumen and diffuse thickening of the valvulae.**
    a. Regional enteritis with its *string sign* due to bowel spasm.
    b. Whipple's disease.
    c. Hemophilia.
    d. Multiple foci of intramural bleeding from any cause.
        (1) Picket fencing and the stacked coin appearance are often associated.
    e. Lymphangiectasia is associated with serration of the ileum especially.
    f. Edema from any cause (the lumen may be somewhat dilated): renal failure; ascites.
    g. Protein-losing enteropathy.
    h. Eosinophilic (allergic) gastroenteritis.

6. **Thickened valvulae with interspersed foci of nodulation.**
    a. Lymphoid hyperplasia.
    b. Dysgammaglobulinemia.
    c. Amyloidosis.
    d. Systemic mastocytosis.
    e. Intramural hemorrhage secondary to trauma, anticoagulants or bleeding tendency.
   These may include regional ischemia and hemorrhage secondary to vasculitis, embolism, and thrombosis or hypoproteinemia.

7. **Few consistently narrowed segments with complete loss of the normal architecture at the site of narrowness.**
    a. Regional enteritis.
    b. Adenocarcinoma.
    c. Lymphosarcoma.
    d. Leiomyosarcoma.
    e. Eosinophilic granuloma.

8. **Diminished caliber of the bowel wall with some increased smoothness of the bowel.**
    a. Angioneurotic edema, or edema from other causes such as renal failure, ascites, hepatic failure.
    b. Mesenteritis (panniculitis; retractile mesenteritis).

9. **Impressions on the bowel wall, single, hard, and immobile.**
    a. Metastatic carcinoma, or malignancy of the mesenteric border of the bowel wall.
    b. Ileocarcinoid tumors (carcinoid of the appendix).

10. **Impressions on the bowel wall, somewhat mobile, tending to be single, mobile and pliable.**
    a. Submucosal lymphatic cysts (Fleming and Carlson).
    b. Intramural lipoma.

11. **Permanency of bizarre disposition of narrowed loops.**
    a. Mesenteric panniculitis (retractile mesenteritis) (Clemett and Tracht; Dietz).

12. **The fixed kink of bowel. Stenosing ulcers of the bowel** (following potassium enteric-coated capsule therapy or methysergide therapy when retroperitoneal fibrosis may develop).

13. **Segmentation, scattering, moulage. Malabsorption syndrome.**

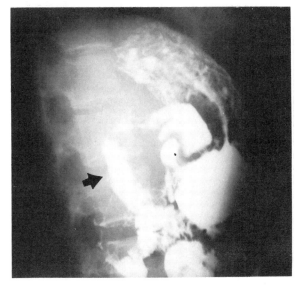

Figure 29–9 Radiograph illustrating loss of villi in the small intestine.

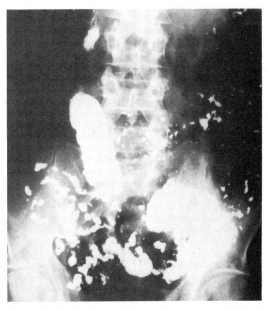

Figure 29–10 Radiograph illustrating segmentation and clumping of the small intestine.

Figure 29–11 Considerable scattering and clumping in the small intestine following intramural and intraluminal hemorrhage in a patient on dicumarol therapy. This demonstrates the "moulage" appearance.

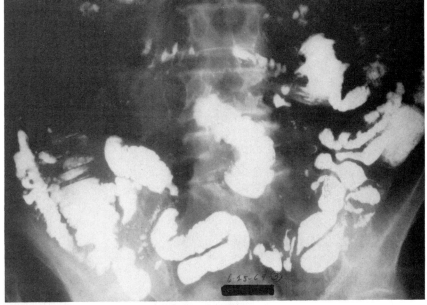

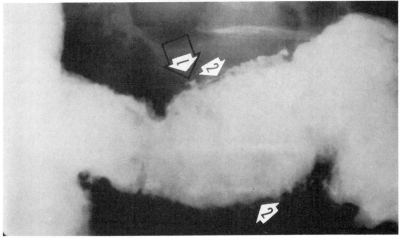

Figure 29–12 Appearance of the small intestine with longitudinal and transverse ulceration. Arrow 1 indicates a collar button type ulceration; arrow 2 shows a longitudinal ulceration.

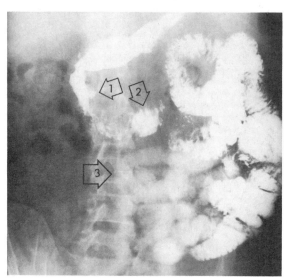

Figure 29-13 Zollinger-Ellison syndrome. Demonstrates three of the roentgen signs: (1) a duodenal ulcer in the second part of the duodenum with complete loss of the normal rugae in this part of the duodenum; (2) the coarsened rugae of the distal duodenum and jejunum; (3) the marked dilution of the barium in the distal jejunum as the secretions "chase" the barium into the more distal loops of small intestine.

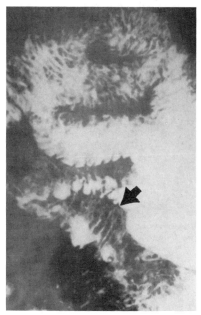

Figure 29-14 Appearance of the small intestine with the "stacked coin" sign caused, in this instance, by intramural hemorrhage in the wall of the jejunum in a patient with hemophilia.

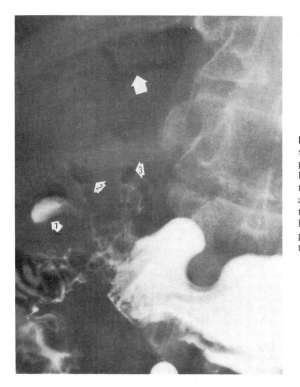

Figure 29-15 Pseudodiverticula of the duodenal bulb resulting from a duodenum that has been markedly scarred by previous ulceration. Note that at Arrow 1 there is both barium and air in this pseudodiverticulum. Arrow 2 shows that mostly air is contained in the pseudodiverticulum, and adjoining Arrow 3 there is a communication with the air in the biliary tree indicating that communication with the biliary tree has occurred by penetration and perforation of previous ulceration. The unnumbered large arrow indicates the free air in the biliary tree.

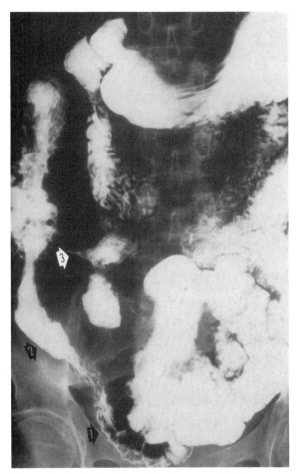

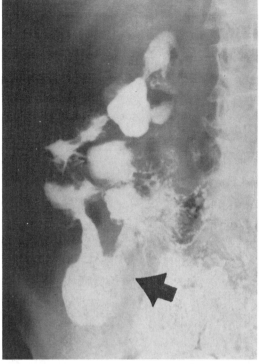

Figure 29–17   Ulceration, rigidity and saw-toothing in the distal ileum in a patient with regional enteritis.

Figure 29–16   Regional enteritis demonstrating the "cobblestone" appearance. The distal small intestine is diffusely involved. Arrow 1 shows the pseudo-papillary appearance of the distal small intestine and ileum called "cobblestone." Arrow 2 shows the somewhat dilated irregular terminal ileum with complete lack of normal mucosal pattern. Arrow 3 indicates the probable fistulation between cecum and distal ileum.

Figure 29–18   The scout roentgenograms (not shown) were normal in this patient with symptoms of mechanical obstruction of the small intestine. Barium sulfate was given orally.

A roentgenogram taken thirty minutes later showed normal loops of small bowel, but two hours later a striking "snakehead" configuration (arrows) of one of the loops of ileum is demonstrated. An adhesion was found at operation. (From Nelson, S. W. et al.: Radiology, *84*:881, 1965.)

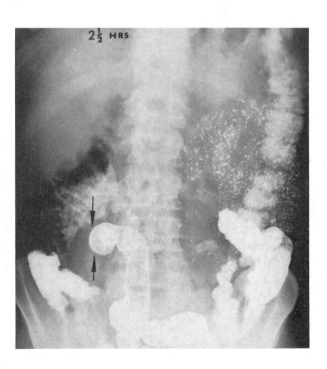

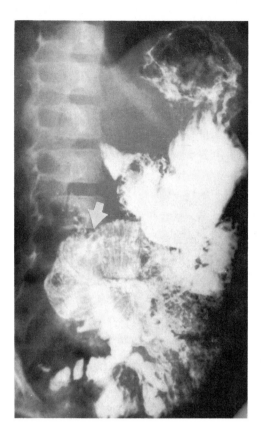

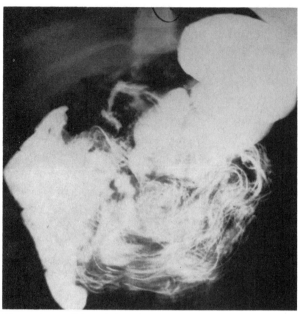

Figure 29–19 Radiograph demonstrating the coiled spring and "stalk" within a sign. This was a patient with Peutz-Jegher's syndrome. Note the multiple polyps and the several areas of intussusception in the small intestine.

Figure 29–20 Worm infestation in the small intestine: note that there is barium, not only surrounding the worms, but also occupying the enteric canals of the worms.

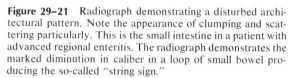

Figure 29–21 Radiograph demonstrating a disturbed architectural pattern. Note the appearance of clumping and scattering particularly. This is the small intestine in a patient with advanced regional enteritis. The radiograph demonstrates the marked diminution in caliber in a loop of small bowel producing the so-called "string sign."

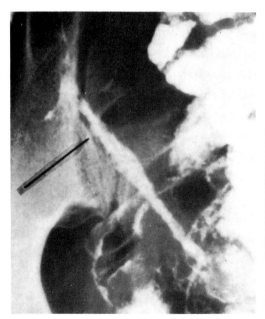

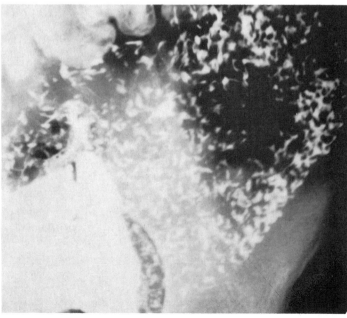

Figure 29–22 Scattering and clumping with a lacelike reticulation in a patient with nontropical sprue.

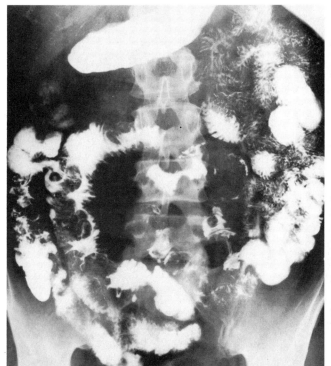

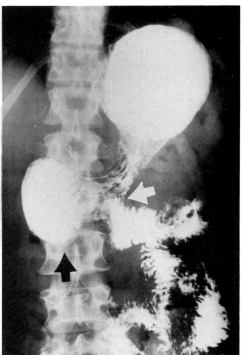

Figure 29–23 Carcinoid tumors involving the small intestine. Barium study of the jejunum and ileum shows multiple round filling defects in a patient with carcinoid tumors. (Courtesy of Dr. Paul E. Shorb, Jr., George Washington University.)

Figure 29–24 Marked thickening of the rugae of an afferent loop in a patient with a "blind loop" syndrome (designated by the dark arrow). There is dilatation and retention of the barium with widening of the mucosal pattern and thickening of the valvulae conniventes, suggesting edematous infiltration in the wall of this loop.

Abnormalities of Density of the Bowel

Increased Density Due to Calcification

Hemangioma of the Small Intestine. This may appear as multiple small phleboliths in the bowel wall (Carlson and Good). More than half of the hemangiomas of the small bowel occur in the jejunum (Bandler; Copple and Kingsbury; Good, 1963).

Foreign Bodies in the Small Intestine

Most Foreign Bodies which pass through the pylorus will pass through the small intestine, at least until the ileocecal junction is reached. Some elongated objects, however, may be detained at the duodenojejunal flexure. Perforation may occur.

Gallstones, when extruded from the biliary tract into the small intestine via choledochojejunal or choledochoduodenal fistulae, behave as do foreign bodies and may cause a partial or complete obstruction at the ileocecal junction (gallstone ileus). When the gallstone is partially calcified it will appear opaque within the gastrointestinal tract.

Worm Infestations may at times be so extensive that they behave like foreign bodies and produce obstruction in the ileocecal junction also. The worm shadows themselves will produce an abnormal air density within the gastrointestinal tract.

Primary Enterolithiasis (Brettner and Euphrat). This is a laminated calculus resulting usually from chronic stasis. It occurs in a diverticulum or proximal to an area of chronic partial obstruction and a favorable chemical milieu. It may be situated in Meckel's diverticulum.

Meconium Ileus in Infants (mucoviscidosis) (see Chapters 17 and 24)

Meconium ileus occurs in approximately 5 to 10 per cent of patients with intestinal obstruction or peritonitis at birth. This is a manifestation of a genetically inherited disorder of glandular structures in several parts of the body.

In the gastrointestinal tract, the inspissated meconium tends to cause early obstruction in the newborn infant. Meconium classically appears as an inspissated mass with a bubble appearance, suggesting inspissated fecal material.

In the respiratory passages a sticky mucus accumulates, causing obstruction and a predisposition to infection, pneumonia, and patchy atelectasis. Emphysema, cor pulmonale, and associated complications frequently ensue.

In older children and in adults, the roentgen pattern of pancreatic insufficiency may closely resemble that of the malabsorption syndrome to be described below.

Diminished Density in the Wall of the Bowel (Chapter 24)

Pneumatosis Cystoides Intestinalis. In this condition multiple small gas cysts are found within the wall of the bowel. The cause is unknown. There may be a break in the mucosal continuity with a dissection of air under the mucosa of the gastrointestinal tract (Nitch and Shattock). Some instances have been reported as occurring with pulmonary disease, harsh cough, and pneumomediastinum (Keyting et al.; Shapiro et al.).

In children the gas pockets are frequently found in the submucosa, whereas in adults these pockets are most frequently in the subserosa.

In the newborn, it may be a manifestation of an exudative necrotizing enterocolitis and is a reflection of severe disease (Rabinowitz et al.).

Spontaneous pneumoperitoneum sometimes occurs as a complication (Lerner and Gazin).

The condition may be found in association with other diseases such as mesenteric occlusion, scleroderma, Whipple's disease and other diarrheal states (see Chapter 30).

Abnormalities in Function of the Small Intestine

Delay in the time of barium passage through the small intestine (greater than four to six hours in the adult, or nine hours in the infant) is usually indicative of small intestinal malfunction and may accompany many diseases. Also, evidence of gas in the small bowel is usually an indication of abnormality except in children and in patients past 60 years of age. Apart from mesenteric abnormalities, alterations in motor function occur in Zollinger-Ellison syndrome (increased transit time with hypersecretion), scleroderma, hypermotility with spasm, atony with ileus, malabsorption syndromes in which the transit time may be either increased or decreased, regional enteritis, protein-losing enteropathies and Whipple's disease.

Usually it is the disordered function which brings the patient to the physician. With the advent of intestinal intubation biopsy, correlated with increased knowledge and skill of roentgen examination many of the disorders which, in earlier years, were merely dismissed as disordered function can now find more specific diagnosis and treatment.

SPECIFIC DISEASE EXAMPLES

The Malabsorption Syndrome
(Samloff et al.; Yardley et al.; Preger and Amberg)

1. *Major roentgenologic findings*—dilatation, segmentation, fragmentation, scattering, thickening of the mucosal folds, flocculation of barium due to hypersecretion.
2. This may be correlated with the histologic demonstration of diminution in number of crypts of Lieberkühn and flattening of the mucosal surface with loss of villi (Figure 29–25).
3. With recovery, gradual return of villi is noted.
4. Children with celiac disease are similarly affected.
5. Characteristic radiographs from the small bowel are shown in Figure 29–25 and comparisons are made with protein-losing enteropathy when there is a definite lymphangiectasis (Figure 29–26).
6. Manifestations of malabsorption also occur in relation to certain lactose or sucrose sensitivities. These may be shown radiologically by obtaining studies after lactose barium ingestion (diagnosis hypolactasia and hyposucrasia). Disaccharide is also similarly involved.

    The radiologic manifestations in these patients are in part due to the osmotic effect of unsplit disaccharide within the gut lumen (Laws, Spencer, and Neale; Pink; Preger and Amberg).
7. The principal small bowel disaccharidases are lactase, sucrase, and maltase. In patients with lactase deficiency, lactose cannot be hydrolized. A barium lactose mixture is necessary to demonstrate characteristic *roentgen findings*—barium dilution, bowel dilatation, and rapidity of intestinal emptying.

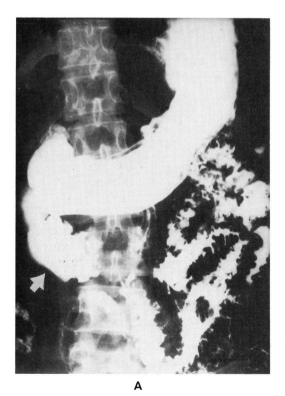

A

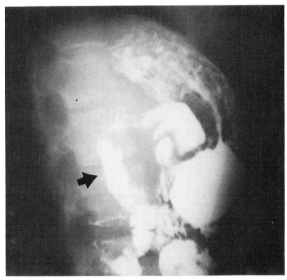

B

Figure 29–25 Nontropical sprue. *A*. The markedly dilated duodenum in nontropical sprue. Note the amorphous appearance of the duodenum with a tendency to "saccular or aneurysmal dilatation." The coarse rugal pattern of the jejunum is also noteworthy. *B*. Lateral view of the stomach and duodenum showing the amorphous and saccular appearance of the duodenum.

Protein-Losing Disorders of the Gastrointestinal Tract
(Marshak et al., Pock-Steen)

1. **Classification**
   a. Primary exudative gastropathy (Menetrier's disease) — mucosal hyperplasia and giant folds of the stomach. It may involve the small intestine and colon also.
   b. Exudative enteropathy of Gordon.
   c. Secondary protein-losing disorders — regional enteritis, carcinoma of the gastrointestinal tract, ulcerative colitis, primary or nontropical sprue, mesenteric vascular occlusion, intestinal malignant lymphoma, congestive heart failure, necrosis, and Whipple's disease (Kalser).
2. **Roentgenologic Manifestations** (Figure 29–26)
   a. Gordon enteropathy: coarsened rugal folds with minimal dilatation and increased secretions (Figure 29–26 A and B). Usually no segmentation or fragmentation.
   b. In the secondary type of protein-losing disorder no special roentgen changes may be seen.

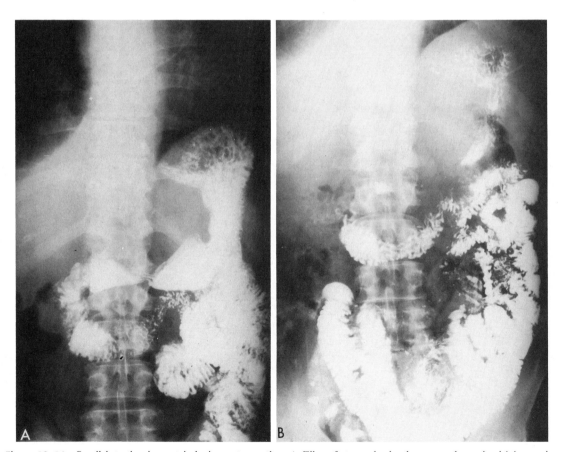

Figure 29–26   Small intestine in protein-losing enteropathy. *A*. Film of stomach, duodenum, and proximal jejunum immediately after the oral administration of the barium. It is noted that the jejunal loops are moderately coarsened. *B*. Film of the small intestine one hour after the oral administration of the barium. The coarsened jejunal pattern is more readily identified.

Small Intestinal Diverticula (Figure 29–27)
(Irwin; Caplan and Jacobson; Cross et al.).

1. Small bowel diverticula usually occur in the duodenum but may occur more distally.
2. Meckel's diverticulum (Figure 29–28) is an embryonic remnant of the vitelline or omphalomesenteric duct as it joins the antimesenteric margin of the distal ileum.
   a. It appears as a blunt pouch, two to four feet proximal to the ileocecal valve.
   b. It may contain heterotopic gastric mucosa (15 per cent) or pancreatic tissue (5 per cent), but rarely calculi and duodenal mucosa.
   c. Inflammation, ulceration, hemorrhage, intussusception, prolapse of the intestine through the umbilical fistula, aberrant gastric mucosa with ulceration causing intestinal hemorrhage, and occasional tumors are the chief complications.
   d. It may measure as much as 10 or 12 cm. in diameter and be associated with a blind loop syndrome.
   e. It may be involved with regional enteritis or even gallstones.
3. Intraluminal diverticulum is described in Chapter 28, since all reported cases originate in the descending duodenum (Marshak and Lindner). The clear zone surrounding this kind of diverticulum has been called the "comma sign."

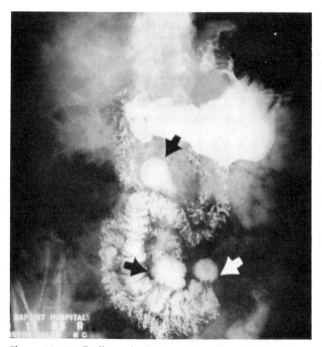

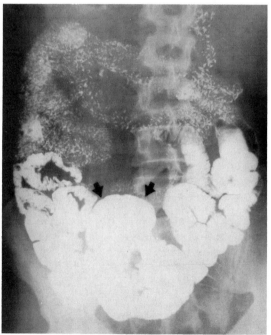

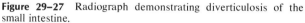

Figure 29–27 Radiograph demonstrating diverticulosis of the small intestine.

Figure 29–28 Meckel's diverticulum.

Scleroderma of the Small Intestine (Figure 29–29)
(Meiercort and Merrill; Bluestone et al.)

1. Gastrointestinal involvement is found in approximately two-thirds of cases (Treacy et al. — 306 cases).
   a. Esophagus, 58.5 per cent.
   b. Small intestine, 4.9 per cent (all with esophageal involvement as well).
2. Roentgenologic manifestations
   a. Slight to great dilatation, which is earliest and most frequent in the duodenum and jejunum.
   b. Loss of tone and motility of the intestine.
   c. Sacculations may occur as in the colon.
   d. Atony of the bowel and absent peristalsis are frequently observed.
3. It is possible that it is related to calcinosis with progressive systemic sclerosis (Gondos).

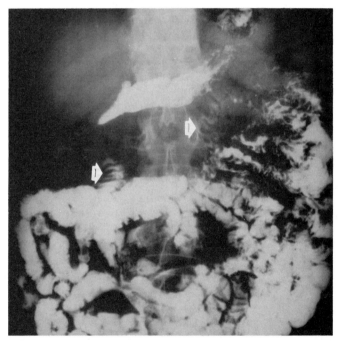

Figure 29–29 Scleroderma of the small intestine, demonstrating the edematous and thickened folds of the proximal small intestine. This patient also had sclerodermatous involvement of the esophagus.

Regional Enteritis (Crohn's Disease)

1. Roentgenologic Manifestations (Figure 29–30)
   a. Blunting, flattening, and thickening of the valvulae conniventes.
   b. Bowel lumen becomes narrow and its contour irregular.
   c. Ulceration with longitudinal streaking of the barium is frequent.
   d. Cobblestone appearance.
   e. Rigid and castlike bowel.
   f. Foci of stenosis and partial or complete obstruction, with complete loss of pliability.
   g. "Skip areas" are characteristic.
   h. Penetration, fistulation, and abscess formation are common.
   i. The string sign probably indicates an area of spasm and irritability.
   j. The colon may also be involved, as may the esophagus and stomach.
   k. The distal 9 to 12 inches of the terminal ileum was the site of involvement in approximately two-thirds of the 700 cases observed over a period of 1 to 12 years (Marshak).
      (1) The entire ileum was involved in 16 per cent of the cases.
      (2) The distal half of the jejunum was involved in 14 per cent, usually including half of the ileum.
      (3) The duodenum was involved in only four cases.
2. Regional ileitis can compress and obstruct one or both ureters (Goldman and Glickman).
3. Pathology
   It is primarily a disease of the submucosa involving the mucosa secondarily.

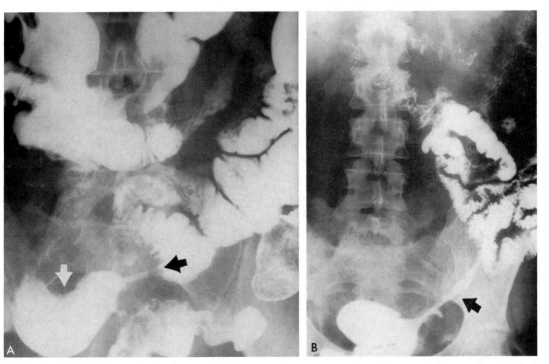

Figure 29–30   *A.* Regional enteritis of the small intestine (Crohn's disease). The white arrow points to a "moulage" sign, whereas the dark arrow points to a fistulation between two loops of small intestine. There is an additional fistula between the ileum and sigmoid colon. *B.* Regional enteritis with fistula formation between jejunum and sigmoid colon.

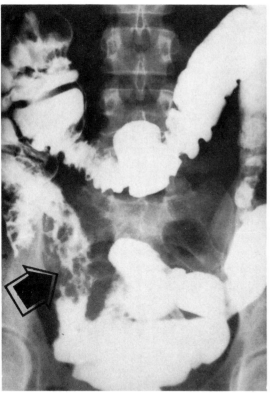

Figure 29-31 Coarsened rugal pattern of the distal ileum producing a cobblestone appearance. This was a patient with regional enteritis.

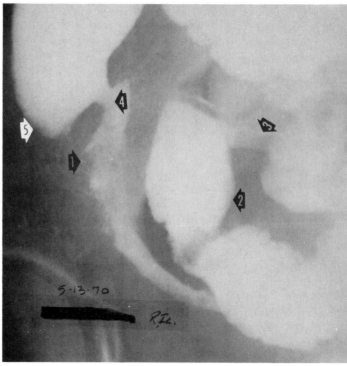

Figure 29-32 The small intestine and cecum in regional enteritis (Crohn's disease). (1) Distal ileum demonstrating irregular thickened mucosa. (2) Markedly dilated segment of distal ileum. (3) Markedly constricted area of distal ileum—(we cannot be certain that this could not have represented a small fistulation). (4) Widely patent ileocecal junction. (5) The thickened shrunken cecum with a "conelike" appearance.

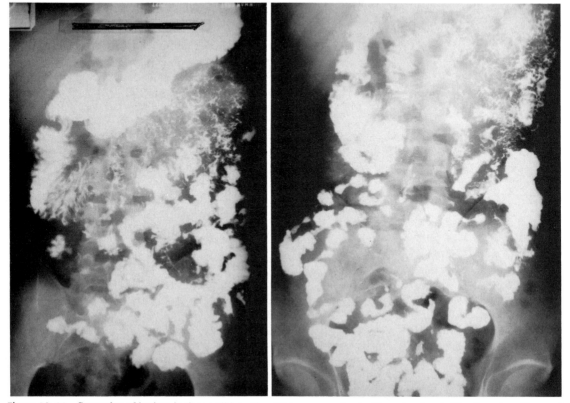

Figure 29-33 Scattering of barium in the small intestine. This was a patient with regional enteritis; there is evidence of disruption of mucosal pattern, some evidence of clumping, and loss of normal mucosal pattern.

Intramural Intestinal Hemorrhage
(Khilnani et al.; Dodds et al.; Wiot et al.; Grossman et al.)

Roentgenologic Manifestations (Figure 29–34)

1. On plain films increased density or displacement of loops of small or large bowel with varying degrees of paralytic ileus and narrowness of the bowel lumen can be seen. Small defects may be seen within the air produced by scalloping of the bowel.
2. Barium studies of small intestine:
    (a) Varying degrees of rigidity and uncoiling of loops.
    (b) Separation of the loops of bowel occasionally.
    (c) Transient intussusception occasionally.
    (d) Uniform regular thickening of the folds with sharp delineation of their margins and parallel arrangement, producing spikelike configuration simulating a stack of coins.
3. In Henoch's purpura and idiopathic thrombocytopenic purpura, increased secretions and edema may blur the sharpness and symmetry of the folds.
4. Scalloping and thumbprinting due to localized hemorrhage or edema may also be seen.
5. Evidence of a mass due to bleeding into mesentery may flatten the folds on the mesenteric side of the bowel. If large, the bowel assumes a hammocklike configuration.

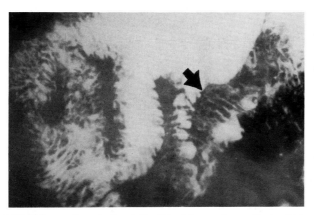

Figure 29–34 Intramural hemorrhage in the wall of the jejunum in a patient with hemophilia. The mucosal pattern assumes the "stacked coin" appearance.

Radiation Enteropathy of the Small Intestine
(Rosen and Shapiro)

Roentgenologic Manifestations (Figure 29–35)

1. Nonspecific. Kinklike adhesions or irregular sawtooth pattern with ulceration in the acute phase.
2. Ordinarily maximum tolerance of small intestine is considered to be 5000 rads in a period of five weeks for orthovoltage radiation. With this dosage it is possible for as many as 10 per cent of patients to have disturbing changes in the small intestine, involving even perforation, obstruction, or fistulation.
3. In the differential diagnosis it is important to relate the findings to the region irradiated, since the roentgenologic alterations are localized to this region (for example, pelvis or renal bed).

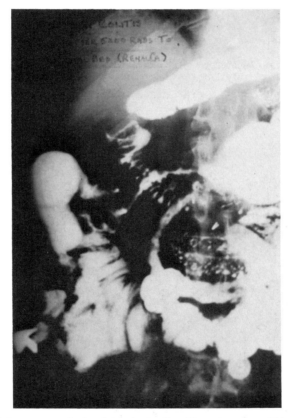

Figure 29–35 Radiation enteropathy involving the small and large intestines. This patient had received, two years previously, 5000 rads to the right renal bed in treatment of a right renal carcinoma. The marked narrowness and irregularity of the rugal pattern are demonstrated.

Whipple's Disease — Intestinal Lipodystrophy Syndrome

(Figure 29–36) (Haubrick et al.; Martel and Hodges; Schatzki; Triano; Rice et al.)

Pathology

Diffuse infiltration of mucosa with large mononuclear macrophages—positive reaction to periodic acid-Schiff stain. There is an accumulation of variable amounts of lipoid substances within the lymphatics and in extracellular cystic spaces in the intestinal mucosa and regional lymph nodes. This is followed by chronic endolymphangitis and fibrosis.

Roentgenologic Manifestations

1. May resemble malabsorption syndrome with scattering, clumping, segmentation, and flocculation of the barium.
2. Extraintestinal manifestations—mediastinal lymph node enlargement, and marked arthritic changes closely resembling advanced rheumatoid arthritis.
3. Retroperitoneal lymph masses may produce marked displacement of intestinal loops.
4. The moulage sign is very seldom present and there is no dilatation of the small or large intestine.
5. Remissions have occurred following treatment with antibiotics, especially Chloromycetin and steroids.

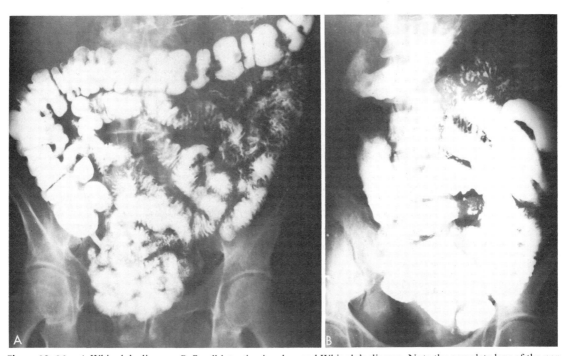

Figure 29–36 *A.* Whipple's disease. *B.* Small intestine in advanced Whipple's disease. Note the complete loss of the normal feathery pattern of the jejunum. Nondescript amorphous clumps and clusters of barium are arrayed one on top of the other.

Benign Tumors of the Small Intestine
(Pearce et al.; Carlson and Good; Marshak and Lindner)

1. Benign tumors usually escape recognition unless complications develop such as: (a) intussusception (Figure 29–37), (b) obstruction, (c) ulceration producing either fistulation or a cavity with gas. (The fistulae are usually short in length—less than 1½ cm.)
2. Approximately half of the benign tumors escape recognition clinically and are discovered at operation or necropsy (Olsson et al.; Good). Radiologic demonstration is obtained in less than two-thirds of the cases studied.
3. The two most frequent types of tumors are adenomas and leiomyomas. Leiomyomas may be recognized by (a) central ulceration, and (b) faint flakes of calcification.
4. The distribution of benign tumors of the small intestine is approximately: duodenum, 20 per cent; jejunum, 40 per cent; ileum, 40 per cent.
5. When obstruction or intussusception is noted, and with it a filling defect in the opacified intestinal lumen, the tumor is usually of regular contour and does not destroy the intestinal mucosa. Obstruction to the small intestine may be associated with extrinsic adhesions if the tumor is largely serosal.
6. Multiple phlebectasias (hereditary hemorrhagic telangiectasia—Rendu-Weber-Osler disease) may produce focal cavernous dilatations of intestinal venous arcades giving rise to the appearance of multiple benign tumors of the small intestine.
7. Submucosal leiomyosarcomas of small intestine may also occur (Dodds et al.).

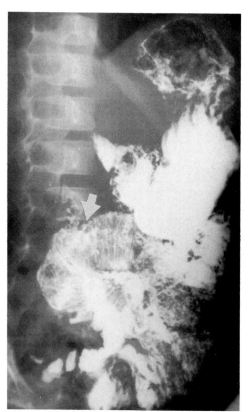

Figure 29–37 Peutz-Jeghers syndrome. Note the multiple polypi and the several areas of intussusception in the small intestine.

Intussusception
(Wiot and Spitz; Hemmingsson, Ruoff et al.)

1. The most frequent causes in the small intestine are
   a. Peutz-Jeghers syndrome (Figure 29–37): multiple polyposis of the gastrointestinal tract with circumoral pigmentation.
   b. Aganglionosis of the small intestine (Lawrence and Van Wormer).
      Intussusception here is ordinarily ileocolic.
   c. Intussusception of a Meckel's diverticulum.
2. Peutz-Jeghers syndrome consists of purple melena pigmentation involving the lips, buccal mucosa, hard palate, and digits, as well as gastrointestinal polypi with recurrent intussusception (Figure 29–37). True malignancy is rare (Bartholomew et al.; Staley and Schwarz; Bailey; Achord and Proctor).

Intestinal Edema
(Marshak et al., 1967; Ellis and McConnell)

Roentgenologic Findings

1. Excessive intestinal secretions.
2. Folds are thickened and appear blunted, incomplete, and irregular.
3. The barium column is fragmented with segmentation.
4. Occasionally it resembles sprue except that in sprue, folds are thin and dilatation is marked.
5. The bowel wall is thickened by edema and its motor activity is irregular and altered.
6. Ascites is frequent.
7. Episodic regional edema of the small intestine and colon may occur with hereditary angioneurotic edema.

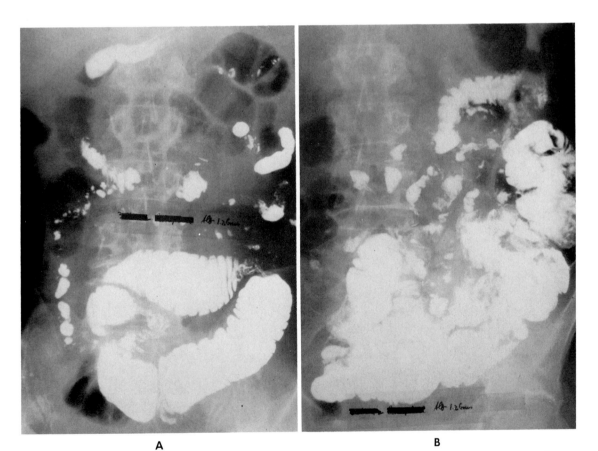

A   B

Figure 29–38 *A* and *B*. Marked edema, scattering, and clumping of the small intestine with hypoalbuminemia.

Blind Loop Syndrome
(Figure 29–39) (Irwin)

1. Any intestinal lesion that produces stasis within a lumen of the gut as a result of either stricture or a redundant loop of bowel may lead to this syndrome.
2. Steatorrhea is often associated.
3. Diverticula are often associated.
4. Pathogenesis—bacterial proliferation within the blind loop. These bacteria suppress the formation of essential substances such as biotin, folic acid, nicotinic acid, riboflavin, thiamine, and vitamin K. A macrocytic megaloblastic anemia is produced.
5. Intestinal biopsy is useful in differentiating the blind loop syndrome from other causes of steatorrhea.

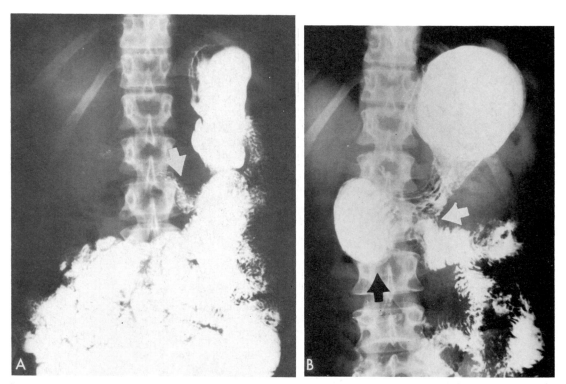

Figure 29–39   *A*. Film of the remaining portion of the stomach and anastomosed portion of jejunum demonstrating the normal filling of an afferent loop. This afferent loop became part of a blind loop syndrome as shown subsequently. *B*. Blind loop syndrome. The jejunum is anastomosed to the stomach at the site of the white arrow. The afferent loop, designated by the dark arrow, behaved as a blind loop in this instance and shows evidence of dilatation and retention of the barium with widening of the mucosal pattern, further suggesting edematous infiltration in the wall of this loop.

Intestinal Lymphangiectasia
(Waldmann et al.; Nugent and Ross; Mistilis et al.)

1. Roentgenologic findings (Figure 29–40):
    a. Thickening of mucosal folds with marked tendency to diffuse involvement.
    b. Fragmentation and scattering of barium.
    c. Dilatation is minimal or absent.
    d. No ulceration or separation of loops of bowel is seen.
    e. Nodular mucosal defects may be present and occasionally an irregular serrated margin of ileum is noted.
2. Important clinical aspects
    a. Familial tendency.
    b. Peripheral edema and diarrhea constitute the two most important symptoms.
3. May also be due to lymphatic obstruction by malignant tumors, especially lymphoma.

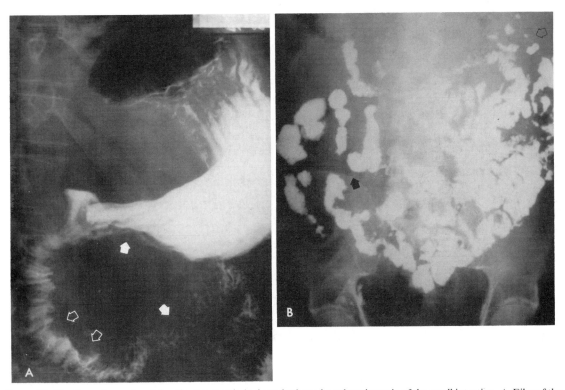

Figure 29–40   Lymphoma involving the pancreatic bed producing a lymphangiectasia of the small intestine. *A*. Film of the stomach and duodenum demonstrating the large filling defect impressing itself on the antrum and duodenum. (Closed arrows show the mass effect upon the antrum and fourth part of the duodenum; open arrows show the irregular scalloped appearance of the second and third parts of the duodenum produced by the mass in the pancreatic bed.) *B*. Demonstrates the marked scattering of the barium owing to the lymphangiectasia. There are also some edematous swollen folds in the small intestine.

Lymphosarcoma of the Small Intestine (Figure 29–41)
(Marshak, Wolf, and Eliasoph; Balikian et al.; Cups et al.)

Roentgenologic Manifestations

1. Multiple small nodular defects.
2. May be an infiltrative type in which the bowel becomes diffusely thickened for variable lengths and the mucosa in these cases is coarsened and infiltrated (Figure 29–41).
3. A polypoid form may be associated with intussusception.
4. An endoexoenteric form may be associated with ulceration, fistulation, and extrinsic mass formation (Figure 29–42).
5. There may be an associated invasion of the mesentery with a large mass displacing adjoining abdominal organs and causing intestinal obstruction.
6. The sprue pattern may be present and diagnosis must ultimately be based on histology (Kent; Deeb and Stilson; Pollock).

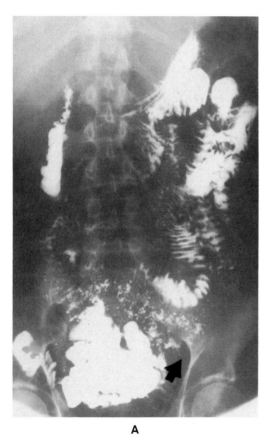
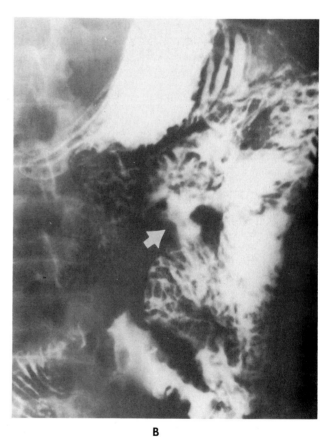

A   B

Figure 29–41 *A* and *B*. Malignant lymphoma of the small intestine. *A*. "Stacked-coin" appearance of infiltrative jejunum. A somewhat similar appearance may also be produced by intramural hematoma of the small intestine. *B*. Ulceration and infiltration with complete loss of normal mucosal pattern of the jejunum with malignant lymphoma.

Adenocarcinoma of the Small Intestine (Figure 29–42)

1. Usually there are short, sharply demarcated napkin-ringlike defects in the column of barium with an obliteration of the normal mucosal pattern.
2. This may be associated with partial or complete obstruction.
3. It is most frequent in the duodenum and proximal jejunum but may occur more distally.

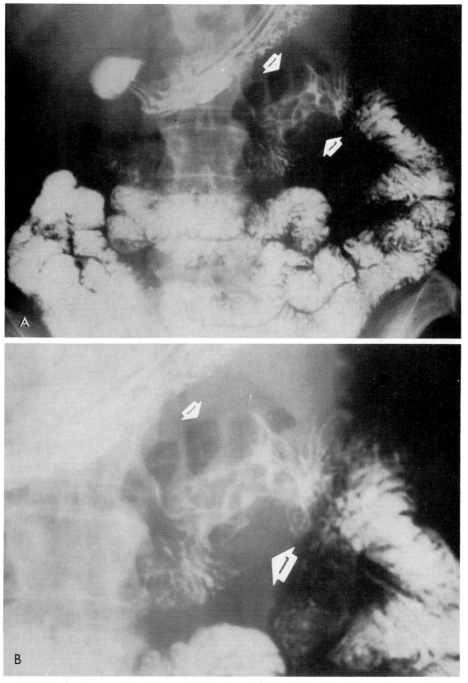

Figure 29–42   Carcinoma of the jejunum. *A*. Film showing the relationship of the carcinoma to the stomach and small intestine. *B*. Magnified view of the carcinoma itself. The thickness of the small bowel is demonstrated at (1).

Metastatic Carcinoma to the Mesentery and Gut
(Figure 29–43) (Zboralske et al., Marshak et al., 1965.)

1. Roentgenologic Findings

    a. The "tacked-down" sign representing the formation in adhesions due to a fibrotic response of the intestinal wall.

        (1) The folds are angulated at their tips. They are distorted but not destroyed.

    b. Thickening of the bowel wall due to malignancy and associated inflammatory exudate and edema.

    c. Immediately adjoining valvulae may appear "spiked."

    d. Small nodular masses give the margins of the gut a scalloped appearance, but if they are large they displace the bowel around it owing to extensions from the primary lesion.

    e. If the metastasis invades the mucosa, ulceration is produced.

    f. The bowel may appear shortened owing to involvement of the mesentery.

    g. If peritoneum is involved, ascites may also be present.

2. In Differential Diagnosis, it is important to recall that Kaposi's sarcoma, when it involves the gastrointestinal tract, most often appears as multiple nodular masses in the small bowel.

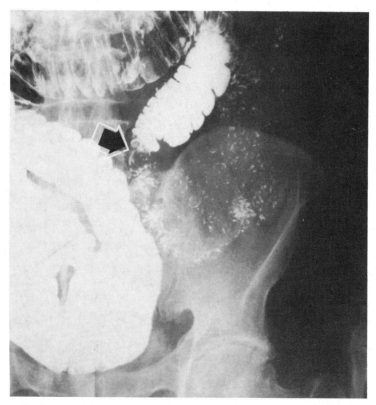

Figure 29–43 Radiograph demonstrating partial small intestinal obstruction produced by an adhesive band. Note the dilated segment of small intestine proximal to the point of partial obstruction. Note also the difference in mucosal pattern between the markedly dilated small intestine and the colon immediately cephalad.

Carcinoid Tumors of the Small Intestine (Figure 29–44)
(Grondin et al.; Biörck et al.; Lembeck; Steele, Shorb and McCune)

1. Roentgenologic Features
    a. Carcinoid tumors occur as small nodules in the submucosa but may grow to large size (Humphreys).

    b. The main filling defects in the small bowel are found in the ileum but may also involve the appendix or cecum.

2. Carcinoid Syndrome (Biörck et al., Lembeck)
    a. Paroxysmal erythematous flushing, mainly of the head and neck.

    b. Recurrent bouts of abdominal cramps and diarrhea unaccompanied by blood, pus, or mucus.

    c. Various inconstant symptoms such as attacks of asthma, personality changes, even psychotic episodes.

    d. Usually metastases are demonstrable in the liver and occasionally in other organs.

    e. The disease is due to a faulty metabolism in tryptophan and the syndrome is caused by excessive serotonin in the body.

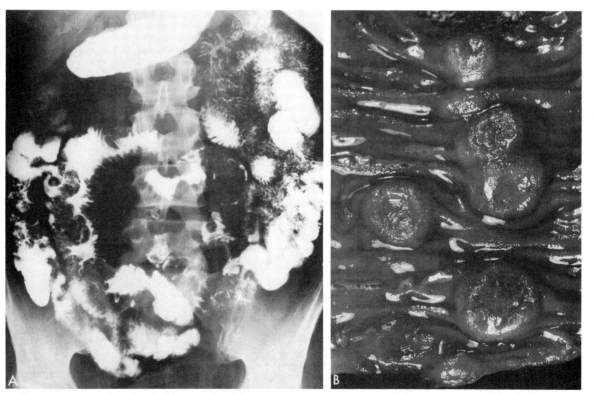

Figure 29–44 *A* and *B*. Carcinoid tumors involving the small intestine. *A*. Barium study of the jejunum and ileum showing multiple round filling defects in a patient with carcinoid tumors. *B*. Resected specimen showing circumscribed elevated umbilicated carcinoid tumors. (Courtesy of Dr. Paul S. Shorb, Jr., George Washington University.)

Volvulus of the Small Intestine (Figure 29–45)

1. Faulty rotation of bowel and embryonic development or faulty fixation of the mesentery or both are usually responsible.
2. The plain film diagnosis may be made by evidence of mechanical intestinal obstruction, particularly if followed by a barium enema and if evidence of hyperrotation or abnormal rotation of the large intestine or cecum is demonstrated.
3. *Abnormalities in rotation of the cecum in an infant with clinical manifestations of obstruction are usually indicative of volvulus of the small intestine.*

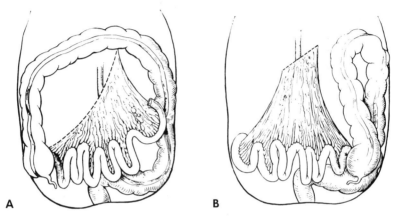

Figure 29–45   *A.* The normal mesenteric fixation is broad, runs from the left upper to right lower quadrant, and anchors the midgut. *B.* Narrow fixation of the midgut with malrotation can predispose to volvulus. (*A* and *B* from Snyder, C. H., and Chaffin, L.: Malrotation of the intestine. In *Pediatric Surgery*, Vol. 2. Chicago, Year Book Medical Publishers, 1969.)

Eosinophilic (Allergic) Gastroenteritis
(Edelman and March; Ureles et al.; McCune et al.; Burhenne and Carbone)

1. Roentgenologic Findings
   a. Resembles regional enteritis closely and is often misdiagnosed as such.
   b. When the stomach is involved along with the small intestine or alone, carcinoma may be suspected by the appearance of eosinophilic gastroenteritis.
2. Characteristic clinical features include the high prominent eosinophilia—as high as 63 per cent in eosinophilic gastroenteritis—and also the self limitation of this disease entity. It responds well to cortisone therapy.

Dysgammaglobulinemia With Nodular Lymphoid Hyperplasia of Small Intestine
(Grise, Hodgson et al.)

Roentgenologic Aspects
   Small nodularities of the intestinal mucosa that are particularly prominent in the duodenum and less prominent in the jejunum but extend all the way to the ileum.

The greatest involvement may be in the jejunum. The small polypoid masses range from 1 to 3 mm. in diameter. The filling defects are round and regular in outline.

Amyloidosis of the Small Intestine
(Golden, 1954; Herskovic et al., Brody et al.; Ritvo and Litner, Marshak and Lindner; Legge et al.)

1. The gastrointestinal tract is the second most frequent site of amyloidosis; the usual sites of occurrence are stomach, small intestine, colon, and esophagus. In 30 per cent amyloidosis is associated with multiple myeloma.
2. *Roentgenologic Features:*
   a. Thickened mucosal folds.
   b. Narrowing and irregularity of the lumen.
   c. Gaseous distention.
   d. Nodular filling defects.
3. Rectal biopsy recommended (Green et al.)

Questions—Chapter 29

1. What features in gross anatomy distinguish the small intestine from the large intestine and how are these manifested radiologically?
2. In what part of the small intestine are the villi most numerous and how is this important radiologically?
3. Where are the lymphoid patches most numerous? Indicate the radiologic importance of this anatomic detail.
4. What are the normal transit times for barium to reach the ileocecal region?
5. What technique of examination of the small intestine is most generally used? How may this technique be modified in order to study the postoperative, partially resected stomach?
6. What are some of the basic differences in roentgen appearances of the small intestine between adults and infants?
7. Describe the abnormalities of intestinal rotation. Why are these of considerable significance radiologically? In what age groups?
8. How would you recognize the normal and abnormal relationships of the small intestine?
9. Describe the roentgen findings with paralytic ileus.
10. Describe the roentgen findings with mechanical obstruction.
11. What are the most frequent causes of small intestinal obstruction in adults?
12. What are the most frequent causes of neonatal intestinal mechanical obstruction?
13. When there is a loss of villi morphologically, how is it manifested roentgenologically?
14. When there is a denudation or ulceration of the mucosa of the small intestine, how is it manifested radiologically?
15. When increased secretions are found in the bowel lumen, what is the roentgenologic appearance? In what disease entity particularly is this an important roentgenologic feature?
16. When there is infiltration of the mucosa as by hemorrhage or hematoma, what are the chief roentgen appearances?
17. What are the chief roentgen changes in scleroderma?
18. When there is a nodular infiltrative involvement of the wall of the bowel how is it manifested radiologically? (Example: amyloid; lymphocytic hyperplastic or neoplastic change; granulomatous infiltration.)

19. When there is an ulceration and diffuse infiltration of the bowel what roentgen appearance is produced?

20. What is meant by the term "skip areas" of involvement and in what disease entities do they especially appear?

21. Under what circumstances is an immobile kink seen in the small intestine?

22. Under what circumstances are concentric rings found mushrooming outward with a thin streak in the canal?

23. What is the meaning of the bull's eye appearance as utilized roentgenologically?

24. What is the roentgenologic significance of coiled linear streaking in the small intestine?

25. What is the significance of the string sign roentgenologically? In what disease entity is this particularly apt to appear? What is its significance?

26. In what connection is the term cobweb or lacelike reticulation utilized?

27. Name some of the disease entities characterized by focal areas of dilated bowel with splayed-out valvulae conniventes.

28. Where are paraduodenal or other internal hernias most apt to occur?

29. What is meant by the blind loop syndrome?

30. Describe the roentgen appearance of abrupt kinking of the bowel and its pathologic significance.

31. Describe the roentgenologic appearance of volvulus of the small intestine.

32. What are the most frequent causes and appearances of intussusception?

33. What are the most frequent roentgenologic appearances of mesenteric thrombosis?

34. When scattered filling defects are manifest in a barium study of the small intestine with no dilatation, what entities come to mind?

35. When there is considerable narrowness of the bowel and lumen, and diffuse thickening of the valvulae throughout the entire small bowel, what entities come to mind?

36. What is the roentgenologic appearance of regional enteritis?

37. What is the roentgenologic appearance of Whipple's disease?

38. What are the roentgenologic appearances associated with multiple foci of intramural bleeding from any cause?

39. What is the roentgenologic appearance of protein-losing enteropathy?

40. What is the roentgenologic appearance of eosinophilic gastroenteritis?

41. What are the various roentgenologic appearances of lymphosarcoma of the small intestine?

42. What are the roentgenologic appearances of adenocarcinoma of the small intestine?

43. What are the roentgenologic appearances of metastatic carcinoma to the small intestine?

44. What are some of the medications which may produce stenosing ulcers of the bowel and resultant mechanical obstruction?

45. Describe the typical roentgen appearances of the malabsorption syndrome and indicate some of the disease entities causing this.

46. What is the significance of meconium ileus in infants?

47. What are some of the disease entities characterized by diminished density in the wall of the bowel? What is the significance of this finding in the newborn?

30

Radiology of the Colon

BASIC RADIOGRAPHIC ANATOMY

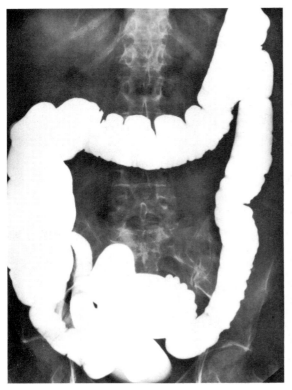

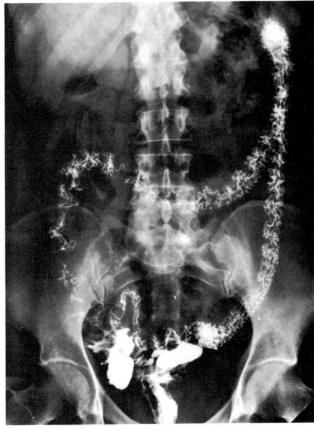

B

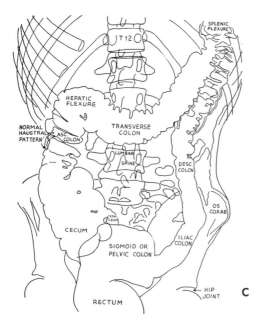

C

Figure 30–1 *A.* Colon distended with barium. *B.* Radiograph of colon after evacuation of barium. *C.* Line drawing with anatomic parts labelled.

591

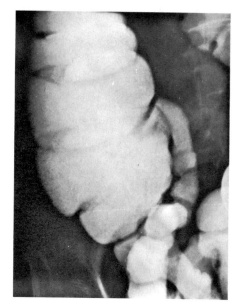

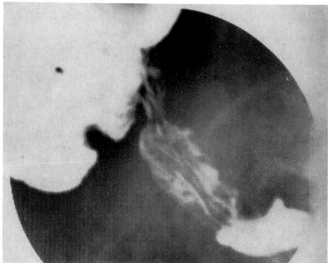

Figure 30–2   Ileocecal junction.

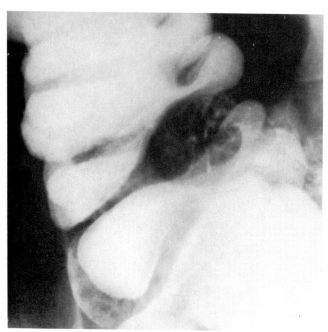

Figure 30–3   En face view of the ileocecal valve demonstrating the star shape of the mucosal folds.

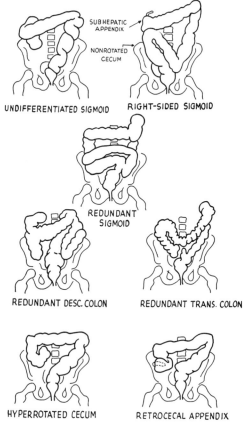

Figure 30–4   Variations in contour of the normal colon.

VARIATIONS OF NORMAL RADIOGRAPHIC APPEARANCES

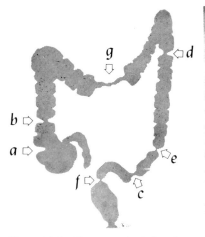

Figure 30–5 The approximate locations of inconstant segmental contractions which may simulate disease in the barium-filled colon. They are designated by the names of their describers; *a*, Busi; *b*, Hirsch; *c*, Moultier; *d*, Payr-Strauss; *e*, Balli; *f*, Rossi; *g*, Cannon's ring. (After Templeton, 1960. *In* Bockus, H. L.: *Gastroenterology*, Vol. 2, 2d Ed. Philadelphia, W. B. Saunders Co., 1964.)

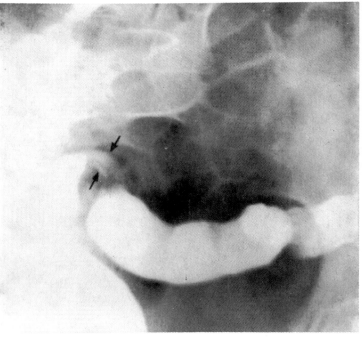

Figure 30–6 Oblique study of the rectosigmoid junction demonstrating a frequently encountered normal narrowness.

ORDER OF THE BARIUM ENEMA EXAMINATION

It has been our preference to perform the barium enema examination *prior* to the study of the upper gastrointestinal tract to avoid any possibility of barium lodging above an unsuspected obstruction in the colon.

We prefer also to examine the urinary tract and biliary system *prior* to the administration of barium orally or by rectum. Telepaque will, of course, introduce opaque material into the colon, and for best study, the examination of the colon cannot be carried forward on the same day as oral cholecystograms (with Telepaque).

LIMITATIONS OF THE ROUTINE BARIUM ENEMA

The barium enema examination should not be considered a substitute for the digital or sigmoidoscopic examination of the rectum. The rectum is often obscured by its voluminous barium content, or by a balloon, if such was employed, and in the post-evacuation study the sigmoid and rectal loops may fold over one another in such a way as to mask a lesion.

Redundancy and overlapping of portions of the colon may obscure one of the anatomic parts, hence, a complete examination of all flexures in the fluoroscopic visualization is essential. Occasionally, such complete examination is virtually impossible and careful notation of this inadequacy should be made.

Haustral points of narrowness and the rectosigmoid junction may give the impression of abnormal areas of narrowness unless the examiner is thoroughly conversant with the wide variation in the normal appearance of the colon.

Unless the terminal ileum or appendix has been visualized, it is difficult to be completely certain that the cecum has been seen, and for that reason caution must be exercised in assuming that the colon has been completely filled when the terminal ileum and appendix have not been visualized. Unfortunately, it is sometimes impossible to fill the terminal ileum and appendix, so experience must dictate when the colon has been entirely distended with barium.

Fluoroscopy is not as accurate as film studies for revealing minute mucosal changes such as those seen in the earliest aberrations of mucosal structure.

When patients are unable to retain the enema and evacuation is forced before complete filling of the colon and cecum, it must not be assumed that an obstructive abnormality of an organic type necessarily exists in the colon. A repeat examination, especially with the aid of a carefully inserted rectal balloon, may be necessary.

The diagnosis of small polyps is difficult, and requires double contrast technique. This double contrast technique is best done with high density barium with the patient in the prone position; care should be taken to avoid reflux into the terminal ileum.

Barium-Air Double Contrast Enema. There are two types of double contrast barium-air enemas. After a conventional barium enema with a nonflocculating Barotrast-type mixture and after evacuation of the conventional barium enema, air may be insufflated. Results from this type of enema are not usually as good as those from a double contrast enema performed as a separate examination as follows:

The preparation of the patient must be especially carefully done under these circumstances. We have preferred placing the patient on a low-residue diet for a period of two days, and on *two* successive nights prior to the morning of the examination we have recommended the administration of one and a half ounces of X-Prep liquid or other aperient. *If two ounces of castor oil is used, it should be given on only one occasion, the evening before the examination as in the routine barium enema examination.*

The colloidal barium mixture (high density) is introduced to the mid-descending colon or lower descending colon, and this is followed immediately by forceful insufflation of air, with rotation of the patient first to the left prone position and then to the right prone to accomplish proper dispersion of the heavy barium mixture.

Another variant of this technique requires that the colloidal barium mixture be introduced into the splenic flexure or the middle of the transverse colon and aspirated into a special bag, after which air is injected. The patient at outset is in the *prone* position.

It is our preference to utilize this special method of double contrast visualization of the colon only if the routine examination of the colon does not yield all information necessary.

It is unfortunate that both the routine barium enema examination and this special double contrast type cannot be done on the same day to best advantage. They are best done one or two days apart as indicated by clinical history.

ROUTINE FOR RADIOGRAPHIC EXAMINATION OF THE COLON

The Full Colon

    a. During fluoroscopy, any impediments to flow are carefully studied and filmed.

    b. The size, contour, and position of the full colon are visualized.

    c. The haustrations are clearly identified.

    d. Each flexure and site of narrowness is screened for any detectable abnormality.

    e. The ileocecal junction is filmed in several projections, and the appendix and terminal ileum are filled and studied if possible.

The Colon After Evacuation

    a. The degree of evacuation is assayed.

    b. Any site of obstruction to evacuation is restudied with the fluoroscope and spot films are taken of the area in question.

    c. The mucosal pattern of each section of the colon is reviewed for any architectural abnormalities.

    d. The terminal ileum is evaluated to the extent that the refluxed barium permits. Pressure spot film studies are obtained.

    e. A decision is made as to whether any suspected abnormality requires further study by the introduction of air or of more barium.

The Double-Contrast Barium-Air Study of the Colon

    a. Each film is reviewed for filling defects—circumscribed by the double contrast.

    b. The mucosal surface is studied throughout.

The technique of this examination differs from that of the routine study in that the patient is first placed in the *prone* position. (1) With the patient lying on his right side, spot films of the rectosigmoid junction are obtained. (2) The patient is then lowered slightly, and a spot film of the entire sigmoid colon is obtained. The rectum and sigmoid colon are studied carefully. (3) High density barium (HD 85) is introduced into the middle of the descending colon (or splenic flexure); the descending colon is then studied. (4) The flow of barium then ceases, and air is substituted for barium. The introduction of air and rotation of the patient force the barium column to the region of the cecum, but reflux into the terminal ileum is carefully avoided. (5) The patient is encouraged to evacuate all the barium, or it is withdrawn into a barium bag used for this purpose. (6) Routine films are obtained in the prone position, both oblique positions, and both lateral decubitus positions; a special oblique view of the sigmoid is obtained, with the central ray pointing cephalad. (7) Spot films are obtained of all suspicious areas in any projection necessary, including tilting the tube 30 to 45 degrees toward the head to bring out detail in the rectum and sigmoid if required.

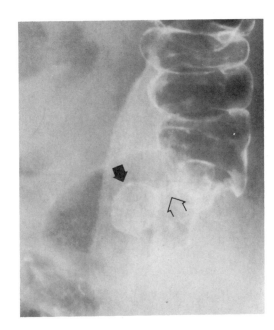

Figure 30–7 Polyp in the colon as seen by double contrast. The closed arrow demonstrates the polyp, and the open arrow shows the stalk.

ROENTGEN SIGNS OF ABNORMALITY IN THE CONTRAST STUDIES OF THE COLON (OMITTING ANGIOGRAMS)

Size

A Diffusely Enlarged Barium-filled Colon (Figure 30–8)

The colon may be *diffusely enlarged above a point of low partial obstruction,* or it is *diffusely enlarged without a detectable obstruction.*

In either case the haustrations appear markedly distended in the proximal part of the colon, but the distal one-half of the colon may no longer have visible haustrations.

Usually, fecal material is retained in these colons, since evacuation is limited and cleansing is poor.

There may be a *fine sawtoothed margin to the barium.* This must be carefully adjudged as to whether it represents retained fecal material or is due to ulceration of the mucosa. (Necrotizing ulcerative colitis may be associated with congenital megacolon. Ulceration may be associated with the cathartic colon also, but rarely.)

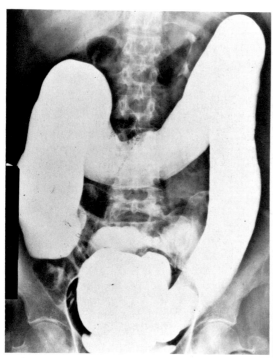

Figure 30–8 Barium-filled colon demonstrating the "cathartic colon." Note the normal distensibility but the complete absence of the haustral markings on the right side of the colon.

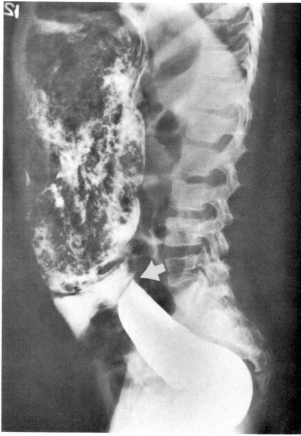

Figure 30–9 Lateral view of rectum and sigmoid colon in Hirschsprung's disease, showing the rectum to be of normal caliber with the marked dilatation of the sigmoid colon above the area of aganglionosis.

A Segmentally Enlarged Barium-filled Colon

This is most frequent at the sigmoid colon, where *redundancy* is encountered. *Hirschsprung's disease* may be focal, in which case a narrowness below the area of dilatation is encountered. Evacuation may be successful below the area of narrowness, but not above. The area of narrowness is the aganglionic segment (Figure 30–9).

Idiopathic segmental dilatation of a portion of the bowel may be encountered—the bowel appearing normal in every respect except that it is dilated.

Toxic dilatation of a segment of bowel may occur with idiopathic ulcerative colitis (Figure 30–10). If recognized on plain films by pneumatosis coli, dilatation, and loss of haustration, barium filling should be avoided. The walls are paper thin and may be readily penetrated by barium. (Sawtoothing due to mucosal ulceration can often be identified when filled with barium.)

If there is *complete obstruction* accounting for the segmental dilatation of the bowel, the obstruction pattern will be studied and very little, if any, bowel above it filled (Figure 30–11).

VARIOUS TYPES OF OBSTRUCTION TO THE HEAD
OF BARIUM COLUMN IN BARIUM ENEMA EXAMINATION

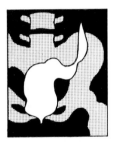
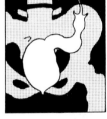
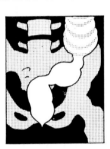

SPASM   CARCINOMATOUS "SHELF"   INTUSSUSCEPTION

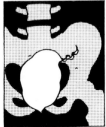

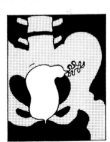

VOLVULUS   DIVERTICULITIS

Figure 30–11

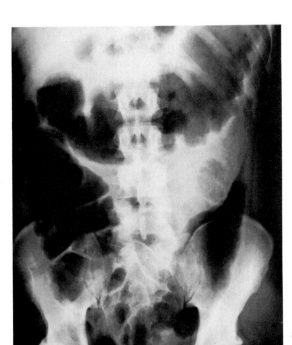

Figure 30–10 Plain film of the abdomen in a patient with ulcerative colitis in its toxic phase. Note the marked tendency to dilatation of the ascending and transverse colons, with irregularity of the haustration, particularly in the transverse colon.

A Diffusely Small Barium-filled Colon

In the newborn, the *"unused colon."*

In the newborn, *"aganglionosis"* of the entire colon.

In both of these, haustrations may be identified, but the colon is small in caliber, thin, and tubular.

When the entire colon is aganglionic, it is foreshortened, flexures are lacking, and the obstruction may be in the small bowel.

In the case of the "unused colon," the obstruction is usually above the level of the colon (jejunal or ileal atresia).

Congenital microcolon also may occur.

In the adult, there are two major causes of diffusely small colon: (1) surgical resection, or (2) long-standing, burned-out "stovepipe" idiopathic ulcerative colitis.

WITH SURGICAL RESECTION there is usually an end-to-end or end-to-side anastomosis and the small intestine is recognized. When half or more of the colon is resected without necessitating a colostomy the anastomotic site is usually in the middle of the transverse colon or in the rectosigmoid junction. A site of narrowness at this juncture may be seen and the architecture of the small bowel is then recognized (Figure 30–12). In some instances of resection of the proximal half of the colon, the colon tends to increase in length and after many years resembles a complete colon.

THE "STOVEPIPE" COLON of long-standing idiopathic ulcerative colitis is a markedly shortened tubular colon of small caliber, its flexures almost absent, and having direct and easy reflux into the ileum. The ileum may in some instances show evidence of backwash disease (ulceration and irregularity). Irregularity and stringiness may be seen in the mucosal pattern on the postevacuation film. The mucosa may also have a pseudopolypoid appearance, producing a cobblestone effect (Figure 30–13).

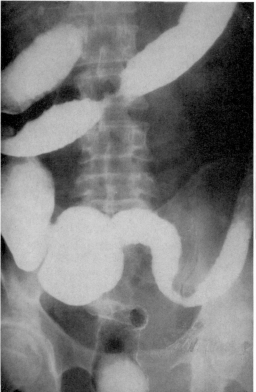

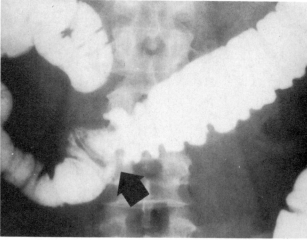

Figure 30–12 The appearance of the bowel following resection and anastomosis. End-to-end anastomosis of ileum to the midtransverse colon.

Figure 30–13 Colon in patient with ulcerative colitis, demonstrating the pipestem changes in long-standing ulcerative colitis.

Narrowness of the Colon, Segmental or Localized

If the margins and internal architecture of the area of narrowness are smooth:

1. The probable diagnosis in an infant is *atresia* or *stricture*, or *aganglionosis.*
2. In the adult the probabilities are:
   a. *Fibrosis* from scar formation from a prior inflammation. This may result from a focalized granulomatous process, now healed, an endometrial implant on the colon in association with endometriosis, or a healed irradiation injury.
   b. *Impression by an extrinsic mass,* often a malignant tumor in a contiguous organ.
   c. *Retroperitoneal fibrosis* resulting from *methysergide therapy.*
   d. *Granuloma inguinale venereum.*
   e. *Volvulus or pseudovolvulus*—here the site of obstruction may assume a pointed and corkscrew appearance.

If the margins and internal architecture of the area of narrowness have a localized ragged or irregular margin the diagnosis may be:

1. *Carcinoma.* This may be polypoid, infiltrative, ulcerative, or linitis plastica. These several varieties will be demonstrated later in the text.
2. *An inflammatory lesion,* especially infectious granuloma or granulomatous colitis, diverticulitis, or ulcerative colitis (Figures 30–14 and 30–15).
3. *Mesenteric vascular occlusion.* This will usually be associated with other findings and will not demonstrate complete obstruction by barium enema. (Other findings may be alterations in architecture and contour such as "thumbprinting" or intramural type irregularity.

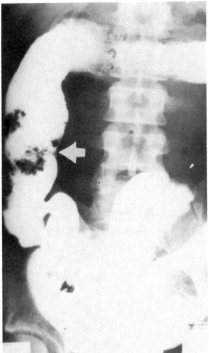

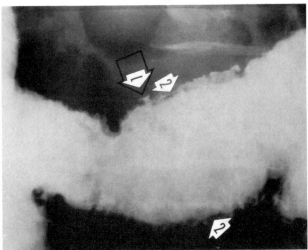

Figure 30–15 Ulcerative colitis. Radiograph demonstrating collar-button ulcers (arrow 1) and longitudinal ulcers (arrow 2) such as are found in some cases of long-standing ulcerative colitis. Such changes simulate closely the findings in granulomatous colitis and differentiation is very difficult. Some refer to this as transitional colitis.

Figure 30–14 Polypoid mass in ascending colon in patient with ulcerative colitis. In this instance the polypoid mass proved not to be malignant. Occasionally such masses are malignant. Usually malignant transformation in ulcerative colitis is associated with annular constriction.

If the Margins of the Colon Show Outpouching

Diverticulosis. Diverticula may occur anywhere in the colon, but are most prevalent in the sigmoid colon. They may be of any size and may be associated with spasm, tenderness, mass, fistulation, or ulceration, in which case the diagnosis of diverticulitis is made.

The pseudodiverticula of scleroderma can be identified especially on the antimesenteric border of the transverse colon as asymmetrical saccular outpouchings several centimeters in diameter.

If There Is a Flow of Barium Outside the Confines of the Colon

1. *Fistulation*
2. *Abscess* adjoining the colon.

If the Flow of the Barium Is in Abnormal Position for the Colon and Is Still Confined to the Colon

Abnormalities in rotation or descent of the colon.

The simplest variety is the hyperrotated or nonrotated cecum, and the most complicated form is the common mesentery deformity (Chapter 29).

Any manifestation of malrotation in the infant, even if localized to the cecum, is highly significant in the presence of any symptoms of obstruction, since it may point to small bowel volvulus.

Displacement of the colon by an adjoining mass lesion. The colon may be adherent or even invaded serosally, but the mucosa will not be altered if it is not itself invaded by the adjoining neoplasm (Figure 30–16).

Herniation of the colon, either into the inguinal region, internally into one of the anatomic fossae, or through the diaphragm into the chest.

Interposition of the colon beneath the diaphragm.

Organoaxial rotation of the stomach, in which case the transverse colon assumes an inverted V appearance.

Herniation of the greater omentum through the diaphragm, in which case the transverse colon is deformed accordingly.

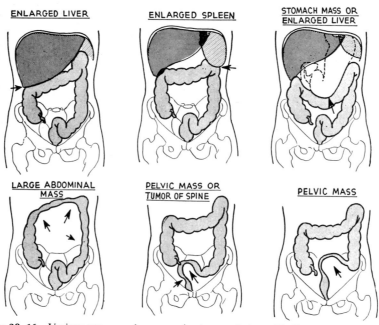

Figure 30–16 Various causes and appearances in association with displacement of the colon.

If an Obstruction to the Flow of the Barium Is Encountered (Figure 30–10), a detailed study of the area of obstruction must be made, and if possible, a small amount of the barium must be allowed to flow past the obstruction to give the full picture. This may be:

"Twisted taper" or corkscrew: volvulus.

"Inverted mushroom and stem" surrounded by coiled spring appearance: intussusception.

Polypoid mass: with an irregular surface, usually points to a malignancy (Figure 30–17).

Napkin ring, irregular channel: usually points to a malignancy of the invasive or ulcerative type (Figure 30–17).

If a smooth-pointed obstruction is encountered: mesenteric occlusion is possible, or spasm.

If the obstructing channel is markedly eccentric and ragged, there may be an extrinsic mass invading the colon and extending down through the mucosa (Figure 30–17).

Carcinoma of Colon — Example of Impairment of Flow Pattern

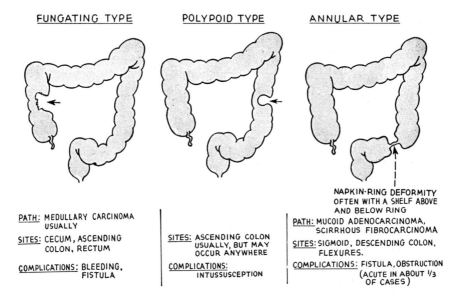

FUNGATING TYPE   POLYPOID TYPE   ANNULAR TYPE

NAPKIN-RING DEFORMITY OFTEN WITH A SHELF ABOVE AND BELOW RING

PATH: MEDULLARY CARCINOMA USUALLY

SITES: CECUM, ASCENDING COLON, RECTUM

COMPLICATIONS: BLEEDING, FISTULA

SITES: ASCENDING COLON USUALLY, BUT MAY OCCUR ANYWHERE

COMPLICATIONS: INTUSSUSCEPTION

PATH: MUCOID ADENOCARCINOMA, SCIRRHOUS FIBROCARCINOMA

SITES: SIGMOID, DESCENDING COLON, FLEXURES.

COMPLICATIONS: FISTULA, OBSTRUCTION (ACUTE IN ABOUT 1/3 OF CASES)

SITE: MORE THAN 1/2 CASES, IN MANY SIZES 3/4 INVOLVE SIGMOID, RECTUM AND RECTO-SIGMOID; RARELY MULTIPLE.

Figure 30–17 Diagram illustrating various radiographic types of carcinoma of the colon and some of the more pertinent features.

If the Architecture Internal to the Colon Is Disturbed on Either the Full Colon Study or After Evacuation the various appearances may be:*

Polypoid filling defect: smooth margins, either sessile or pedunculated of any size.

Polypoid defect, markedly irregular on its surface:
1. Polypoid carcinoma.
2. Villous adenoma—cecal and rectosigmoid especially (Figure 30–18).

Multiple small polypoid defects, frondlike, throughout the colon in a child: familial polyposis.

Slightly lucent, mobile and pliable polypoid defect: lipoma.

Marked irregularity of the colon for a long stretch of the colon, *diminished size of lumen:* idiopathic ulcerative colitis or granulomatous colitis.
1. Granulomatous colitis is characterized by "skip areas" and a greater tendency to involve the proximal colon and the terminal ileum. The colon wall, if identified, tends to be thick and there may be associated fistulation (Figure 30–19).
2. There may be carcinoma in long-standing ulcerative colitis.

Smooth impression upon the cecum (and possibly adjoining ileum):
1. Carcinoid.
2. Adjoining abscess or inflammation.
3. Hypertrophic changes in ileocecal valve.

Irregular and conized transfiguration of the cecum, often with irregularity of the ileum adjoining:
1. Infectious granuloma (tuberculosis, actinomycosis).
2. Regional enteritis.

Sawtoothing of the margin of the colon:
1. Idiopathic ulcerative colitis.
2. Granulomatous colitis.
3. Necrotizing enterocolitis.

Cobblestone appearance of the colon
1. Long-standing old ulcerative colitis.
2. Granulomatous colitis.
3. Amyloidosis.
4. Vascular occlusion.
5. Mucoviscidosis affecting the colon.

Thumbprinting of the barium column
1. Vascular occlusion.
2. Lymphosarcoma.
3. Amyloidosis.

Linear streaking, circular or longitudinal
1. Usually implies ulceration—linear with granulomatous colitis; circular with idiopathic ulcerative colitis.

---

*The student is referred to Volume 3 of *Analysis of Roentgen Signs* for specific illustrations: Figures 30–15, 30–26, and 30–36 to 30–46. Some of these findings will be illustrated in this text.

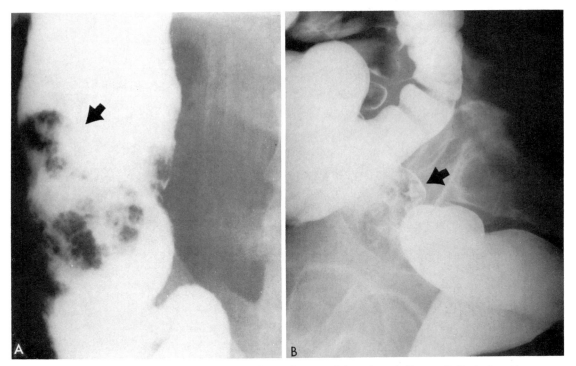

Figure 30–18 Radiograph demonstrating villous adenoma of the colon. *A*. Cecum. *B*. Rectosigmoid.

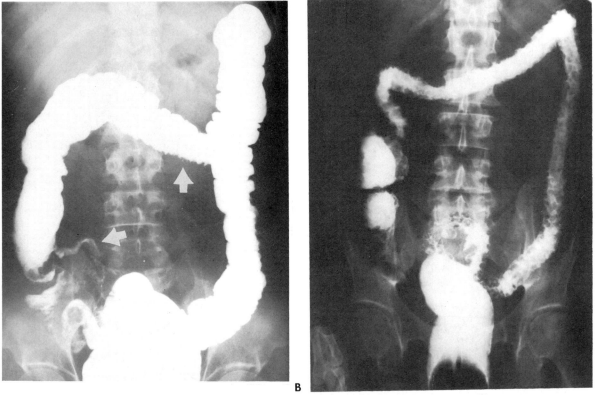

Figure 30–19 *A*. Granulomatous colitis (of Crohn). There is a fistula between the ileum and cecum. There are numerous ulcerations in the midtransverse colon as designated. Skip areas of normal-appearing large intestine are also noteworthy. *B*. Generalized idiopathic ulcerative colitis in an advanced stage. Appearance immediately following barium enema showing maximum distention of the colon with barium.

Air in Bubbles or Streaks in the Wall of the Bowel (Figure 30–20)

Pneumatosis coli.
Necrotizing enterocolitis.
Rupture of bowel due to trauma.

Calcium in the Wall of the Bowel

Calcifying tumors: adenocarcinoma (mucinous) or leiomyosarcoma.
Hemangiomas: appearance suggests multiple phleboliths.
Calcified appendices epiploicae.

Persistence of Fecal Filling Defects Despite Every Effort

Congenital megacolon (Hirschsprung's disease).
Meconium ileus.
"Cathartic colon"
Nonvisualized obstructing lesion.
Eraserophagia or bezoar.

Spastic Colon

Barium appears in long strings on postevacuation films but there are no other alterations from the normal.

Irritability of the colon, and more complete evacuation without extra stimulation.

May appear normal roentgenologically.

The Postoperative Colon

Transverse colon changes following partial gastric resection.
Partial colonic resection.
Hemicolectomy – proximal.
Gastrocolic fistulae.

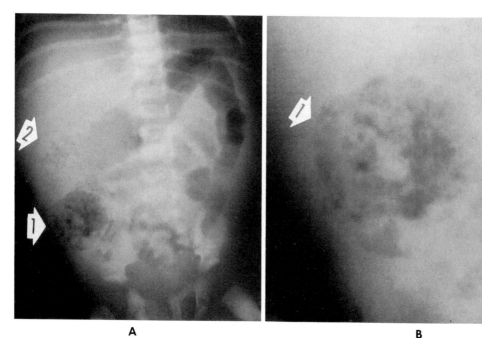

A   **B**

Figure 30–20 *A.* Toxic enterocolitis. (1) Demonstrates the free air in the wall of the bowel, and (2) air, probably also free, in the right upper quadrant, representing an abscess. *B.* Close-up view of the free air permeating the wall of the bowel in toxic enterocolitis.

ROENTGEN SIGNS OF ABNORMALITY OF THE COLON AS MANIFEST IN SPECIFIC DISEASES

ABNORMALITIES IN SIZE

1. Diffuse Increase in Size
   a. The "cathartic colon"
   b. The idiopathic symptomatic megacolon
   c. Hirschsprung's disease (aganglionosis, congenital megacolon)
   d. Dilatation of the colon due to low obstruction
        (1) Imperforate anus
        (2) Anal or rectal stricture
        (3) Carcinoma
   e. Reflex ileus
   f. Myxedema ileus

2. Segmental or Localized Increase in Size
   a. Redundancy
   b. Hirschsprung's disease, localized
   c. Idiopathic segmental dilatation
   d. Neoplastic obstruction of the more proximal parts of the colon
   e. Volvulus
   f. Mesenteric vascular occlusion
   g. Meconium ileus and meconium plug syndrome
   h. Intussusception
   i. Pseudovolvulus
   j. Toxic dilatation of the colon — usually transverse colon — in ulcerative colitis

Megacolon (Hirschsprung's Disease)

Roentgenologic Considerations (Congenital Megacolon)

With sigmoidal or rectal involvement, the colon above the area of involvement is usually tremendously distended. In a lateral view of the rectum and sigmoid following evacuation, the area below the aganglionic segment appears to be of normal caliber and empties normally, whereas above this level there is considerable retention of barium and feces (Figure 30–8).

Small bowel distention may also be present.

Stasis (with fluid levels) in the small intestine of the newborn is a more definitive sign of aganglionosis than the colon diameter at a transition point (Frech, Berdon and Baker).

Ulcerations in the bowel above the aganglionic segment may be seen, with clinical evidence of a secondary exudative enteropathy in as many as 50 per cent of cases that are not diagnosed in the first year of life (Berdon and Baker). (Death may occur from this complication in about 25 to 50 per cent of cases [Feinberg et al.].)

The wall is thickened with pseudopolypoid irregularities, and evidence of sawtoothing in the presence of ulcerations. These may best be identified on postevacuation studies in the lateral projection.

The roentgen manifestations are reversible if treatment is instituted at an early age and if the localized aganglionic segment is excised.

Acquired Megacolon may be due either to a functional disorder (chronic constipation) or to an obstructing lesion somewhere in the distal bowel.

Roentgen Findings in Imperforate Anus

The true nature of anorectal malformation must be established.
A "low" lesion must be differentiated from a "high" lesion.

- a. First film: inverted KUB film in A-P and lateral after holding infant upside down three to five minutes. Lead marker is placed on perineum at site thought to be anus (Figure 30–21).
- b. In the lateral film a pubococcygeal line is drawn. If gas is cephalad to this line only, a high lesion is present; if gas extends caudad to this line to ischial bones or lower, the lesion is of the low type (Figure 30–21).

Further classification requires knowledge of sex and presence of air in region of urinary bladder or dilated vagina (Table 30–1).

Associated anomalies of spine or urologic abnormalities must be evaluated.

Lesion may be evaluated in accordance with the Shopfner classification of ectopic anus with imperforate anus.

TABLE 30–1   SIMPLIFIED RADIOLOGIC APPROACH IN EVALUATING IMPERFORATE ANUS (Berdon et al.)

Sex	Physical Examination	Presumptive Classification	Plain Film Evidence of Site of Fistula	Plain Film Sign of Spinal Anomalies	Urologic Abnormalities on IVP Voiding Cystogram
Male	No perineal orifice	High	Air in bladder	Two-thirds	Two-thirds
Female	No perineal orifice	High	Rarely air in dilated vagina	Two-thirds	Two-thirds
Male	Perineal orifice	Low	None	One-third	One-third
Female	Perineal orifice	Low	None	None*	None*

*Although over 75 "low" females have been evaluated and found to have no spinal or genitourinary anomalies, intravenous urography and voiding cystography are still performed in all such patients (as in any infant with any type of imperforate anus).

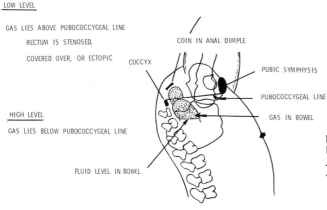

LOW LEVEL

GAS LIES ABOVE PUBOCOCCYGEAL LINE

RECTUM IS STENOSED,

COVERED OVER, OR ECTOPIC

HIGH LEVEL

GAS LIES BELOW PUBOCOCCYGEAL LINE

COIN IN ANAL DIMPLE

COCCYX

PUBIC SYMPHYSIS

PUBOCOCCYGEAL LINE

GAS IN BOWEL

FLUID LEVEL IN BOWEL

INFANT IN INVERTED POSITION

Figure 30–21 Classification of imperforate anus by pubococcygeal line. (Diagram after Scott, J. E. S., and Swenson, O.: Ann. Surg., *150*:477–487, 1959.)

Disease Entities Producing Distention of the Large Intestine by Obstruction

Reflex Ileus (adynamic or paralytic ileus).   Radiographically, the small intestine is usually diffusely distended, as is the large intestine, and there may be fluid levels within both. Generally, fluid levels are not as frequent as with mechanical obstruction. In the upright position, the distended loops of bowel arrange themselves in a stepladder fashion.

Myxedema Ileus.   Atony and hypomotility of the gastrointestinal tract structures may occur with myxedema, manifesting themselves clinically as distention, flatulence, and stubborn constipation. The ultimate expression of this dysfunction is an intestinal obstruction (Hohl and Nixon).

Mechanical Ileus (dynamic ileus).   The site of the obstruction can be determined by the pattern of the obstructed loops of bowel and their position. Ordinarily, the distention of the small intestine especially is very marked, considerably more marked than in paralytic ileus. Difficulty in distinguishing the large from the small intestine is encountered, particularly in the ileum, where distention of the ileum may closely resemble distention of the large intestine.

THE MOST FREQUENT CAUSES of mechanical obstruction in the *adult* are (Chapter 24) adhesions and strangulation of hernias. In the *newborn infant*, atresias, webs, stenoses, bands and volvulus are probably the most frequent causes of obstruction. In the *young infant*, past the early newborn period, intussusception is a frequent cause. In *later childhood and adolescence* the most frequent causes are abscesses and other inflammatory bands occurring in the peritoneal space.

Many of these appearances can be recognized on plain films of the abdomen without additional contrast (see Chapter 24). Some of the entities producing mechanical obstruction are to be described later.

Volvulus (Figure 30–22)

GENERAL COMMENT.   In the adult, the sigmoid and the cecum are the two areas most frequently involved by volvulus; the sigmoid, however, is involved in at least three quarters of the cases. Males are more frequently affected than females (in a 2 to 1 ratio), and the ages of most frequent incidence are 20 to 50 years.

In the child, the most frequent site of volvulus is the small intestine, usually caused by abnormal rotation of the bowel on an anomalous basis (see Chapter 23). In the infant, the administration of oral barium will show the obstruction to be high in the small intestine, very often at the duodenal or jejunal level.

ROENTGENOLOGIC FINDINGS

The specific radiographic findings on plain films of the abdomen without contrast have been described in Chapter 24.

In view of the fact that the twisted bowel may be necrotic, the barium enema is omitted unless some question about the diagnosis exists.

By barium enema, in infant or adult, the twisted taper or corkscrew ending of the barium-filled column at the site of obstruction is virtually pathognomonic, particularly if the plain film findings are taken into consideration.

In view of the danger of perforation of bowel, once the diagnosis is made there should be no effort made to fill the bowel above the site of obstruction.

Occasionally, if the twist is 100 degrees or less, spontaneous reduction may be obtained at the time of evacuation.

VOLVULUS - COLON

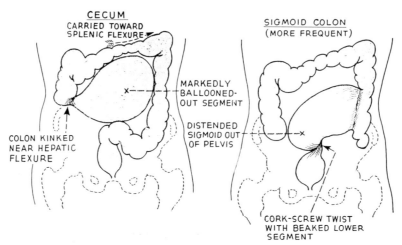

CECUM
CARRIED TOWARD
SPLENIC FLEXURE

MARKEDLY
BALLOONED-
OUT SEGMENT

COLON KINKED
NEAR HEPATIC
FLEXURE

DISTENDED
SIGMOID OUT
OF PELVIS

SIGMOID COLON
(MORE FREQUENT)

CORK-SCREW TWIST
WITH BEAKED LOWER
SEGMENT

ETIOLOGY: 1. ABNORMAL MESENTERY.
2. CHRONIC HYPOTONICITY AND REDUNDANCY.
3. ABNORMAL MOBILITY OF CECUM OR SIGMOID.
ROTATION: 180° OR MORE — SEVERAL TURNS; MAY BE LOOSELY
OR TIGHTLY TWISTED; MAY RECUR.
AGE & SEX: MALE : FEMALE = 2:1; 20-50 YRS.

A

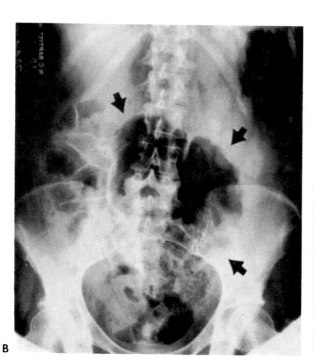

B

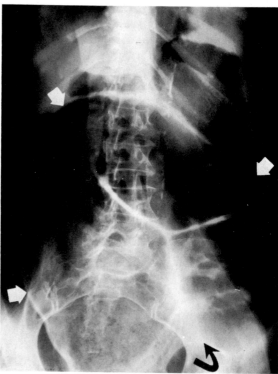

C

Figure 30–22 *A.* Diagrams illustrating rather typical appearances of volvulus of the cecum and of the sigmoid colon. *B.* Radiograph demonstrating volvulus of the cecum. *C.* Volvulus of the sigmoid by barium study. Note the beaked appearance of the superior aspect of the column of barium. The inverted U appearance suggests sigmoid involvement.

Mesenteric Vascular Occlusion (see Chapter 23)

Roentgen Findings in Ischemic Colitis (Figure 30–23)

Dilated colon

Extensive loss of mucosa with large penetrating ulcers

Pseudopolyp formation (Miller et al.)

Irregular thickening of bowel wall

Intramural gas (Rigler and Pogue; Schorr), but this is uncommon (Tomchik)

In transient ischemic colitis, the colon is narrowed; when gangrenous, it is widened.

Involvement of the splenic flexure and not the rectum (thus differing from ulcerative colitis)

"Thumbprinting" (Schwarz et al.)

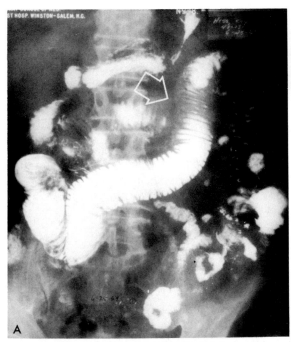

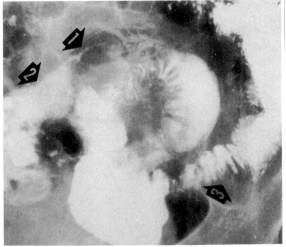

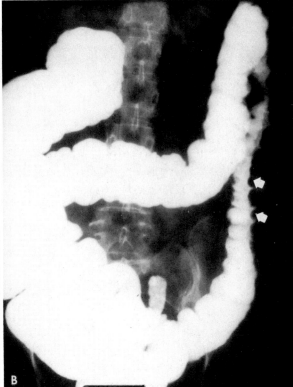

Figure 30–23 Dicumarol bleeding in the gastrointestinal tract: *A*. The jejunum; *B*. The descending colon immediately after the barium enema; *C*. Infarction of the small intestine. Generally, the roentgen signs are: (a) "stacked coin" appearance (open arrow in *A*; 3 in *C*); (b) scalloped filling defects (arrow 1 in *C*) along the margin of the bowel; (c) irregular streaking of the bowel (arrow 2 in *C*). Not demonstrated but occasionally seen are air dissections in the wall of the bowel.

Meconium Ileus and the Meconium Plug Syndrome. These are two distinct syndromes.

MECONIUM ILEUS is one of the complications of mucoviscidosis occurring in the neonatal period. The inspissated mass of meconium produces obstruction, usually in the lower small intestine, with the resulting roentgen picture described in Chapter 24 of low small intestinal mechanical obstruction. It is distinguished from ileal atresia or stenosis on the following *roentgen signs:*

There is great variation in the degree of distention of the loops of bowel—some loops being normal in size.

The distal intestinal contents have a mottled appearance due to the intermixture of gas with the meconium.

In the erect KUB film fluid levels are few or absent.

By barium enema, the colon is relatively normal in length but the "unused colon" is small in diameter (microcolon). This demonstrates that the obstruction is in the small intestine.

The inspissated meconium may be demonstrated in the colon. In occasional cases the colon may evacuate most of this meconium, and the barium will encircle and intermix with the remaining meconium (Grossman et al.).

There may be retrograde filling of the terminal ileum, further demonstrating the inspissated meconium in the distal ileum (Keats and Smith).

THE MECONIUM PLUG SYNDROME (Swischuk) differs from the preceding condition as follows (Clatworthy et al.; Ellis and Clatworthy):

The infants are unable, from inherent weakness or prematurity, to dislodge and evacuate the initial meconium, which leads to obstruction. After successful treatment they show no evidence of a bowel disorder or mucoviscidosis.

Plain films of the abdomen show that the obstruction is a low intestinal one with inspissated meconium throughout the large intestine, which has numerous distended loops.

Many fluid levels are present in the distended bowel.

The *barium enema* outlines the continuous meconium cast in the colon. If the patient has passed the plug, the barium may show a small tapered meconium plug near the terminal ileum. This may, then, resemble mucoviscidosis, but such cases are rare.

IN THE CASE OF EITHER MECONIUM ILEUS OR MECONIUM PLUG SYNDROME, if there has been a rupture of bowel antenatally with escape of meconium into the peritoneal cavity, abdominal calcification may be visualized. This is indicative only of a perforated bowel, but is called "meconium peritonitis."

Intussusception (Figure 30–24)

GENERAL COMMENT. Intussusception refers to an invagination of one segment of intestine into another. About 90 per cent of cases of intussusception are in male infants and usually these occur in infants under two years of age. Intussusception is usually seen in healthy robust children with a very short history of sharp colicky pain and melena. About 70 per cent of these have a palpable tumor. The most common demonstrable cause is a Meckel's diverticulum, but other lesions responsible include a pedunculated tumor, a long mesentery, hypertrophied Peyer's patches, ileal duplication, hematoma of the ileum and lymphosarcoma. A definite responsible lesion may be found in about 5 per cent of patients, mostly children past infancy.

Intussusception may be classified as enteroenteric, 15 per cent of cases, mostly in adults; ileocecal or ileocolic, about 75 per cent of cases, mostly in infants; colicocolic, usually in the proximal colon, 10 per cent of cases. The retrograde type of intussusception is extremely rare.

ROENTGENOLOGIC CONSIDERATIONS

By barium enema examination, when the obstructed head of barium is examined, a polypoid defect is seen within a distended area of colon and this in turn is surrounded by a coiled spring appearance (Figure 30–24). If barium enters the invaginated loop, a small "stem inside a mushroom" appearance is obtained. On the postevacuation film, the findings are usually quite characteristic in that the coiled spring and "stem" become more apparent.

Early, a therapeutic as well as diagnostic barium enema is indicated. Reduction of the intussusception may be accomplished under fluoroscopic control. If recurrence or resistance is encountered, surgery is indicated. The danger of relying upon barium enema for reduction is the fact that devitalized bowel may be overlooked and a peritonitis may result. In children less than three years old, hydrostatic reduction of intussusception should be safe and practical (Singleton). Surgical treatment in older children may be necessary because of the possibility of an associated neoplastic lesion.

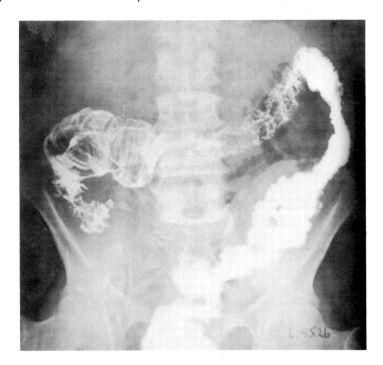

Figure 30–24 Radiograph demonstrating a frequent appearance obtained with enterocolic intussusception.

ROENTGEN SIGNS OF ABNORMALITY OF THE COLON AS MANIFEST IN SPECIFIC DISEASES *(Continued)*

ABNORMALITIES IN SIZE *(Continued)*

3. **Narrowness of the colon lumen — diffuse**
    a. The "unused colon" of the newborn
    b. Aganglionosis of the entire colon in the newborn
    c. Long-standing ulcerative colitis — the "pipestem colon"
    d. Congenital microcolon
4. **Narrowness of the colon — segmental or localized**
    a. Congenital stricture or atresia
    b. Inflammatory lesions such as
        (1) Idiopathic ulcerative colitis
        (2) Granulomatous colitis
        (3) Amebic colitis
        (4) Tuberculosis
        (5) Actinomycosis
        (6) Diverticulitis
        (7) Peridiverticulitis
        (8) Lymphogranuloma inguinale venereum
    c. Carcinoma of the colon
        (1) Fungating
        (2) Polypoid
        (3) Annular
        (4) Linitis plastica
    d. Endometrial implants on the colon
    e. Torsion, thrombosis, infarction, gangrene, inflammation or intussusception of appendices epiploicae
    f. Irradiation bowel injury
    g. Retroperitoneal fibrosis (methysergide therapy)

Irradiation Injury to the Bowel (Figure 30–25)

PATHOGENESIS.   The mucosa of the gastrointestinal tract is moderately radio-sensitive. The rectosigmoid region may be seriously damaged in the course of ir-radiation for any pelvic malignancy (particularly carcinoma of the cervix), espe-cially when dose levels exceed 5000 rads in a period of approximately six weeks. In any case, the mucosal cells are distorted and may become shrunken and necro-tic. The mucosal cells may slough, producing ulcerative changes, and inflammation of the underlying submucosal connective tissue becomes prominent, with edema and inflammation. The vessels of the bowel wall are also damaged, with degenera-tion and intravascular thrombosis. In later stages, fibrous thickening of the vessel walls and bowel wall supervenes, with narrowness of the lumina of both.

Secondary infection may also supervene by bacterial contamination.

Regeneration may reconstitute the bowel wall, or the bowel wall may be vul-nerable to any other trauma. Scarring is common, and cicatricial stenosis with ob-struction may also occur.

ROENTGENOLOGIC ASPECTS.   These will depend upon the phase of the study.

Early, the mucosa will be edematous and distorted, irritable and spastic.

Later, stenosis may supervene, with evidence of thickening of the bowel wall.

The evidence of partial or total obstruction may also supervene.

Fistulation resulting from superimposed bacterial infection rarely occurs as long as radiation is carried forward within tolerable limits for the normal bowel.

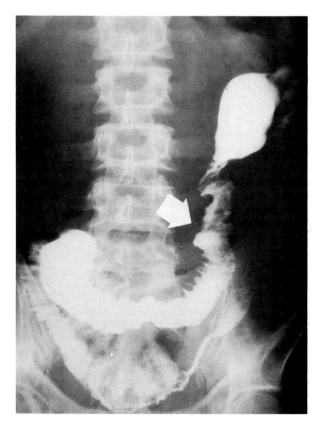

Figure 30–25 Radiation colitis following irradiation of the abdomen for retroperitoneal fibrosarcoma.

Abnormalities of Contour

> 1. Diverticula
> 2. The pseudodiverticula of scleroderma
> 3. Mass displacement (see later under *Abnormality of Position*)

Diverticulosis of the Large Intestine (Figure 30–27)

General Comment. True or complete diverticula of the colon involving all layers of the wall of the large intestine are rare. Most diverticula are of the false variety representing protrusions of the mucosa and submucosa through a defect in the wall of the bowel. These are frequently found in persons past the age of 40, and occur in about 5 per cent of autopsy cases past the age of 50 (Robbins). They are most abundant (95 per cent) in the sigmoid. Usually, they are aligned along the margins of the taenia coli. Massive hemorrhage does occur, but rarely. Usually diverticulosis is asymptomatic unless complicated.

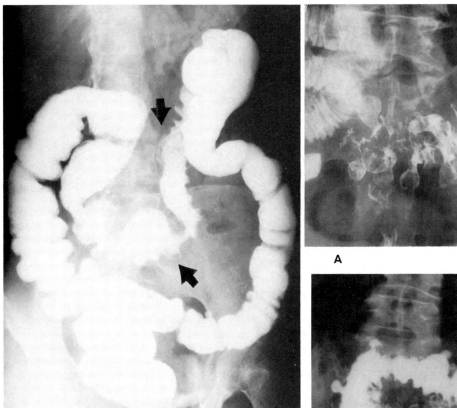

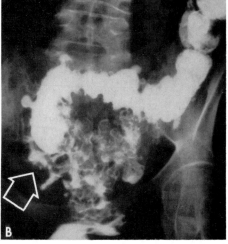

Figure 30–26 Radiographic appearance of the colon in scleroderma. Note the "wide mouth" diverticula and sacculated appearance, particularly in the transverse colon.

Figure 30–27 *A* and *B*. Diverticulosis of the sigmoid. In *B*, not only are the diverticula demonstrated, but there are irregular fistulations into the adjoining soft tissues.

ROENTGEN SIGNS OF ABNORMALITY OF THE COLON AS MANIFEST IN SPECIFIC DISEASES (Continued)

Abnormalities of Position

1. Abnormalities in rotation and descent of the colon
2. Interposition of the colon
3. Displacement of the colon
4. Enteroptosis
5. Hernias of the colon
6. With organoaxial rotation or volvulus of the stomach
7. With herniation of greater omentum through the diaphragm

Abnormalities of Density

1. Pneumatosis coli
2. Necrotizing enterocolitis
3. Meconium ileus
4. Calcified appendices epiploicae
5. Hemangiomas of the gastrointestinal tract
6. Calcified tumors: adenocarcinoma, leiomyosarcoma
7. Calcified appendiceal fecaliths
8. Eraserophagia
9. Bezoars and inspissated fecal material

Abnormalities of Architecture of the Colon

1. Idiopathic ulcerative colitis
2. Granulomatous colitis
3. Amebiasis
4. Tuberculosis
5. Actinomycosis
    a. Review of lesions affecting the cecum
6. Lymphogranuloma inguinale venereum
7. Polyps of the colon (Gardner syndrome; Turcot syndrome; polyps in children)
    a. The villous adenoma
    b. Familial polyposis of the colon
    c. Peutz-Jeghers syndrome
8. Lipomas of the colon
9. Carcinoid of the colon
10. Carcinoma of the colon
11. Lymphosarcoma of the colon
12. Amyloidosis of the colon
13. Vascular occlusion; intramural hemorrhage
14. Colitis cystica profunda
15. Schistosomiasis mansoni
16. Lymphoid hyperplasia
17. Metastases to the colon

Abnormalities of Architecture of the Colon

Idiopathic Ulcerative Colitis

General Comment. This is an inflammatory disease of the colon which begins in the rectosigmoid region and eventually involves the entire colon and long stretches of the ileum in some cases.

It may begin in segments other than the rectum.

Anatomic Distribution

1. Distal colon in 80 per cent of cases.
2. Entire colon in approximately 50 per cent of cases.
3. Limited to proximal colon in approximately 20 per cent of cases.
4. Segmental colitis (with uninvolved areas on either side) occurs in only 5 per cent of cases (Reeves et al.).
5. May "backwash" into the terminal ileum for as much as twelve inches, producing superficial ulcers characteristic of "backwash ileitis."
6. Toxic dilatation tends to involve the transverse colon especially severely, but usually there is extensive involvement of the colon elsewhere as well.

Radiologic Manifestations

Superficial ulceration occurs especially in the rectosigmoid region but eventually involves the entire colon, imparting a sawtooth appearance to the mucosal pattern.

As the disease progresses, there is a loss of haustration and considerable spasm, irritability, and numerous mass movements along the entire colon.

On the postevacuation study, the mucosal pattern often has a cobblestone and stringy appearance (because of excess mucus).

After further progress, the colon becomes shortened, rigid, and moderately thickened ("stovepipe" colon). Pseudopolyps are especially visible at this time.

Strictures may form as concentric areas of narrowness, with low-grade

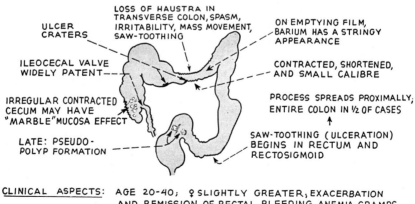

Figure 30-28 Diagram of ulcerative colitis summarizing major features of this disease in the colon.

obstruction. They are, on occasion, reversible (Kolodny). These may even resemble the "napkin ring" of carcinoma—which leads to confusion since carcinoma may form after the disease has been present for 10 years or longer.

Toxic megacolon and pneumatosis coli (already described) may occur at any time in the course of the disease (Madison and Bargen; Lumb et al.).

Granulomatous Colitis (Crohn's disease)

General Comments. Although regional enteritis was originally described as affecting the terminal ileum (Crohn et al.), it has been known for some time that it may also affect virtually all other portions of the gastrointestinal tract (Harris, F. I. et al.; Brown et al.; Colp). In many patients both the ileum and colon are affected (Rappaport, 55 per cent; Janowitz, 70 per cent). In some the condition may be confined to the colon alone (Janowitz, 18 per cent).

Roentgenologic Features

The involvement of the colon is usually segmental with skip areas; the segment least frequently involved is the rectum. The segments most frequently involved are the transverse colon, cecum, and ascending colon, often in association with regional enteritis in the distal ileum.

Longitudinal ulcerations and a cobblestone appearance to the mucosa in the involved areas where inflammatory polypoid appearance is common. Strictures and thickened areas give rise to an appearance of pseudodiverticulum formation.

Fistulation with sinus tract formation is common.

General Summary of Findings. The six most important hallmarks (Borland et al.) of granulomatous colitis are a history of abdominal pain, marked weight loss, and arthralgia; and proximal involvement of the colon only, stricture formation, and rectal complications in the radiographic findings.

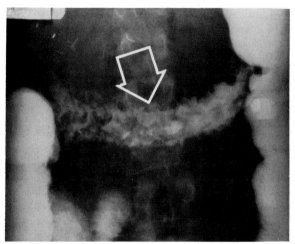
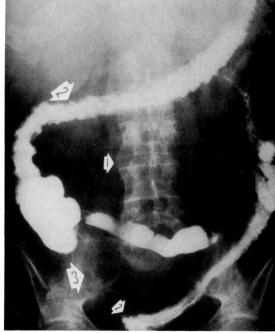

Figure 30–29 *(Left)* Granulomatous colitis demonstrating the "cobblestone" pattern of the transverse colon. *(Right)* Ulcerative colitis in conjunction with ankylosing spondylitis: (1) paraspinous ligamentous calcification; (2) ulcerations of the sigmoid and transverse colon; (3) obliterated sacroiliac joints.

Tuberculosis of the Colon.   Tuberculosis of the terminal ileum and colon is difficult to differentiate from other forms of granulomatous disease involving this area. The ileocecal region is the primary site of involvement in over 90 per cent of cases, with frequent involvement of the appendix also. Intestinal tuberculosis occurs in about 30 per cent of cases of pulmonary tuberculosis, but primary intestinal tuberculosis without pulmonary involvement is quite rare at this time.

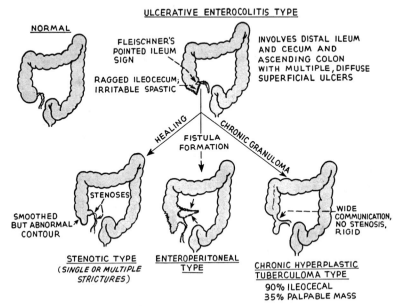

SITE: 1. ILEOCECAL IN OVER 90% OF CASES
2. OCCASIONALLY WIDESPREAD
3. APPENDIX FREQUENTLY INVOLVED ALSO.

CLINICAL ASPECTS: NO PATHOGNOMONIC CLINICAL
EVIDENCE. ANY PATIENT WITH KNOWN
TUBERCULOSIS ELSEWHERE WHO HAS
DIARRHEA, INTERMITTENT ABDOMINAL
PAIN AND TENDERNESS (PARTICULARLY
IN RIGHT LOWER QUADRANT), LOW
GRADE FEVER AND PALPABLE TUMOR
MUST BE SUSPECTED. THERE MAY BE
FINDINGS SIMULATING APPENDICITIS
OR ILEUS.

COMPLICATIONS: 1. PERFORATION → FISTULAS
2. PERITONITIS IN 10%
3. OBSTRUCTION

ROENTGEN
METHODS: 1. SMALL INTESTINAL SERIES
2. ROUTINE BARIUM ENEMA
3. DOUBLE CONTRAST ENEMA

ROENTGEN ASPECTS:
1. HYPERMOTILITY
2. IRREGULAR ILEOCECAL
FILLING DEFECTS
3. SPASM - ILEOCECAL REGION
4. "PLASTIC PERITONITIS"
5. SEGMENTATION, DILATATION,
MATTING, STASIS IN
ILEAL LOOPS
6. STIERLIN'S SIGN: ILEUM
AND TRANSVERSE COLON
FILLED BUT BARIUM
DOES NOT REMAIN IN
CECUM AND ASCENDING
COLON.

INCIDENCE:
1. INTESTINAL TUBERCULOSIS
OCCURS IN ABOUT 30% OR
MORE OF CASES OF PULMO-
NARY TUBERCULOSIS
2. PRIMARY TYPE RARE

Figure 30–30   Pertinent features of tuberculosis of the colon.

Figure 30–31   *(Continued)*
Granulomas of cecum.
Appendiceal disease including appendiceal stump.
Intussusception with or without mass (*C* only).
    PART 3. *Narrowing.* (*A*) Shortening; smooth edges; ileum involved. (*B*) Smooth; conical cecal tip; ileum not involved.
(*C*) Shortening; irregular; ileum not involved.
Chronic inflammatory and granulomatous disease: amebiasis, tuberculosis, regional enterocolitis.
Malignant lesions: carcinoma.

A Review of Roentgen Signs and Lesions Affecting the Cecum
(Figure 30–31) (Bartone et al.)

Bartone et al. have classified lesions and roentgen signs in and around the cecum, terminal ileum, and ascending colon as shown in the accompanying illustration.

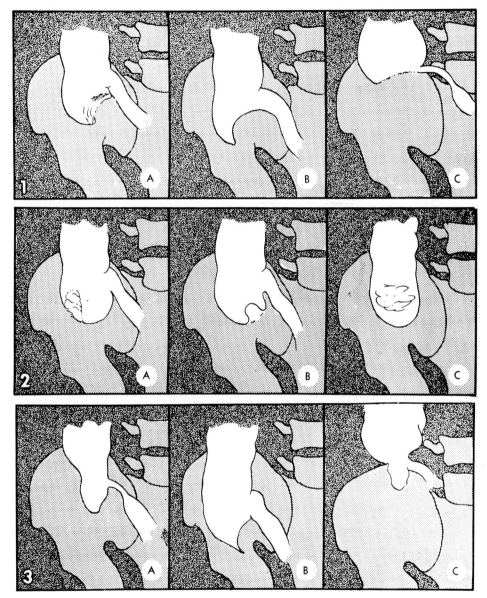

Figure 30–31 PART 1. *Local wall displacement and/or filling defect.* (*A*) Irregular margin. (*B*) Smooth margin; ileum displaced. (*C*) Irregular margin; ileum displaced and narrowed.

Appendiceal mass lesions: abscess, mucocele, carcinoid, carcinoma.

Cecal benign neoplasms: adenoma, leiomyoma, fibroma, carcinoid, lipoma.

Cecal malignant neoplasms: carcinoma, lymphosarcoma.

Cecal granulomatous masses: amebic granuloma, actinomycosis, hyperplastic tuberculosis.

Other extrinsic or extramucosal masses: ovarian, uterine, sigmoid colon, congenital cysts.

Postoperative defects.

PART 2. *Filling defect.* (*A*) Contour irregular; peripheral. (*B*) Contour smooth near base of appendix. (*C*) Central type irregular contour near valve region with ileum not filled.

Benign neoplasms of cecum: polyps, carcinoid, lipoma, fibroma.

Malignant neoplasms of cecum.

Legend continued on the opposite page *Illustration continued on the following page*

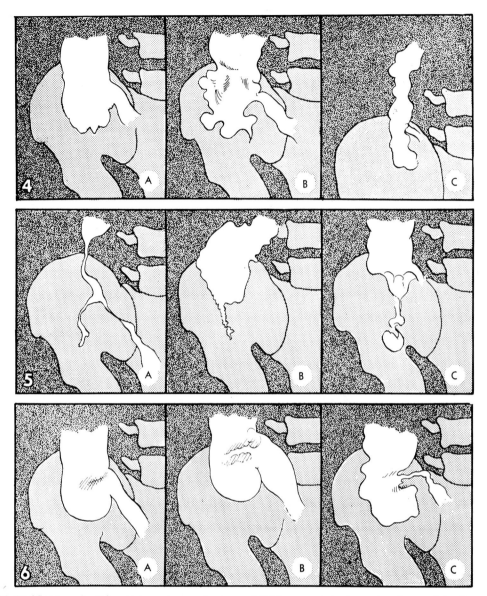

Figure 30–31 (*Continued*) PART 4. *Irregular cecal contour.* (*A*) Fine serrated edge; primarily cecal tip; ileum not involved. (*B*) Slight involvement of ascending colon; ileum not involved. (*C*) Narrowing; marked involvement of ascending colon; ileum involved.

    Malignancy: carcinoma or lymphosarcoma.

    Chronic inflammatory and granulomatous diseases: ulcerative colitis, regional enterocolitis, segmental colitis, tuberculosis, amebiasis, diverticulitis.

    PART 5. *Marked irregular narrowing.* (*A*) Fistula formation; fixation; ileum extremely involved. (*B*) Marked serrated edge; ileum not filled. (*C*) Abrupt transition with shelf formation. Advanced chronic inflammatory and granulomatous disease: tuberculosis, regional enterocolitis, ameboma.

    Malignant lesion.

    Appendiceal disease.

    PART 6. *Ileocecal region and valve.* (*A*) Ill-defined margins. (*B*) Lobulated margins; ileum involved. (*C*) Irregular margins; body of cecum and ileum involved.

    Prominent valve: normal, hypertrophy, edema, prolapse of ileal mucosa.

    Benign tumors.

    Malignant tumors.

    Granulomas and chronic inflammation.

    Intussusception: minimal stage, or incompletely reduced. (From Bartone, N. F., Grieco, R. V., and Vasilas, A.: Amer. J. Roentgenol., *84*:285, 1960.)

Polyps of the Colon

General Comment. A polyp may be defined as any outgrowth from a mucosal surface (Robbins). There are many different classifications (Turell) but perhaps the simplest is the following:

1. The sporadic pedunculated or sessile adenoma.
2. The villous adenoma.
3. Heredofamilial or congenital familial polyposis of the colon. In the latter entity there is a profusion of polyps scattered throughout the colon and sometimes the entire intestinal tract.

The *familial polyposis* in children must not be confused with other isolated (or occasionally multiple) polyps which may occur in children. These may occur infrequently in the region of the rectosigmoid and disappear spontaneously in many instances following puberty. They are called juvenile polyps.

POLYPOSIS SYNDROMES OF THE COLON

1. Hereditary

   a. Familial multiple polyposis.

   b. Gardner's syndrome: multiple soft tissue tumors, osteomatosis, polyposis coli, and a potential for colon malignancy.

   c. Peutz-Jeghers syndrome: mucocutaneous pigmentation, especially circumoral, buccal, or on tongue; and gastrointestinal polyposis. Transient intussusceptions are common, especially in the small intestine. The small bowel is involved in more than 95 per cent of cases; the colon and rectum in about 30 per cent; and the stomach in about 25 per cent. These lesions are benign hamartomas, although the incidence of carcinoma in these patients is greater than that in the general population.

   d. Turcot syndrome: Polyposis coli and central nervous system tumors. These polyps are usually limited to the rectum and colon, and appear to be benign adenomas. The brain tumors have usually been supratentorial glioblastomas.

2. Nonhereditary

   a. Cronkhite-Canada syndrome: generalized gastrointestinal polyposis and ectodermal abnormalities. Usually these are inflammatory juvenile type polyps.

   b. Juvenile polyposis (sometimes hereditary): non-neoplastic and not associated with malignancy. The polyps are usually solitary (about 75 per cent) and benign, and have a tendency to autoamputation. They may, however, be highly variable and may resemble other types of polyposis.

TABLE 30–2 SUMMARY OF FEATURES CHARACTERIZING GASTROINTESTINAL POLYPOSIS SYNDROMES*

Syndrome	Symptom Onset Usual Age (yrs.)	Hereditary Transmission	Distribution			Histology	Additional Features	Prognosis
			STOMACH	SMALL BOWEL	COLON			
Multiple polyposis	15 to 30	Dominant	Less than 5%	Less than 5%	100%	Adenomas		Colon carcinoma
Gardner's	15 to 30	Dominant	~ 5%	~ 5%	100%	Adenomas	Soft tissue tumors, osteomatosis	Colon carcinoma
Peutz-Jeghers	10 to 30	Dominant	25%	95%	30%	Cellular hamartomas	Pigmented skin lesions	With or without G.I. tract carcinoma
Turcot's	Teens	Recessive	—	—	100%	Adenomas	C.N.S. tumors	C.N.S. tumors
Cronkhite-Canada	40 to 70	None	100%	Less than 50%	100%	Inflammatory glandular dilatation	Alopecia, onychia, hyperpigmentation / Diarrhea with protein and electrolyte losses	Death often of cachexia
Juvenile polyps (common type)	Less than 10	Usually none	—	—	100%	Inflammatory	Diarrhea with protein loss possible	Regression, autoamputation

*From Youker, J. E., Dodds, W. J., and Welin, S.: Colonic polyps. *In* Margulis, A. R., and Burhenne, H. J. (eds.): *Alimentary Tract Roentgenology,* 2nd Ed. St. Louis, C. V. Mosby Co., 1972.

The Adenomatous Pedunculated Polyp

RELATIONSHIP TO MALIGNANCY.   The relationship of polyps of the colon to malignancy is a matter of controversy. The pedunculated lesion, however, rarely if ever recurs, irrespective of the microscopic findings over the head of the polyp (Castleman and Krickstein; Bockus et al., 1961; Grinnell and Lane). Since frank invasion of the core of the polyp and stalk of the pedunculated lesion sometimes occurs with extension to the underlying colonic wall, some investigators have recommended that the diameter of the polyp be used as an important criterion. Accordingly, when the diameter is greater than 1.25 cm., nonintervention carries a greater risk than colotomy with polypectomy or segmental colectomy. Sessile growths require radical segmental resection, but there is no agreement as to how much of the colon should be removed.

The Villous Adenoma

GENERAL COMMENT.   The villous adenoma is a papillary soft tumor occurring predominantly in the rectum and sigmoid with numerous frondlike projections actively secreting mucus. Electrolyte depletion may result (Cooperman and Lowman). It is attached to the colonic mucosa by a broad base. The incidence of malignancy in these tumors varies in different reports from 7.4 per cent to 74 per cent (Grinnell and Lane; Swinton et al.; Wheat and Ackerman).

Lesions over 5 cm. in diameter and even up to 15 or 20 cm. are not uncommon. They are about one-twentieth the frequency of pedunculated adenomas. They secrete copious quantities of mucoid material and potassium and cause significant losses of fluid and electrolytes (Davis et al; Kaye and Bragg).

Familial (Heredofamilial) Polyposis of the Colon

GENERAL COMMENT. Familial polyposis is a hereditary disorder characterized by innumerable closely packed polyps studding the entire mucosal surface of the colon (Figure 30–19). It is apparently an autosomal nonsex-linked dominant characteristic. McKusick has described six distinct syndromes which are apparently genetically separate: (1) congenital familial polyposis of the colon; (2) occasional discrete polyps of the colon and rectum; (3) the Peutz-Jeghers syndrome which includes generalized intestinal polyposis with melanin spots of the bronchial mucosa, lips, and digits; (4) the Gardner syndrome which implies colonic polyposis with osteomas; (5) the Turcot syndrome which involves brain tumor as well as colonic polyposis. (Medulloblastoma of the spinal cord and glioblastoma of the frontal lobe with pigmentation of the skin and atrophy of the fingernails and toenails also occur.) (6) Multiple endocrine adenomatosis embracing the Zollinger-Ellison syndrome.

Lipomas of the Colon

Common sites: colon, 61.1 per cent to 73.1 per cent; rectum, 1.3 to 5.2 per cent; ileum, probably 11.5 to 21 per cent; esophagus, stomach, and duodenum, 10 to 20 per cent.

Carcinoma

Carcinoma of the colon may be either fungating, polypoid, annular, or scirrhous.

In a series of 102 carcinomas of the colon reported by Hodges and MacMillan (Figure 30–32), 75 per cent of the lesions were described as annular in character and 23 per cent were polypoid. Evidence of dilatation of the gut proximal to the lesions was recorded in a quarter of the cases. Retrograde obstruction to the introduction of the barium enema occurred in 40 per cent, but complete obstruction was encountered in only 10 per cent of the cases. The lesions ranged in length from 1 to 12 cm., with an average of 5 cm.

The Linitis Plastica type (Wolf and Marshak, 1963; McQueeney et al.) may occur in patients with long-standing ulcerative colitis, or it may simulate ulcerative colitis.

Roentgenologic Findings (Figure 30–33)

Involvement of a long segment without clearly demarcated margins.

Bizarre mucosal pattern which does not appear to be completely effaced.

Narrowness of the lumen with flat irregular scalloped margins of the tumor.

Tapering or trumpet-shaped transition to adjacent normally distensible bowel.

Shortening of the involved segment and mesentery with acute looping when the sigmoid is involved.

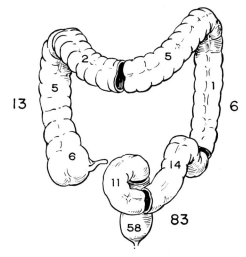

Figure 30–32   Distribution of lesions in 102 carcinomas of the colon. Eighty-three were situated in the rectum, proximal, and distal sigmoid; 6 in the descending colon; 5 in the distal one-half of the transverse colon; and 13 in the proximal one-half of the colon, with 6 of these latter 13 being situated in the cecum. For further description of this study see text. (From Hodges, F., and MacMillan, H. C.: J.A.M.A., *147*:1191, 1951.)

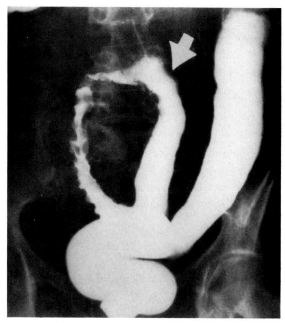

Figure 30–33   Scirrhous or diffusely infiltrating carcinoma of the sigmoid colon of the linitis plastica type. The distal limb is markedly narrowed with an extremely coarse mucosal pattern. The proximal limb is more distensible but shows numerous fine spiculations and coarse scalloping along its contours. The barium column in the apical portion of the sigmoid loop (arrow) has an amorphous, nonhomogeneous appearance.

ROENTGEN SIGNS OF GASTROINTESTINAL OBSTRUCTION ON PLAIN FILMS OF THE ABDOMEN

1. The cardinal sign is dilatation of the gastrointestinal tract proximal to the lesion and the collapse of the distal bowel.
2. The gross morphology of the organ determines its roentgen appearance. The air may be partially trapped in folds or rugae.
3. Stomach dilatation: The shape of the distended stomach closely resembles that of the barium-filled stomach. There may be deformity of the stomach by an intrinsic or extrinsic lesion.
4. Duodenal obstruction.
   1. The stomach is distended.
   2. The duodenum proximal to the obstruction is also distended. The gas pattern may not reveal its C shape.
      a. In infants the characteristic double bubble may be found.
5. Small intestinal obstruction.
   1. Coiled spring appearance.
   2. "Staircase" in erect studies with fluid levels.
   3. "Herringbone" pattern.
   4. Ileal loops when distended may resemble the large intestine but can be differentiated by position and lack of serosal involvement in valvulae.

6. Large intestinal obstruction.
   1. The dilated loops tend to be in the distribution of the colon.
   2. The haustral pattern of the colon may be identified.
   3. The colon has a "cut-off" sign at the site of obstruction.
   4. Isolated loop distention with volvulus.

Roentgen Features of Metastases to the Colon (Khilnani et al., 1966). There may be colonic involvement by extension from an extracolonic mass, or primarily intramural involvement.

Roentgenologic Findings

Narrowing of the lumen with occasional obstruction.
Nodular defects.
Fixed transverse or radiating folds.
Rigidity of the involved segment, similar to linitis plastica or scirrhous carcinoma.
Although ulceration is rare, certain metastases do characteristically undergo central necrosis. Melanoma is an example of a tumor which has great propensity to ulceration—and to association with a "bull's eye" sign (Figure 30–34).

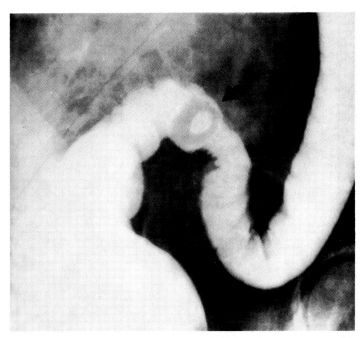

Figure 30–34 Bull's eye appearance of an ulcerating polypoid metastasis involving the sigmoid colon. This appearance may occur with any polypoid lesion with a tendency to undergo central necrosis. Similar appearances may be produced by melanoma, carcinoid, and leiomyosarcoma. (Intensified.)

THE VERMIFORM APPENDIX (Figure 30–35)

Concretions or Coproliths of the Appendix. The association of coproliths of the appendix with appendicitis is well established (Kelly, Berg and Berg; Shaw). Such concretions in the appendix may be very faint (Figure 30–36) but their demonstration in patients with inflammations of the abdomen or right lower quadrant should signal a tentative diagnosis of appendicitis. They are frequently laminated and demonstrable in about 10 per cent of adult patients with acute appendicitis, and they may be multiple (Felson and Bernhard).

A barium enema examination is not contraindicated in the presence of appendicitis if it is done carefully. The inflamed appendix ordinarily will not fill with barium (Chrom and Gudbjerg; Figiel and Figiel). When outright evidence of appendicitis is present clinically, however, or when perforation is suspected, it is probably best to omit this examination (Figure 30–35).

Roentgenologic Findings with Acute Appendicitis (Beneventano et al.)

Ileus, more localized to the right lower quadrant ("sentinel loop" ileus).

Obliteration of the right psoas shadow, with a distinct haziness over the right lower quadrant.

Abscess gas bubbles in the right lower quadrant, perhaps causing a slight bulging of the flank immediately adjoining.

Coproliths which may be projected in the vicinity of the vermiform appendix.

Air fluid levels in the cecum.

Evidence of peritonitis coupled with the above (Chapter 24).

Fluid density interposed between the right flank stripe and the ascending colon (Casper; McCort; Frimann-Dahl).

The appendix fails to fill ordinarily by barium enema examination when it is inflamed.

Barium may enter an abscess cavity.

There may be contour defects on the cecum adjacent to an appendiceal abscess (Figiel and Figiel) or any other organ contiguous with the inflammatory process.

A soft tissue mass which displaces the cecum and right colon may be identified by barium enema.

The terminal ileum may show evidence of spiculation, irregularity, spasm, and irritability.

Postappendectomy Deformities

Evidence of inversion of the stump.

Persistence of a small stump.

A Roentgen Sign of Gangrenous Appendicitis. The normal appendix contains gas only transiently and occasionally. A constant gas collection without fluid level may be seen in the subhepatic appendix or with marked cecal distention. A dilated fixed gas-filled appendix with a fluid level has been described as a sign of gangrenous nonperforated appendicitis (Fisher).

Other Diseases of the Appendix

Appendiceal intussusception, or prolapse of an appendiceal stump (Figiel and Figiel; Paul and Ferraro).

Tumors of the appendix. The most frequent of these are (1) mucoceles, producing small filling defects if impressed upon the cecum, (2) carcinoids, (3) carcinomas.

Regional enteritis (Cohen and Denbesten).

Infectious granulomas such as amebiasis.

THE APPENDIX

PATHOLOGIC CONDITIONS DETECTED RADIOGRAPHICALLY

1. LACK OF FILLING - MAY OR MAY NOT BE OF SIGNIFICANCE
2. RETENTION MORE THAN 48 HRS. - NOT NECESSARILY SURGICAL
3. CONCRETIONS (COPROLITHS)
4. FIXATION (INDICATING ADHESIONS)
5. KINKING
6. APPENDICEAL ABSCESS   (a) 85% PERICECAL
                              (b) PRESSURE DEFECT - ASSOCIATED

Figure 30-35 Pertinent features regarding the vermiform appendix from the radiologic standpoint.

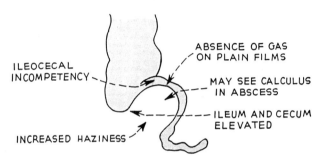

Figure 30-36 Radiograph demonstrating a coprolith of the appendix with an associated inflammatory process and obstructive appendicitis.

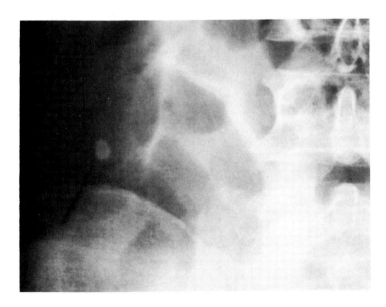

Questions—Chapter 30

1. What are the distinguishing anatomic features of the large intestine as reflected roentgenologically?

2. Describe the normal anatomy of the ileocecal valve and how it is portrayed radiologically.

3. What are some of the variations of the normal colon?

4. What is meant by hyperrotation and incomplete rotation of the cecum and what is the clinical significance of this anomaly?

5. What is the scope of the barium enema examination and what are its limitations? How does the routine barium enema examination differ from the barium-air double contrast enema and what is the scope of the double contrast enema in comparison with the routine procedure?

6. Indicate the importance of the lateral view of the rectum and sigmoid colon.

7. What are some of the complications of a barium enema and how may they best be avoided?

8. In summary, what are the roentgen signs of the normal barium study of the colon?

9. What are the two main categories of etiology responsible for the diffusely enlarged barium-filled colon?

10. What are some of the causes of the segmentally enlarged barium-filled colon? What is meant by toxic dilatation of the colon and what is its roentgenologic and clinical significance?

11. What are some of the causes of the diffusely small barium-filled colon? How does aganglionosis of the entire colon appear roentgenologically? What are the major causes of the diffusely small colon in the adult? What are the roentgen appearances which differentiate these two processes?

12. What are some of the main causes of narrowness of the colon, segmental or localized?

13. If the margins and internal architecture of an area of narrowness in the colon have a localized but smooth appearance, what are the main causes to be considered?

14. If the margins and internal architecture of the area of narrowness have a localized ragged and irregular appearance, what are the main causes? If the margins of the colon show outpouchings, what are the main causes? If there is a flow of barium outside the confines of the colon, what are the main causes?

15. If the flow of barium is in abnormal position for the colon but is still confined to the colon, what are some of the main causes?

16. If an obstruction to the flow of barium is encountered, what are some of the appearances to be closely investigated? What are the clinical significances?

17. If the architecture internal to the colon is disturbed either on the full colon study or after evacuation, what are some of the causes considered?

18. If there is a conical appearance of the cecum with irregularity of the adjoining ileum what are some of the causes?

19. If there is a cobblestone appearance of the colon, what are some of the causes?

20. If there is a thumbprinting of the barium column, what are some of the causes? If there is a linear streaking, either circular, transverse, or longitudinal, what are some of the causes? If there are air bubbles or streaks of air in the wall of the bowel, what are some of the causes?

21. If there is a persistence of feces within the colon after every effort for cleansing and evacuation, what are some of the causes considered?

22. What are the general appearances of the postoperative colon and what are some of the complications that might be seen in the postoperative colon?

23. Describe the roentgen appearance of the "cathartic" colon.

24. Describe the roentgen appearance of Hirschsprung's disease.

25. Describe the roentgen appearances of imperforate anus. What is meant by ectopic anus and how may this be determined roentgenologically?

26. How would you differentiate reflex ileus from a mechanical obstruction?

27. What is the roentgen appearance of volvulus? Where are the most frequent sites of volvulus in the colon?

28. What is the roentgen appearance of a mesenteric vascular occlusion?

29. What is meant by meconium ileus and meconium plug syndrome and how are these different? How do these entities in turn differ from meconium peritonitis?

30. What are the roentgen appearances of intussusception?

31. What is the roentgen appearance of toxic dilatation of the colon and in what pathologic entity is it most apt to occur?

32. How would you evaluate imperforate anus roentgenologically in respect to a simple classification and what is the significance of the so-called high type imperforate anus group?

33. What is the pathogenesis and what are the roentgenologic aspects of irradiation injury to the bowel?

34. Describe the roentgenologic considerations in respect to diverticulosis of the large intestine.

35. What is the roentgen appearance of scleroderma involving the large intestine?

36. What is the significance of necrotizing enterocolitis especially in the newborn infant?

37. What is the appearance of pneumoperitoneum in the newborn infant?

38. Describe the roentgen appearances of idiopathic ulcerative colitis and indicate how this differs from granulomatous colitis.

39. Describe the roentgen appearances of amebiasis of the colon. How would you differentiate granulomatous colitis from amebiasis?

40. Describe the roentgen appearances of various lesions which affect the terminal ileum and cecum. How do they resemble one another and how do they differ?

41. Indicate the roentgenologic aspects of lymphogranuloma inguinale venereum.

42. What is meant by the term Gardner's syndrome?

43. What is meant by the term Turcot's syndrome?

44. Describe the roentgen appearances of the villous adenoma involving the colon. Where is it most frequently found and what is its clinical significance?

45. How does familial polyposis of the colon differ from multiple polypi of the colon in children?

46. Describe the clinical and roentgenologic aspects of Peutz-Jeghers syndrome.

47. What is meant by the term carcinoid syndrome?

48. What are some of the roentgen appearances of carcinoma of the colon?

49. What are some of the roentgen appearances of lymphosarcoma of the colon?

50. What is the importance and what are the roentgenologic aspects of metastases to the colon?

51. What are the abnormalities to be looked for in a study of the postoperative colon?

52. Define "coprolith" of the appendix and indicate its clinical significance.

53. Describe the roentgenologic findings with acute appendicitis. How does gangrenous appendicitis manifest itself roentgenologically?

31

Roentgen Diagnosis in Obstetrics and Gynecology

PURPOSES OF STUDY

The purposes of roentgen study of the female patient in obstetrics and gynecology may be outlined as follows.

1. A study of the pregnant mother in respect to the fetus; the purposes of such a study may include
   a. Determination of the presence of a fetal skeleton in utero or intra-abdominally.
   b. Determination of multiple fetuses.
   c. Determination of fetal normalcy, age, and development.
   d. Determination of fetal viability or death.
   e. Description of the accurate presentation of the fetus.
2. A study of the uterus apart from its fetus, including
   a. The placenta—its size, position, and density.
   b. The amniotic space. (The amniotic space may be entered to withdraw fluid for special study, or may serve as a guide to fetal transfusion.)
   c. General uterine density and normality of appearance.
3. The study of the maternal abdomen apart from the pregnant uterus, including
   a. The determination of extrauterine pregnancy.
   b. The study of pelvic soft tissues outside the uterus, particularly to determine if interference to parturition may result.
   c. Pelvic mensuration and description of the maternal pelvis as a guide to determine cephalopelvic disproportion.
4. Special gynecologic study of the nonpregnant female for
   a. Hysterosalpingography.
   b. Pelvic pneumography.
   c. Pelvic arteriography.
5. Genitography of the infant or child.

INTRODUCTION

Protection from radiation and potential radiation hazards take on greater significance in this field, since there are two or more lives involved (mother and fetuses) and not just that of the patient. **The hazards of radiation must be carefully weighed against the benefits to be achieved.**

Study of the Pregnant Mother

Determination of a Fetal Skeleton in Utero

The fetal skeleton does not occur prior to the third month of gestation, and radiographically detectable fetal skeletal parts are difficult to find prior to the thirteenth or fourteenth week.

The indications for seeking fetal skeletal parts are:

1. An enlarging uterus without other evidence of pregnancy;

2. An enlarging tumor mass of the pelvis that could conceivably be teratomatous or represent an extra-uterine pregnancy.

3. A previously suspected gravid uterus when the clinical situation has changed and pregnancy tests have ceased to be positive.

4. An abnormal fetus that is strongly suggested by clinical appearances (hydrocephalus; anencephaly).

The fetal parts that lend themselves most readily to early detection are the segmental structures such as those of the spine and ribs; occasionally the extremities and head may be seen in faint outline.

The oblique views of the pelvis are often more helpful than straight anteroposterior views, since the fetal ossified parts may be projected over the sacrum and lost to view.

Determination of Multiple Fetuses. Study for multiple fetuses is not undertaken prior to the later stages of pregnancy, preferably late in the last trimester when radiation hazard to the fetus is minimal.

Fetal Normalcy. Fetal normalcy is best studied late in the last trimester.

Fetal Age and Development. Fetal age determination should rarely be required prior to the third trimester of pregnancy. There are many different bases upon which fetal age can be estimated, but probably the most reliable are estimation of actual fetal length and determination of average fetal head diameter.

Prediction of Fetal Maturity. The following criteria are perhaps most important.

1. An ossification center is present in the distal end of the femur in 90 per cent of term fetuses.

2. Proximal tibial epiphysial ossification is noted at term in 70 to 80 per cent of the newborn.

3. A fetal lumbar vertebral length of 52 mm. or more indicates that 95 per cent of the group weigh over 2500 grams, with an actual total length of 49 cm. or more (Margolis and Voss).

Determination of Fetal Viability or Death. Fetal death is indicated by several roentgen signs (Figure 31–1).

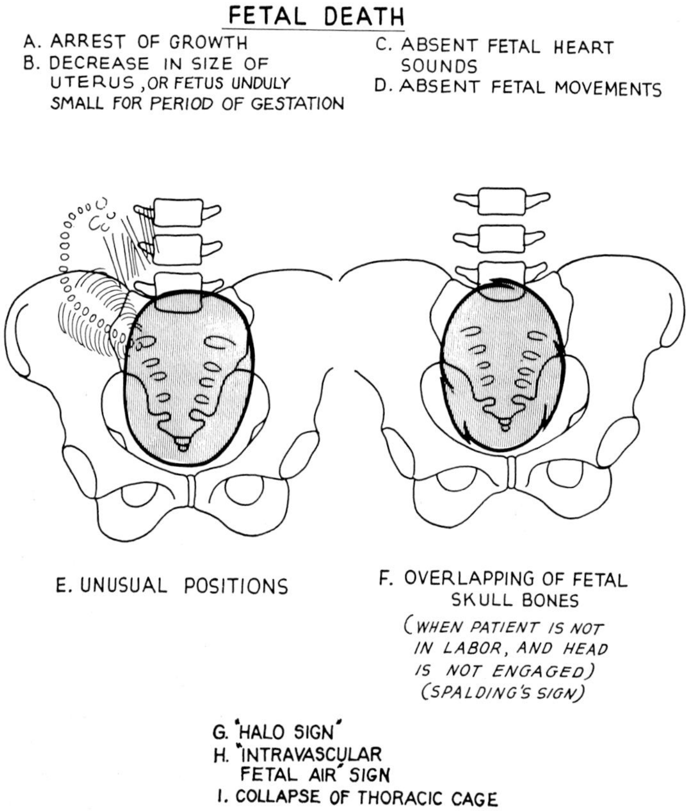

FETAL DEATH

A. ARREST OF GROWTH
B. DECREASE IN SIZE OF UTERUS, OR FETUS UNDULY SMALL FOR PERIOD OF GESTATION
C. ABSENT FETAL HEART SOUNDS
D. ABSENT FETAL MOVEMENTS

E. UNUSUAL POSITIONS

F. OVERLAPPING OF FETAL SKULL BONES (WHEN PATIENT IS NOT IN LABOR, AND HEAD IS NOT ENGAGED) (SPALDING'S SIGN)

G. "HALO SIGN"
H. "INTRAVASCULAR FETAL AIR" SIGN
I. COLLAPSE OF THORACIC CAGE

Figure 31–1 Diagram illustrating radiographic findings in fetal death.

During Amniography, a viable fetus will ingest an opaque medium from amniotic fluid, and the water soluble contrast agent will be demonstrated in the gastrointestinal tract of the fetus. This phenomenon has not been demonstrated in a nonviable fetus.

To detect true stillbirth, an examination is conducted for the presence of air in the lungs or intestines. Absence of air is an indication of stillbirth. On the other hand, the presence of air in the intestines may be the result of putrefaction in a fetus which has been dead for some time.

Fetal Abnormalities. These have been classified in antenatal recognition as follows:

1. Abnormal changes in the fetal soft tissues
    a. Hydrops fetalis
    b. Thyroid tumors
    c. Abdominal tumors
2. Pathologic changes in fetal skeleton
    a. Syphilitic osteochondritis
    b. Osteogenesis imperfecta
    c. Osteopetrosis
    d. Achondroplasia
3. Abnormalities of skeletal development
    a. Cranial-vertebral anencephaly, hydrocephaly, spina bifida, craniolacunia
    b. Limb deformities (or absence of limb)
    c. Miscellaneous deformities (teratoid development)

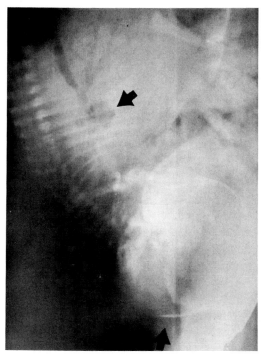

Figure 31-2 Close-up view of dead fetus *in utero*, near term. The lower arrow points to the halo sign around the fetal head; the upper arrow points to gas in the vascular system of the fetus.

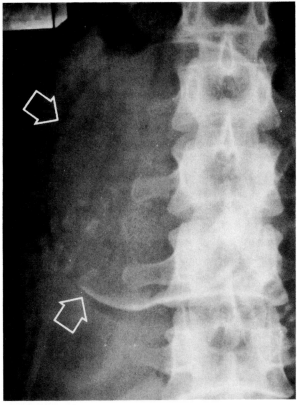

Figure 31-3 Halo sign in erythroblastosis fetalis surrounding the fetal head (magnified view).

Presentation of Fetus (Figure 31–4)

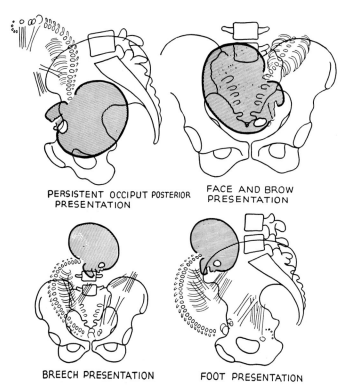

PERSISTENT OCCIPUT POSTERIOR
PRESENTATION

FACE AND BROW
PRESENTATION

BREECH PRESENTATION

FOOT PRESENTATION

Figure 31–4   Diagrams illustrating various types of atypical presentation as seen radiographically.

When the head is not engaged in a prima gravida, some possibilities to be considered are: obstructing masses in the pelvis such as ovarian cysts or fibroids; placenta praevia centralis; a short umbilical cord, or more often a cord twisted around the fetus; fetal malformation such as hydrocephalus and cystic hygroma of the neck; or a pendulous uterus impairing the direction of uterine force.

Study of the Pregnant Mother for Uterine Detail Outside the Fetus

Placenta

ROENTGEN STUDY OF THE PLACENTA

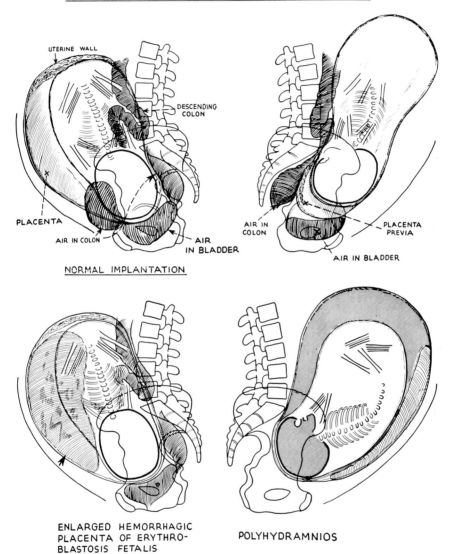

Figure 31–5 Radiographic appearance of normal placental implantation compared with appearances of abnormal implantations. The placenta praevia is shown in good contrast by means of air distention of both the bladder and the rectum. Ultrasound depiction is significant in this area of diagnosis.

Radiographic Criteria for Placenta Praevia

Lack of demonstration of a placental shadow on plain film studies in the usual locations.

Asymmetry of the presenting parts with respect to the pubic symphysis and sacrum.

Displacement of the presenting part away from the pubic symphysis.

Information obtained from special contrast studies of the urinary bladder and rectum (Figure 31–5)—so-called "air rectograms and cystograms."

Amniography

Purposes of Procedure

1. It provides a positive contrast outline of all structures within or impinging upon the amniotic sac. Thus the method may be used to detect placenta praevia.
2. Fetal death can be distinguished with reasonable certainty. In films taken after two hours, some of the contrast agent should be detected in the fetal stomach or intestine. In a dead fetus, no swallowing will have occurred.
3. It can be a guide to fetography and intrauterine fetal transfusion.
4. It assists in diagnosis of uterine or fetal abnormalities.
5. Premature membrane rupture may be diagnosed by leakage of the contrast medium into the vagina.
6. Extrauterine pregnancy can be demonstrated.
7. Removal of the amniotic fluid under fluoroscopic guidance prior to delivery has also been very helpful in determining the onset of deterioration from erythroblastosis fetalis in the fetus.

Study of the Pregnant Mother for Intra-abdominal Abnormalities Outside the Uterus

Extrauterine Fetus

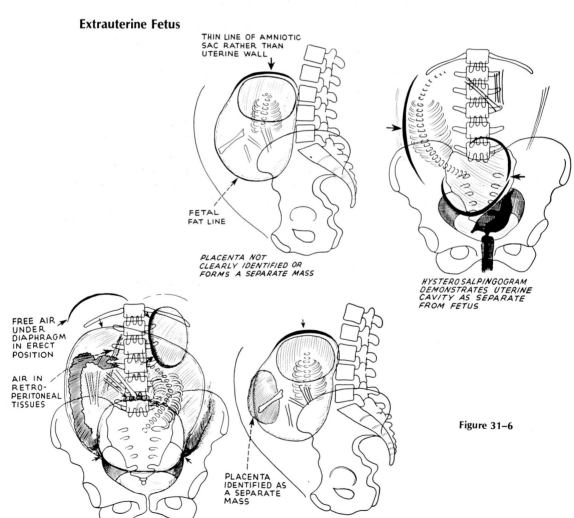

THIN LINE OF AMNIOTIC SAC RATHER THAN UTERINE WALL

FETAL FAT LINE

PLACENTA NOT CLEARLY IDENTIFIED OR FORMS A SEPARATE MASS

HYSTEROSALPINGOGRAM DEMONSTRATES UTERINE CAVITY AS SEPARATE FROM FETUS

FREE AIR UNDER DIAPHRAGM IN ERECT POSITION

AIR IN RETROPERITONEAL TISSUES

PLACENTA IDENTIFIED AS A SEPARATE MASS

FREE AIR IN ABDOMEN

Figure 31–6

Study of Pelvic Soft Tissue Structures Outside the Uterus

Retroperitoneal Soft Tissues.   The main retroperitoneal abnormalities which might interfere with parturition are tumors of the sacrum, inflammatory swellings involving extensions along the psoas muscle or the obturator muscle, and ureteral abnormalities.

Urinary Bladder.   Abnormalities of the urinary bladder have been described in Chapter 24.

Abnormalities of the Intestine.   The rectum, sigmoid colon, and terminal ileum are the intestinal structures most frequently encountered in the pelvis. Abnormalities contained within the pelvis may displace bowel either to one side, as in the case of the rectum, or upward.

Neoplasms of the Pelvis

Fibromyoma of the Uterus

Ovarian Cysts

Salpingolithiasis

Cephalopelvic Disproportion and Pelvic Measurement*

In all these proposed methods the *basic concepts and objectives are to measure the important diameters of the pelvis and head,* eliminating as much as possible the elements of magnification and distortion; *to describe the pelvic architecture* as accurately as possible from the standpoint of parturition; and to *describe any other factors* in relation to the pelvis, fetus, or placenta such as have been previously indicated in this section.

1. Roentgen pelvic encephalometry should not be considered a routine procedure. It must be employed only after thorough obstetrical examination and evaluation, and the information to be obtained must be of critical value. Nevertheless, this procedure must be undertaken with the full understanding that the radiologist cannot and should not by himself attempt to predict the outcome of delivery. The data obtained should permit a thorough study of the maternal pelvis in all its aspects and should provide some idea of the relative size, shape, and position of the fetal skull in relation to the maternal pelvis.

2. The optimal time for roentgen pelvic encephalometry is during the last 2 weeks of pregnancy. Under these circumstances, with a cephalic presentation the fetal gonads may actually lie outside the primary beam of radiation if one concentrates on the maternal pelvis.

---

*Use of ultrasound has not been considered part of this text.

Study of Pelvic Architecture

TYPICAL GYNECOID PELVIS

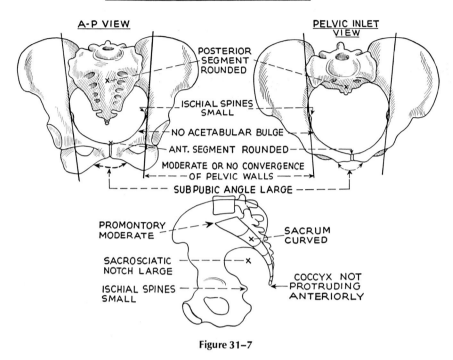

Figure 31-7

DIFFERENT PELVIC TYPES
(PELVIC INLET VIEW)

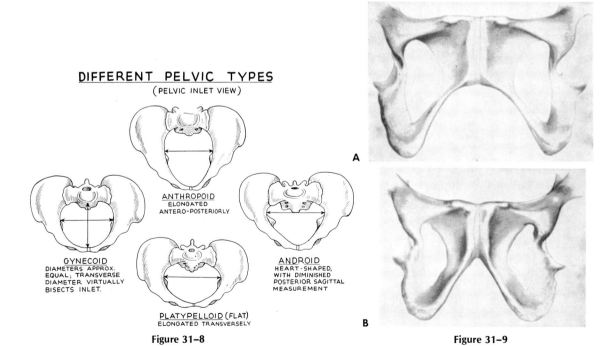

Figure 31-8

Figure 31-9

Figure 31-9   Variations in size and shape of the subpubic arch. *A.* Delicate bones; wide angle; well-curved female type of pubic rami. *B.* Heavy bones; narrow angle, straight masculine type of pubic rami. (From Golden: *Diagnostic Roentgenology*, Vol. 2. Baltimore, Williams and Wilkins Co., 1963–1969.)

FACTORS STUDIED IN PELVIC ARCHITECTURE

1. PELVIC INLET STUDY (*SEE DIAGRAMS OF DIFFERENT PELVIC TYPES*)

2. PROMINENCE OF ISCHIAL SPINES

3. CONVERGENCE OF LATERAL PELVIC WALLS

4. SUBPUBIC ANGLE

5. CURVATURE OF SACRUM

6. COCCYX VARIATIONS, PELVIC FLOOR AND GREATER SCIATIC NOTCH

7. UTERINE AXIS FACTOR IN RELATION TO SACRUM AND SACRAL PROMONTORY

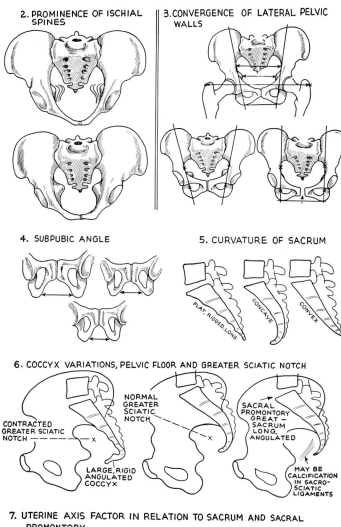

A. AXIS OF UTERUS NEAR SPINE, GOOD FLEXION OF HEAD

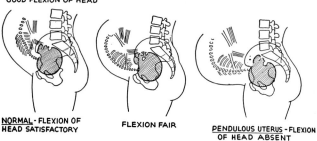

Figure 31–10

Study of the Nonpregnant Female — Gynecologic Radiology

X-ray Appearance of Intrauterine Contraceptive Devices

Hysterosalpingography

Introduction. The main uses of this procedure are:
1. Study of sterility problems.
2. Investigation of uterine bleeding.
3. Re-establishment of tubal patency.
4. Visualization of abnormalities of the uterine cavity or oviducts.
5. Visualization of sinus tracts communicating with the female genital tract.

Although practically all patients are examined for sterility or habitual abortion, the following abnormalities may be visualized:

1. Anomalies varying between a completely double vagina, cervix, and uterus, to a slight dimpling of the dome of the uterus
2. Fibroids
3. Polyps
4. Endometrial hyperplasia
5. Adenomyosis
6. Intrauterine synechiae
7. Tubal disease and defects such as hydrosalpinx, tubo-ovarian cavities, kinking and adhesions, nodular salpingitis, endometriosis, tubal occlusion from infection, and tubal amputation and closure
8. Carcinoma of the uterus
9. Cervical lesions, varying from stenosis to polyps and adenomyosis
10. Lesions of the internal os such as stenosis, polyposis, dilatation or widening, scarring and extreme spasm.
11. Ovarian tumors. Here the 24-hour follow-up is of some advantage since the outline of pelvic masses is thereby obtained.

Figure 31–12 *A*. Position of patient (after instillation of gas) for radiography. Pneumoperitoneum of the female pelvis in postero-anterior (*B*) and lateral (*C*) projections. This patient was a 29 year old female with a Stein-Leventhal syndrome proved by surgery, but her ovaries are considered normal in size for a young woman. (Courtesy of Dr. Wilma C. Diner, Department of Radiology, University of Arkansas Medical Center, Little Rock, Arkansas.)

THE NORMAL HYSTEROSALPINGOGRAM

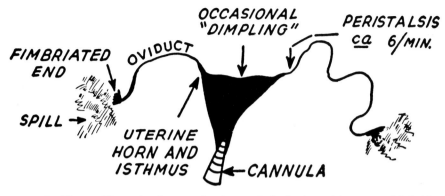

Figure 31–11   Diagram illustrating the normal antero-posterior hysterosalpingogram—labeled tracing.

THE NORMAL GYNECOGRAM

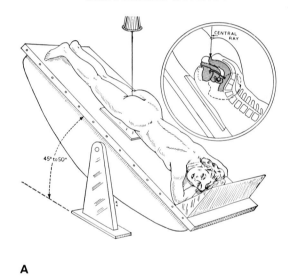

A

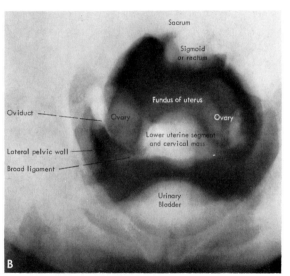

B

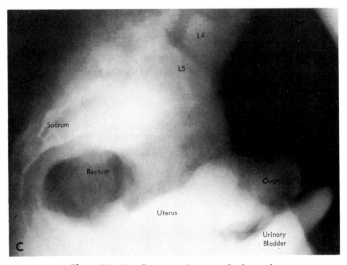

C

Figure 31–12   *See opposite page for legend.*

Questions—Chapter 31

1. Indicate some of the purposes of the roentgenologic examination of a pregnant mother in respect to the fetus.

2. Indicate some of the roentgenologic purposes of studying the pregnant uterus apart from the fetus.

3. Indicate some of the roentgenologic purposes of studying the maternal pregnant abdomen apart from the pregnant uterus.

4. Indicate some of the roentgenologic methods of study of the nonpregnant female in reference to gynecologic problems.

5. What are some of the indications for seeking fetal skeletal parts roentgenologically? In what phase of pregnancy must radiologic exposure be avoided?

6. Which fetal parts in the pregnant uterus lend themselves most readily to early roentgenologic detection?

7. When is the fetus best studied for normalcy? What roentgenologic features generally indicate a normal fetus?

8. How does one determine fetal age and development in utero? What is the most accurate method in your estimation?

9. What are the best indicators of fetal maturity at the time of term or immediately following delivery? Discuss the relative accuracy of these indicators.

10. What are some of the roentgenologic methods for determination of fetal death?

11. What precaution must be utilized in the interpretation of the "Horner-Spalding sign"? What are some of the unequivocal determinates of fetal death roentgenologically?

12. What is meant by the term "halo sign" and what is its significance pathologically?

13. In what clinical condition is hydrops fetalis apt to occur?

14. What is meant by the "Buddha attitude" of the fetus and what is its clinical significance?

15. Indicate some of the fetal skeletal abnormalities that may be detected in utero.

16. What part does the roentgenologic technique play in determination of the presentation of the fetus? What significance does this have in respect to the overall process of parturition?

17. Describe the roentgenologic techniques for study of the placenta. What are some of the radiographic criteria for abnormalities?

18. Describe at least two radiologically oriented techniques for determination of placenta praevia.

19. Describe the technique of amniography. What are its main hazards and what are its main purposes?

20. What is the main purpose of intrauterine fetal transfusion?

21. What are some of the roentgenologic features which suggest extrauterine pregnancy?

22. Indicate some of the important pelvic soft tissue structures outside the uterus for identification roentgenologically in respect to parturition.

23. Describe a useful teleroentgenographic technique for determination of cephalopelvic disproportion and pelvic measurement.

24. What features of pelvic architecture are important in respect to normal parturition?

25. Indicate some of the abnormalities which might be visualized by hysterosalpingography.

26. What is meant by the term gynecography?

Index

Note: Page numbers in **boldface** indicate major discussions; numbers in *italic* indicate illustrations.